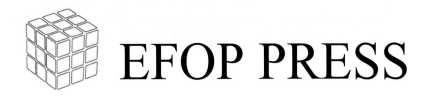

EFOP PRESS

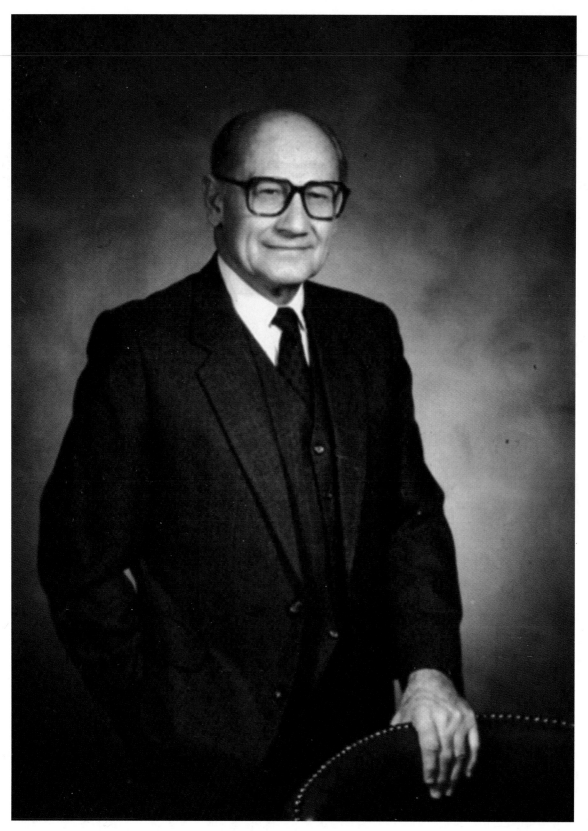

Robert Edison Moyers

This book is dedicated to the memory of

Robert Edison Moyers, D.D.S., Ph.D., D.Sc. (Honorary), D.Sc. (Honorary)

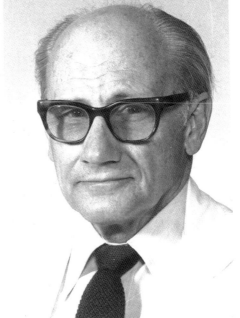

Bob Moyers was born on September 12, 1919. He grew up in a small rural Iowa town, where his father was a high school principal and teacher. In grade school, his father told him that he could choose only one: a bicycle or a horse. He chose the horse over the bicycle, and went on to become a competitive equestrian. Along with his many high school academic highlights, Bob participated in track, winning the Iowa State high school championship in the 440-yard event.

Bob stayed in Iowa to attend dental school at the University of Iowa. After earning his dental degree, he enlisted in the U.S. Army and became the chief medical liaison officer of the military mission to the Greek resistance movement. He parachuted behind the Nazi lines and played a critical role in liberating Greece from the Nazis. For his efforts in the Office of Strategic Services (OSS), he was awarded the Bronze Star, the Legion of Merit, the Order of the British Empire and the Order of the Greek Phoenix. He was also wounded, and received the Purple Heart.

After World War II, he returned to the University of Iowa for orthodontic specialty training and a Ph.D. degree in physiology. During that period he preached at a Welch Church outside of Iowa City, earning the nickname of "Deacon". In 1948, he was appointed as chairman of the Department of Orthodontics at the University of Toronto. He served in that capacity for four years, and then accepted the chairmanship of the Department of Orthodontics at the University of Michigan. He held that position until 1966. While at the University of Michigan, he conceived, organized and became the founding director of the Center for Human Growth and Development. He served as its director until 1980, at which time he became head of the Craniofacial Biology Group at the Center for Human Growth and Development for another ten years.

He retired in 1990 and became Fellow Emeritus of the Center and Professor Emeritus of the School of Dentistry. He also retired from his clinical practice at that time. Dr. Moyers was an avid gardener, specializing in creating hybrids of rhododendrons. He won a number of international awards for his hybrids. He was also interested in faceting, and would create specially cut stones for jewelry he crafted. He had widespread interests and gained international prominence in developmental biology, public health and nutrition, anthropology, morphometrics and pediatrics. One of the highlights each year has been the "Moyers Symposium" on subjects of orthodontics and craniofacial biology, started by gifts from grateful students. The Symposium is still an annual winter event after 36 years.

Dr. Moyers' main academic interest was orthodontics, and his contributions to this specialty were immense. His doctoral investigations and subsequent clinical research provided us with a better understanding of the neuromuscular function in facial growth. Throughout his career he received NIH-supported program project grants. Bob was twice a Fulbright Scholar. He also wrote a textbook of orthodontics that was published through four editions.

Despite the many awards and honors he had received over his career, including two honorary doctorate degrees, he indicated that the thing that gave him great pleasure was stimulating students to pursue careers in academic orthodontics. He took pride in the 35 students he helped mentor and who later became departmental chairs throughout the world. We will always be grateful for his encouragement to seek greater heights, and yet he allowed us the freedom to seek our own goals.

MLR
JKA

Essentials for Orthodontic Practice

First Edition

Michael L. Riolo, D.D.S., M.S.
Adjunct Clinical Professor of Orthodontics
Department of Orthodontics
School of Dentistry
University of Detroit Mercy
Detroit, Michigan, USA

James K. Avery, D.D.S., Ph.D.
Professor Emeritus, Dentistry and Anatomy
Schools of Dentistry and Medicine
University of Michigan
Ann Arbor, Michigan, USA

Editorial Staff
Lorel A. Bradshaw R.D.A., R.D.H., B.S.
Elizabeth A. Van Tubergen B.S.

Cover Design
Michelle J. Thornberg D.D.S., M.S.

1124 Illustrations, 868 in color

EFOP, LLC
EFOP Press
Ann Arbor & Grand Haven, Michigan, USA

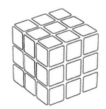

Library of Congress Catalog-in-Publication Data

Essentials for Orthodontic Practice/ editors, Michael L. Riolo, James K. Avery, 1st ed.

Includes bibliographical references and glossary and index.
ISNBN 0-9720546-0-X
The Library of Congress Control Numer is
2002107942
1. Orthodontics, 2. Facial Growth, 3. Facial Development, 4. Prenatal Facial Development, 5. Postnatal Facial Development, 6. Embryology, 7. Orthodontic Treatment and Diagnosis for Orthodontics, 8. Treatment Planning, 9. Retention, Relapse, 10. Development of the Dentition, 11. Force Systems and Tissue Engineering, 12. Clinical Epidemiology and Orthodontics, Human.
I. Michael L. Riolo; II. James K. Avery
2003
First Edition
by EFOP Press, of EFOP, LLC
Grand Haven, Michigan, USA
PO Box 374
Grand Haven, MI 49417

1-866-431-3311

Important Note: Medicine and dentistry are ever-changing sciences that are undergoing continual development. Research and clinical experience are continually expanding our knowledge, in particular our knowledge of proper treatment. Insofar as this book mentions any treatment, readers may rest assured that the authors, editors and publishers have made every effort to assure that such references are in accordance with the state of knowledge at the time of production of the book.

Nevertheless, this does not express, imply or involve any guarantee or responsibility on the part of the publishers with respect to any instructions and forms of treatments stated in the book. Every form of treatment used is entirely at the user's own risk and responsibility.

The objective of this book is to enable the student or practitioner of dentistry to learn the essentials and fundamentals underlying the diagnosis, treatment planning and treatment of basic orthodontic target disorders. The book is divided into sections to roughly coincide with the four years of dental education. This does not imply any absolute necessity of sequencing of studies but is meant only to represent, by way of an outline, one sequence of viewing the orthodontic heuristic process.

Section I, Growth and Development, contains five basic growth and development chapters, encompassing Developmental, Psychosocial, Behavioral and Compliance Aspects of Care, Prenatal Craniofacial Development, Postnatal Craniofacial Development, Growth of the Craniofacial Skeleton and Development of the Dentition and Occlusion. These chapters represent typical courses that relate to orthodontics found in the first or second years of dental school.

Section II, Foundations for Orthodontics, covers Classification and Terminology, Etiology of Malocclusion, Force Systems and Tissue Response, Tissue Engineering in Orthodontics, and Clinical Epidemiology and Malocclusion. This material is typically taught in the first, second or third years of dental school.

Section III, titled Examination and Diagnosis, covers Orthodontic Exam and Diagnosis, Analysis of Orofacial and Jaw Musculature, Analysis of Dentition and Occlusion, Dental Dysmorphogenesis, Analysis of the Orofacial Skeleton and Planning Orthodontic Treatment. This material is usually taught in the second or third years of dental school previous to clinical rotations.

Section IV, titled Treatment and Effects, covers Preadolescent Treatment, Adolescent Treatment, Adult Treatment, Treatment of Patients with Craniofacial Anomalies, Retention, Relapse, and The Recurrence of Malocclusion, and The Adverse Effects of Orthodontic Treatment. Each chapter author has tried to create a chapter that represents a balanced approach to their topic while emphasizing facts in light of any substantive new approaches to their topic area.

The book's contributors are made up of a well-known group of university-based professionals who represent 13 schools and 19 departments. The book was two years in its design and the last one and a half years in production and editing. During this time each author continued to follow the literature to ensure that new important information was incorporated into the text. Every chapter has been constructed and sequenced to integrally fit the text. The authors recognize the weaknesses of a multiple author text: a lack of continuity of thought and format. We have worked hard to achieve the mind-meld of the "Unimind". Each of the authors has worked tirelessly to create an error-free text, but with little expectation that this miracle will occur.

The format of the text is unique in that the chapter outlines are paginated, the glossary terms are emboldened in every chapter of the text and the chapter headings are graphically tied to each section, giving a positive visual reference to the chapters. A full color presentation adds to the book by enhancing the clinical cases and clarifying the histologic sections. All chapter authors have followed the suggestion to place all figures on facing pages with text to make the book's use easier. Chapters and topics that are unique for an orthodontic text are 1, 5, 9, 10, 14, 21 and 22. (Developmental, Psychosocial, Behavioral and Compliance Aspects of Care, Development of the Dentition and Occlusion, Tissue Engineering in Orthodontics, Clinical Epidemiology and Malocclusion, Dental Dysmorphogenesis, Retention, Relapse, and The Recurrence of Malocclusion, and The Adverse Effects of Orthodontic Treatment).

Within the constraints of time and personalities, we give you "The Essentials for Orthodontic Practice". The aim of the text is to serve to stimulate students' investigation through various demonstrations, which may tend to lead students to further explore by themselves. No book will satisfy every need, though we hope you find that this text's depth and breadth offer an excellent foundation for the study of orthodontics. Please send any questions that may arise directly to the chapter authors.

MLR
JKA

Acknowledgements

The first edition of this text was developed by way of a collaboration of researchers, teachers and clinicians who felt there was a need for a text tailored for educational methods by which a student undergoing a dental education can review all of the essentials and foundations for orthodontic practice.

The contributor list on the following pages acknowledge the broad cross-section of talent who came together to create this book. Chapter co-authors contributed to the text by proofreading and making suggestions for other chapters' content, format and sequencing. Lorel A. Bradshaw, RDA, RDH, BS and Elizabeth Anne "Betsy" Van Tubergen, BS, worked as staff editors for specific chapters of the text. Lorel interfaced with the chapter co-authors for chapter 2, 3, 4, 8, 9, 12, and 15. Betsy managed the editing for chapters 1, 5, 6, 7, 10, 11, 13, 14, 16, 17, 18, 19 20, 21, and 22. Lorel's language skills and eye for detail were challenged as she proofread each page of the book in the final weeks of its construction. Dr. Michelle J. Thornberg mastered the Quark XPress software to establish our protocol for reformatting the text to a photo-ready condition. Dr. Thornberg also designed the front and back covers of the book, as well as the announcement booklet. Betsy additionally mastered the Quark XPress software and worked daily to convert chapter files and interfaced with all chapter co-authors as required in the final editing process.

We are grateful to Dr. G. Frans Currier for his extra effort in the final editing process. The basic Glossary was produced by the consensus of the chapter authors. Its final construction was the result of exemplary efforts by Dr. Michelle J. Thornberg and Elizabeth A. Van Tubergen. Additionally, Dr. Michelle J. Thornberg created the index of terms. Dr. James A. McNamara Jr. furnished the photos for the Dedication to Dr. Robert E. Moyers. Dr. McNamara also helped furnish information and details for Dr. Moyers' dedication. Dr. William Harrell, Jr. contributed pages 405-410, titled "The Future of Imaging for Orthodontics".

Bonding and re-bonding occurs within this author group. The project seemed like a slow burn exercise experience for 90% of the time and the last 10% was like the last 100 yards of a 440 yard dash. I am sure that everyone who has finished a paper, chapter or book can relate to the feelings that accompany the completion of a text such as this one. I am also aware of how happy all of our families are to see this project completed.

MLR
JKA

Contributors

James K. Avery, D.D.S., Ph.D.
Professor Emeritus, Dentistry and Anatomy
Schools of Dentistry and Medicine
University of Michigan
Ann Arbor, Michigan, USA

Burcu Bayirli D.D.S., M.S.
Assistant Professor
Department of Orthodontics
School of Dentistry
University of Detroit Mercy
Detroit, Michigan, USA
Postdoctoral Fellow, School of Public Health
University of Michigan
Ann Arbor, Michigan, USA

Anne-Marie Bollen D.D.S., M.S., Ph.D.
Director of Undergraduate Orthodontics
Associate Professor of Orthodontics
Adjunct Associate Professor of Orthopaedics
School of Dentistry
University of Washington
Seattle, Washington, USA

Joseph Damone II D.M.D.
Associate Professor
Department of Orthodontics
School of Dentistry
University of Pennsylvania
Pittsburgh, Pennsylvania, USA

Thomas J. Cangialosi D.D.S.
Professor of Orthodontics
Chairman Orthodontic Division
Associate Dean for Advanced and Postdoctoral Education
School of Dentistry and Oral Surgery
Columbia University
New York City, New York, USA

Steven J. Ceresnie Ph.D.
Departments of Patient Management and Orthodontics
School of Dentistry
University of Detroit Mercy
Detroit, Michigan, USA

G. Frans Currier D.D.S., M.S.D., M.Ed.
Director of Graduate Program
Professor of Orthodontics
Department of Orthodontics
Adjunct Professor of Pediatric Dentistry
School of Dentistry
University of Oklahoma
Oklahoma City, Oklahoma, USA

Stella S. Efstratiadis D.D.S, M.S.
Professor, Division of Orthodontics
School of Dentistry and Oral Surgery
Columbia University
New York City, New York, USA

Donald H. Enlow M.S. Ph.D.
Thomas Hill Distinguished Professor Emeritus
Department of Orthodontics
Case Western Reserve University
Cleveland, Ohio, USA

John E. Grubb D.D.S., M.S.D.
Clinical Associate Professor
School of Dentistry
University of Southern California
Los Angeles, California, USA

Mark G. Hans D.D.S., M.S.D.
Associate Professor and Chair
Department of Orthodontics
School of Dentistry
Case Western Reserve University
Cleveland, Ohio, USA

William F. Hohlt D.D.S., M.S.
Associate Professor
Indiana School of Dentistry
Indiana University
Indianapolis, Indiana, USA
Adjunct Professor
School of Dentistry
University of Illinois-Chicago
Chicago, Illinois, USA

W. Stuart Hunter D.D.S., M.S., Ph.D.
Professor Emeritus, Chair Emeritus
Department of Orthodontics
School of Dentistry
University of Western Ontario
London, Ontario, Canada

Bailey N. Jacobson D.D.S., M.S.
Consulting Orthodontist, Cleft Lip and Palate Habilitation
Team, Children's Memorial Hospital
Chicago, Illinois, USA
Clinical Professor of Orthodontics
School of Dentistry
University of Detroit Mercy
Detroit, Michigan, USA
Former Clinical Professor of Orthodontics
School of Dentistry
Northwestern University
Chicago, Illinois, USA

Ronald S. Jacobson D.D.S., M.S.
Consulting Orthodontist, Cleft Lip and Palate Habilitation
Team, Children's Memorial Hospital
Chicago, Illinois, USA
Former Associate Professor of Clinical Orthodontics
School of Dentistry
Northwestern University
Chicago, Illinois, USA
Guest Lecturer
Graduate Orthodontic Division,
University of Detroit Mercy
School of Dentistry
Detroit, Michigan, USA

Contributors

Malcom C. Johnston D.D.S., M.Sc.D., Ph.D.
Professor Emeritus
Department of Orthodontics
School of Dentistry
University of North Carolina
Chapel Hill, North Carolina, USA

Richard Kulbersh D.D.S., M.S.,
Associate Professor and Chair
Department of Orthodontics
School of Dentistry
University of Detroit Mercy
Detroit, Michigan, USA

Colin A. Mayers D.D.S., M.S.
Adjunct Clinical Assistant Professor
Department of Orthodontics
School of Dentistry
University of Michigan
Ann Arbor, Michigan, USA

James Mah D.D.S., M.S.
Assistant Professor
School of Dentistry
University of Southern California
Los Angeles, California, USA

David J. Mooney Ph.D.
Professor of Biomedical Engineering
Professor of Biologic and Materials Science
Associate Professor Of Chemical Engineering
School of Dentistry and College of Engineering
University of Michigan
Ann Arbor, Michigan, USA

William L. Murphy Ph.D.
Graduate Research Assistant
Department of Biologic and Materials Science
School of Dentistry
University of Michigan
Ann Arbor, Michigan, USA

William M. Northway D.D.S., M.S.
Clinical Practice
12776 SW Bay Shore Dr.
Traverse City, Michigan, USA

Valmy Pangrazio-Kulbersh D.D.S., M.S.
Professor
Department of Orthodontics
School of Dentistry
University of Detroit Mercy
Detroit, Michigan, USA

Deborah E. Priestap D.D.S., M.S.
Adjunct Assistant Professor of Dentistry
Department of Orthodontics
University of Detroit Mercy
Detroit, Michigan, USA
Adjunct Assistant Professor of Dentistry
Department of Orthodontics and Pediatric Dentistry
University of Michigan
Ann Arbor, Michigan, USA

Christopher S. Riolo D.D.S., M.S.
Postdoctoral Fellow, School of Public Health
University of Michigan
Ann Arbor, Michigan, USA

Michael L. Riolo D.D.S., M.S.
Adjunct Clinical Professor of Orthodontics
Department of Orthodontics
School of Dentistry
University of Detroit Mercy
Detroit, Michigan, USA

Stephanie A. Riolo M.D., M.P.H
Director, Community and Consultation Psychiatry
Lecturer, Division of Child and Adolescent Psychiatry
School of Medicine
University of Michigan
Ann Arbor, Michigan, USA

Judith B. Rose B.S.
Orthodontic Department
School of Dentistry
Indiana University
Indianapolis, Indiana, USA

Robyn S. Silberstein D.D.S., Ph.D.
Professor
Department of Orthodontics
School of Dentistry
University of Illinois, Chicago
Chicago, Illinois, USA

Daman D. Thanik B.D.S, D.D.S., M.S., M.S.
Associate Professor
Department of Orthodontics
School of Dentistry
University of Detroit Mercy
Detroit, Michigan, USA

Michelle J. Thornberg D.D.S., M.S.
Assistant Professor
Department of Orthodontics
School of Dentistry
University of Detroit Mercy
Detroit, Michigan, USA

James L. Vaden D.D.S., M.S.
Professor and Chair
Department of Orthodontics
School of Dentistry
University of Tennessee
Memphis, Tennessee, USA

Manish Valiathan B.D.S., M.D.S., D.D.S., M.S.D.
Assistant Professor
Department of Orthodontics
School of Dentistry
Case Western Reserve University
Cleveland, Ohio USA

Elizabeth A. Van Tubergen B.S.
Student
School of Dentistry
University of Michigan
Ann Arbor, Michigan, USA

Contents

Section I
Growth and Development

This first section is concerned with the prenatal and postnatal development of the human. As the embryonic human grows, the craniofacial area develops in neural complexity and the skeletal, vascular, muscular and connective tissues specialize for speech and masticatory function.

Chapters:

Section I	Section II	Section III	Section IV
1. Developmental, Psychosocial Behavioral, and Compliance Aspects of Care 2. Prenatal Craniofacial Growth 3. Postnatal Caniofacial Growth 4. Growth of the Craniofacial Skeleton 5. Development of the Dentition and Occlusion	6. Classification and Terminology 7. Etiology of Malocclusion 8. Force Systems and Tissue Response 9. Tissue Engineering in Orthodontics 10. Clinical Epidemiology and Malocclusion	11. Orthodontic Exam and Diagnosis 12. Analysis of Orofacial and Jaw Musculature 13. Analysis of Dentition and Occlusion 14. Dental Dysmorphogenesis 15. Analysis of Orofacial Skeleton 16. Planning Orthodontic Treatment	17. Preadolescent Treatment 18. Adolescent Treatment 19. Adult Treatment 20. Treatment of Patients with Craniofacial Anomalies 21. Retention, Relapse and the Recurrence of Malocclusion 22. The Adverse Effects of Orthodontic Treatment

CHAPTER 1

Developmental, Psychosocial, Behavioral, and Compliance Aspects of Care

Stephanie A. Riolo

Steven J. Ceresnie

1. INTRODUCTION

The goal of this chapter is to familiarize the reader with developmental, psychosocial, and behavioral issues that are necessarily a part of working with children and adolescents in orthodontics. This goal is undertaken with the hope that it will influence the reader through increased awareness of normal development and psychological principles, promoting a change in behavior in relation to colleagues, peers, children, and patients and their families.

2. WHAT IS "NORMAL"?

Throughout this chapter the word "normal" will be used in reference to development. What is meant by "normal" in the context of developmental processes? Can a person be "normal" or "abnormal?" Offer and Sabshin have provided 4 definitions of "normal":

1.) The absence of pathology- health; the lack of illness or disorder.

2.) The ideal- ideals differ by cultural group. An ideal is not necessarily perfect, but something that is considered perfect is often an ideal.

3.) Average- this refers to the mean using a bell curve or so-called normal distribution. A range of normal is commonly used and, in this case, "normal" refers to all those observations that lie within one standard deviation of the mean of the normal distribution.

4.) The usual- in normal development there are predictable patterns which are considered normal. For example, there are predictable stages of cognitive development.

For more information go to www.aacap.org/publications/factsfam/normal.htm to see the American Academy of Child and Adolescent Psychiatry Publication Facts for Families: Normality.

3. PRINCIPLES OF NORMAL GROWTH & DEVELOPMENT

Early child development is commonly discussed in terms of domains of function. These domains are interdependent, but can be classified into eight gross categories defined below:

1.) Physical Development- physical growth and maturation, gross and fine motor development, perceptual/sensory development, and neurodevelopment,

2.) Cognitive Development- development of higher mental processes, including thinking, attention, memory, learning, and intelligence, e.g., logical thinking and conceptualization of space,

3.) Speech and Language Development- development of receptive, expressive, and written language,

4.) Personality Development- inborn temperament and development of mature personality traits,

5.) Social Development- **attachment**, socialization, and development of mature relationships,

6.) Emotional Development- development of psychological defense mechanisms and emotional stability,

7.) Psychosexual Development- sexual identity development,

8.) Moral Development- development of superego, understanding of rules and conventions.

Table 1-1

Major Milestones	
Newborn:	-Has Moro, grasp, and rooting reflexes
2-3 Months:	-Smiles -Tonic neck reflexes
5-6 Months:	-Babbles -Begins to sit up -Moro, grasp, and tonic neck reflex disappear -Holds bottle
9 Months:	-Babbles -Says "mama" and "dada"
12 Months:	-Stands and may walk
15 Months:	-Walks -Says several words -Points to objects
18 Months:	-Says > 6 words -Feeds himself -Points to simple objects/body parts
24 Months:	-Uses 2-3 word sentences -Runs

Table 1-2

Developmental Sequences of Adaptive Behavior	
Levels of Maturity	
Birth	------------
4 weeks	Stares at surroundings. Restricted eye following.
16 weeks	Competent eye following. Regards rattle in hand.
28 weeks	Transfers cube from hand to hand.
40 weeks	Combines two cubes.
12 months	Releases cube in cup.
18 months	Dumps pellets from bottle. Imitates crayon strokes.
2 years	Builds tower of six cubes. Imitates circular stroke.
3 years	Builds bridge of three cubes. Imitates cross.
4 years	Builds gate of five cubes. Draws "man."
5 years	Counts ten pennies.

All health personnel having responsibility for the care of children should be familiar with normal patterns of growth and development and be able to recognize deviations from the norm as soon as possible, so that underlying disorders may be promptly identified and treated.

The term growth and development refers to the entire process of change from gestation to an adult person. Whereas growth generally refers to changes in size of the body, development refers to other aspects of **differentiation** of body form.

Growth and development depend on both genetic and environmental factors. Genetic factors set limits on biological potential of the individual, but these limits are also affected by the individual's environment in a very complex way. The magnitude of physical growth may be increased or decreased by environmental factors, but development may also be modified in a myriad of ways. Nutritional as well as social and emotional factors affect growth and development. Examples of social and emotional factors include the gender of the child, the position of the child in the family, the quality of interaction of the child with parents, siblings, and important others, and the child-rearing patterns of the parents, extended family, and the community. Trauma may be prenatal or postnatal and may take a variety of forms including nutritional, toxic (e.g., through exposure to alcohol or other substances), vascular, infectious, and many others.

3.1 PHYSICAL DEVELOPMENT

Children are not simply small adults. Most obviously, children are dramatically different from adults in their body proportions. Their heads are relatively larger compared to their body size. In general, children also have rounder faces, less developed noses, and smaller mandibles than do adolescents and adults. Their abdomens are relatively more prominent. They also have shorter extremeties and the mid-point of stature in an infant is the umbilicus, compared to midpoint at the symphysis pubis in adults.

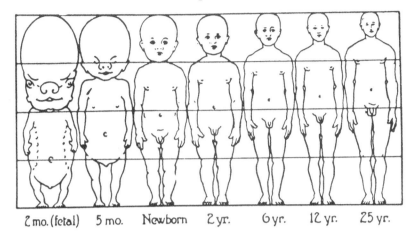

2 mo. (fetal)   5 mo.   Newborn   2 yr.   6 yr.   12 yr.   25 yr.

Figure 1-1: Changes in body proportions from the 2nd fetal month
a to adulthood. (From Robbins WJ, Brody S, Hogan AG, et al:
Growth. New Haven, Yale University Press, 1928.

Children are in a period of rapid growth and have very different energy requirements and metabolic activity than do adults. Measurement of weight, height, and head circumference indicate the status of a child in relation to other children of the same age. Percentile location is commonly used to follow the course of physical development of children with age show curves at positions corresponding to distances from average values, either above or below the mean. Approximately 10% of normal persons fall either above the 95th percentile (5%) or below the 5th percentile (5 %) for any normally distributed measurement (e.g., weight, height, and head circumference). Sequential measurements must be followed to assess whether a child is achieving his or her growth potential. For example, a child below the 10th percentile may be suspected of being undernourished, but (by definition) 10 percent of normal children are below this level. If a child has regular sequential growth in height and weight along a percentile curve above the third to fifth percentile, they are often manifesting normal physical growth. If a child's height and weight are found to cross percentiles in a downward direction, it is most likely that there is an underlying disturbance, e.g., physical illness, nutritional disturbance, or psychosocial difficulty. See sections below on Failure to Thrive and measuring body fat.

The standard height, weight, and head circumference charts are inappropriate for children with intrinsic growth disorders. Special reference growth charts are available for children who have Down, Turner, and Klinefelter syndromes or classic achondroplasia.

3.1.1. Physical Growth- Weight

Fetal weight gain is greatest during the 3rd trimester of pregnancy. Average birth weight is 7 ½ pounds (3.4 kg). Infants normally lose 10% of their birth weight after birth. Subsequently, with usual intake the normal full-term infant will re-gain approximately 30 grams of weight per day and reach its birth weight by 10-14 days of age. By 4-6 months of age, normal infants will double their birth weight. And by one year, the normal infant will triple its birth weight. The increase in subcutaneous tissue in the early months of life reaches its peak at about 9 months. Weight gain slows after the first year of life. The average child gains about 2.5 kg (5-6 lbs) during the second year of life. During the 3rd, 4th, and 5th years of life gains in weight are relatively steady at approximately 2 kg (4.5 lbs). The early school years are a period of relatively steady growth ending in the preadolescent growth spurt by about 10 years in girls and 12 years in boys. The average weight gain during these years is about 3-3.5 kg (7 lbs) per year.

3.1.2. Physical Growth- Height

The average birth height is 20 inches (50 cm.) An average infant's height increases by 50% during the first year (25-30 cm or 10-12 inches) and doubles by 3 to 4 years of age. During the second year of life there is a deceleration in the rate of growth; the average child gains about 12 cm (5 inches) in height during the 2nd year. Height growth continues to slow in the early school years until the growth spurt. Average height gain during these years is 6 cm (2.5 inches) per year. On average, in girls, the growth spurt occurs between 10-12 years. In boys, the growth spurt occurs, on average, between 12-14 years. During the growth spurt, females average an increment in height of 8 cm per year at the mean age of 12 years. Boys average 10 cm per year during their later growth spurt at the mean age of 14 years. There is an orderly progression of skeletal growth from the distal to proximal parts of the body, beginning with growth of the feet, followed by calf and the thigh. Similarly, hands grow before upper parts of the arms. This results in transient disproportionately large hands and feet and contributes to the clumsiness of adolescents. Peak acceleration of the legs and arms is followed by that of the chest and hips. Elongation of the trunk and increase in the anteroposterior diameter of the chest are the last manifestations of the pubertal growth spurt.

3.1.3. Physical Growth- Head Circumference

The increase in head circumference (HC) is proportional to increase in brain mass for at least the first 2 years. The anterior **fontanel** may increase in size after birth but generally diminishes after 6 months. At birth, the average head circumference is 35 cm (13 ¾ inches.) Microcephaly (defined as HC less than 10th percentile for age) occurs for many reason, including prenatal/postnatal insult (ischemia, **TORCH**, shaken baby syndrome), familial predisposition, and genetic predisposition. Macrocephaly (defined as HC greater than 90th percentile for age) is most commonly related to familial predisposition. Other causes of macrocephaly include neoplasm and hydrocephalus.

The growth of the brain decelerates during the second year of life. Head circumference, which increased approximately 12 cm during the first year, increases only 2 cm during the second year. By the end of the first year the brain has reached approximately 2/3 of its adult size. By the end of the second year the brain is approximately 4/5 of adult size. Growth of head circumference slows during the early school years and has reached approximate adult size by the preadolescent growth spurt. The development of the facial bones is active during the school years, particularly with enlargement of the nasal accessory sinuses.

3.1.4. Measuring Body Fat

Body weight is not an accurate measure of body fat content or adiposity. Overweight may be due to excess fat or an excess of other tissue (muscle, bone, water) in relation to height. Obesity is not equivalent to overweight. Obesity specifically denotes an excess of body fat. Age, gender, and sexual maturity are highly correlated with body fatness and therefore must be taken into account when measuring fatness/adiposity.

3.1.5. Growth Curves

Growth curves are the recommended tool to track childhood growth and to screen for overweight and underweight risk in children (See Figures 1-1, 1-2). The Center for Disease Control (CDC), using data collected by the National Center for Health Statistics (NCHS) in the third National Health and Nutritional Examination Survey (NHANES III), has developed revised growth curves to be used by health providers. The revised growth curves use the Body Mass Index plotted according to age and are specific for gender. The **Body Mass Index (BMI)** is an anthropometric index of weight and height.

$$BMI = \text{weight (kg)} \; / \; [\text{height}]^2$$

BMI is not a direct measure of body fatness, but serves as a proxy for direct measures such as hydrostatic weighing and dual energy x-ray absortiometry (DEXA.)

BMI-for-age curves more accurately track adiposity from age 2 years through adulthood (as compared to using simple weight, weight for age, or weight for height.) It is recommended that BMI-for-age be used for individuals 2-20 years of age. From birth until two years of age simple weight by age, height by age, and weight by height percentiles may be used.

Using the updated CDC growth curves, youths (aged 2-20 years) with BMI between the 85th-95th percentile for age are classified as "at risk for obesity." Youth with BMI greater than or equal to the 95th percentile of BMI-for-age are classified as "obese." For adults, BMI is used without adjusting for age or gender. Adults with BMI >= 30 are considered obese. Adults with BMI between 25-29.9 are considered overweight.

The Prevalence of Overweight in U.S. Children and Adolescents
(1988-94, NHANES III)

Gender	85th Percentile	95th Percentile
both sexes	22.0	10.9
boys	21.3	11.7
girls	24.2	13.7

from Troiano, RP, et al   Arch Pediatr Adolesc Med 149:1085-1091, 1995

Figure 1-2

The latest findings from the Centers for Disease Control (CDC) and the National Health and Nutrition Examination Survey (NHANES) show that increasing numbers of children and adolescents are overweight. Between 1963-1991, there was a doubling of the prevalence of children with a BMI of more than 95th percentile. There was a 50% increase in the prevalence of children with a BMI of more than 85th percentile over this same period.

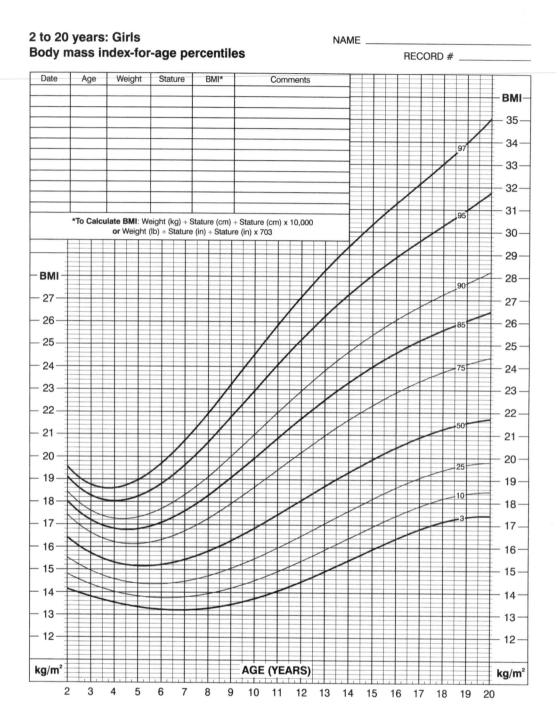

2 to 20 years: Girls
Body mass index-for-age percentiles

NAME _____

RECORD # _____

Date	Age	Weight	Stature	BMI*	Comments

*To Calculate BMI: Weight (kg) ÷ Stature (cm) ÷ Stature (cm) x 10,000
or Weight (lb) ÷ Stature (in) ÷ Stature (in) x 703

SOURCE: Developed by the National Center for Health Statistics in collaboration with
the National Center for Chronic Disease Prevention and Health Promotion (2000).
http://www.cdc.gov/growthcharts

Figure 1-3A

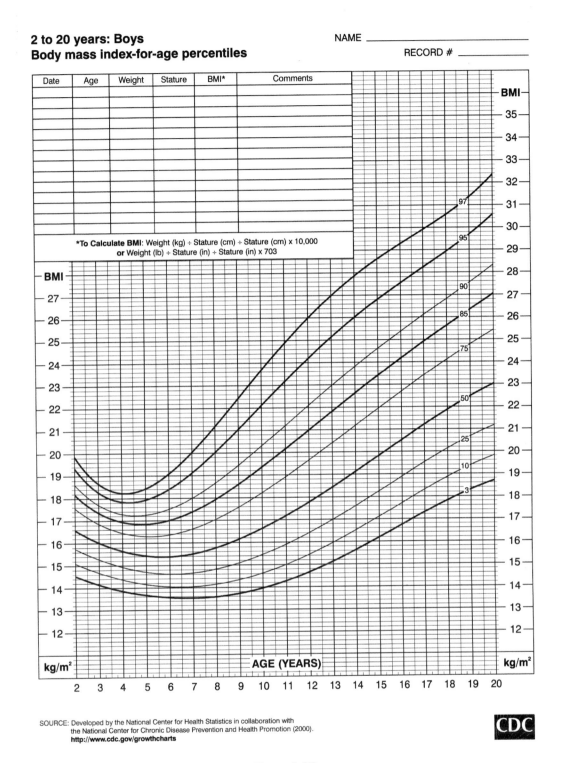

2 to 20 years: Boys
Body mass index-for-age percentiles

NAME _____

RECORD # _____

*To Calculate BMI: Weight (kg) ÷ Stature (cm) ÷ Stature (cm) x 10,000
or Weight (lb) ÷ Stature (in) ÷ Stature (in) x 703

SOURCE: Developed by the National Center for Health Statistics in collaboration with
the National Center for Chronic Disease Prevention and Health Promotion (2000).
http://www.cdc.gov/growthcharts

CDC

Figure 1-3B

3.1.6. Gross and Fine Motor Skills

Gross motor skills involve large body movements such as running, climbing, jumping, and throwing (See Table 1-3). **Fine motor skills** involve small body movements such as those of the hands and fingers. Fine motor skills are much more difficult to master than gross motor skills. Examples include accurate penmanship, pouring liquids into a glass, cutting with scissors, and tying a shoelace. The chief reason why many children experience difficulty with fine motor skills is that they have not yet developed the necessary muscular control, patience, and/or judgement, in part because the central nervous system is not yet sufficiently myelinated. The difficulty of early fine motor coordination is often compounded by short, stubby fingers. Adults can assist and prevent unnecessary frustration by knowledge of normal development (and variation) and by providing appropriate tools, time, and encouragement.

3.1.7. Failure to Thrive

Failure to Thrive (FTT) is defined as growth rate less than the 3rd percentile for height or weight or a drop in weight/height that crosses two percentiles on the growth curve. The most common cause of failure to thrive is non-organic and is due to psychosocial factors.   Improper feeding accounts for 50-60% of cases of FTT. Other causes of failure to thrive include gastrointestinal problems (inflammatory bowel disease, severe gastroesophageal reflux, malabsorption), respiratory problems (e.g., bronchopulmonary **dysplasia**, cystic fibrosis), renal problems (e.g., chronic renal failure, renal tubular acidosis), endocrine/metabolic problems (e.g., diabetes mellitus, hypothyroidism), and infectious illness (e.g., HIV.)

Developmental Sequences of Motor Behavior	
Levels of Maturity	
Birth	------------
4 weeks	Head sags. Tonic neck reflex. Hands fisted.
16 weeks	Head steady. Symmetrical postures. Hands open.
28 weeks	Sits, leaning forward on hands. Grasps cube. Rakes at pellet.
40 weeks	Sits alone. Creeps. Pulls to feet. Crude prehensory release.
12 months	Walks with help. Cruises. Prehends pellet with precision.
18 months	Walks without falling. Seats self. Tower of three cubes.
2 years	Runs. Builds tower of six cubes.
3 years	Stands on one foot. Builds tower of ten cubes.
4 years	Skips on one foot.
5 years	Skips on alternate feet.

Table 1-3

3.2 NEURODEVELOPMENT

Brain development begins before birth. Between the 7th month of gestation and the 2nd year of postnatal life, more than half of the future adult brain mass is formed. An individual's full complement of **neurons** (nerve cells) is present before birth. In fact, the total number of neurons actually begins to decrease in late pregnancy. The developing brain has a maximum number of neurons at the end of the 2nd trimester of pregnancy, with 100-200 billion neurons. At birth there are only 100 billion remaining neurons. Approximately 1/2 the total neurons die between birth and one year of life.

Brain development proceeds sequentially. There are critical periods of neurodevelopment in which a set of signals must be present in order for neurons to differentiate normally. In this way, environmental stimulation directly affects the architecture (and therefore function) of the brain. The increase in brain mass seen in early childhood corresponds to **synaptogenesis** and **myelination.** An individual's experiences lead to neural changes (by synaptic pruning and synaptogenesis.) The remolded brain then facilitates new experiences, and so the process goes on.

During brain development, patterns of neural activity define patterns of synaptic connectivity, and thereby, the brain's functional capacity. The brain is the ultimate use-it-or-lose-it machine. The brain matches all incoming sensory signals against previously stored patterns. Patterns of neural activity that are repeated or familiar are categorized. Patterns that are novel cause central nervous system arousal and focus the organism's attention, and sometimes cause alarm. **Synapses** are pruned and made accordingly. In adults, experience can alter pre-existing neural organization. In children, experience literally provides the organizing template for neural systems.

Thus the brain is always changing, or "plastic". While the first few years of life are very important and provide a foundation for brain development, the process of change continues throughout life. The plasticity is not uniform across all brain areas or ages, however; the frontal and limbic areas are particularly sensitive. It takes less time, intensity, and repetition to organize the developing neural systems during early life than to re-organize the already developed neural systems in the older brain. Also, the organizational and functional capacity of the brain is sequentially developed. Optimally, developmentally appropriate experiences should be made available to children in early life.

3.3 COGNITIVE DEVELOPMENT

As with motor development, a child's cognitive development proceeds in an orderly fashion. Simple observation of a child's use of toys or objects can help to determine the child's cognitive progress.

3.3.1. Object Permanence

By six months of age, children usually exhibit the early capacity for the concept of **object permanence**. For example, the child who drops a toy from his high chair and is able to track the toy through the vertical fall and search for it on the floor even though his gaze has been interrupted. To test for the concept of object permanence, induce the infant or child to look for a hidden toy or play a game of peek-a-boo. The child's anticipation of reappearance of the object indicates the child's development of the concept of object permanence. By 9 to 12 months of age, children often demonstrate full capacity of the concept of object permanence. For example, the child who is able to locate a small, hidden object even though no part of it remains visible. By 18 months of age, children normally can deduce the location of an object even if they did not see it hidden from view.

3.3.2. **Pre-Operational Logic**

In the second year of life the child demonstrates mental activity independent of sensory processing or motor manipulation. This was referred to as the pre-operational stage by **Piaget**. Thinking during the pre-operational stage is **egocentric**, or self-centered, as the child is unable to put himself in another's place. Also, perceptual evaluation dominates over cognitive or intellectual evaluation during this stage. In other words, the child's logic is largely influenced by the appearance of objects. One example of this is that a preschooler may assume that people on a plane have become smaller as a plane takes off and flies away because the size of the plane has gotten smaller. Suppose a child in this stage is asked to compare two rows of pennies with one row of seven and one row of nine pennies. If the row of seven is spaced so that it is longer in total length than the row of nine pennies, then the child will say the row of seven has more pennies than the row of nine, even if the child understands that nine is more than seven.

Thinking during the pre-operational period is also limited by inability to focus on more than one aspect of a situation. In addition, children in pre-operational period do not understand cause and effect. A child in this phase often assumes causality between two things that are closely connected in time. For example, the child may believe that he got sick as a punishment for bad behavior or thoughts. The child may believe that a person died because the child was bad or at some point the child wished that person were dead.

The pre-operational child does not possess the ability to understand the concept of reversibility. For example, if the child breaks a toy, he cannot understand that it can be fixed again. Children in the pre-operational stage learn that a name stands for an object and is the symbol for the object. However, the child may also believe that the name he assigns an object (e.g., "fuzzy" for a blanket) is the real name and may not understand why others do not also know the name. A toddler's ability to play with a toy telephone indicates the emergence of **symbolic thought**. Full development of symbolic thought is exemplified by the child's capacity for symbolic play. For example, a child who observes a TV super-hero in a rescue mission and then, hours later, reenacts the scene in detail.

During the late pre-operational phase the child develops the concept of conservation and realizes the amount or quantity of matter stays the same, regardless of changes in shape or position. For example, the child now realizes that people in planes do not shrink in size after take-off. Another example is that the child realizes that an amount of liquid is the same in two different shape containers (particularly if liquid is poured from one to the other.)

In addition to limited cognitive ability, children in the pre-operation phase have not yet developed emotional stability. If a child during the pre-operational phase becomes frustrated or upset, a response of empathy is likely to soothe more effectively than a response of reason, since rational reasoning is limited during this cognitive period.

3.3.3. Logical Thinking

By mid to late elementary school, cognitive development has progressed toward abstract and hypothetical thinking such that the child is able to reflect self-consciously about him/herself and others. Children of this stage begin to develop a **Theory of Mind** and **self-awareness**. Self-awareness is a person's sense of him/herself as being distinct from other people. Self-awareness makes many new self-conscious emotions possible, such as shame, guilt, embarrassment, and pride. While first and second graders struggle to understand causes of conflict and their emotional reactions to it, older elementary school children and adolescents are developmentally able to analyze situations, reasons, and reactions. Although older children may not be fully able to regulate their emotional reactions to events, they are beginning to understand their own motivations and environmental triggers of their emotional responses.

3.3.4. Intelligence

The following is the Policy Statement of the American Academy of Child and Adolescent Psychiatry (AACAP). This policy statement was revised and adopted by council on 6/14/96. For further information regarding the AACAP go to http://www.aacap.org.

"Multiple factors contribute to the development of intelligence. It is a grave error when heredity is promulgated as the sole or primary **factor**(s) indicative of intelligence and then is coupled with race or ethnicity. As clinicians, researchers, and teachers, child and adolescent psychiatrists are acutely aware of the multiple influences that impact (negatively or positively) on the make-up of a child. All should deplore the call by supporters of heredity as a sole basis for intelligence and use [of this argument] for the political/physical dissolution of remediation and social programs. The value and effectiveness of many such programs are well documented [e.g., the documented value of head start programs]; we urge when indicated the continuation of such services and programs and when reasoned evidence suggest transition to new and better programs."

Please see the glossary for definitions of **IQ tests, achievement tests,** and **aptitude tests.**

3.4 SPEECH AND LANGUAGE DEVELOPMENT

Table 1-4

Language is defined as any symbolic system for storage and exchange of information. When assessing language ability, there are two main domains: auditory expressive ability and auditory receptive ability. However, language is also conveyed visually in the form of gestures and through formal systems of sign language.

Human infants produce a uniform sequence of pre-linguistic utterances, regardless of the language spoken by their adult caretakers. Cooing, which consists of musical, open vowel sounds, is the first spoken language by infants and should be well established by 4 to 6 weeks of life. Next infants produce bilabial sounds: blowing bubbles or the producing the "raspberry". By 5 months, laughing and a variety of monosyllables appear, such as "ba" or "ga". By 10 months, infants say "mama" or "dada" spontaneously and consistently to label the appropriate parent. By 12 months, infants have acquired 1-2 words other than "mama" and "dada." Vocabulary growth accelerates throughout the second year. The typical 2-year-old has a vocabulary of at least 50 words. Vocabulary growth continues to accelerate during the third year and children begin to put words together in sentences and learn grammar. By 36 months, the normal child is able to produce grammatically correct sentences in the present tense. Along with increased language complexity comes increased intelligibility. A normal child's speech should be ½ intelligible at 2 years, ¾ intelligible by 3 years, and completely intelligible by 4 years of age (See Table 1-4).

Developmental Sequences of Language Behavior	
Levels of Maturity	
Birth	——————-
4 weeks	Small throaty sounds. Heeds bell.
16 weeks	Coos. Laughs. Vocalizes socially.
28 weeks	Crows. Vocalizes eagerness. Listens to own vocalizations.
40 weeks	Says one word. Responds to name.
12 months	Says two or more words. Basic single word comprehension. Responds to simple commands. 10-50 word vocabulary. Begins word combinations.
18 months	Jargons. Names pictures.
2 years	Uses phrases. 2-3 word sentences. 50-200 word vocabulary. Identifies body parts. Understands "in" and "on."
3 years	Talks in sentences. Answers simple questions. Asks "why" questions. Uses pronouns. Uses past and present tenses. 4-5 word sentences. Understands opposites. 200-1500 word vocabulary.
4 years	Uses conjunctions. Understands prepositions. Understands comparatives. 2700 word vocabulary.
5 years	Speaks without infantile articulation. Correctly uses all parts of speech. 5000 word vocabulary. Enjoys jokes and riddles.

3.5 EMOTIONAL DEVELOPMENT

3.5.1. Emotions

John Watson first suggested the existence of innate emotions. Watson proposed 3 basic innate emotions: fear, rage, and love. Subsequently, evidence has supported the existence of the universal emotions of sadness, anger, happiness, and surprise. The evidence that love, fear, disgust, and contempt are universal emotions is more variable and expression and experience of these emotions varies by culture.

Self-awareness develops in the second year of life and allows a new set of emotions, including pride, embarrassment, and jealousy. At this time the infant becomes less predictable and less compliant but more interesting.

3.5.2. Development of Emotional Security

3.5.2.1. Transitional Objects- "Binkies" & "Blankies"

Transitional object is a concept coined by D.W. Winnicott to refer to an object to which a child confers emotional meaning and becomes temporarily attached. These objects are usually soft toys or pieces of cloth (e.g., blanket, pillow, doll, piece of mother's clothing, stuffed animal) that the child carries with him/her for comfort, particularly before going to sleep. The object is typically held close the child's face/mouth (See photo in Figure 1-4), and often is rubbed on the skin (especially against the face). Perhaps the most famous example is Linus (Charlie Brown's friend) and his blanket, which he dragged everywhere (See Figure 1-6).

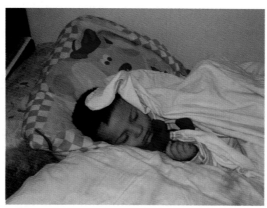

Figure 1-4

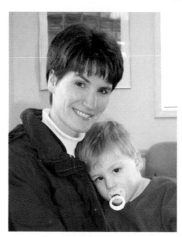

Figure 1-5

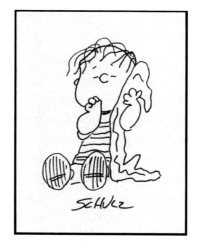

Figure 1-6

The transitional object starts acquiring importance when the child begins to distinguish between him/herself and others. During the first few months of life, an infant experiences his/her mother (main caretaker) as an extension of his/herself. Gradually, the child realizes that he and his mother are separate people and becomes frightened when she is out of sight. The object reminds the child of his mother. The object allows increased independence. A transitional object need not be a blanket ("blankie", "lovie") but may be any object (pacifier "binkie", photo, or object of the loved one) (See photo in Figure 1-5). It can also be metaphorical (e.g., an ideology or group of people who share the same belief, (such as a clique of preadolescent children.) The "security blanket" is a mother substitute that has the mother's smell, but stays with the child. In fact, children often choose a transitional object more by smell or touch than by sight. It remains firmly under the child's control especially when the child's mother is absent.

Despite myths to the contrary, transitional objects are not a sign of weakness or insecurity. In fact, these objects can be very helpful. Parents may wish to encourage such objects and even help their child choose one and build it into a nighttime ritual. They can keep a small soft toy or blanket in the crib from infancy. The child may initially ignore it but will probably take to it eventually. It may be helpful to actually have two or more identical security objects- this will allow you to clean one. Rotate them early or else the second may feel "too new" and may not be accepted by the child.

Transitional objects can be very useful for children in foreign situations or undergoing stressful procedures (dental/orthodontic office, dental/orthodontic exam/procedures). It may be helpful to encourage parents of young children to bring such objects to the office.

3.5.2.2. Normal Emotional Regression

Throughout childhood and **adolescence** (and indeed for many throughout early adulthood) the desire to grow up and for independence is in continued conflict with the desire to remain a child or remain dependent and cared for by someone else. During times of stress, temporary regressions to earlier, safer levels of functioning may occur. It is important to view these lapses as normal and temporary phases of development rather than as intentional lapses on the part of the child or adolescent. For example, it is not uncommon for a preschooler to have temporary behavioral/emotional regression after the birth of a new child. The preschooler may become clingy and "immature" and may even have a lapse in toilet training. In later years, it is not uncommon for pre-adolescent children to develop increased feelings of loneliness and even to develop fears of being alone or mild **separation anxiety** symptoms.

3.5.3. Emotional Regulation

Perhaps the most important domain of development during early childhood is development of emotional regulation (See Table 1-5). **Emotional regulation** is the ability to direct or modify one's feelings of fear, frustration, and anger. It is the ability to inhibit, enhance, maintain, and modulate emotional arousal to accomplish one's goals. **Emotional lability** is defined as rapidly changing emotions or emotional instability. Pride is tempered by guilt (and vice versa), joy by sadness, anger by fear, and fear by rituals. Because of brain maturation, emotional regulation becomes more possible during the preschool years. How does emotional regulation develop? Part of it is neurological. The ability to regulate one's emotions, to think before acting, is related to the frontal cortex. This area is immature in toddlers but develops during preschool years. A child's brain may be damaged in utero (by alcohol, drugs, infection, anoxia, or other insult), stunted during infancy and early childhood (by malnutrition or lack of stimulation or neglect), or injured during infancy or early childhood (by head injury or infection). As a result the child may be intellectually intact in most ways but unable to regulate his of her emotions or may have other relatively subtle deficits in executive functioning.

Table 1-5

Emotional Milestones
1. Innate/Basic emotions 2. Development of self-conscious emotions 3. Development of emotional self-regulation 4. Development of capacity to respond to others' emotions

3.6 PERSONALITY DEVELOPMENT

The combined affects of biological factors, environmental factors, and individual experience on a child's development is perhaps best illustrated by the transactional model of development. According to the transactional model, described by *Sameroff* (1993), a child's individual perceptions, innate patterns of responses, and individual strengths and weaknesses combine with the perceptions, responses, and strengths and weaknesses of that child's caretakers to determine the course of a child's development and ultimately the child's adult personality. The "Big Five" major clusters of **personality** found in adults are extroversion, agreeableness, conscientiousness, neuroticism, and openness.

A child's experience is critical to his/her development and occurs in the context of bi-directional relationships. Thus, a child's development is the result of a continuous dynamic interaction between the child and the experience provided by his/her family and social context.

3.6.1. Nature vs. Nurture

"Nature" refers to a child's genetic or biological endowment and includes that child's innate **temperament**. "Nurture" refers to early childhood environment and experiences; it consists of many variables, including nutrition, physical and emotional security, stimulation and quality and quantity of interactions with parents and important others. There is no such thing as "nature vs. nurture" in the sense that a particular cognitive, behavioral, or emotional characteristic is solely caused by either genetic or environmental factors. All behavior and development has to do with the brain. And brain development is dependent on the genetics, the environment, and the experiences of the developing individual.

3.6.2. Temperament

Chess and Alexander (1977) described 9 traits within 3 categories of temperament in their New York Longitudinal Study (See Tables 1-6 and 1-7). Temperament is each child's individual and innate pattern of response to the environment. Temperament is largely biologically determined but influences developmental outcome because it influences how a child is perceived by others. Temperament affects how a child fits in a social situation.

Table 1-6

Table 1-7

Temperamental dimensions/traits identifiable in infancy
1.) Activity level 2.) Rhythmicity (regularity and predictability of biologic functions) 3.) Approach or withdrawal to novel stimuli 4.) Adaptability to environmental changes 5.) Intensity of reaction 6.) Threshold of responsiveness (intensity of stimulation required to evoke a response) 7.) Quality of mood (positive, neutral or negative) 8.) Distractibility 9.) Attention span and persistence

Temperamental Clusters
1. Easy 　　-Positive mood 　　-Regular biologic rhythms 　　-Adaptable 　　-Low intensity 　　-Positive approach to novelty 2. Difficult 　　-Negative mood 　　-Irregular biologic rhythms 　　-Slow to adapt 　　-Intense reactions 　　-Negative response to novelty 3. Slow to Warm Up 　　-Negative responses to new stimuli 　　-Mild intensity 　　-Gradual adaptation after repeated contact

3.6.3. Development of Sense of Self

Self-awareness develops gradually through childhood. Emerging self-awareness can usually be seen between 6 to 8 months, when infants first display interest in looking at their own image in a mirror. After approximately one year of age, toddlers rapidly expand their sense of self. They can explore and function with independence. They are able to feed themselves and have clear ideas about what they do and do not like. Between 1 and 2 years of age, toddlers begin to enjoy their own company- as demonstrated by the child who claps for his own successes. These developments come with increasing discipline concerns.

3.6.4. Development of **Body Image**

An individual's perceived physical appearance or **body image** is not a reflection of their body as it is, but an interpretation of it. This interpretation is emotionally charged and is influenced by many factors, both individual (biological and psychological) and contextual (social and cultural). Body image is one part of an individual's entire self-image and begins to develop in the earliest stages of awareness of self.

Although development of body image begins with the early development of sense of self (during the first year of life), a coherent and constant body image is not fully developed until 5-7 years of age. Conversely, cognitive ability influences an individual's perception of his/her body. **Mental retardation** significantly limits the development of body image because of the inability to form abstract concepts and relate self-perceptions with the bodies of others.

Children and adolescents are accurate in perception of "ideal" occlusion and facial form (Graber 1980, Cohen and Horowitz 1970, Hulsey 1970, Peck and Peck 1970, Gochman 1972, 1975, Foster 1973, Prahl-Anderson *et al,* 1975). Even relatively minor deviations from "normal body" or ideal or facial form are self-perceived and are over-valued in perception of self as well as perception of others (Wright 1960, Graber 1980).

Development of body image is greatly impacted by variation from average physical appearance (i.e., physical deformity.) Both the timing and degree of the variation is important. For example, whether a deformity is inborn or acquired can have a dramatic effect on development of body image and self-image. Data is available that demonstrates that children with significant disfigurement, such as a **cleft palate**, have normal cognitive and emotional development until they enter school. Thereafter, their cognitive and emotional development depends on their social support.

3.6.5. Social Norms for Physical Appearance and their Effect on Body Image and Self Image/Self Esteem

Even in early childhood, a child's self image is strongly influenced by their physical appearance and how his/her appearance is perceived by others. All children, regardless of their actual physical 'normalcy,' compare their bodies with others. First with their family, then with their peers and contacts, and finally with those that are presented by the culture as ideal, e.g., fashion models, film stars, athletes. Simmons and Rosenberg (1975) evaluated 1988 children between 3 - 12 years and found that children who were dissatisfied with their appearance are more self conscious, emotionally unstable, and have lower self-esteem. The outward physical appearance of children influences their self-perception, which in turn influences their inner psychological state (both their body image and self image or self esteem).

There is evidence that children as young as 6 years of age understand the importance of being thin

(Flannery-Schroeder and Chrisler 1996). Stigmatization of obese individuals is established in early childhood (Goldfield and Chrisler 1995).

3.7 SOCIAL DEVELOPMENT

Table 1-8

Developmental Sequences of Personal-Social Behavior
Levels of Maturity
Birth ------------
4 weeks	Regards faces.
6 weeks	Social smile
16 weeks	Plays with hands and dress. Recognizes bottle. Poises mouth for food.
28 weeks	Plays with feet and toys. Expectant in feeding situations.
40 weeks	Plays simple nursery games. Feeds him/herself a cracker.
12 months	Cooperates in dressing. Gives toy. Finger feeds.
18 months	Uses spoon with moderate spilling. Toilet regulated.
2 years	Verbalizes toilet needs. Plays with dolls.
3 years	Uses spoon well. Puts on shoes. Takes turns.
4 years	Washes and dries face. Goes on errands. Plays cooperatively.
5 years	Dresses without assistance. Asks meanings of words.

3.7.1. Attachment

Attachment, according to Mary Ainsworth (1973), is defined as "an affectional tie that one person or animal forms between him/herself and another specific one (usually an important caregiver)- a tie that binds them together in space and endures over time." When people are attached to each other, they try to be near one another and they interact with each other often. The drive for attachment is thought to be innate. Children and adults who are attached demonstrate proximity seeking behaviors and contact maintaining behaviors. Examples include a child following a parent or sibling (See Figure 1-7) or a child climbing into a parent's lap, a parent tiptoeing into their sleeping child's room to watch them sleep or smoothing a toddler's hair. Attachment deepens the parent-child relationship and has likely contributed to human survival.

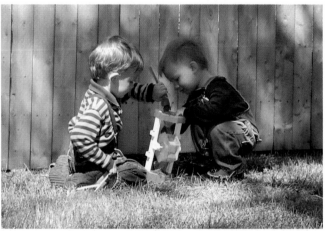

Figure 1-7

A **secure attachment** is one in which an infant derives comfort and confidence from a caregiver, as evidenced first by the infants attempts to be close to the caregiver and then, equally important, by the infant's readiness to explore the environment in the presence of the caregiver. The caregiver acts as a secure base for exploration, from which the child is willing to venture forth. In response to separation from their caregiver, a securely attached child shows some degree of distress at separation, varying in severity from a pause or woeful look to a loud cry. On being reunited after a limited period of time, the securely attached toddler is unambivalent and welcoming in their behavior toward the caregiver and is soothed by contact with the caregiver. Approximately 2/3 of all toddlers are securely attached to their caregivers.

By contrast, **insecure attachment** is characterized by an infant's fear, anxiety, anger, or seeming indifference toward a caregiver. The insecurely attached child has much less confidence for exploration when compared to a securely attached infant. In response to separation from their caregiver, the insecurely attached child may show no apparent distress or may have extreme distress on separation. When reunited (even after a brief period) insecurely attached children may avoid their caregiver, show ambivalence in their response to the caregiver, or continue to be very distressed despite attempts of the caregiver to soothe them.

There are three types of insecure attachments in toddlers:

1.) Insecure-avoidant type- The toddler appears minimally interested in the caregiver, explores busily, show minimal distress at separation, and ignores or avoids the caregiver on reunion. Approximately 15-25% of toddlers are classified as Insecure-avoidant type when tested.
2.) Insecure-resistant type- The toddler does minimal exploration and is preoccupied with their caregiver. When reunited after separation the child has difficulty settling down and is ambivalent in their response to the caregiver- both seeks and resists contact. The child may be angry or very passive. Approximately 10-15% of toddlers are classified as Insecure-resistant when tested.
3.) Insecure-disorganized/disoriented/ambivalent type- These toddlers exhibit disorganized and/or disoriented behavior in the caregiver's presence (e.g., approaches with head averted, engages in trance-like freezing, adopts anomalous postures). Approximately 10-20% of toddlers are Insecure-disorganized when tested.

Adults can also be classified based on their attachment to their childhood caregivers. There are four categories of adult attachment:

1.) Autonomous- These adults value close relationships and regard them as influential. They are not overwhelmed by emotions when they think about or discuss their childhood caregivers. They can see both positive and negative aspects of past caregivers.
2.) Dismissing- These adults tend to devalue the importance and influence of their attachment relationships. They sometimes idealize their early relationships with their parents without ability to provide specific supporting examples.
3.) Preoccupied- These adults are still very emotionally involved with their childhood experiences. They are unable to discuss their childhood relationships objectively and often show excessive emotion when discussing their parents.
4.) Unresolved- These adults are not (yet) reconciled about their past attachments. They are struggling to understand troublesome past experiences/losses.

Childhood experiences, even those of early infancy, affect adult attitudes and behavior. However, understanding childhood, as may come through psychotherapy, can overcome damage that may have occurred. Current attitudes about past experiences are crucial in determining emotions, behavior, and relationships. Researchers have discovered that mothers' current adult attachment classifications closely parallel the kind of attachment their children form with them. Autonomous mothers tend to have securely attached children; dismissing mothers tend to have insecure-avoidant children; and preoccupied mothers tend to have insecure-resistant children. Mothers with unresolved attachment have children with variable attachment.

3.7.2. Goodness of Fit

"**Goodness of fit**" results when properties of the environment and its expectations and demands are in accord with a child's own capacities, motivations, and style of behavior (temperament). Although there is no such thing as 'normal' or 'abnormal' temperament, a child's temperament can fit well or poorly with cultural norms or with the expectations and behavioral style of the child's parents, teachers, and other significant caregivers. When a child's behavior violates expectations, caregivers often react negatively, pressuring the child to change their behavior that was perceived as distressing. With consonance between a child and his/her environment, optimal development is possible. "Goodness of fit" does not imply lack of stress and conflict. Stress and conflict, when in keeping with the child's developmental potential and capacity for mastery, can have quite positive developmental consequences (See Figure 1-8).

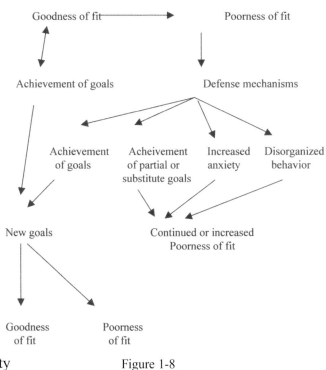

Figure 1-8

3.8 SUMMARY: NEURODEVELOPMENTAL CORRELATES OF CHILD DEVELOPMENT

All behavioral and emotional development in childhood correlates with the underlying development of the child's brain. **Neonatal biobehavioral state** shifts correspond directly to early brain development. The typical newborn spends 3-6 hours in a quiet or actively alert state, 1-3 hours crying, and the remainder of each day in some stage of sleep. By 2-3 months of age the average child, because of rapid synaptogenesis, cries much less, is able to settle his/herself, has a diurnal sleep-wake cycle, and smiles socially. Early development of object permanence, inhibitory control, social referencing, social judgement, and crawling at 7-9 months correspond to myelination of the corticolimbic interconnections to the prefrontal cortex. Similarly, the language burst and the development of pretend play seen between 18-20 months of age corresponds to the completion of limbic maturation and myelination of the language areas. By seven years of age, the brain's anatomical structures and myelination are largely, but not entirely, complete. The 7-year-old brain is nearly the size of that of the adult. During **adolescence**, myelination of higher brain centers continues, resulting in faster information processing and the ability for abstract thought. Also during adolescence, synaptic pruning in the prefrontal cortex continues through age 20, resulting in increased strategic planning ability and improved social judgement. Functional development of the cerebral cortex is evident in the characteristic changes seen in the developing child's electroencephalogram (EEG).

Table 1-9 summarizes the neurodevelopmental correlates of motor, language, cognitive, social-emotional, and behavioral development.

Table 1-9
Neurodevelopmental Correlates of Child Development

Age (yrs)	Brain Myelination	EEG (Metcalf)	Motor (Gesell)	Language (Lennenberg)	Drawing (DiLeo)	Attachment (Bowlby)	Cognitive (Piaget)	Environment
0-1		0 cps	Reflexes	babbles		Signaling (0-3 mo.)	Sensori-motor	Mothering Person
1-2		5 cps	Pincer Grasp Walks	2 words		Proximity Seeking		
2-3				200 words	○		Pre-Operational	Parents
3-4		8 cps				Goal-Directed		
4-7		11 cps	Uses Scissors		□	Partner-ship	Concrete Operational	School & Peers
7-12				Normal Language	◊			
12+		10 cps	Rides Bike				Formal Operations	Peers & Adults

3.9 NEWBORN REFLEXES

A **reflex** is an automatic reaction to a stimulus, mediated by the spinal cord or lower brain. Some examples of reflexes common to children and adults include blinking, sneezing, coughing, yawning, and gagging.

Newborn reflexes are mechanisms for survival, indicators of brain maturation, and vestiges of evolutionary history. There are three sets of newborn reflexes that are critical for survival:

1.) Reflexes that maintain the oxygen supply. The **breathing reflex** begins in normal newborns even before the umbilical cord, with its supply of oxygen from the mother, is cut. Additional reflexes that maintain oxygen supply are hiccups and sneezes, as well as thrashing (moving arms and legs about) to escape something that covers the face.
2.) Reflexes that maintain constant body temperature. When infants are cold, they cry, shiver, and tuck their legs close to their body. When they are hot, they cry and try to push blankets away.
3.) Reflexes that manage feeding. The **sucking reflex** causes newborns to suck anything that touches their lips- fingers, toes, blankets, rattles, as well as natural and artificial nipples of various sizes and shapes. The **rooting reflex** causes babies to turn their mouths toward anything that brushes against their cheeks, a reflexive search for a nipple, and start to suck. Swallowing is another important reflex that aids feeding. By crying when their stomach is empty, infants also manage feeding. Spitting up is another reflex, and occurs when too much has been swallowed too quickly.

There are also vestigial newborn reflexes that are no longer necessary for survival, but continue to be important signs of normal brain and body functioning. These reflexes only persist for a limited period of time and include:

1.) **Babinski reflex**- When the infant's feet are stroked, their toes fan upward.

2.) Palmar grasp reflex- When something touches the infant's palms, they grip it tightly.

3.) Stepping reflex- When infants are held upright with their feet touching a flat surface, they move their legs as if to walk.

4.) Moro reflex- When someone bangs on the table the infant is lying on, or moves the infant vertically/suddenly, the infants flings their arms upward to their chest as if holding onto something, while crying and with wide open eyes.

The Moro and grasp reflexes historically assisted with holding tightly to their mother. The stepping reflex is a precursor of voluntary movement, and if practiced daily probably leads to earlier walking.

3.10 ORAL PHARYNGEAL DEVELOPMENT

The oral pharyngeal reflexes that are present at birth are the underpinnings for future feeding and swallowing maturation. The main oral reflexes present at birth are summarized in Table 1-10.

Table 1-10

Oral Reflexes Present in the Full-term Infant			
Reflex	Stimulus	Involved Cranial Nerves	Age of Disappearance
Gag	Touch posterior 3/4 tongue or pharynx	IX, X	Persists
Phasic Bite	Pressure on gums	V	9-12 months
Tongue Protrusion	Touch anterior tongue	XII	4-6 months
Rooting	Touching cheek near mouth	V, VII, XI, XII	3-6 months
Suckling	Nipple in mouth or stroking tongue	V, VII, IX, XII	6-12 months
Swallowing	Bolus of food in mouth	V, VII, IX, X, XII	Persists

3.11 GAG REFLEXES

The **gag reflex**, also known as a laryngeal spasm, consists of tongue protrusion, head and jaw protrusion, and pharyngeal contractions. A gag reflex is evident in the developing fetus at 26-27 weeks gestation and is usually strong in the newborn infant. The gag reflex may occur when the posterior tongue or pharynx is stimulated. It can also be stimulated in response to strong, aversive smells and sometimes by intense emotional responses. Sensitivity of the gag reflex varies among individuals. The gag and swallowing reflexes are not the same and have no relationship. There does not appear to be a direct relationship between the presence of a gag reflex and swallowing ability. The gag reflex is not a protection against aspiration (as are coughing and choking), but the body's protection against ingesting spoiled food.

Parents often mistake choking for gagging. Gagging is very common and is a part of the process of learning how to chew and swallow. Gagging occurs when some pieces of food fall to the back of the tongue and trigger the gag reflex. Choking occurs when food is too hard or large when swallowed or when food slips to the back of the tongue, falls down the throat, and gets lodged in the trachea. The individual may be unable to breathe or cough the food out. If the individual is unable to vocalize, unable to cough, or turns red/blue in the face, the Heimlich maneuver should be performed.

It is not uncommon to gag during a dental examination, dental impressions, throat culture, or similar procedures. Breathing slowly and deeply through your nose is a simple way to prevent gagging. This method works well for most people, but may be difficult for small children to employ. Other techniques that have been used to prevent or diminish a gag reflex include: application of a topical anesthetic near the back of mouth, distracting the patient, hypnosis, and forced respiration. In theory, sensory stimulation of the superior laryngeal nerve branch would block the physiological gag response. This is an extreme measure that may be employed when patients have a very sensitive gag reflex and have not benefited from other methods. General anesthesia may also be required in extreme cases in order to perform oral procedures.

3.12 HYPERACTIVE GAG REFLEX

Children and adults with a hyperactive gag reflex gag at the slightest provocation. For example, an infant with a hyperactive gag reflex may gag in response to different tastes, textures, and even smells. They may avoid oral play (e.g., mouthing toys). Because of the hyperactive gag response, the infant may restrict the variety of food textures in their mouth, which further perpetuates their sensory deprivation and oral sensitivity.

A hyperactive gag may be noted in some neurologically impaired children, although with severe neurological or motor involvement it may be difficult to elicit.

Treatment is needed to decrease hypersensitivity in order to change feeding behavior and improve nutritional intake. Treatment is usually multidimensional and may involve the assistance of a pediatrician, an occupational, speech, and/or physical therapist, as well as a clinical dietician.

3.13 GASTROESOPHAGEAL REFLUX

Gastroesophageal reflux (GER) is defined as the regurgitation of gastric contents into the esophagus. GER is a common, generally self-limited, condition in infants. Fifty percent of two-month old infants regurgitate twice a day or more, compared to only 1% of twelve-month old infants. Regurgitation by an infant, even when frequent, generally is not a concern if the infant is otherwise healthy, because most cases spontaneously remit. A small percentage of infants develop pathogenic gastroesophageal reflux disease (GERD), with esophagitis, stricture, Barrett's esophagus, respiratory disease, apnea, or failure to thrive.

While older children, like adults, with GERD often have heartburn, regurgitation with reswallowing, and a chronically acid taste, GERD may be difficult to diagnose in pre-verbal infants or young children on the basis of symptoms and signs. Because a number of disorders can present with chronic regurgitation, GERD is often a diagnosis of exclusion. For example, cyclic vomiting may be the only manifestation of common migraine in children. In addition, various respiratory disorders may present with vomiting. Vomiting in the older child must be distinguished from an eating disorder.

3.14 FEEDING AVERSION

Difficulties with food acceptance and feeding may result from an aversion to swallowing which is called "feeding aversion" or "conditioned dysphagia". Feeding aversion is a learned disorder, acquired and maintained through a behavioral conditioning process that can occur when a noxious stimulus is paired with the act of swallowing. When an intrusive/noxious stimulus (e.g., suctioning of the mouth/**nasopharynx**, passage of a nasogastric tube, bronchoscopy, upper endoscopy, tracheostomy) is paired with swallowing the patient may respond with conditioned avoidance to swallowing. Approximately 40% of children with cleft palate continue to have food aversion even after corrective **pharyngeal flap** surgery.

Children who suffer a choking episode can develop a post-traumatic food aversion. Children who have a mechanical, behavioral, or social-emotional interruption of normal feeding development are at risk for developing food aversion. Continued avoidance of stimuli can reduce sensory input to the oral cavity. The avoidance behavior becomes self-perpetuating. Some other examples of conditions that may predispose to a feeding disturbance include: cleft palate syndromes, cerebral palsy, traumatic brain injury, neurodegenerative disease, mental retardation, **autism**, bronchopulmonary dysplasia, gastro-esophageal reflux, supplemental feeding tube dependence, prematurity, inflammatory bowel disease, cystic fibrosis, parent-child relational difficulties, **child abuse**/neglect, "poor fit" between parent and child temperament. Abnormalities of motor tone (of the facial, oro-pharyngeal, as well as head and trunk regions) can result in abnormal feeding development and food aversion. Similarly, tactile hypersensitivity (which may be localized to a hyperactive gag reflex or may be manifested in more general body tactile hypersensitivity "defensiveness") is not uncommon. Children with multiple handicaps are at risk for tactile hypersenstivity.

3.15 DROOLING

Approximately 0.5 to 1.0 liters of saliva are produced daily in the adult. **Sialorrhea**, or excessive drooling, is the unintentional loss of saliva and other oral contents from the mouth. Drooling, which is normal in infancy, generally resolves by 15-18 months of age. Although occasional drooling can occur after this age, persistence of drooling beyond 4 years of age is considered abnormal. In children with drooling, the primary problem is usually related to oral motor dysfunction rather than excessive production of saliva. Certain psychiatric medications (such as Clozaril and Depakote) may cause sialorrhea as a side effect, however, it is much more common to have dry mouth as a side effect of psychotrophic medication.

3.16 ORAL MOTOR DYSFUNCTION

Eating and swallowing are highly integrated sensory motor functions. Coordination of the lips, tongue, jaw, cheeks, and soft palate are necessary to manipulate the food while protecting the airway. Swallowing requires a large area of the brain stem, six cranial nerves, a large number of sensory receptors, and 31 pairs of muscles. Oral motor dysfunction in children most often occurs as a result of neurological impairment, which leads to abnormal muscle tone, persistent oral reflexes, and sensory-perceptual deficits. Other conditions such as craniofacial anomalies, gastrointestinal disorders, and chronic pulmonary disease may be associated with oral motor dysfunction.

3.17 TONGUE THRUST

Pathological persistence of oral motor reflexes beyond 6 months of age interferes with normal oral motor development and, in combination with other postural tone abnormalities, may result in a variety of problems such as exaggerated **tongue thrust**, jaw thrust, jaw clenching, as well as persistent tonic bite. These problems may in turn result in malocclusion.

4. SELECTED COGNITIVE, EMOTIONAL, AND BEHAVIORAL PROBLEMS IN CHILDREN AND ADOLESCENTS

4.1 MENTAL RETARDATION

Table 1-11

The term mental retardation is often misunderstood and is generally considered as derogatory. Many think that mental retardation is diagnosed solely on the basis of below-normal intelligence. Actually, in order to be diagnosed as mentally retarded, a person must have both significantly low IQ and considerable problems in adapting to everyday life. There must be problems concurrently in two or more of the following applicable adaptive skill areas: communication, self-care, home living, social skills, community use, self-direction, health and safety, functional academics,

Classification of IQ for Mental Retardation	
Average	90-109
Below Average	80-89
Borderline	70-79
Mild (educable)	52-69
Moderate (trainable)	36-51
Severe	21-35
Profound	Below 20

leisure, and work. The accepted convention is to view intelligence in a distribution, with mild mental retardation classified as two standard deviations below the median. Mental retardation manifests before age 18 years of age. Most children with mental retardation can learn a great deal, and as adults can lead at least partially independent lives. More importantly, people with mental retardation can enjoy their lives just as everyone else does.

Mental retardation may be complicated by physical and emotional problems. Mentally retarded children have an increased risk of hearing, vision, or speech problems. There is an increased incidence of **cleft lip**/palate, syndrome-related dysmorphic features, and malocclusion in mentally retarded individuals. Mentally retarded children also have an increased risk for behavioral and emotional problems and increased incidence of psychiatric disorders as well. There is an increased risk of mood disorders, both depression and bipolar disorder. Most children with mental retardation recognize that they are behind others (cognitively, socially, and often physically.) They may become frustrated, withdrawn, or anxious. They may manifest externalizing behaviors (i.e., "bad behavior") as a means to express their emotions, to get attention, and sometimes to withdraw themselves from the stress of interacting with others. Mentally retarded children may not have sufficient cognitive development and/or language skills to express their feelings and, therefore, may demonstrate their emotions (and demonstrate signs/symptoms of mental illness) through their behavior, such as through **aggressive** behavior, eating problems, sleeping problems, etc.

4.2 **DISORDERS OF SPEECH**

4.2.1. Disorders of Articulation

Dysarthria or articulation disorder refers to a physical dysfunction of the muscles of speech production; symbolic aspects of language function are intact. This diagnosis is applied to children who misarticulate sounds by substition of one sound for another (e.g., "wabbit" for "rabbit"), omission of a sound ("kool" for "school"), distortion or nonstandard production of a sound, or addition of a sound. A useful guide to assessing development of articulation is the so-called Rule of Fourths. The average 2-year-old child should be intelligible to strangers half the time (2/4), a 3-year-old child, three quarters of the time, and a 4-year-old, all the time. Dysarthria is caused by an impairment of the upper motor neurons or brainstem motor nuclei that govern the muscles of the face, oropharynx, and larynx. Cerebral Palsy (CP) frequently results in dysarthria; however, most children with dysarthria do not have CP.

4.2.2. Disorders of Voice

Disorders of voice may be functional and/or anatomical in origin. and may be congenital or acquired. For example a child may be born with a paralyzed vocal cord or with congenital stenosis (anatomical defect in the larynx that results in a narrowed airway). The child may also have a congenital subglottic hemangioma. These lesions generally go unnoticed, but with progressive enlargement of the hemangioma the child will present with airway distress.

The vocal cord may be damaged by trauma, such as after repeated intubation and/or mechanical ventilation. Glottic and subglottic stenosis are most commonly the result of prolonged intubation. Individuals may damage their vocal cords by overuse- screaming, singing. Children may also develop tumors of the larynx. The most common benign tumor of the larynx is the papilloma, which accounts for more than 80% of laryngeal growths.

4.2.3. Disorders of Fluency- Stuttering

Dysfluencies include pauses, hesitations, interjections, prolongations, and repetitions that interrupt or disrupt the flow of speech. Speech dysfluency is a normal part of communication. Most speakers are dysfluent to some extent. Dysfluent speech often begins in early childhood between the ages of 2 1/2 and 4 years. During this time, a certain amount of repeating, stopping, or pausing is to be expected and is normal. When the frequency of these behaviors becomes excessive or when the types of behaviors seem different from other children, the child may be demonstrating early signs of stuttering. Stuttering is a form of dysfluency that is characterized by high frequency of sound repetition, sound prolongation, and visible struggle behavior. Stuttering affects approximately 1% of the general population, with 85% of cases beginning in the preschool years (ages 2-5.) Although the incidence of stuttering in preschool is equal for boys and girls, girls more frequently recover so that for persistent stuttering, boys outnumber girls by a ratio of 3:1-4:1 in frequency of persistent stuttering. Recent data suggest that about 90% of children who begin to stutter in the preschool years will recover with minimal or no treatment.

The following are signs are associated with development of stuttering and indicate the need for evaluation:

1.) Repetitions- Repetition of more than 50 per 1,000 words is considered too frequent.
2.) Prolongation- occurs with pulling out a sound with prolonged attention and forcing the initial sound of a word, e.g., "ffffffffish".
3.) Struggle- Examples of struggle behaviors include facial contortions, jaw jerks, wide open mouth, protrusion of the tongue, or rolling of the eyes.
4.) Avoidances- Children may engage in complex behaviors to cope with and hide stuttering behavior.

4.3 LANGUAGE DISORDERS

Developmental Language Disorders

Developmental Language Disorders (DLD) are a clinically heterogeneous group of disorders characterized by selective impairment of speech and/or language development, with relative sparing of other developmental domains. Overall intelligence is usually normal, or not sufficiently affected to account for the degree of language impairment. There are no universally accepted criteria for diagnosing DLD. Estimated prevalence is 5-10% of preschool children. Boys are more commonly affected than girls in a ratio of 3:1.

Auditory Processing Disorders

A child with a language and learning disorder who has difficulty with listening tasks may have an auditory processing disorder. This means that the child may have difficulty with transmission, analysis, organization, transformation, elaboration, storage, and/or retrieval of auditory signals. Children with behavioral and emotional problems are difficult to assess for auditory skills. Because of their emotional state, they may have difficulty attending and listening to auditory stimuli. A child with depression or anxiety will have decreased attention secondary to worries. A child with a thought disorder will be confused and distracted. A child with attention deficit disorder has shifting thoughts making sustained focus difficult.

Non-Causes of Language Disorders

Birth order, bilingualism, tongue tie, "laziness", and uncomplicated twinning are NOT causes of language delay. Later-born children speak no later than first-born. Normal twins speak no later than singletons. Toddlers, while frequently noncompliant, are not developmentally capable of being "lazy." Children raised in bilingual homes generally intermix languages for the first 24-30 months, but usually by 36 months are truly bilingual, such that communication ability may be assessed as usual for each language. Tongue tie does affect articulation but does not produce a true language disorder in children. In the majority of cases of DLD, the etiology remains unknown. Family history is frequently positive for speech delay, but there is generally no clear pattern of Mendelian inheritance, suggesting polygenic inheritance interacting with gender and environmental factors.

Other Causes of Language Disorders

Other causes of language disorders in children include hearing loss, auditory processing disorders, autistic spectrum disorders, and mental retardation. One infant per thousand is born with severe to profound hearing loss (HL). One third of congenital HL is genetic in origin, one third is non-genetic, and one third is of unknown etiology. Otitis media with effusion causes mild-moderate hearing loss that is transient with proper treatment but, if untreated, may result in scarring of the tympanic membrane and permanent hearing loss. Meningitis is also a cause of acquired hearing loss in children, but fortunately is less common with the availability of antibiotic treatment. Three percent of all children are mentally retarded. All children who are mentally retarded are language delayed. Moreover, mentally retarded children manifest delay in all language areas: auditory expressive, auditory receptive, and visual language (refers to gestures, facial expressions and interaction.) Most mentally retarded children are mildly retarded and often have mild language delay. All children with **autism** have a language disorder, because autism is characterized by delayed and deviant language development. Language is deviant in that many of the typical language features seen in autistic children are not normal for children of any age. The hallmark of the autistic type of language disorder is impaired pragmatics, e.g., failure to use language as a medium of social interaction. The abnormality is often evident from an early age, with failure to make eye contact, engage in reciprocal vocalization, or point to objects. In autistic disorder, speech consists mainly of naming of objects and repetition of others' speech (called echolalia.) Speech inflection (prosody) may be sing-song, robot-like, or stilted.

There is a high frequency of speech and language disorders among children in treatment for psychiatric disorders. Research has consistently documented the high co-morbidity of psychiatric disorders and communication impairments. Cantwell and Baker (1987) reported that 67% of children admitted to an inpatient psychiatric unit failed speech and language screening. The documented frequency of children with speech and language problems among outpatients in psychiatric or behavioral pediatric clinics varies from 30% to 50+ %. The etiologic relationship between communication and psychiatric disorders continues to be ambiguous. Several hypotheses have been proposed in the literature, but regardless, there has been consistent data to support that children with communication impairments are vulnerable to social and emotional difficulties, and children with psychiatric disorders are found to have higher than average prevalence of language disorders.

4.4 AUTISTIC SPECTRUM DISORDERS

4.4.1. Autistic Disorder

Autistic Disorder, or "**autism**," is a complex, life-long biological disorder of development that results in social interaction problems, communication difficulties, and restrictive or repetitive interests and behaviors. The prevalence of autistic spectrum disorders is 1/500-1/1,000. The symptoms of autism vary in both occurrence and severity, making the diagnosis difficult.

DSM IV Diagnostic Criteria for Autistic Disorder:

A.) Qualitative impairment in social interaction, as manifested by at least two of the following:

1.) Marked impairment in the use of multiple nonverbal behaviors such as eye-to-eye gaze, facial expression, body postures, and gestures to regulate social interaction
2.) Failure to develop peer relationships appropriate to developmental level
3.) Lack of spontaneous seeking to share enjoyment, interests, or achievements with other people (e.g., by a lack of showing, bringing, or pointing out objects of interest to other people).
4.) Lack of social or emotional reciprocity.

B.) Qualitative impairments in communication as manifested by at least one of the following:

1.) Delay in, or total lack of, the development of spoken language (not accompanied by an attempt to compensate through alternative modes of communication such as gestures or pantomime).
2.) In individuals with adequate speech, marked impairment in the ability to initiate or sustain a conversation with others.
3.) Stereotyped and repetitive use of language or idiosyncratic language.
4.) Lack of varied, spontaneous make-believe play or social imitative play appropriate to developmental level.

C.) Restricted repetitive and stereotyped patterns of behavior, interests, and activities, as manifested by at least one of the following:

1.) Encompassing preoccupation with one or more stereotyped and restricted patterns of interest that is abnormal either in intensity or focus.

2.) Inflexible adherence to specific, nonfunctional routines or rituals.

3.) Stereotyped and repetitive motor mannerisms (e.g., hand or finger flapping or twisting, or complex whole-body movements).

4.) Persistent preoccupation with parts of objects.

D.) Delays or abnormal functioning in at least one of the following areas with onset prior to age 3 years: 1.) social interaction; 2.) language as used in social communication; or 3.) symbolic or imaginative play.

E.) The disturbance is not better accounted for by Rett's Disorder or Childhood Disintegrative Disorder.

Autism can be reliably diagnosed by age 3. Although experts, and often parents, can detect symptoms during infancy, a formal diagnosis is generally not made until approximately age 2 when the child fails to develop functional/normal language. Approximately 20 percent of children with autism reportedly experience a "regression" of normal development, in which they were apparently normal and then lost communication and social skills. Boys are 3 – 4 times as likely to be affected as girls. Autism occurs in all racial, ethnic, and social groups.

Although there is currently no known cure for autism, autism is treatable. Persons with autism can make progress if they receive appropriate, individual intervention. Pre-school children who receive intensive, individualized behavioral interventions have shown remarkable progress. In addition, pharmacological treatment is available to treat specific symptoms of autism.

In the majority of cases, no specific underlying cause of autism can be identified. A variety of infectious, metabolic, genetic, and environmental factors are being investigated. In 1995 a work group of the National Institute of Health reached a consensus that autism probably results from genetic susceptibility that involves multiple genes. To date, there is no conclusive evidence that any vaccine increases the risk of developing autism or any other behavior disorder.

4.4.2. Pervasive Developmental Disorder

For years, psychiatrists have debated how to classify and subdivide the category of Pervasive Developmental Disorder (PDD). Pervasive Developmental Disorder is a category that contains several specific diagnoses that can be seen on a spectrum, including Autistic Disorder, Asperger's Disorder, and Pervasive Developmental Disorder not otherwise specified. Individuals with PDD have problems with social interaction, and often show delays in several other areas. These other areas may include language, coordination, imaginative activities, and intellectual functioning. The degree of severity can vary tremendously in the various forms of PDD. Autism is the most severe form of PDD. An individual with autism has marked difficulty relating to other human beings. He or she frequently has delayed or absent speech and may be mentally retarded. Asperger's Disorder is on the milder end of PDD. Individuals with Asperger's generally have normal intelligence and normal early language acquisition. However, they show difficulties with social interactions and non-verbal communications. They may also show perseverative or repetitive behaviors.

According to the DSM IV, a diagnosis of "Pervasive Developmental Disorder Not Otherwise Specified" should be made when an individual has a severe and pervasive impairment in the development of reciprocal social interaction or verbal and nonverbal communication skills, or when stereotyped behavior, interests, and activities are present, but the individual does not meet criteria for Autistic Disorder, Asperger's Disorder, Schizophrenia, or a personality disorder.

4.4.3. Asperger's Disorder

Asperger's Disorder or **Asperger's Syndrome** is not widely recognized by the public or by health care providers. As discussed above, Asperger's Disorder is classified as part of a larger spectrum of Autistic Disorders called Pervasive Developmental Disorder. It is on the milder end of PDD. Individuals with Asperger's generally have normal intelligence and normal early language acquisition. However, they show difficulties with social interactions and non-verbal communications. They may also show perseverative or repetitive behaviors.

A preschool-aged child with Asperger's Disorder might show difficulty understanding the basics of social interaction. He or she may have difficulty picking up social cues. He or she may want friends but be unable to make or keep any friends. Children and adults with Asperger's Disorder often have poor pragmatic language skills. This means that the individual cannot use the right tone and volume of speech. He may stand too close or make poor eye contact. He may have trouble understanding age-appropriate humor and slang expressions. Many people with Asperger's Disorder are clumsy and have visual-perceptual difficulties. Learning difficulties, subtle or severe, are common. Persons with Asperger's Disorder may become fixated on a particular topic and bore others with frequent or repetitive talk even when the other children have given clear signals that they are no longer interested in the topic. Some have difficulties tolerating changes in their daily routine. Change must be introduced gradually. Individuals with Asperger's have difficulty understanding which of their peers might want to be a friend. A socially marginal boy might try to date the most popular girl in his class. He will probably experience rejection. He is unaware that some other girl might accept his invitation. Because of his social naiveté, he may not realize when someone is trying to take advantage of him. He can be especially vulnerable to manipulation and peer pressure.

There is less information on Asperger's Disorder in adulthood. Some individuals with mild Asperger's Disorder are able to learn to compensate. Some individuals may seem indistinguishable from everyone else. They may marry, hold a job, and have children. Other individuals live an isolated existence with continuing severe difficulties in social and occupational functioning. Individuals with Asperger's often do well in jobs that require technical skill but little social finesse. Some do well with predictable repetitive work. Others relish the challenge of intricate technical problem solving.

Asperger's Disorder may be associated with learning difficulties and attention deficit disorder. Indeed, many children and adolescents with Asperger's have previously been diagnosed with **ADHD** instead of Asperger's. Individuals with ADHD may have difficulty with social interaction, but the primary difficulties are inattention, hyperactivity and impulsivity. In individuals with Asperger's, the social awkwardness is a greater concern. As individuals with Asperger's enter **adolescence**, they become acutely aware of their differences. This may lead to depression and anxiety. The depression, if not treated, may persist into adulthood.

There is no one specific medication for Asperger's Syndrome, but medication may be prescribed to treat specific target symptoms. One might use a stimulant for inattention and hyperactivity. An SSRI such as Paxil, Prozac or Zoloft might help with obsessions or perseveration. The SSRIs can also help associated depression and anxiety. In individuals with stereotyped movements, agitation and idiosyncratic thinking, we may use a low dose antipsychotic such as Risperidone.

Social skills training is one of the most important parts of treatment for Asperger's Disorder. The individual with Asperger's Disorder often must to learn read nonverbal social cues ("body language") as others learn a foreign language. The individual with Asperger's must learn concrete rules for eye contact, social distance and the use of slang. Global empathy is difficult, but they can learn to look for specific signs that indicate another individual's emotional state. Social skills are often best practiced in a small group setting. Such groups serve more than one function. They give people a chance to learn and practice concrete rules of interpersonal engagement. They may also be a way for the participant to meet others like himself. Individuals with Asperger's do best in groups with similar individuals. If the group consists of street-wise, antisocial peers, the Asperger's individual may retreat into himself or be dominated by the other members.

Because Asperger's covers a wide range of ability levels, the school must individualize programming for each student with Asperger's Disorder. Teachers need to be aware that the student may mumble or refuse to look him in the eye. Teachers should notify the student in advance about changes in the school routine. The student may need to have a safe place where he can retreat if he becomes overstimulated. It may be difficult to program for a very bright student with greater deficits. In one case, a student attended gifted classes but also had an aide to help her with interpersonal issues. That student is now in college. Children with Asperger's are often socially naive. They may not do well in an "emotionally disturbed" class if most of the other students are **aggressive**, street-wise and manipulative. I have seen some do well when placed with other students with pervasive developmental disorders. Some do well in a regular classroom with extra support. This extra help might include an instructional assistant, resource room, or extra training for the primary teacher.

Individuals with Asperger's Disorder may have trouble with a therapist who insists that they make an early intense emotional contact. The therapist may need to proceed slowly and avoid more emotional intensity than the patient can handle. Concrete, behavioral techniques often work best. Play can be helpful in a limited way if the therapist uses it to teach ways of interaction, if it is used to lower emotional tension. Adults and children may do well in group therapy. Support groups can also be helpful.

Parents play an important role in helping their child or adolescent with Asperger's Disorder. This child or adolescent will require time and extra nurturing.

It is important to distinguish between willful disobedience and misunderstanding of social cues. It is also important to sense when the child is entering emotional overload so that one can reduce tension. They may need to prepare the child for changes in the daily routine. One must choose babysitters carefully. Parents may have to take an active role in arranging appropriate play dates for the younger child. Some parents seek out families with similar children. Children with Asperger's often get along with similar playmates. Parents should help teachers understand the world from the child's unique point of view. Parenting an adolescent with Asperger's can be a great challenge. The socially naive adolescent may not be ready for the same degree of freedom as his peers. Often parents can find a slightly older adolescent who can be a mentor. This person can help the adolescent understand how to dress, and how to use the current slang. If the mentor attends the same school, he can often give clues about the cliques in that particular setting.

Adults may benefit from group therapy or individual behavioral therapy. Some speech therapists have experience working with adults on pragmatic language skills. Behavioral coaching, a relatively new type of intervention, can help the adult with Asperger's Disorder organize and prioritize his daily activities. Adults may need medication for associated problems such as depression or anxiety. Some adults do not need treatment. They may find jobs that fit their areas of strength. They may have smaller social circles, and some idiosyncratic behaviors, but they may still be productive and fulfilled.

DSM IV Diagnostic Criteria for Asperger's Disorder

A.) Qualitative impairment in social interaction, as manifested by at least two of the following:

1.) Marked impairment in the use of multiple nonverbal behaviors such as eye-to-eye gaze, facial expression, body postures, and gestures to regulate social interaction.

2.) Failure to develop peer relationships appropriate to developmental level.

3.) Lack of spontaneous seeking to share enjoyment, interests, or achievements with other people (e.g., by a lack of showing, bringing, or pointing out objects of interest to other people).

4.) Lack of social or emotional reciprocity.

B.) Restricted repetitive and stereotyped patterns of behavior, interests, and activities, as manifested by at least one of the following:

1.) Encompassing preoccupation with one or more stereotyped and restricted patterns of interest that is abnormal either in intensity or focus.

2.) Inflexible adherence to specific, nonfunctional routines or rituals.

3.) Stereotyped and repetitive motor mannerisms (e.g., hand or finger flapping or twisting, or complex whole-body movements).

4.) Persistent preoccupation with parts of objects.

C.) The disturbance causes clinically significant impairment in social, occupational, or other important areas of functioning.

D.) There is no clinically significant delay in language (e.g., single words used by 2 years, communicative phrases used by 3 years).

E.) There is no clinically significant delay in cognitive development or in the development of age-appropriate self-help skills, adaptive behavior (other than in social interaction), and curiosity about the environment in childhood.

4.5 ATTENTION DEFICIT HYPERACTIVITY DISORDER

Neurodevelopmental dysfunction of attention is a very common problem in children. Clinicians are seeing increased numbers of children, adolescents, and even adults who are suspected of having attention deficits, or **Attention Deficit Hyperactivity Disorder** (ADHD). This diagnosis refers to a specific constellation of difficulties with attention, organization, and impulsivity.

Many, but not all, children with attention deficits also have difficulty with hyperactivity. Depending on the presence and degree of hyperactivity, the diagnosis will be Attention Deficit Disorder, predominantly inattentive type, Attention Deficit Disorder, predominantly hyperactive type, or Attention Deficit Disorder, combined type.

It is important to recognize that Attention Deficit Disorder is not a simple lack of attention. Individuals with ADD almost always demonstrate intermittent attention and inconsistent performance. They can be alert and productive at times, but at other times display mental fatigue and apparent lack of effort. This inconsistency of performance is frequently misinterpreted by others. Because the affected individual can succeed some of the time, when they are out of focus and unsuccessful at tasks they may seem to be "not really trying" or "lazy" or even "defiant". It is important not to mistakenly expect that consistent performance is totally within the control of individuals with ADD.

People with deficits of attention have frequently had difficulty with other associated "executive functions". For example, individuals with ADD often have problems with distractibility (the inability to filter irrelevant stimuli or ignore irrelevant information), task analysis (the ability to organize information and plan ahead to complete a complex task), rank ordering (the ability to prioritize information and activities), vigilance (the ability to remain alert to rarely occurring stimuli), divided attention (the ability to focus on multiple simultaneous tasks), experience analysis (the ability to learn from experience), and **working memory**.

DSM IV Diagnostic Criteria for Attention Deficit Hyperactivity Disorder

A.) Either (1) or (2)

  1.) Six (or more) of the following symptoms of inattention have persisted for at least 6 months
       to a degree that is maladaptive and inconsistent with developmental level:

Inattention

  a.) Often fails to give close attention to details or makes careless mistakes in schoolwork,
       work or other activities.
  b.) Often has difficulty sustaining attention in tasks or play activities.

  c.) Often does not seem to listen when spoken to directly.

  d.) Often does not follow through on instructions and fails to finish schoolwork, chores,
       or duties in the workplace (not due to oppositional behavior or failure to understand
       instructions).

  e.) Often has difficulty organizing tasks and activities.

  f.) Often avoids, dislikes, or is reluctant to engage in tasks that require sustained mental
       effort (such as schoolwork or homework).

  g.) Often loses things necessary for tasks or activities (e.g, toys, school assignments,
       pencils, books, or tools).

h.) Often easily distracted by extraneous stimuli.

i.) Often forgetful in daily activities.

2.) Six (or more) of the following symptoms of hyperactivity-impulsivity have persisted for at least 6 months to a degree that is maladaptive and inconsistent with developmental level:

Hyperactivity

a.) Often fidgets with hands or feet or squirms in seat.

b.) Often leaves seat in classroom or in other situations in which remaining seated is expected.

c.) Often runs about or climbs excessively in situations in which it is inappropriate (in adolescents or adults, may be limited to subjective feelings of restlessness.)

d.) Often has difficulty playing or engaging in leisure activities quietly.

e.) Often "on the go" or often acts as if "driven by a motor."

f.) Often talks excessively.

Impulsivity

g.) Often blurts out answers before questions have been completed.

h.) Often has difficulty waiting turn.

i.) Often interrupts or intrudes on others (e.g., butts into conversations or games.)

B.) Some hyperactive-impulsive or inattentive symptoms that caused impairment were present before age 7 years.

C.) Some impairment from the symptoms is present in two or more settings (e.g., at school or work and at home.)

D.) There must be clear evidence of clinically significant impairment in social, academic, or occupational functioning.

4.6 MOOD DISORDERS

4.6.1 Major Depressive Disorder

Depression is not simply sadness. It is more than just "feeling blue" or having a bad day, and it is different from the feelings of grief or sorrow that might follow a major loss, such as a death in the family. Depression does not result from a personal weakness or a character flaw. Depression is diagnosed when feelings of sadness or depression persist and, in combination with other symptoms, interfere with a person's ability to function. See DSM IV diagnostic criteria below. Major Depressive Disorder

(MDD), also known as "unipolar depression" (in contrast to bipolar depression), is commonly referred to as "clinical depression".

Not only adults become depressed. Children and adolescents may also suffer from depression. The point prevalence of depression for children and adolescents is 5%. As many as 1 in every 33 children—and 1 in 8 adolescents—may have depression. (Source - According to Center for Mental Health Services.)

MDD is a prevalent, episodic, and often recurrent disorder. It has both short- and long-term negative consequences. Consequences of depression can include social isolation, academic underachievement, and strained family interactions. Depression in children is also associated with an increased risk for suicidal behaviors. Once a young person has experienced an episode of depression, he or she is at an increased risk for developing another episode of depression within the next 5 years. Children who experience a depressive episode are 5 times more likely to have depression as an adult, and depression in childhood may predict a more severe depressive illness in adulthood.

No one thing causes depression. Biological, environmental, and psychological factors occurring individually or in combination seem to contribute to the onset of the disorder. Children who develop depression are likely to have a family history of the disorder. Episodes are often precipitated by traumatic life events, such as the death of a loved one or interpersonal loss. Children under stress, who experience loss, or who have attention, learning, conduct, or anxiety disorders are at higher risk for depression. Children who have a chronic illness or who experience abuse, neglect, or other trauma are also at a higher risk for depression. Depression in children frequently occurs with other mental disorders such as anxiety disorders or disruptive behavior disorders. Adolescents who are depressed are also at risk for substance abuse.

People with clinical depression can't simply "snap out of it"; depression is a real medical illness that is treatable and requires professional help. Early diagnosis and treatment are essential for children and adolescents who are depressed, as the burden of untreated symptoms on the developing child is tremendous.

The signs and symptoms of depression in children differ from those seen in adults. When asked directly, these children may or may not state that they are sad or depressed. Because the diagnosis of Depressive Disorders can be especially difficult in children, it is essential that all children suspected of suffering depression are evaluated by an experienced mental health professional, preferably a child psychiatrist. The depressed child may not always seem sad, but may instead demonstrate behavioral problems at school and/or home. Parents and teachers may not realize that the troublesome behavior is a sign of depression. The child or adolescent who is depressed may become irritable, angry, or withdrawn. They may be less interested in activities they used to enjoy. Other symptoms to watch for include:

> -Change in eating or sleeping habits
> -Violent actions, rebellious behavior, or running away
> -Drug and alcohol use
> -Marked personality change
> -Unusual neglect of personal appearance
> -Frequent complaints or physical symptoms

Suicides among youth have increased dramatically over the past decades. Suicide is the third leading cause of death for 15 to 24-year-olds and the sixth leading cause of death for 5 to 14-year-olds. Children who are depressed may talk about death, say no one loves/likes them, or say they wish they were dead. Depressed children and adolescents are at increased risk of suicide and any suicide threats or attempts should be taken seriously. Although parents sometimes feel that expressed wishes to die, threats or attempts of suicide are an attempt "to get their own way," such behavior should always be viewed as a clear cry for help by the child. All children and adolescents who express suicidal thoughts or intent should be brought for a complete evaluation.

DSM IV Diagnostic Criteria for Major Depressive Episode

Five (or more) of the following symptoms have been present during the same 2-week period and represent a change from previous functioning. At least one of the symptoms is either depressed mood or loss of interest or pleasure:

1.) Depressed mood most of the day, nearly every day, as indicated by either subjective report (e.g., feels sad or empty) or observation made by others (e.g., appears tearful). Note: In children and adolescents, can be irritable mood.

2.) Markedly diminished interest or pleasure in all (or almost all) activities most of the day, nearly every day (as indicated by either subjective account or observation made by others.)

3.) Significant weight loss when not dieting or weight gain (e.g.. a change of more than 5% of body weight in a month), or decrease or increase in appetite nearly every day. Note: In children, consider failure to make expected weight gains.

4.) Insomnia or hypersomnia nearly every day.

5.) Psychomotor agitation or retardation nearly every day (observable by others, not merely subjective feelings of restlessness or being slowed down).

6.) Fatigue or loss of energy nearly every day.

7.) Feelings of worthlessness, or excessive or inappropriate guilt (which may be delusional) nearly every day (not merely self-reproach or guilt about being sick).

8.) Diminished ability to think or concentrate, or indecisiveness, nearly every day (either by subjective account or as observed by others).

9.) Recurrent thoughts of death (not just fear of dying), recurrent suicidal ideation without a specific plan, or a suicide attempt or a specific plan for committing suicide.

4.6.2. Bipolar Disorder

Bipolar Disorder, also known as manic-depression, is a less frequent but serious mental illness. It is a mental disorder marked by extreme changes in mood, energy levels, and behavior. Bipolar Disorder usually starts in adult life. Although less common, it does occur in teenagers and even rarely in young children. Until recently, a diagnosis of the disorder was rarely made in childhood. Doctors now recognize and treat Bipolar Disorder in children and adolescents.

Bipolar Disorder can affect anyone; however, if one or both parents have Bipolar Disorder, the chances are greater that their children will develop the disorder. Family history of drug or alcohol abuse may also be associated with Bipolar Disorder in teens.

Up to one third of the 3.4 million children and adolescents with depression in the United States may actually be experiencing the early onset of Bipolar Disorder. However, the illness is different in children than it is in adults. Children with Bipolar Disorder typically alternate rapidly between mania (high energy) and depression. These rapid mood shifts may take the form of irritability, followed by withdrawal, with few clear periods of wellness between episodes.

Bipolar Disorder is a life-long illness but can be effectively treated. Treatment is critical to prevent the potentially devastating psychosocial consequences of the illness as well as development of co-morbid psychiatric illness. Individuals with Bipolar Disorder are at great risk for substance abuse and suicide. Treatment usually includes patient and family education, mood stabilizing medication (such as Lithium, Depakote, Tegretol, or Neurontin), and psychotherapy. Medications often reduce the number and severity of manic episodes and also help prevent depression.

Signs to look for include:

-A persistent irritable mood
-Depression
-Rapidly changing moods lasting a few hours to a few days
-Explosive, lengthy, and often destructive rages
-Defiance of authority
-Hyperactivity, agitation, and distractibility
-Sleeping little or sleeping too much
-Delusions and hallucinations
-Strong and frequent cravings, often for carbohydrates and sweets
-Excessive involvement in multiple projects and activities
-Impaired judgment, impulsivity, racing thoughts, and pressure to keep talking
-Dare-devil behaviors
-Grandiose belief in own abilities (ability to fly, for example)

DMSM IV Diagnostic Criteria for Manic Episode

A distinct period of abnormally and persistently elevated, expansive, or irritable mood, lasting at least one week (or any duration if hospitalization is necessary). During the period of mood disturbance, three (or more) of the following symptoms have persisted (four if the mood is only irritable) and have been present to a significant degree:

1.) Inflated self-esteem or grandiosity.
2.) Decreased need for sleep (e.g., feels rested after only 3 hours of sleep).
3.) More talkative than usual or pressure to keep talking.
4.) Flight of ideas or subjective experience that thoughts are racing.
5.) Distractibility (i.e., attention too easily drawn to unimportant or irrelevant external stimuli).
6.) Increase in goal-directed activity (either socially, at work or school, or sexually) or psychomotor agitation.
7.) Excessive involvement in pleasurable activities that have a high potential for painful consequences (e.g., engaging in unrestrained buying sprees, sexual indiscretions, or foolish business investments).

The mood disturbance is sufficiently severe to cause marked impairment in occupational functioning or in usual social activities or relationships with others, or to necessitate hospitalization to prevent harm to self or others, or there are psychotic features.

The symptoms are not due to the direct physiological effects of a substance (e.g., a drug of abuse, a medication, or other treatment) or a general medical condition (e.g., hyperthyroidism).

Note: Manic-like episodes that are clearly caused by somatic antidepressant treatment (e.g., medication, electroconvulsive therapy, light therapy) should not count toward a diagnosis of Bipolar Disorder.

4.7 FEAR AND ANXIETY   Table 1-12

Fear and anxiety are normal and useful when the right level of fear/anxiety is aroused for the right duration in response to the right cue. Fear is defined as an unpleasant emotion that is caused by psycho-physiological changes in the body in response to a realistic threat or danger. In contrast to fear, in anxiety the danger or threat is unreal and is produced by intrapsychic conflict. Both fear and anxiety are adaptive and essential for survival. Fear serves as a warning and is associated with heightened awareness and readiness to respond to a threat. Just as individuals who have impaired pain (as seen in leprosy or diabetes) are at increased risk of harm, individuals with too little fear are at risk.

Most Common Human Fears
public speaking
making mistakes/failure/disapproval/rejection
embarrassment
angry people
being alone
darkness
dentists
injections
hospitals
open wounds
blood
taking tests
police
dogs
spiders
deformed people

Crossculturally, similar fears are common in healthy adults. Fear of dentists ranks among the top 10 most common fears. See Table of 1-12 for the most common human fears.

Normal Childhood Fears

Fears and anxieties have a predictable developmental course and are linked with normal cognitive and psychological development. Fears in the first 12 months of life are based on both vulnerability (actual environmental threat) and biology (innate fears). These fears surface around separation from primary caregivers, exposure to strangers, sudden noises, loss of support (falling), sleep, animals, and medical visits. Early childhood fears cross cultural barriers. Bright children tend to have precocious fears whereas developmentally delayed children have fears consistent with their (delayed) mental age. Children and teenagers who watch a lot of movie or television violence are relatively more fearful than those who do not.

Separation anxiety is a part of normal development. The key to understanding and alleviating separation anxiety lies in understanding the developmental stage at which it occurs. Separation anxiety normally peaks at 8, 13, 20, and 24 months of age. These peaks are linked to the child's developmental level. For example, before 8 months babies have no capacity for understanding object permanence and therefore believe that if their mother disappears she will never return. As the baby matures cognitively, the image of the mother becomes more permanent and separation anxiety decreases. At one year of life, as children begin walking, they realize that they can wander away from mother, thus creating a resurgence of separation anxiety that is now based in part on personal responsibility. After its final peak around 20-24 months of age, separation anxiety usually begins to decline. It then disappears but may resurface between 6-10 years of age when it is usually associated with going to school (so-called school phobia.) Sometimes separation anxiety can re-occur around 12 years of age, usually when precipitated by stress (illness or death of a loved one) or loneliness.

Like separation anxiety, stranger anxiety is a normal phenomenon. Stranger anxiety normally surfaces shortly after development of specific and secure attachment of the child to their primary caregiver(s). Children that have not formed such an attachment (e.g., institutionalized children) show no stranger anxiety, and therefore are indiscriminant in their friendliness with others.

Between 24-36 months children are attempting to master many physical, emotional, and cognitive skills: development of secure attachment to caregiver, appropriate interaction with strangers, control of bodily functions, control of intense emotions, and control of aggression. Toddlers experience a significant fear of losing emotional control. A parent can help their toddler maintain control by using calm, consistent discipline and setting firm and appropriate limits. Typical fears of three year olds include: dark, dogs, scary noises (e.g., fire engines), monsters, scary images (e.g., seen on TV), death, feeding, toilet training (fear of falling in the toilet and being flushed down the drain, fear of losing control of feces and/or urine), fear of drains/baths. Adult strangers who approach quickly in a strange situation especially without an attachment figure present arouse intense fear. Parents and doctors should not attempt to break down the normal and appropriate stranger fear with admonitions. A toddler should not be expected to pet every dog or kiss every stranger. Strangers and clinicians should wait until the child makes an approach before moving close to dissipate the child's fear. Prolonged separation from caregivers, particularly in a strange setting, should be avoided because toddlers do not have the cognitive skills necessary to tolerate the anxiety that is evoked. When separation from the caregiver is absolutely necessary, the child should be told who will be there for them, when the caregiver will return, and what to expect during the separation. During illness, fears increase, cognitive skills regress, and coping strategies are diminished. Childeren need more structure and emotional support during illness and in strange situations, such as a dental office.

Many fears are prompted by the times in which we live. Terrorism, muggings, car thefts, and house break-ins have become sufficiently common that no one can avoid thinking about them. Because divorce now ends 50% of marriages, most children worry when they hear their parents arguing. But why do people worry about the 'wrong' things? For example, some anxieties are not warranted when one considers the probability of the threat in question. For example, statistically people are more than 2.5 times more likely to be injured in their home or car than to be the victim of a violent crime or be involved in an air crash. Fear of bombing attacks and "being invaded" has been in the top ten list of childhood fears for the past three decades. Seventy percent of children also report fears of being followed by strange people and being kidnapped. There must be some sense of personal control to avoid overwhelming anxiety. Therefore, people assume mastery of common things (safety in their home and while driving) in order to adjust psychologically. Individuals who are persistently anxious of common things usually suffer from an anxiety disorder.

4.8 ANXIETY DISORDERS

Anxiety disorders are the most common psychiatric disorders in childhood and **adolescence**. Large representative studies of pediatric clinic populations have revealed 8-9% of elementary age and adolescent patients have at least one anxiety disorder. Several epidemiological studies also report a high prevalence of anxiety in non-referred children (Anderson 1987, Bird 1988, Bowen 1990):

    2.5-4.5% separation anxiety disorder
    3.0-4.5% generalized anxiety disorder
    2.5%   simple phobia
    0.5-1.0% social phobia

4.8.1. Phobias

A **phobia** is a type of anxiety disorder consisting of morbid and irrational fear of a specific object or situation associated with severe anxiety. The feared object or situation must be avoided or can be endured only with marked distress. In phobias, fear is recognized as unreasonable or unwarranted, but the affected individual is unable to prevent the anxiety response.

Three major forms of phobias are recognized:

1.) Specific Phobia- Also known as simple phobia. The most frequent specific phobia are the natural environmental type, e.g., animals, insects, storms, water. Also common are medical phobias (blood, injection, injury) and situational phobias (bridges, elevators, cars, planes, tunnels, escalators).

2.) Social Phobia- Social phobia was formerly called avoidant disorder. It consists of avoidance of situations in which the person may be subjected to scrutiny by others and in which he/she fears he/she will act in a way that will be humiliating or embarrassing. Included is performance type (unable to speak, play an instrument, or sing in front of others; unable to write or eat in front of others.) Also includes interactional type (fear is restricted to specific situations such as speaking with authority figures, dating), as well as generalized type (where most social situations are avoided).

3.) Agoraphobia- the most severe phobia. This is the phobia for which professional help is most often sought. It consists of anxiety about being in places or situations from which escape might be difficult or embarassing or in which help may not be available in the event of a panic attack. Examples include fear of leaving home alone, being in a crowd, standing in line, crossing bridges, being in a car, bus, or train. The feared situation or place is avoided, endured with marked distress, or requires the presence of a trusted companion.

4.8.2. Panic Attacks   Table 1-13

Panic attacks can occur in childhood, but increase in frequency after puberty. Panic attacks are variously described as a sense of dread, intense fear, fear of losing control, going crazy, or dying. (See Table 1-13 for **DSM-IV** criteria for Panic Attacks.) Panic attacks are frequently mistaken as medical problems. It may be difficult to distinguish a panic attack from medical conditions that cause similar symptoms. Some medical problems that should be included in the differential diagnosis for panic attacks include: hyper- or hypo-thyroidism, hypoglycemia, myocardial infarction, arrythmia, partial complex seizure, asthma attack, anemia, medication side effect, or drug-related symptoms (caffeine, stimulants, alcohol/sedative withdrawal, etc.)

DSM-IV   Criteria for Panic Attack

A discrete period of intense fear or discomfort, in which four (or more) of the following symptoms developed abruptly and reached a peak within 10 minutes:

(1) palpitations, pounding heart, or accelerated heart rate
(2) sweating
(3) trembling or shaking
(4) sensations of shortness of breath or smothering
(5) feeling of choking
(6) chest pain or discomfort
(7) nausea or abdominal distress
(8) feeling dizzy, unsteady, lightheaded, or faint
(9) derealization (feelings of unreality) or depersonalization (being detached from oneself)
(10) fear of losing control or going crazy
(11) fear of dying
(12) paresthesias (numbness or tingling sensations)
(13) chills or hot flashes

Post Traumatic Stress Disorder

All children and adolescents experience stressful events that can affect them both emotionally and phys-ically. Their reactions to stress are usually brief so that they recover without further problems. A child or adolescent who experiences a catastrophic event may develop ongoing difficulties known as post-traumatic stress disorder (PTSD). The stressful or traumatic event involves a situation where someone's life has been threatened or severe injury has occurred. For example, the child may be the victim or a witness of physical abuse, sexual abuse, violence in the home or in the community. They may be involved in an automobile accident, natural disaster, or be diagnosed with a life threatening illness. A child's risk of developing PTSD is related to the seriousness of the trauma, whether the trauma is repeat-ed, the child's proximity to the trauma, and his/her relationship to the victim(s). Approximately 20% of children/adolescents who experience a severe trauma will develop PTSD.

Following trauma, children may initially show agitated or confused behavior. They may also show intense fear, helplessness, anger, sadness, horror or denial. Children who experience repeated trauma may develop a kind of emotional numbing to deaden or block the pain and trauma. This is called dis-sociation. Children with PTSD avoid situations or places that remind them of the trauma. They may also become less responsive emotionally, depressed, withdrawn, and more detached from their feelings.

A child with PTSD may also re-experience the traumatic event by:
-having frequent memories of the event, or in young children, play in which some or all of the trauma is repeated over and over
-having upsetting and frightening dreams
-acting or feeling like the experience is happening again
-developing repeated physical or emotional symptoms when the child is reminded of the event

Children with PTSD may also show the following symptoms:
-worry about dying at an early age
-losing interest in activities
-having physical symptoms such as headaches and stomachaches
-showing more sudden and extreme emotional reactions
-having problems falling or staying asleep
-showing irritability or angry outbursts
-having problems concentrating
-acting younger than their age, e.g., clingy or whiny behavior.
-showing increased alertness to the environment
-repeating behavior that reminds them of the trauma

The symptoms of PTSD may last from several months to many years. The best approach is prevention of the trauma. Once the trauma has occurred, however, early intervention is essential. Support from par-ents, school, and peers is important. Emphasis needs to be placed upon establishing a feeling of safe-ty. Child and adolescent psychiatrists can be very helpful in diagnosing and treating children with PTSD. Psychotherapy (individual, group, or family) which allows the child to speak, draw, play, or write about the event is helpful. Behavior modification techniques and cognitive therapy may help reduce fears and worries. Medication may also be useful to deal with agitation, anxiety, or depression. With the sensitivity and support of families and professionals, youngsters with PTSD can learn to cope with the memories of the trauma and go on to lead healthy and productive lives.

4.9 REPETITIVE BEHAVIORS

Repetitive behaviors are repeated, purposeless, and sometimes rhythmic actions. Some examples of repetitive behaviors are: 1.) lip, hand, finger, thumb sucking, 2.) lip, skin, nail biting, 3.) banging head, hand(s), object(s), 4.) foot kicking, 5.) hair pulling, 6.) skin, scab, nose picking, 7.) hand or arm flapping, 8.) body rocking, 9.) teeth grinding (bruxism), 10.) psychogenic/habitual coughing, 11.) and breath holding. These behaviors are common during childhood and are usually benign and self-limited. Most children with repetitive behaviors are of normal intelligence and development. Nevertheless, children with repetitive behaviors deserve special consideration in this text for several reasons: 1.) repetitive behaviors occur with increased frequency in children with developmental, emotional, or physical problems and may therefore be a red-flag for further testing, 2.) repetitive behaviors may cause tissue damage, 3.) they may be socially undesirable, 4.) and they may cause subjective stress to the individual and/or their family.

Repetitive behaviors are adaptive, at least initially, as they provide stimulation and/or soothing to the child. There is strong evidence that repetitive behaviors are biologically driven actions that develop into a habit in some children.

Table 1-14 Onset and longitudinal prevalence of some repetitive behaviors in early childhood

Percentage of Children

Repetitive Behavior	Mean Age of Onset (months)	0-1 year	1-2 year	2-6 year
Hand, finger, thumb-sucking*	Birth	100%	40-50%	14-19% at 5 yr.
Lip biting or sucking**	4-5	93%		1-10%
Foot kicking***	2-3	99%		
Body rocking****	6	91%	9-30%	3%
Head banging*****	8-9	7%	5-19%	1-3%

*   Kravitz and Boehm (1971); Mahalski and Stanton (1992)

**   Kravitz and Boehm (1971); Troster (1994)

*** Kravitz and Boehm (1971)

****   Kravitz and Boehm (1971)

*****Abe et al (1984); Kravitz and Boehm (1971); Sallustro and Atwell (1978)
     Male to female ratio of 3:1; 9% of those with head banging at age 3 had persistent banging at age 7

4.9.1. Hand/Digit Sucking

Sucking of the hand, fingers, or thumb has been observed in utero as early as 29 weeks of gestation and is a nearly universal phenomenon in healthy newborns. Hand or digit sucking is usually harmless, but if it persists, can be associated with a number of problematic sequelae.

The most frequent sequelae of persistent digit sucking are social. Children who suck their thumbs are often nagged and reprimanded by their parents and other adults, which may lead to family conflict and/or unhappiness or insecurity in the child. In a 1993 study, Friman showed 1st grade children pictures of their peers who were thumb sucking and pictures of the same peers when they were not thumb sucking. The children rated their peers who were sucking their thumbs as less intelligent, less happy, less attractive, less likable, and less fun, as well as less desirable as a friend or playmate. The next most frequent sequelae of persistent digit sucking are dental problems such as **anterior open bite**, decreased **alveolar bone** growth, mucosal trauma, and even altered growth of the facial bones.

Treatment of thumb sucking is rarely indicated in children younger than age 4 years. In older children, if the sucking occurs infrequently (only at night) or is a transient response to a stressor, then treatment is also rarely indicated. Treatment may be indicated if the sucking causes dental problems, digit malformation, tissue damage, distress to the child, or excessive family conflict.

Treatment for hand/digit sucking usually involves some combination of reinforcement for not sucking (e.g., praise, tangible rewards), application of aversive taste to the nail/skin (e.g., Stop-Zit from Purepac Pharmaceutical Co.), or physical barriers to sucking (e.g., gloves, hand socks, thumb splints.) Firman and Leibowitz (1990) combined a reward system with aversive taste treatment and achieved cessation of thumb sucking in 12/22 children within 3 months and 20/22 within one year.

When necessary, intraoral dental appliances can be effective treatments. Such appliances provide a reminder not to suck and interfere with the seal that sucking creates. When a fixed maxillary appliance is placed the clinician may find a desired cessation of a digital habit because the appliance has unbalanced the pattern of satisfaction from sucking.

4.9.2. Nail-Biting

Nail-biting is uncommon in preschool children, but is common in grade school, occurring in 30-60% of children (boys=girls) at age 10 years. The incidence then decreases to 20% during **adolescence** and 10% during adulthood. During adolescence and adulthood (vs. in younger ages), more males than females bite their nails.

Most individuals confine their nail-biting habit to the fingernails, usually biting all 10 nails equally. Occasionally, toe nails are bitten. Sometimes the margins of the nailbeds and/or cuticles are bitten.

When severe, nail-biting may be harmful to the dentition, resulting in apical **root resorption**, fractures in the edges of incisors, and gingivitis. Nail-biting may also result in paronychia or extensive tissue damage.

Efforts should be made to be supportive of the nail-biter, because punishment, nagging, and ridicule often only serve to worsen the problem or create further difficulties in parent-child or other relationships. The Habit Reversal Procedure has been effective in reducing nail-biting (Azrin, Nunn, and Frantz 1980, see description below.)

4.9.3. **Bruxism**

Bruxism refers to grinding and clenching of teeth. It may occur during sleep, during the day, or both. It is common in both children and adults. The incidence in children has been variably reported from 7-88%, however most studies report 15-30% incidence (Cash 1988).

The frequency of bruxism increases during childhood, reaching its peak incidence between 7-10 years of age. The etiology of bruxism remains unclear, but it is believed to be multifactorial. The peak in incidence of bruxism between 7-10 years is attributed to the mixture of deciduous and permanent teeth present at this time. The role of occlusal discrepancies in bruxism remains controversial, however evaluation of the occlusion is important in individuals with bruxism because occlusion affects the distribution of forces generated by the bruxism. Various psychological factors have been postulated to be associated with bruxism. For example, bruxism is thought to be associated with emotions such as frustration, anger, anxiety, or fear. Vanderas (1995) demonstrated that children aged 6-10 years who experienced unpleasant life events were more likely to have bruxism than controls, however this study does not differentiate between diurnal and nocturnal bruxism. According to Cash (1988), when studies are limited to nocturnal bruxism, the relationship of bruxism to emotional stressors is less clear.

The decision of whether or not to treat bruxism is complex. Bruxism is often transient and causes less frequent symptoms in children compared to adults. Reassurance may be the only indicated treatment in many cases. The most common symptom of bruxism in children is pain on palpation over the muscles of mastication (Cash 1988.) Other symptoms such as temporomandibular joint dysfunction and recurrent headaches may occur. The most common sign of bruxism is abnormal wearing of the teeth. Hypermobility of the teeth, injury to the peridontium, fractured teeth, and pulpitis may also occur.

Psychological treatments may be helpful for some individuals with bruxism. These are aimed at decreasing stress and/or teaching stress management. For example, relaxation training and biofeedback have been reported to have at least short-term benefits in treatment of adults with bruxism. These techniques have not been studied in children with bruxism. Nocturnal alarms have been demonstrated to decrease the frequency and duration of bruxism, but gains may not be maintained after the discontinuation of use of the alarm.

Physical therapists may be involved in the treatment of pain associated with bruxism. A variety of physical therapy techniques may be used such as facial/jaw exercises, application of heat, and transcutaneous electrical stimulation.

Non-steroidal anti-inflammatory agents may also be helpful for pain management. Muscle relaxants may decrease bruxism or associated pain/muscle spasm, but have significant side effects (not the least of which is development of physical dependence) and therefore should not be used as a long-term treatment.

4.9.4. Tics

Tics are involuntary, brief, rapid, repetitive, non-rhythmic movements or vocalizations. They may be classified as transient or chronic, simple or complex, and motor or vocal. Simple motor tics involve an individual muscle group. Examples of simple motor tics are eye blinking, shoulder shrugging, lip smacking, eye squinting. Simple vocal tics consist of simple sounds. Examples include throat clearing, grunting, (psychogenic/habitual) coughing, sniffing. A tic that consists of a cough may also be referred to as psychogenic coughing. Complex motor tics involve a cluster of simple motor tics or a more coordinated pattern of movements and may be difficult to recognize and/or distinguish from compulsive behavior. Examples of complex motor tics include touching, jumping, manipulating clothing, facial grimacing. Complex vocal tics (also known as Tourette's Syndrome) involve saying words, parts of words, phrases, palolalia (repeating one's own words), or echolalia (repeating other's words).

Most tics are simple and motor. The average age of onset for motor tics is 7 years and of vocal tics is 9 years, however, tics may occurs as early as 2 years of age and/or may have new onset in adulthood.

Most tics are transient. They usually have a waxing and waning course and may be exacerbated by anxiety, stress, excitement, and/or fatigue. Tics may be hugely variable in severity and frequency. Tics are often associated with other behavioral, emotional, or learning problems. Obsessive compulsive behaviors occur in 90% of individuals with Tourette's Syndrome. 40-50% of people with Tourette's Syndrome meet full criteria for Obsessive Compulsive Disorder (OCD). Attention Deficit Disorder is often co-morbid with tics/tic disorders.

The presence of tics may not be a sufficient reason for treatment. Treatment is indicated when the tics cause significant disruption in function (speech, motor, time-displacement) or are interfering with a child's social or emotional development or interpersonal relationships. Pharmacological treatment for tics has the best scientifically documented efficacy. Clonidin, Haldol, and newer antipsychotic medications are often used (See Section 7, Psychiatric medication in children and adolescents). There are several nonpharmacological treatments for tics including the Habit Reversal Procedure (see description below), relaxation training, biofeedback, and hypnosis. More research needs to be done to demonstrate whether these treatments are efficacious before they can be widely recommended.

4.9.5. Habit Reversal Procedure

The original habit reversal procedure was described by Azrin and Nunn (1973). It is a multicomponent behavioral treatment that has been demonstrated to be effective for a wide variety of repetitive behaviors including digit sucking, nail biting, and tics (Woods and Miltenberger 1995). The treatment goals of this procedure are 1.) increase the individual's awareness of the problem, 2.) teach the individual a competing response to engage in when they feel they are about to engage in the habit, 3.) help the individual sustain compliance and facilitate generalization of the response. Most studies have targeted adolescents and adults. Treatment of children requires motivation (which may be developmentally challenging), simplification of the procedure, and a high degree of cooperation between the parent and child.

4.10 SELF-INJURIOUS BEHAVIOR

Self-injury is the act of deliberately destroying body tissue. Some common forms of self-injury include:

-Head banging
-Hitting
-Biting skin, nails, cuticles
-Picking skin or scabs
-Pulling hair
-Burning or branding skin
-Carving or scratching skin
-Excessive body piercing
-Tattooing

Excessive body piercing is that which is in excess of what is sanctioned by the individual's culture. For example, currently for most groups in the United States, a single pierce per ear lobe is considered normal, however there remain sub-groups in the U.S. (e.g., Amish communities) in which even a single ear pierce is not culturally accepted.

The causes and severity of self-injury can vary. In addition, the meaning and acceptability of self-injury varies depending on one's group and culture within society. Self-injurious behaviors are viewed by some clinicians/researchers as an extension of self-stimulatory behaviors such as hand flapping, spinning, or finger flicking. Sometimes people injure themselves to change the way they feel (both physically and emotionally.) For example, people who engage in recurrent superficial cutting of their skin sometimes report experiencing a relief of pain, tension, anger, anxiety, and/or distress after the self-injury.

Some adolescents may self-mutilate to take risks, rebel, reject their parents' values, state their individuality, or merely be accepted. Others, however, may injure themselves out of desperation or anger; in order to seek attention, to demonstrate their feelings of worthlessness or hopelessness, or because of suicidal thoughts. These children and adolescents may suffer from serious psychiatric illness such as depression, psychosis, post traumatic stress disorder, or bipolar disorder. Self-injurious behavior is 50 times more common in persons with a psychiatric diagnosis versus the general population. Adolescents who have difficulty talking about their feelings may show their emotional tension, physical discomfort, pain, and low self-esteem with self-injurious behaviors.

Self-injurious behavior appears to be more popular recently, especially in adolescents. The effects of peer pressure or contagion can also influence adolescents to injure themselves (e.g., carving words into arms, self-tattooing.) Although repetitive behaviors are very common in children of normal development, truly self-injurious behavior is more common in adolescents. Severely self-injurious behavior is most common in the mentally retarded population. In some individuals, self-injury may be so severe as to be disfiguring (e.g., complete loss of external ear secondary to scratch.)

4.11 RISK TAKING BEHAVIOR

4.11.1. History of Tattooing and Body Piercing

Throughout history tattooing and body piercing have been practiced by many cultures for many centuries. Egyptians identified tattooing with fertility and nobility. The Japanese have used tattooing for ornamental, cosmetic, and religious purposes as well as for identification and punishment of criminals. Many cultural groups have used body piercing as a rite of passage, including Egyptian Pharaohs, Roman soldiers, and Native American warriors.

More recently in Western culture, tattoos have been traditionally associated with particular groups, such as gang members, criminal populations, motorcycle group members, and military personnel. There has been a dramatic increase in the practice of tattooing and body piercing over the past 10 years. Tattoos and body piercing are now much more commonly seen, such that the previous associations may no longer apply.

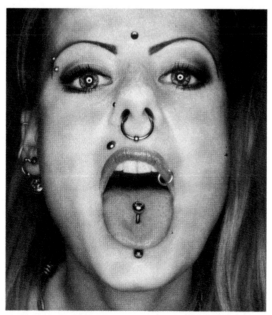

Figure 1-10 Photograph by Erwin Olaf, boomerang freecards, www.boomerang.nl

4.11.2. Body Piercing

The popularity of body piercing has skyrocketed over the past ten years. The earlobe and ear cartilage remain the most frequently pierced sites. Almost any body site can be pierced, for example nostril, nasal septum, nasal bridge, eyebrow, lip, tongue, navel, nipple, and various genital sites.

Complications from body piercing relate to the body part pierced. Ear cartilage piercings do not heal as quickly as lobe piercings because of the different type of tissue and pressure on the pierce area during sleep. Tongue piercings initially swell dramatically but heal quickly because of the tongue's profuse blood supply. Nipple piercings may burrow through some of the milk-producing ducts and cause infection or problems with later breast feeding. Navel piercings become infected easily because tight-fitting clothes do not allow enough air to circulate and collect moisture around the piercing site. Piercing guns should not be used because they crush the tissue that is pierced and cannot be properly re-sterilized.

There may be problems related to the size, weight, and fit of the jewelry worn. For example, if the jewelry is too large or heavy, the skin may stretch/rip. If the jewelry is too tight, the blood supply may be cut off to the pierce site causing swelling and pain. People with body piercings can also have an allergic reaction to the jewelry material used (contact dermatitis.) Non-toxic metals such as surgical steel, solid 14K gold, niobium, and titanium are often recommended to avoid this. Gold-plated jewelry should not be used.

The healing time required after piercing will depend on the body site pierced (See Table 1-15).

Table 1-15

Healing Times of Body Pierce by Site	
Ear lobe	6-8 weeks
Ear cartilage	4 months - 1 year
Nostril	2-4 months
Nasal septum	6-8 months
Nasal bridge	8-10 weeks
Tongue	4 weeks
Lip	2-3 months
Nipple	3-6 months
Navel	4 months - 1 year
Female genitalia	4-10 weeks
Male genitalia	4 weeks - 6 months

For tongue piercing, barbell jewelry is usually worn. In the event that the barbell end comes loose, the patient may swallow the barbell or damage a tooth. One should avoid fingering the pierce site to minimize the risk of infection. The tissue around a new pierce should be kept clean using antibacterial soap. Alcohol and peroxide should not be used as they will dry the skin. Betadine may discolor gold jewelry. The patient with a new pierce should avoid public pools and hot tubs until the piercing has healed. An antibacterial mouthwash can be used following tongue or lip piercing. Occasionally the patient may experience tongue discoloration and/or bad breath. This may indicate that the normal flora of the mouth has been killed, in which case the patient should use salt water rinses rather than antibacterial mouthwash. Pain, prolonged swelling, and bad breath may indicate infection.

4.11.3. Tattoos

Some important complications of tattoos:

-Increased susceptibility to infections including, but not limited to, Streptococcus, Tetanus, Hepatitis B, Hepatitis C, and HIV.
-Tattoos are not easy to remove and in some cases may cause permanent discoloration.
-Tattoo removal is very expensive. A tattoo that cost $50 to apply may cost over $1,000 to remove.
-Some people are allergic to tattoo dye and their body will work to reject the tattoo. Even 5

minutes of direct sunlight on a healing tattoo may trigger an allergic reaction.

-Blood donations cannot be made for one year after getting a tattoo, body piercing, or permanent make-up.

Two different surveys conducted in urban high schools in 1993 and 1995 revealed an increasing number of adolescents engaging in tattooing at a younger age. The 1993 study of 642 adolescents from six suburban high schools in Texas revealed 8.6% of students had a tattoo with the youngest being 11 years old when their tattoo was obtained. Very few tattoos were identified as gang-related. Sixty-five percent of the students with tattoos had grades of A's and B's. Sixty-five percent of students with tattoos were male and 35% were female. In 1995 the study surveyed 1,762 adolescents in eight high schools across the U.S. Fifty-five percent (versus 33% in 1993) of students expressed an interest in tattooing. The total percent of adolescents with tattoos was higher at 9%, and the youngest was 8 years old when their tattoo was obtained. More gang affiliation was reported. There was a slightly lower percentage of A/B students (60%).

Substance Abuse & Motor Vehicle Accidents

1.) The use of psychoactive substances is increasing in all age groups of children and adolescents. Of particular concern is that the first drug experiences are at increasingly young ages. The percentage of students using drugs by the time they have reached 6th grade has tripled over the past decade. One in twenty high school seniors drink alcohol daily; nearly 37% drink five or more drinks during a single drinking episode. At least 1 out of every 25 high school seniors smokes marijuana on a daily basis. 1 in 25 high school seniors has used "crack" cocaine at least once. Three-fourths of all deaths in the 15-24 age group are attributable to traffic accidents, other accidental traumas, suicide, and homicide. The contribution of alcohol and drugs to this tragedy is significant. Alcohol and other **drug abuse** can interfere with the developmental process in children and adolescents and can have long-term physical, psychological, and sociological consequences. Youthful users are more prone to develop accelerated onset of both tolerance and **addiction**. They are more vulnerable to life-threatening accidents and injuries, impulsive risk taking behaviors, physical complications, illegal activity, sexually transmitted diseases including AIDS, impairment of memory, and impairment of cognitive and motor performance. See the glossary for definitions of **drug use, drug abuse,** and **drug addiction.**

2.) Alcohol and other **drug use** in children and youth should be regarded as harmful. Any non-prescription use of psychoactive drugs by a child or adolescent requires appropriate concern by family and community. Although some use of alcohol, nicotine, and marijuana is so common in older age groups as to be normative, it is dangerous for health care providers and other role models to represent such behavior as "normal" as this may delay recognition of dependence.

3.) A comprehensive professional evaluation regarding the nature, extent, and pattern of substance use, as well as any related problems and consequences, is a necessary prerequisite for accurate diagnosis and appropriate intervention.

4.12 SLEEP APNEA

Apnea is defined as lack of oronasal airflow lasting more than 10 seconds. In adults, sleep apnea is currently diagnosed when there are five or more apneic episodes per hour on polysomnography ("sleep study"). The definition of sleep apnea in children is more controversial because children experience oxygen desaturation more readily than adults. In children, one should have a low threshold for obtaining polysomnography.

Sleep apnea frequently goes unrecognized in both adults and children. The currently reported prevalence of sleep apnea in adults is 1-2%, but it is probably more frequent. When discovered, it is often because of loud snoring and/or observed pauses in beathing during sleep. It is also sometimes discovered during evaluation of excessive daytime sleepiness.

Apnea may be obstructive or central (i.e., central nervous system) in origin. Tissue hypertrophy (tonsils and/or adenoids) and septal deviation are common causes/contributors of obstructive sleep apnea. Children with craniofacial abnormalities, Down Syndrome, hydrocephalus, cerebral palsy, degenerative or neuromuscular disorders, and obesity are at increased risk for apnea and sleep apnea. Polysomnography ("sleep study") is the definitive tool for diagnosis of sleep apnea.

Treatment of sleep apnea can be complex and depends on the etiology and severity of the problem. For some people with obstructive sleep apnea, changes in sleep positioning can be helpful. Dental devices are also effective in selected cases. For others, tonsillectomy and adenoidectomy may be indicated and is often curative. Continuous positive airway pressure (CPAP) or bi-level positive airway pressure (BiPAP) devices may be required for treatment in others with sleep apnea (both obstructive and central). Rarely, extreme measures such as tracheotomy may be required.

5. DISCIPLINE

Physical/Sexual/Emotional Abuse and Neglect

The rate of child maltreatment is alarmingly high. In the United States, since 1993, the number of reported cases of child maltreatment has been approximately 3 million per year and the number of substantiated cases has been approximately 1 million per year. The number of substantiated cases of child maltreatment in the US translates to approximately 1 in every 70 children. Orthodontists are well positioned to identify emotional and physical signs of child abuse due to the frequency of their contact with children and their parents.

Neither age nor race of children correlates with maltreatment. However, rates of child neglect skyrocket as family income falls. In contrast to child neglect, the frequency of physical and sexual abuse does not differ by socioeconomic status. Single mothers are most likely to be neglectful of their children, whereas fathers are more likely to be perpetrators of abuse. Familial alcohol and drug abuse is a significant factor in up to 90% of child abuse cases.

Definitions

Child Maltreatment- Any intentional harm to a person under 18 years of age.

Child Abuse- Any action that is harmful (physically, sexually, or psychologically) to a child's wellbeing. The harm incurred by the abuse (i.e., severity and duration of physical and psychological effects) depends in part on the specific type of abuse inflicted, the severity of the abuse, and the frequency and duration of occurrence. The severity of harm (both physical and psychological) also depends greatly on the vulnerability/resilience of the victim.

Some specific signs of child physical abuse are bruises or welts about the face or head, on the trunk, back, thighs, or genitals. The skin findings are often on multiple body surfaces or planes and may be in the shape of a hand or object such as a belt or electrical cord. Any bruises on the body of non-ambulatory infants are highly suspicious. Burns and scalding, usually second or third-degree, may result from immersion, non-accidental splashing of hot liquids, or contact with hot objects (e.g., irons, heaters, or cigarettes). Fractures, especially bucket-handle or corner fractures (metaphyseal fractures), rib fractures, scapular fractures, vertebrae fractures, spiral fractures in non-weight bearing infants, or multiple fractures in various stages of healing should be regarded as strongly suggestive of physical abuse. Subdural, subarachnoid, and retinal hemorrhages with or without skull fractures that cannot be adequately explained by history are most strongly suggestive of non-accidental trauma. The shaken baby syndrome is not an uncommon form of abuse but often results in significant morbidity and mortality. Signs and symptoms of shaken baby syndrome may vary from irritability, lethargy, poor feeding, vomiting (with or without diarrhea), temperature instability, developmental delay, gasping respiration, apnea, acute loss of consciousness, or seizures. A skeletal survey must be done in all suspected cases of child abuse and neglect in children less than two years old. Head CT or MRI and ophthalmology consultation should be obtained to rule out intracranial bleeding and retinal hemorrhages.

Emotional Abuse- Emotional maltreatment may be the result of psychological unavailability of the caregiver. Children may suffer frequent humiliation and scapegoating. Parents may show inconsistent and/or unrealistic expectations. Manifestations of emotional abuse include excessive anxiety (worries, fears, phobias), impulse control problems, aggression, somatic complaints, nightmares, low self-esteem, failure to thrive, school or peer problems.

Neglect- Any interaction that harms or endangers a person. **Child neglect** can involve not providing for physical needs (food, shelter, clothing, warmth, medical care, education, and appropriate supervision) or psychological needs (love, language, and appropriate interaction/stimulation.) Child neglect is as lethal as physical abuse. Some studies have shown that as many children die from neglect as physical abuse. Some indicators of neglect include lack of appropriate child supervision, lack of medical attention (e.g., immunizations not up to date) and developmental delay. Obviously, not all children who are developmentally delayed have been neglected, but many children who have been neglected are developmentally delayed.

Child Sexual Abuse- the involvement of a child in any act or situation, the purpose of which is to provide sexual gratification or financial benefit for the perpetrator. While it often involves physical contact (fondling, penetration) there need be no physical contact for an act to be considered child sexual abuse. For example, showing a child pornographic material or exhibiting one's genitals to a child are considered child sexual abuse. Behavioral indicators of child sexual abuse include shame or guilt, sexually explicit play, promiscuity, runaway behavior, pseudomaturity, change in behavior, drop in school performance, nightmares, panic attacks, periods of "spacing out" (dissociation), bedwetting, soiling underwear, substance abuse, depression, and suicidal behavior. While sexual abuse may be discovered through routine physical examinations, it most often leaves no physical evidence of harm.

Child abuse should be considered as a possibility in all children who present with recurrent injuries or injuries that are inconsistent with their developmental age or inconsistent with the story of the injury. Burn marks, bruises with unusual shapes or sharp margins (e.g., hand mark, cord mark) should be considered suspicious. Unaccountable lesions or bruising of the soft palate should be considered suspicious. The finding of certain sexually transmitted infections (e.g., gonorrhea on genital culture) is almost certainly evidence of sexual abuse in a young child, as children are emotionally and cognitively unable to consent to sexual relations (even with other children.) Remember, however, that HIV may be acquired prenatally or by blood transfusions therefore its finding is ambiguous. Similarly, HSV I is ubiquitous and therefore not at all definitive.

Corporal Punishment

Corporal punishment involves the application of some form of physical pain in response to undesirable behavior. Corporal punishment ranges from slapping the hand of a child about to touch a hot stove to identifiable child abuse, such as beating, scalding, or burning a child as a form of punishment. Spanking refers to striking a child with an open hand on the buttocks or extremities with the intention of modifying behavior and without the intention to produce physical injury.

Other Forms of Physical Punishment

Spanking is one of the most commonly used discipline strategies. More than 90% of families report having used spanking at least one time. Despite its common acceptance, and even advocacy for its use by some, spanking has been demonstrated to be a less effective strategy than time-out or removal of privileges for reducing undesired behavior. The American Academy of Pediatrics (AAP) does not endorse the use of spanking as a discipline strategy. Rather, the AAP recommends that parents be encouraged and assisted in developing methods other than spanking in response to undesirable behavior. At best, spanking is only effective when used in selective and infrequent situations. Be aware that most adults were spanked when they were children. Encouraging alternative discipline methods to spanking may evoke strong responses from some parents and even some pediatricians and other medical professionals.

Spanking children less than 18 months of age increases the chance of physical injury to the child. Children less than 18 months are unlikely to understand the connection between the behavior and the punishment. Spanking may immediately reduce or stop an undesired behavior, but its effectiveness decreases with subsequent use. The only way to maintain the initial effect of spanking is to systematically increase the intensity with which it is delivered, which can quickly escalate into frank child abuse. Time-out and positive reinforcement of other behaviors are more difficult to implement and take longer to become effective when spanking has previously been a primary method of discipline. Because the act of spanking a child as punishment may provide some relief of the parent's anger, the likelihood that that parent will use spanking in the future is increased. Moreover, parents who use spanking are more likely to use other unacceptable forms of corporal punishment.

Studies have demonstrated that children who are spanked report more anger as adults and are more likely to spank their own children, more likely to have marital conflict, and more likely to approve of hitting a spouse. Spanking models **aggressive** behavior as a solution to conflict. Spanking has been associated with increased aggression in pre-school and school-aged children. Spanking has been associated with higher rates of physical aggression, more substance abuse, and increased risk of crime and violence when used with older children and adolescents.

Mandatory Reporting of Child Abuse and Neglect

Health care providers (physicians, dentists, nurses, social workers, etc.) have an ethical responsibility to report <u>all suspected </u>cases of child maltreatment to child protective services. Many states have made failing to report an incident a crime. Note that you need only have a reasonable suspicion; it is the responsibility of the child protective services to investigate and determine whether the allegations are substantiated.

6. DEVELOPMENTAL ASPECTS OF PAIN

Table 1-16

Pain in neonates and children is misunderstood, underreported, and undertreated. Some clinicians have proposed that infants and young children have an elevated pain threshold compared with older children or adults. This view was initially supported by the observation that some neonates slept comfortably following major surgery, even without analgesic medication. Recent observations of facial expressions, motor response, physiological stress responses (blood pressure, heart rate, respiratory rate), crying, suggest a significant adverse response to pain in infants. (See Table 11-16: Developmental Sequence of Children's Understanding of Pain.) The perception of pain

Developmental Sequence of Children's Understanding of Pain	
0 - 3 months	No apparent understanding of pain; memory for pain not understood; likely not conclusively demonstrated; responses appear reflexive and are perceptually dominated.
3 - 6 months	Pain response supplemented by sadness and anger response.
6 - 18 months	Developing fear of painful situations; use of common words for pain, e.g., owie, ouchie, boo-boo; localization of pain develops.
18 - 24 months	Use of the word "hurt" to describe pain; beginning to use noncognitive coping strategies.
24 - 36 months	Begins to describe pain and attribute an external cause to the pain
36 - 60 months	Can give a gross indication of the intensity of the pain and beginning to use more descriptive adjectives and attach emotional terms such as "sad" or "mad" to the pain.
5 - 7 years	Can more clearly differentiate levels of pain intensity; beginning to use cognitive coping strategies.
7 - 10 years	Can explain why the pain hurts.
> 11 years	Can explain the value of pain.

involves both sensory and affective/cognitive components. The sensory component consists of activation of neural pathways in response to a noxious stimulus. The affective/cognitive component involves a variety of secondary behavioral responses. A generalized motor and vocal response occurs to pain. Because infants, young children, and cognitively impaired individuals lack the communication skills of adults, their response to pain differs from that of the cognitively intact adult. It may be difficult to determine whether young children and cognitively impaired individuals "feel pain." Several physiological parameters have been used to assess pain in infants and children, including changes in heart rate and blood pressure, serum cortisol level, transcutaneous oxygen tension, and palmar sweating.

7. PSYCHIATRIC MEDICATION IN CHILDREN AND ADOLESCENTS

In recent years there have been an increasing number of children and adolescents treated with psychiatric medications. Medication can be a very effective part of treatment for psychiatric disorders of childhood and adolescence but should only be prescribed after a thorough evaluation and as a part of a comprehensive treatment plan. Prescribing psychiatric medications for children and adolescents requires the judgement of a physician with training and qualifications in the use of psychiatric medication in this age group. With the possible exception of stimulant medication prescribed to a child with clear and uncomplicated Attention Deficit Disorder, psychiatric medication should ideally be prescribed by a (board-certified) Child and Adolescent Psychiatrist. All children under the age of five should be carefully evaluated by a physician with special training and experience working with young children prior to receiving psychiatric medication. The American Academy of Child and Adolescent Psychiatry (AACAP) opposes the use of brief medication visits (e.g., 15-minute medication checks) as the accepted standard of care by the insurance industry and managed care organizations. Psychosocial interventions, such as parent training and individual and family psychotherapy should be considered as part of a comprehensive treatment plan.

There is an increasing number of psychiatric medications that have been shown to be effective in treatment of mental illness in adults. Most psychiatric medications have not yet received specific approval by the Federal Drug Administration (FDA) for use in children under the age of 12. Unfortunately, pharmacological research lags far behind clinical practice in child and adolescent psychiatry. Child and adolescent psychiatrists must, for now, rely on data from studies with adults, studies conducted outside the United States, case reports of use in children and adolescents, and their own clinical experience as well of that of their colleagues. Research studies are underway to establish which medications are most effective for use in children.

Stimulant Medications: Primary indication for stimulant medication is treatment of Attention Deficit Hyperactivity Disorder. Examples include *Dextroamphetamine (Dexedrine) Adderal and Methylphenidate (Ritalin, Concerta, Methidate)*.

Antidepressant Medications: Primary indications are treatment of depression, anxiety disorders (such as Post Traumatic Stress Disorder, Panic Disorder, Obsessive Compulsive Disorder, school phobia, separation anxiety, and others.) There are several classes of antidepressant medications. Examples of selective serotonin reuptake inhibitors (SSRIs) are *Fluoxetine (Prozac)*, *Sertraline (Zoloft), Paroxetine (Paxil), Venlafaxine (Effexor), Citalopram (Celexa), and Fluvoxamine (Luvox)*. Examples of *tricyclic antidepressants* include *Amitriptyline (Elavil), Nortriptyline (Pamelor), Imipramine (Tofranil), and Clomipramine (Anafranil)*. Examples of atypical antidepressants include *Bupropion (Wellbutrin), Nefazodone (Serzone), Trazodone (Desyrel), and Mirtazapine (Remeron)*. Examples of *monoamine oxidase inhibitors* include Phenelzine (Nardil) and Tranylcypromine (Parnate).

Antipsychotic Medications: Main indications are for treatment of delusions, hallucinations, or disordered thinking. May also be helpful for treatment of tic disorders and stuttering. Also useful for (rapid) mood stabilization and treatment of agitation and aggression. Newer medications include *Risperidone (Risperdal), Olanzapine (Zyprexa), Quetiapine (Seroquel), Clozapine (Clozaril), and Ziprasidone (Geodon)*. Older medications include *Haloperidol (Haldol), Fluphenazine (Prolixin), Chlorpromazine (Thorazine), Thioridazine (Mellaril), Thiothixixene (Navane), and Trifluoperazine (Stelazine)*.

Mood Stabilizers and Anticonvulsant Medications: Main indication is Bipolar Disorder (Manic Depression) but helpful in treating excessive mood swings, aggressive behavior, and impulse control problems. Examples include *Valproic Acid (Depakote, Depakene), Carbamazepine (Tegretol, Carbitrol), Trileptal, Gabapentin (Neurontin), and Lamotrigine (Lamictil)*.

Anti-anxiety Medications: Also see antidepressant medications. There are several types of medications used to treat anxiety. Examples include SSRIs, tricyclic antidepressants, *benzodiazepines (Diazepam/Valium, Lorazepam/Ativan, Clonazepam/Klonopin, Alprazolam/Xanax), antihistamines (Diphenhydramine/Benadryl, Hydroxyzine/Vistaril)*, and others such as *Buspirone (BuSpar)*.

Sleep Medications: Generally used for short term treatment of sleep problems. Examples include: *Trazodone (Desyrel), Zolpidem (Ambien), and Diphenhydramine (Benadryl)*.

Miscellaneous Medications: Examples include *Clonidine (Catapress)* for Post Traumatic Stress Disorder, Attention Deficit Disorder, or Tic Disorder; *Guanfacine (Tenex)* for Attention Deficit Disorder or Post Traumatic Stress Disorder.

8. A CLINICAL PERSPECTIVE AND SUMMING UP

A Clinical Perspective:

The orthodontist has the privilege, opportunity, and challenge to improve the esthetics and malocclusions of pre-adolescent and adolescent patients. No list of psychiatric symptoms is sufficient to fully capture the complexities of the lively, energetic adolescent who unconsciously and consciously charts the way through the internal and external difficulties associated with growing up. The orthodontist has a unique window into the mind of the adolescent, offering the adolescent both a potential boost to self-image and self-respect, and the benefits of an ongoing relationship with a trusted adult. It is easy for the orthodontist to underestimate the potential to have a lasting, positive influence on adolescent patients.

Most of the approximately 30 million 13 – 19 year olds are normal, even though almost all go through periods of sometimes-intense crises and change. In studies of adolescent samples, 10 – 25% of the youngsters meet the criteria for psychiatric disorders. Anxiety, depression – and other mood disorders, attention deficit hyperactivity disorder, and conduct problems account for most of the problems (Lewis and Volkmar, 1990).

Since **adolescence** is a time of crises and change, orthodontists enter the lives of their adolescent patients when much psychological growth is churning at and below the surface. This psychological growth of the adolescent takes the form of at least four major universal tasks:

1.) Defining one's own self or identity with sometimes-intense self-centeredness.
2.) Achieving psychological separation from parents and coming to terms with specific feelings about one's family. There is a rebellion against and withdrawal from adults and their values. The peer group serves the important role as a way station during the transition from childhood to adulthood.
3.) Developing love relationships.
4.) Achieving mastery over one's intense sexual and **aggressive** impulses and fantasies, bodily functions, and developing one's intellectual and emotional capacities.

Although some adults romanticize their lost youth, for many adolescents high school is filled with tension, turmoil, and humiliation. A constant concern with peer status, fitting in, feeling left out, coupled with an intense self-consciousness and awareness of one's magnified and distorted personal deficiencies are often the norm for adolescents.

Successful orthodontic treatment depends, in part, on the severity of the patient's dental facial deformity, on the orthodontist's ability to form a treatment alliance through an understanding of the real world experiences of adolescents, and on the capacity of the orthodontist to understand the influence of the dental problem on the unique personality of the patient. The orthodontist's task is to create a set of conditions that will enhance the patient's motivation for effective orthodontic treatment.

To do this, the orthodontist must at least express 1.) empathy and respect, 2.) develop a discrepancy, 3.) avoid arguments, 4.) roll with resistance, and 5.) support self-efficacy (Miller and Rollnick, 2002; this model offers a thoughtful, sensitive approach to working with patients, but must be subject to clinical study and **hypothesis** testing with dental patients).

1.) The orthodontist seeks to communicate empathy and respect, blending the role of supportive professional and knowledgeable consultant—-not talking down to the patient. Forming the treatment alliance means that the orthodontist listens to and understands the patient not being too eager to inform or persuade, cultivating an attitude of acceptance of the patient — not necessarily the same as agreement or approval.

- "In the most general terms, we are all much more simply human than otherwise, be we happy and successful, contented and detached, miserable and mentally disordered, or whatever."
—Harry Stack Sullivan

- "The belief that medicine involves the application of impersonal facts to an objective problem that can be seen separately from the person who has it is the cardinal and emblematic error of twentieth-century medicine."
—Eric J. Cassell

2.) The orthodontist helps the patient develop an understanding of the discrepancy between the presenting malocclusion and the proposed orthodontic outcome of esthetic and functional improvement, helping the patient carry out what is required for successful treatment. Motivation for change happens when the patient perceives a discrepancy between the current dental deformity and what is required for cosmetic improvement. The orthodontist seeks to clarify important treatment goals, give reasons for specific procedures and treatments – using an appliance – and explores the benefits or potential benefits of going along with wearing that "weird looking contraption." The most effective general approach is to let the patient in his own words tell his understanding of the reasons for a specific treatment in collaboration with the orthodontist's support and knowledge.

3.) The orthodontist should avoid arguments with the adolescent and the family. For some parents and their adolescents, orthodontic treatment takes on psychological meanings associated with anxiety and conflicts that can interfere with treatment. For example, some parents feel guilty that they have created a child with an obvious inherited defect, some parents are angry that they did not stop their child from thumb-sucking, and still others may view orthodontic treatment as a sign of the family's tense struggle for economic success. If the orthodontist needs to be right regardless of the attitudes and concerns of the patient and the family, uses jargon where plain words will do, and blames the patient or parents for treatment difficulties, the treatment will be compromised. Whatever the patient's reasons for coming to "get braces" and the parents' unconscious or conscious conflicts about orthodontic care, the orthodontist who is sensitive to how these conflicts get played out during the start of treatment will no doubt achieve more successful outcomes.

- "Don't be too sweet, lest you be eaten up; don't be too bitter, lest you be spewed out."
Jewish proverb

4.) To avoid or minimize these potential treatment snags, consider adopting a roll with resistance approach. Here the orthodontist uses a kind of psychological judo, a strategy that does not meet patient resistance head on but rather rolls with the flow, hoping to listen and accept (not necessarily agree) the patient's views, with the goal of shifting the patient's perceptions in the process. The orthodontist is aware that there are many reasons for seeking orthodontic care and invites the patient to consider new ways of viewing the specific treatment approach. That the patient and family may feel ambivalent about the treatment is viewed as normal, not pathological, and is openly explored, acknowledged, and respected. The orthodontist keeps in mind that what to do in a particular treatment case is ultimately the patient's and family's decision.

- "When you find yourself in a hole, stop digging."
-Will Rogers

5.) The orthodontist persuades his patients that there is hope for successful treatment. To support self-efficacy means to gently promote a patient's belief in his ability to benefit and comply with the treatment. The patient is reminded that he is responsible for choosing and carrying out his commitment to orthodontic treatment.

A Summing Up:

We have documented an array of complex child and adolescent psychiatric disorders, rendering detailed descriptions of psychosocial, developmental and behavioral principles. In this section, we offer some perspectives (McHugh and Slavney, 1998) to further promote the orthodontist's understanding of the psychology of his patients, taking into account the gaps in our knowledge about how minds and brains work together.

Our knowledge about the workings of the mind and brain sparks a central question: How does the brain produce the mind – or – how does consciousness flow from brain tissue? This brain-mind discontinuity is unlike conceptual dilemmas faced by other medical and dental professionals who stay at the level of physical understanding, relying on knowledge of biology, chemistry, anatomy, physical development, and so on.

Psychiatrists and psychologists cannot go directly from understanding the elements of the physical brain (e.g., neurons, neurotransmitters) to explaining a patient's conscious mental experience. Despite our advances in neuroscience, genetics, development and so on, we have no idea how the brain produces the "I" of our personality and how this "I" "tells" the brain what to pay attention to. This unique gap in our knowledge connecting brain to mind disrupts our explanatory paths from the physical to the psychological states of mind.

To circumvent this brain-mind gap in our knowledge and to organize and clarify our knowledge and treatment approaches to the complexity of our patients, we can approach people from four perspectives, offering a variety of complementary explanations to account for psychiatric disorders: 1.) diseases; 2.) dimensions; 3.) behaviors; and 4.) life stories (McHugh and Slaveney, 1998). These perspectives can help guide the orthodontist to a more accurate understanding of the mental life of patients.

The perspective of diseases (Autism; Bipolar Disorder) or disorders (Asperger's Disorder; Attention Deficit Hyperactivity Disorder) resulting from a faulty "hard drive", where "broken" brain-based problems are assumed to cause the symptoms. The assumption here is that psychiatric disease – often intangible and sometimes causing misunderstanding for those professionals trained to rely on such familiar diagnostic tangibles as studying blood chemistry, taking X-rays, and so on – is provoked by some as yet unknown bodily abnormality of structure or function. The disease perspective is sometimes overlooked no doubt because of its diagnostic intangibility, with many preferring to view mental states as the result of trauma, life experience, or personality traits. There is a caution with this approach —- because the disease perspective sometimes runs the risk of looking for a "broken" brain for every sign of mental distress, assuming a twisted neuron for every twisted thought and neglecting other more accurate explanations for disordered minds.

The perspective of dimensions or differences between people along a continuum highlights personality traits discussed in a previous section (See Section 3.6 PERSONALITY DEVELOPMENT. Sameroff, 1993). Most human personalities can be described by estimating positions along each of the following five continua:

-Agreeableness – likeable/pleasant to aggressive/unfriendly.
-Conscientiousness – organized/responsible to careless/impulsive.
-Extraversion – outgoing/lively to shy/reserved.
-Neuroticism – doesn't worry/stable to worries/unstable.
-Openness – imaginative/novelty-seeking to narrow/harm-avoiding.

People on the extremes of a dimension – very shy – may be more easily provoked to psychological distress. Coming to understand where a patient is positioned along these personality dimensions does much to foster effective orthodontic care.

The perspective of abnormalities in goal-directed behaviors, such as eating or drinking, including problems with addictions. We all grow up learning ways to channel our basic drives into socially accepted behaviors. Regardless of the etiology of a psychiatric disorder, the adult outcome of a childhood disorder is a combination of risk and protective factors, and therapeutic forces. Family and peer influences on behavior are often mind saving. These influences can amplify or minimize a child's difficulties. Some people can even learn to turn childhood symptoms into adult strengths - the energetic, enthusiastic adult with a history of Attention Deficit (Hyperactivity) Disorder, or the excessively sensitive adult with past symptoms of Separation Anxiety Disorder. Orthodontic treatment is sometimes an important positive influence, enhancing a patients looks, self-image, and confidence.

The perspective of life stories or "software problems" – where we look at what happens to people over their lives – for example – divorce of parents, poverty, physical and sexual abuse, death of a parent – that leaves some people with "faulty directions" about how to cope. This perspective relies on the most natural method of reasoning humans have – they explain problems by telling a story. We see patients responding to a set of circumstances and explain the patient's reactions as a response to distressing events of past and present. A common problem of the life-story perspective is for a patient —- and those around him – to mistakenly describe his problems with a "story," rather than with a disease such as Bipolar Disorder or Attention Deficit Hyperactivity Disorder. Using the life-story perspective instead of the more accurate disease explanation may lead to ineffective treatments and missed opportunities to reroute development back to a more normal course.

The orthodontist is in the unique role of treating the adolescent patient over an extended time, gathering a wealth of observations, and becoming a part of the patient's life-story. Sometimes this unique role offers the orthodontist an opportunity to contribute to helping the patient get psychiatric help. For example, an orthodontist who observes an adolescent patient during several months of appointments in a relatively depressed state and then months later sees the adolescent patient in an overly cheerful, enthusiastic state, has much to contribute to the psychiatric diagnostic picture of the patient.

These perspectives are complementary ways of looking at people with psychiatric problems – each requiring a different treatment approach. For example, pharmacotherapy is often effective for patients with Bipolar Disorder and psychological therapies are often the treatments of choice for patients with life-stories that leave them shaken, emotionally unsteady, and discontented.

In sum, we can understand psychiatric disorders as life under altered circumstances (McHugh and Slavney, 1998). Life can be altered by what a patient "has" (disease), what a patient "is" (dimensions), what a patient "does" (behaviors), and what a patient "encounters" (life stories).

Psychiatric medications sometimes offer life-enhancing measures to improve the faulty "hard drive", improving mood stability or self-control. Psychological therapies do much to repair "software," providing supportive settings to help people reroute faulty "instructions," to teach people how to live better, and to promote hope.

> *"...hope takes work. No matter how negative the situation, you seek the positive elements and build on them...Hope is especially important when there is nothing you can do...In American culture there is a powerful equation that says to lose control is to lose everything. But the most serious problems —- a terrible accident, a major disease—-are those in which we are objectively helpless. The best way to cope is to find out how to live with it. It's fine to keep fighting when you can change your situation. But when you can't change the facts, accept them. That's the key to health—-and to wisdom."*
> —Shlomo Breznitz

When Anna Freud - daughter of Sigmund Freud and a gifted therapist in her own right - was eighty-five, a depressed young man sent her a lament about the chaotic state of the world, and she sent him a succinct statement of her credo: *"I agree with you wholeheartedly that things are not as we would like them to be. However, my feeling is that there is only one way to deal with it, namely to try and be all right with oneself, and to create around one at least a small circle where matters are arranged as one wants them to be." (Young Bruehl, 1988)*
—Anna Freud

The profession of orthodontics offers the challenge and opportunity "to create around one at least a small circle where matters are arranged as one wants them to be."

9. SUGGESTED READINGS

Principles of Normal Development

Stassen Berger K. The Developing Person Through Childhood and Adolescence. Fifth Edition Worth Publishers, 2000 pp. 376-84.

American Psychiatric Association, American Psychiatric Association: Diagnostic and Statistical Manual of Mental Disorders, Fourth Edition, Washington, DC, 1994 pp. 55-65.

Coplan J. Normal Speech and Language Development: An Overview, Pediatrics in Review, 1995, 6(3), 91-100

Levine, MD, Carey WB, Crocker AC. Developmental-Behavioral Pediatrics, Third Edition. WB Saunders Company, 1999 Chapter 63

Kain ZN, Rimar S. Management of Chronic Pain in Children. Pediatrics in Review, 1995, 16(6): 218-222

Stassen Berger K. The Developing Person Through Childhood and Adolescence. Fifth Edition Worth Publishers, 2000 pp. 143-46.

Levine, MD, Carey WB, Crocker AC. Developmental-Behavioral Pediatrics, Third Edition. WB Saunders Company, 1999 Chapter 43 and 74.

Stassen Berger K. The Developing Person Through Childhood and Adolescence. Fifth Edition Worth Publishers, 2000 ch. 7, pp. 147-

48 and 308-326.

Cunningham, S., et al., Are Orthognathic Patients Different?, European J of Ortho, 22, 195-2002, 2000.

Mandal, N., et al., Perceived Aesthetic Impact of Malocclusion and Oral Self-Perceptions in 14-15 year old Asian and Caucasian Children in Greater Manchester, European J of Ortho, 21, 175-83, 1999.

Becker, A., et al., Orthodontic Treatment for Disabled Children; Motivation, Expectation, and Satisfaction, European J of Ortho 200;22:151-58.

Stassen Berger K. The Developing Person Through Childhood and Adolescence. Fifth Edition Worth Publishers, 2000, ch. 7, 13 and 16.

Levine, MD, Carey WB, Crocker AC. Developmental-Behavioral Pediatrics, Third Edition. WB Saunders Company, 1999 Chapter 63, ch. 8 .

Stassen Berger K. The Developing Person Through Childhood and Adolescence. Fifth Edition Worth Publishers, 2000 pp. 55-60.

Levine, MD, Carey WB, Crocker AC. Developmental-Behavioral Pediatrics, Third Edition. WB Saunders Company, 1999 Chapter 63, ch. 22.

Stassen Berger K. The Developing Person Through Childhood and

Adolescence. Fifth Edition Worth Publishers, 2000, ch. 3.

Stassen Berger K. The Developing Person Through Childhood and Adolescence. Fifth Edition Worth Publishers, 2000 pp. 137-39 and 341-45.

Levine, MD, Carey WB, Crocker AC. Developmental-Behavioral Pediatrics, Third Edition. WB Saunders Company, 1999 Chapter 38 (Obesity) and 41 (Failure To Thrive) .

Selected Cognitive, Emotional, and Behavioral Problems in Children & Adolescents

Stassen Berger K. The Developing Person Through Childhood and Adolescence. Fifth Edition Worth Publishers, 2000 pp. 148-56.

Levine, MD, Carey WB, Crocker AC. Developmental-Behavioral Pediatrics, Third Edition. WB Saunders Company, 1999 Chapter 47.

Stassen Berger K. The Developing Person Through Childhood and Adolescence. Fifth Edition Worth Publishers, 2000 pp. 148-50.

Levine, MD, Carey WB, Crocker AC. Developmental-Behavioral Pediatrics, Third Edition. WB Saunders Company, 1999 Chapter 68-73.

Stassen Berger K. The Developing Person Through Childhood and Adolescence. Fifth Edition Worth Publishers, 2000, ch. 6 pp. 365-76 and 384-95.

Stassen Berger K. The Developing Person Through Childhood and Adolescence. Fifth Edition Worth Publishers, 2000 pp. 318-26.

Howard B. Advising Parents on Discipline: What Works. Pediatrics Suppl Dec, 1996;98(4):809-17.

Straus M. Spanking and the Making of a Violent Society. Pediatrics Suppl. Oct 1663;98(4):837-44.

McCord J. The Unintended Consequences of Punishment. Pediatrics Suppl Oct. 1996;98(4):833-36.

Larzelere R. A Review of the Outcomes of Parental Use of Non-abusive or Customary Physical Punishment. Pediatrics Suppl Oct 1996;98(4): 824-31.

Subabusive Violence in Child Rearing in Middle-Class American Families. Pediatrics Suppl Oct 1996;98(4): 845-51.

Attitudes of Primary Care Physicians Toward Corporal Punishment. JAMA June 17, 1992;267(23): 3161-65.

Tuchman D, ed. Walter R. Disorders of Feeding and Swallowing in Infants and Children: Pathophysiology, Diagnosis, and Treatment. Singular Publishing Group, 1994.

Hall, K., Pediatric Dysphagia Resource Guide, Singular Thomson Learning.

Arvedson, J. and Brodsky, L. Pediatric Swallowing and Feeding: Assessment and Management, ed., Singular Publishing Group, 1993.

American Psychiatric Association., American Psychiatric Association: Diagnostic and Statistical Manual of Mental Disorders, Fourth Edition, Washington, DC, 1994 pp.352-76.

Levine, MD, Carey WB, Crocker AC. Developmental-Behavioral Pediatrics, Third Edition. WB Saunders Company, 1999 Chapter 60.

American Psychiatric Association., American Psychiatric Association: Diagnostic and Statistical Manual of Mental Disorders, Fourth Edition, Washington, DC, 1994 pp. 65-71.

Stassen Berger K. The Developing Person Through Childhood and Adolescence. Fifth Edition Worth Publishers, 2000 pp. 357-76.

Levine, MD, Carey WB, Crocker AC. Developmental-Behavioral Pediatrics, Third Edition. WB Saunders Company, 1999 pp. 52-53.

American Psychiatric Association., American Psychiatric Association: Diagnostic and Statistical Manual of Mental Disorders, Fourth Edition, Washington, DC, 1994 pp. 78-85.

Levine, MD, Carey WB, Crocker AC. Developmental-Behavioral Pediatrics, Third Edition. WB Saunders Company, 1999 Chapter 56.

American Psychiatric Association., American Psychiatric Association: Diagnostic and Statistical Manual of Mental Disorders, Fourth Edition, Washington, DC, 1994 pp.39-46.

Mood Disorders

Levine, MD, Carey WB, Crocker AC. Developmental-Behavioral Pediatrics, Third Edition. WB Saunders Company, 1999 Chapter 64.

Stassen Berger K. The Developing Person Through Childhood and Adolescence. Fifth Edition Worth Publishers, 2000, ch. 16.

Frielander A and Mahler M. Major Depressive Disorder-Psychopathology, Medical Management, and Dental Implications. J Am Dental Assoc (JADA) May 2001;132, 629-38.

Levine, MD, Carey WB, Crocker AC. Developmental-Behavioral Pediatrics, Third Edition. WB Saunders Company, 1999 Chapter 45.

Levine, MD, Carey WB, Crocker AC. Developmental-Behavioral Pediatrics, Third Edition. WB Saunders Company, 1999 Chapter 44.

Other Relevant References:

"Orthodontic Care of Children with Special Needs," American Association of Orthodontists, Orthodontic Dialogue, 13(1), Spring 2001.

Behavior Management Needs for the Orthodontic Treatment of Children with Disabilities, European Journal of Orthodontics 2000;22:143-9.

American Academy of Child and Adolescent Psychiatry (AACAP) website: www.aacap.org Go to the "Facts for Families." Topics which may be of particular interest include:
#1   Children and Divorce
#2   Teenagers with Eating Disorders
#3   Substance Abuse
#4   The Depressed Child
#5   Child Abuse- The Hidden Bruises
#6   Children Who Can't Pay Attention/ADHD
#9   Child Sexual Abuse
#10 Teen Suicide
#11 Autism
#21 Psychiatric Medication for Children and Adolescents, Part I
#23 Children Who Are Mentally Retarded
#22 Normality
#24 Know When to Seek Help for your Child
#25 Being Prepared: Knowing Where to Find Help for Your Child

#29   Psychiatric Medication for Children and Adolescents

Part II
#35   Tic Disorders
#38   Bipolar Disorder
#41   Substance Abuse
#43   Discipline
#47   The Anxious Child
#50   Panic Disorder
#51   Psychiatric Medication for Children and Adolescents

Part III
#52   Comprehensive Psychiatric Evaluation
#56   Parenting: Preparing for Adolescence
#57   Normal Adolescent Development: Middle School and
       Early High School
#58   Normal Adolescent Development: Late High School and
       Beyond
#69   Asperger's Disorder
#70   Post Traumatic Stress Disorder
#73   Self Injury in Adolescents
#79   Obesity

Also see the AACAP Policy Statements. Statements which may be
of particular interest include:

Substance Abuse- The Nature and Extent of the Problem
HIV and Youth

Prescribing Psychoactive Medications for Children and
Adolescents

Corporal Punishment in Schools

7. Clinical Perspective and Summing Up

Lewis, Melvin, and Volkmar, Fred R. Clinical Aspects of
Developmental Concepts and Clinical Experience. Philadelphia:
Lea and Febiger, 1990.

McHugh, Paul R., and Slavney, Phillip R. The Perspectives of
Psychiatry. Second Edition. Baltimore: The Johns Hopkins
University Press, 1998.

Miller, WR, Rollnick, S. Motivational Interviewing. Second
Edition. New York: The Guilford Press, 2002.

Young-Bruehl, E. Anna Freud. New York: Summit Books, 1988.

CHAPTER 2

Prenatal Craniofacial Development

Malcom C. Johnston

James K. Avery

1. INTRODUCTION

An understanding of the events leading up to the organization of the face in its normal form is critical to the understanding of variations responsible for abnormal development of the face. In this chapter, an attempt will be made to describe both the mechanisms underlying normal development, as well as the alterations leading to developmental abnormalities.

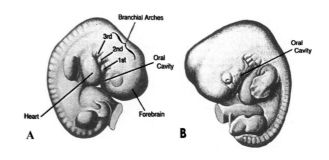

Figure 2-1: Surface morphology of the human embryo at (A) 5 weeks and (B) 7 weeks. The branchial arches illustrated in A are present in all vertebrate embryos, although they are not obvious in surface views of amphibian embryos.

The superficial appearance of all vertebrate embryos, except for amphibian embryos, is very similar to that of the human embryos at the stages of development illustrated in Figure 2-1. In Figure 2-1A (4-5 weeks post-fertilization age), the forebrain, eye, the first three of a series of branchial (visceral, pharyngeal) arches, as well as the heart and limb rudiments, are clearly visible. The first branchial arch becomes the lower jaw and associated structures, while the more caudal arches become the gills of fish and, in higher vertebrates, various ear and neck structures. Previously, the mechanisms underlying embryonic development (e.g., cell migrations and interactions) had been conducted on amphibian embryos, and were largely ignored by those studying higher vertebrate embryos.

The unusual feature of amphibian embryos, making them both attractive for experimental study and very different in appearance, is that each embryonic cell carries its own nutritional supply in the form of yolk platelets. This makes for very large, easily manipulated cells that are capable of surviving in simple salt solutions, but which give the embryo a plump appearance, quite unlike other vertebrate embryos, including the human (Figure 2-1). As new scientific advances occur (e.g., the development of radioisotopically labeled biological compounds), it becomes much more feasible to study developmental mechanisms in higher vertebrate embryos, confirming and extending the findings of studies on amphibian embryos.

2. EMBRYOLOGICAL ORGANIZATION OF THE FACE

Most descriptions of facial development are similar to those illustrated in Figure 2-1A. However, a number of fairly common malformations arise at earlier stages, necessitating at least some description of these stages of development.

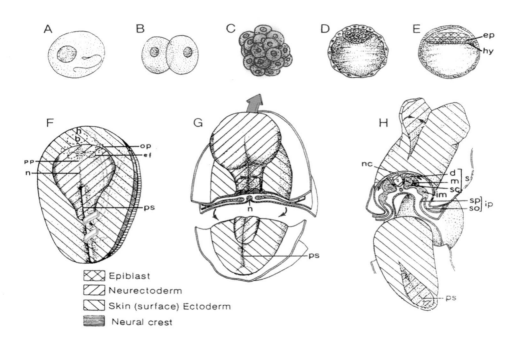

Figure 2-2: Sketches summarizing development of the human embryo from fertilization through neural tube formation. The epiblast (ep) of the two-layered embryonic disc in E will form virtually the entire embryo through a complex series of tissue movements and cell migrations described in the text and illustrated in F. The resulting three-germ-layer embryo is illustrated in G. The notochord (n) and associated mesoderm (the "chorda-mesoderm") induce the neural plate from the overlying ectoderm, which then rolls up to form the neural tube as illustrated in H. Neural crest cells (nc) form at the edges of the neural plate and migrate from the neural folds as illustrated in H to form many types of cells, including almost all of the skeletal and connective tissues of the face. Other abbreviations are as follows: (b), buccal (oral) plate; (ef), eye fields; (h), heart; (ps), primitive streak; (pp), prechordal plate. Different portions of the mesoderm are illustrated in H. The somite(s) with its three layers: the dermatome (d), the myotome (m), and the sclerotome (sc), the intermediate mesoderm (im) and the lateral plate (lp) with its two layers: the splanchnopleure (sp) and somatopleure (so).

2.1 EARLIEST STAGES OF EMBRYONIC DEVELOPMENT

Some of the major features of early embryonic development are illustrated in Figure 2-2. Development begins at fertilization (A) and proceeds through cell division and cavity formation to produce the "embryonic disc" (D). From cell marking (see below), it now appears that the entire embryo arises from the upper layer of the two-layer disc with the lower layer contributing only to the supporting tissues (e.g., the amnion and placenta) of the embryo.

The first major cell movements (F) convert the upper layer into the three-germ-layer embryo. Cells from a midline structure (the primitive streak) of the upper layer insert themselves into the midline of the lower layer, and lateral expansion of these cells pushes those of the lower layer aside. Cells of the new portion of the lower layer become the "endoderm", the lowest layer of the future three-germ-layer embryo, and also form the first "skeletal" element; a midline structure termed the notochord. Another group of cells migrate as individual cells from the primitive streak (arrows in F) into the space between the two layers. These will form the middle germ layer or "mesoderm". The formation of mesoderm is the first example of the transformation of epithelial cells (tightly arranged cell groupings as found in the two layers of the embryonic disc) into **mesenchyme** cells (loosely arranged groupings of cells with considerable space occupied by a fluid containing extracellular molecules), as are the migrating mesodermal cells. The terms "mesenchyme" and "epithelia" are descriptive terms for the two principle embryonic cell populations, which tell little about the functions of the cells. For example, these terms tell nothing about the origins or destinations of the cells. Unfortunately, these terms are often confused with ectoderm and mesoderm, particularly in the clinical literature.

Finally those cells remaining in the upper layer become the third germ layer, the "ectoderm". The ectoderm will form the neural tube and the epidermis of the skin, while the mesoderm will form most of the skeletal and connective tissues as well as muscle, and the endoderm will form the epithelial lining of the gut.

Experimental studies on amphibian embryos indicate that the mesoderm is capable of considerable further **differentiation** on its own, but that the ectoderm requires developmental interactions with the underlying mesoderm. The induction of the neural plate by a portion of the underlying mesoderm and associated notochord (the "chorda-mesoderm") is sometimes called "primary embryonic induction". Induction is a uniquely embryonic phenomenon, the molecular nature of which is now beginning to be understood.

The amphibian studies, which included experimental combinations of cell populations in culture, did show that once an inductive stimulus has passed, the responding tissue is capable of further differentiation on its own without the continued presence of the inducing tissue. As the neural plate continues to differentiate, different cell populations begin to segregate themselves in preparation for the formation of specialized structures (e.g., the eye field indicated as "ef" in Figure 2-2F, which will form most of the eye).

A cell population forming at the edge of the neural plate (horizontal hatching in Figure 2-2F), the **neural crest** cells, is of particular significance to facial development for they will form virtually all the skeletal and connective tissues. Elsewhere in the body, this function is largely confined to mesodermal cells, with neural crest cells forming most of the peripheral nervous system and the pigment cells in the skin. By the time the neural folds have rolled up to make contact, neural crest cells have already begun their migrations in most vertebrate species.

In the meantime, mesodermal cells have continued their differentiation, forming blocks of tissue termed somites (Figure 2-2H). Still continuing independent differentiation, the somite differentiates into three layers: the dermatome which contributes to the dermis, the myotome which contains the only **myoblasts** capable of forming the contractile cells of voluntary skeletal muscle, and the sclerotome which forms skeletal and other tissues. Lateral to the somite (Figure 2-2H), is the intermediate mesoderm, which forms the renal system, and the lateral plate mesoderm, which forms connective and endothelial cells which line blood vessels. The notochord, which is initially part of the endoderm (Figure 2-2G) separates from this layer to lie in the mesodermal plane. Also shown in Figure 2-2G is a regional growth center, the forebrain, that begins to overgrow the underlying embryonic tissues.

2.2 PHARYNGEAL ARCH FORMATION

The overgrowth of the forebrain carries this part of the head over the oral plate and heart (Figure 2-2 G and H, Figure 2-3). This overgrowth creates a pocket, which forms the foregut (Figure 2-3B).

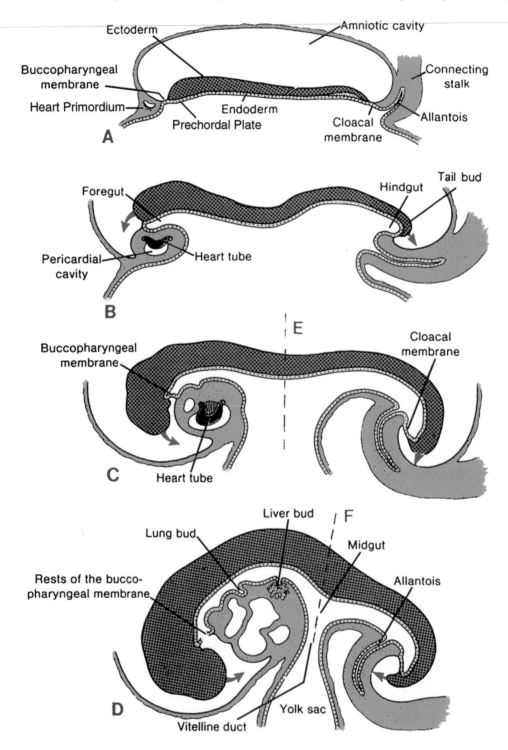

Figure 2-3: Longitudinal sections through the developing embryo illustrating the manner in which differential growth and folding movements from about day 17 to day 36 create the fore- and hindguts (compare to Figure 2-2 G and H). Modified from Sadler, 2000.

The oral plate is a region where the ectoderm and endoderm remain fused together and marks the future position of the oral cavity. Later it is termed the bucco-pharyngeal plate, indicating the fact that it separates the developing oral and pharyngeal cavities, which lie between the expanding forebrain and rapidly growing heart (Figure 2-3 B and C). The lateral wall of the oral and pharyngeal cavities becomes segmented (Figure 2-4) by invaginations of the surface ectoderm (clefts) and out-pouchings of the pharyngeal endoderm (pouches).

As these clefts and pouches approach each other, they partially, or completely in some areas, segment the mesoderm which lies between them. It is not clear whether the segmentation process is controlled by the lateral plate mesoderm or the ectoderm and endoderm. The resulting branchial arches thus consist of mesodermal cores with inner (endodermal) and outer (ectodermal) epithelial coverings. The mesodermal cores in the branchial arches are involved mostly, if not exclusively, in the formation

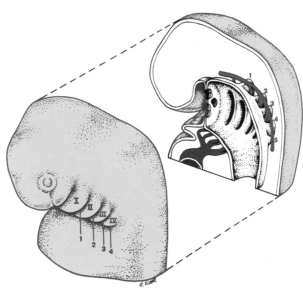

Figure 2-4: Split embryonic head and neck illustrating the outer and inner surfaces of the head. By the stage of development illustrated, the blood vessels (numbered 1 through 5) originating from the heart pass through branchial arches (numbered I through IV) to reach the rest of the body.

of blood-vascular elements. Neural crest cells migrating into the region surround the mesodermal cores (Figures 2-5A, B and D).

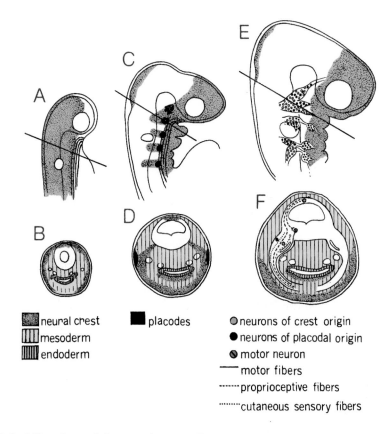

neural crest
mesoderm
endoderm

placodes

○ neurons of crest origin
● neurons of placodal origin
◉ motor neuron
── motor fibers
----- proprioceptive fibers
········· cutaneous sensory fibers

Figure 2-5: Migrations of the neural crest cells (green stipple) as they migrate from the neural folds into the upper part of the face and the branchial arches, where they surround the mesodermal cores already present. Development of the cranial ganglia will be discussed later.

These neural crest cells will form not only the connective tissue components of the aortic arch blood vessels but also the other connective tissues and skeletal elements in the region. The configuration of the aortic arch vessels is illustrated in Figure 2-4 and their relation to other components in the arches in Figure 2-6.

Described in Figure 2-6 are the origins of the pharyngeal glands. The epithelial components are derived from the endoderm of the arches, which invaginates into their underlying neural crest mesenchyme. This mesenchyme will form most of the connective tissue of the glands. After the branchial arch mesenchyme becomes vascularized by capillary buds from the mesodermal cores, the cells remaining in the core undergo cell death and are replaced by myoblasts, which migrate from the myotomes noted above. These myoblasts will form the contractile cells of the branchial arch voluntary skeletal muscles, such as the masseter muscle in the first arch and the muscles of facial expression in the second arch. Each arch also has its own nerve, the motor component of which arrives with the myoblasts. The developmental relations of these are further described in Figure 2-7. This figure also describes their segmental relationships to the developing neuromeres of the hindbrain. The mechanisms involved in both normal and abnormal segmentation will be described later in this chapter.

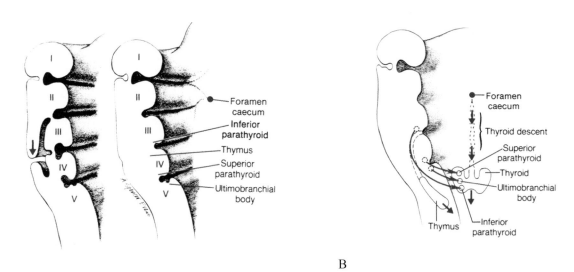

A   B

Figure 2-6: A.) Ventral floor of the pharynx with a frontal section through the branchial arches (compare to Figure 2-9A, which shows the relations of the mesodermal cores to the surrounding crest cells and the aortic arch vessels). B.) Illustration of the sites of origin and movements of the epithelial portions of the pharyngeal glands.

2.3 THE FORMATION, MERGING AND FUSION OF FACIAL GROWTH CENTERS

In addition to forming most of the peripheral nervous system, crest cells migrating farther into the facial region (Figure 2-5) give rise to almost all the skeletal and connective tissues of the face and portions of the cranium, unlike the origins of these tissues from mesoderm elsewhere in the body. When they reach the branchial arches, they surround the lateral plate mesoderm already present; while in the upper facial region they fill all the space between the surface ectoderm and the underlying brain (Figure 2-5). In these regions they interact with the local cell populations to form skeletal and connective tissues. Experimental work on amphibian embryos has shown, for example, that combinations of neural crest cells and pharyngeal endoderm is sufficient to induce the crest cells to form cartilage. The further addition of oral ectoderm is sufficient for tooth formation, where the ectoderm forms the enamel. The last experiment has now been extended to the mouse embryo. In the upper face, the forebrain, eye and surface ectoderm apparently act as the inducing tissues. At the completion of crest cell migration, regional growth centers appear (Figures 2-8 and 2-9).

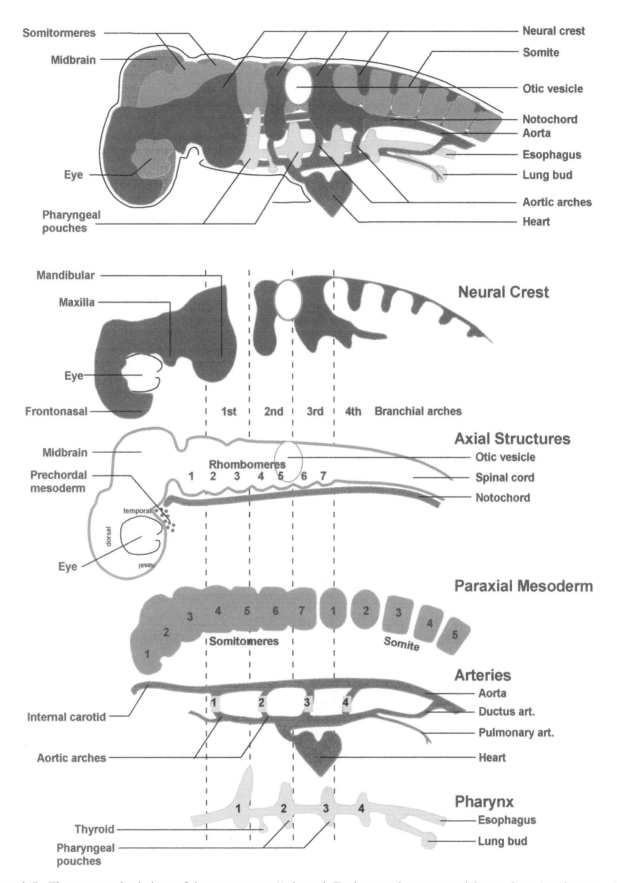

Figure 2-7: The segmental relations of the neuromeres (1 through 7), the neural crest, paraxial mesoderm (somitomeres 1 through 7 and somites 1 through 5) and aortic arch vessels are shown. Also indicated: segmental relations of the branchial arches and the pharyngeal pouches, as well as the position of the otocyst, which will give rise to the epithelial portions of the inner ear.

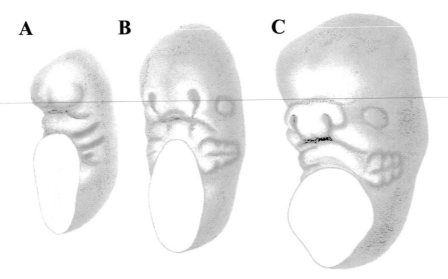

Figure 2-8: The developing face at (A) 4 weeks, (B) 5 weeks, (C) 6 weeks. In A, only the bulging forebrain and branchial arches are apparent, while in B the nasal pits, eye and developing external ear (bulges at the corner the mouth) can be seen. The face has matured further in C and is beginning to be clearly recognized as human.

The mesenchymal process meshwork underlying these epithelia (Figure 2-9C) may be involved in mediating the interactions between epithelia and mesenchyme that will be described below.

2.3.1. Development of Growth Centers in the Branchial Arches and Floor of the Mouth

Growth centers appear at the ends of the branchial arches (Figure 2-9B,C). This is a poorly document-ed aspect of development, but failure of these processes to contact and fuse is apparently responsible for clefts of the chin and mandible. Further development of the floor of the pharynx is depicted in Figure 2-10 A-D. The significance of the various swellings will be discussed later.

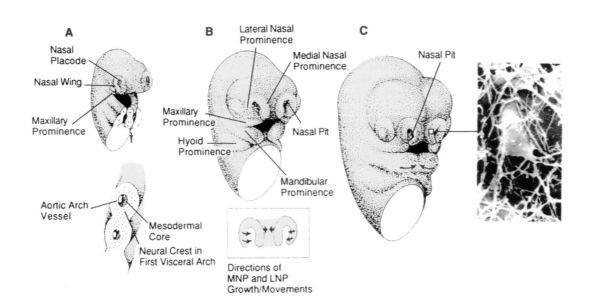

Figure 2-9: More details of the developing face covering roughly the same period. In (A), the onset of primary palate for-mation and the composition of the branchial arches are illustrated. In (B) and (C), growth and apparent morphogenetic movements of the facial processes (prominences) are illustrated, and in (C), the subepithelial cell process meshwork char-acteristic of the growing processes.

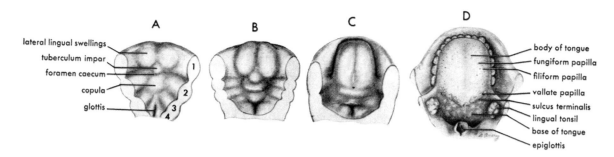

Figure 2-10: Other growth centers also appear in the floor of the mouth, giving rise to the definitive adult structures illustrated in (D). Formation of the lateral lingual swellings in (A) coincides with the arrival of hypoglossal myoblasts, which will be described later. The significance of many of the other growth centers is poorly understood.

2.3.2. Development of the Primary Palate

Some growth centers appear to grow primarily at their tips, such as the maxillary processes, and the ends of the branchial arches noted above. In both these examples, the processes remain fused to the underlying tissues. Thus, when such processes come into contact with each other (as do the mandibular arches, Figure 2-9) or with other structures (as when the maxillary process contacts the lateral nasal process, Figure 2-9B), their underlying mesenchyme is already continuous. This is in contrast to the tip of the medial nasal process, which is growing as a "free- ended" process, much like the limb bud. When the nasal process contacts the combined lateral nasal and maxillary processes (see Figures 2-9, 2-11), a two-layered epithelial plate is formed (Figures 2-11 and 2-12).

In the case of the **primary palate**, the plate remains continuous with the underlying epithelium and is sometimes termed the epithelial "seam" or "nasal fin". A portion of this epithelial seam is replaced by mesenchyme (Figure 2-12) that it is able to strengthen the union greatly through the production of intercellular substances such as **collagen**.

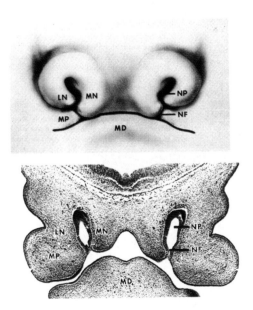

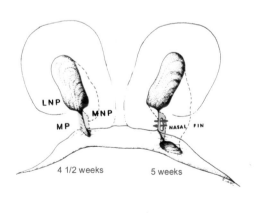

Figure 2-11: Formation of the nasal fin (NF) at the area of contact between the medial nasal process and the combined lateral nasal and maxillary nasal processes (see also Figure 2-14A). Other abbreviations are as follows: (LN) lateral nasal, (MN) medial nasal and (MP) maxillary processes.

Figure 2-12 Diagram depicting the breakdown of the epithelial seam between 4 ½ weeks (right side) and 5 weeks (left side).

The persisting epithelium behind the mesenchymal bridge eventually breaks down to form the connection between the developing nasal cavity (nasal or olfactory pit) and the oral cavity. This phenomenon involving epithelial contact and mesenchymal consolidation is often termed "fusion", in contrast to unions such as those observed between the mandibular arch processes, which is often termed "merging". It now appears that the epithelial changes are more complex than originally thought, involving a sloughing only of specialized surface peridermal cells (See Figure 2-13), with transformation of the remaining peridermal cells to mesenchyme cells.

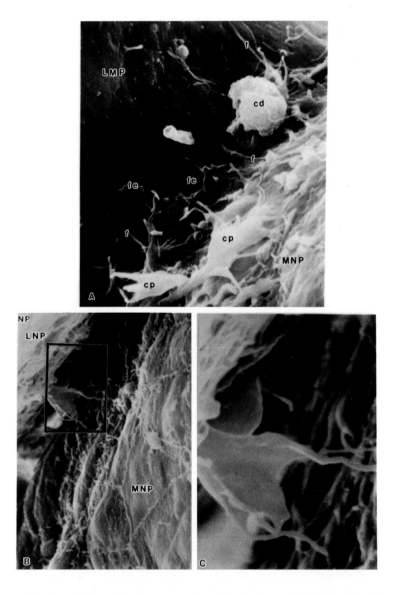

Figure 2-13: Recent studies have indicated a far more active role for the epithelia forming the seam, one aspect of which is depicted in (A). Here, the surface epithelial (peridermal) cells have sloughed off (see "cd", cell debris) while the underlying cells have formed processes (cp) that may be assisting in bringing the processes together. Almost complete failure of these changes is seen in the CL/Fr mouse embryo (B), which shows intact peridermal cells (outlined by microvilli at their edges) with only very occasional attempts to bridge the gap (see higher magnification of cell process extending from LNP toward MNP). This defect in epithelial differentiation is thought to be partly responsible for the approximately 25% incidence of cleft lip and palate in this mouse strain.

Most studies on this phenomenon have been conducted on corresponding epithelial plates involved in **secondary palate** formation and will be further considered below. Contributions of the facial processes to definitive facial structures are illustrated in Figure 2-14.

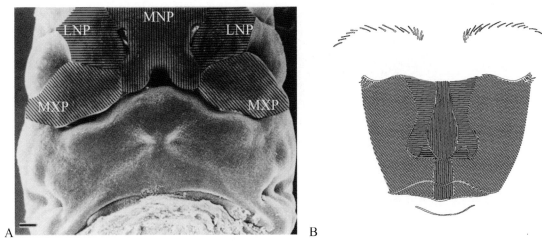

Figure 2-14: A scanning electron micrograph of the primary palate is illustrated in (A), showing contact of the medial nasal process (MNP, pink, vertical hatching) with lateral nasal (LNP, green, horizontal hatching) and maxillary (MXP, gold, diagonal hatching) processes at the completion of primary palate formation (courtesy of KK Sulik). The approximate contributions of the MNP, LNP and MXP processes in the adult face are illustrated in (B).

2.3.3. Development of the Secondary Palate

At the completion of primary palate formation the tongue remains high within the nasal cavity and the palatal shelves, which will form the secondary palate, grow down beside it (Figure 2-15). Again, epithelial-mesenchymal interactions are involved and these have been extensively studied (See Greene and Weston (1996), for review).

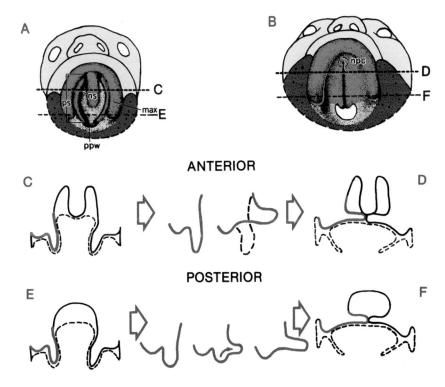

Figure 2-15: Formation of the secondary palate before (A, C, E) and after (B, D, F) palatal shelf elevation. Shelf elevation in the posterior (soft palate) region appears to involve tissue translocation.

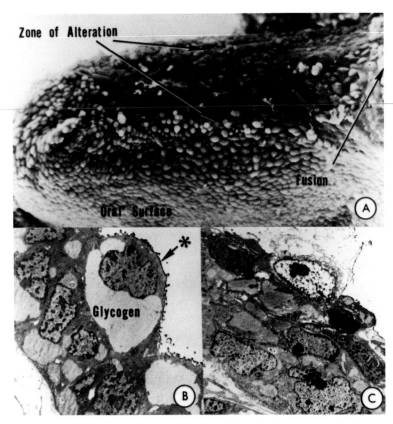

Figure 2-16: Scanning (A) and transmission (B, C) electron micrographs of the same palate shelf at approximately day 56. Sloughing of the peridermal cells just prior to contact is shown in (A) and sections of the epithelia from the oral surface and zone of alteration in (B) and (C).

There is considerable evidence that the tongue must be withdrawn from between the shelves before they can elevate to the horizontal position and fuse, and that inhibition of this movement is probably involved in the pathogenesis of many, if not most, cases of **cleft palate**. The conversion of at least some of the cells in the epithelial seam to mesenchymal cells has been alluded to above. It used to be thought that all the epithelial cells died due to the presence of pyknotic figures (condensed darkly staining cells or fragments of cells) in the epithelial seam, but electron microscopic and cell marking studies now indicate that it is only the peridermal cells that die, and, while most of them are sloughed before (Figure 2-16A,C) and after contact, some are trapped within the fusing epithelium, giving the false impression that all of the cells in the epithelial seam eventually die. In fact there has long been evidence that they actively participate in the contact and adhesion of palatal shelves, and transformation to mesenchyme cells is further evidence of their active participation.

3. DEVELOPMENT OF SYSTEM

Some reference to the development of systems, such as the neural, vascular and muscular systems, has already been made. Here the further development of these systems during the embryonic period will be described. Development of the skeletal system occurs during the fetal period and its description will be delayed until this period is discussed.

3.1 DEVELOPMENT OF THE NERVOUS SYSTEM

The neural crest cells have been noted above (Figures 2-2H and 2-5). In the facial region, they migrate from the neural folds and follow a path under the surface ectoderm (Figure 2-5). They maintain contact with the neural tube where cranial sensory ganglia will form and, in fact, form the initial ganglionic primordia. Placodes are thickenings of the ectoderm not unlike the neural tube. The ganglionic placodes are often found in close **association** with the pharyngeal pouches, which form between the branchial arches and contact the surface ectoderm at their proximal extremities. They overlie the distal portion of the ganglionic primordia (Figure 2-5C, D), and cells migrating from these into the ganglia form the earliest differentiating neurons.

This is in contrast to the trunk region where all neurons are derived from neural crest cells. Crest cells do form many of the later-differentiating neurons in the cranial sensory system and all of the supporting cells. Crest cells also form the peripheral components of the sympathetic and parasympathetic systems, as they do elsewhere in the body. As with the cranial sensory ganglia, they send their axons back into the central nervous system as well as into peripheral portions of the embryo. In contrast, the axons of the motor nerves originate from the central nervous system. Their supporting cells, the cells of the Sheath of Schwann, originate from neural crest, as do all the supporting cells in the peripheral nervous system. Their development is closely related to that of the skeletal voluntary muscles and will be further considered in the section dealing with development of the muscular system.

3.2 DEVELOPMENT OF THE VASCULAR SYSTEM

There are two major types of cells that crest cells cannot form: the endothelial cells that line blood vessels, and the contractile cells of skeletal voluntary muscle. These endothelial cells arise from local mesoderm. In the branchial arches they arise from the mesodermal cores already present in the arches before the crest cells migrate. Vascular tissues first arise as blood islands, which are endothelially-lined sacs containing blood cells. Blood islands link together to form blood vessels. The branchial arch (aortic arch) blood vessels are the first to form, and they link up the developing heart with the dorsal aorta, which carries blood to other parts of the body (Figures 2-17 and 2-4).

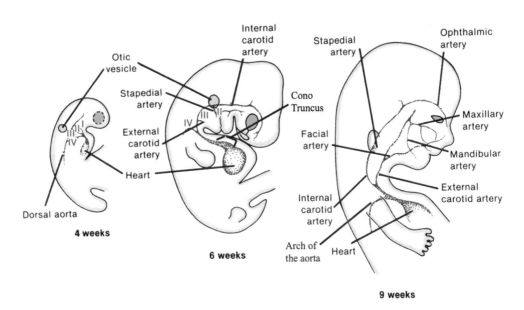

Figure 2-17: Arterial development at three different stages of development. The aortic arch vessels (I – IV) are shown at 4 weeks and their contributions to later vessels at 6 weeks. The stem of the external carotid is formed from the third aortic arch vessel at 6 weeks, grows forward to contact and fuse with the stapedial artery and has taken over much of the arterial supply to the face by 9 weeks. The cono-truncal portion of the developing heart is shown at 6 weeks. Modified from Ross and Johnston.

A branch (capillary bud) from the second aortic arch blood vessel then extends throughout most facial regions initiating the second phase of facial vascular development. This vessel is known as the stapedial artery because it is surrounded by the developing stapes of the middle ear. Finally, a branch of the fourth aortic arch vessel fuses with the stapedial, after which the proximal portion of it regresses and the distal portions form the definitive facial, maxillary and mandibular arteries.

The fourth aortic arch vessel persists on the right side to form a portion of the arch of the aorta. It now appears that defects in the development of crest cells contributing to the aortic arches and to the midline septum of cono-truncus (outflow portion of the developing heart, see Figure 2-17) are involved in a number of craniofacial malformations that are associated with cardiovascular malformations.

After the initial rudiments of the aortic arch vessels are formed, the remaining progenitor cells undergo programmed cell death, much as in the case of excess neuroblasts developing sensory ganglia, and are replaced by myoblasts migrating into the cores of the arches.

When the endothelial progenitor cells of the first arch die prematurely, a genetically determined animal model forms a malformation termed otocephaly, to be described in detail later. The first aortic arch vessels fail to develop and the crest cells are unable to survive. The mandibular arch degenerates leaving disproportionately large ears, which approach the midline.

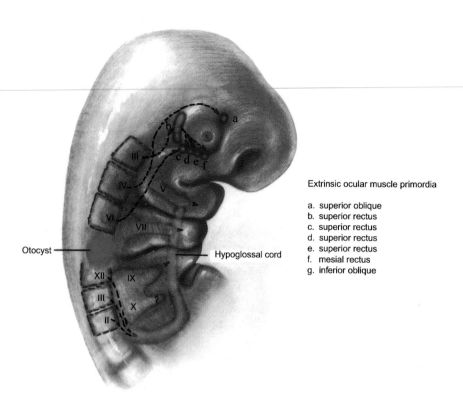

Extrinsic ocular muscle primordia

a. superior oblique
b. superior rectus
c. superior rectus
d. superior rectus
e. superior rectus
f. mesial rectus
g. inferior oblique

Figure 2-18: The myoblasts of all skeletal voluntary muscles are supplied by the myotomes of somites (Figure 2-2H) or by comparable structures (somitomeres) anterior to the otocyst. Both are indicated by the cranial nerves that supply the derived muscles. The myoblasts of muscles served by cranial nerves V and VII are also derived from the somitomeres indicated, while the myoblasts of muscles served by cranial nerves IX and X are derived from the same somites as those giving rise to the myoblasts of muscles innervated by the XIIth cranial nerve. During their primary migrations, myoblasts of muscles innervated by cranial nerves V, VII, IX, and X migrate into the cores of the appropriate branchial arches. At the same time, those of muscles innervated by the XIIth cranial nerve follow a more complicated path behind the branchial arches, and then anteriorly in the floor of the pharynx as the hypoglossal cord.

3.3 DEVELOPMENT OF THE MUSCULATURE IN THE HEAD AND ANTERIOR NECK

As noted earlier, the myoblasts of skeletal voluntary muscle originate from the myotomes of somites (Figure 2-2H). In contrast, smooth muscle cells (which might be considered as modified **fibroblasts**) arise from mesenchyme, which may be of mesodermal or ectodermal (neural crest) origin. For this reason, the smooth muscle cells in the facial vasculature described above originate from neural crest mesenchyme, as do fibroblasts and other connective tissue cells in the blood vessel walls.

Actually, many of the craniofacial muscle myoblasts originate from somite-like structures ("somitomeres") found anterior (rostral) to the primordium of the inner ear (see Figure 2-18). The somitomeres contain myotomes and sclerotomes, but lack the dermatomes found in somites (Figure 2-2H). As was noted earlier, the dermatome forms the dermis of the skin, a function taken over by crest and other cells anterior to the ear. Even before the myoblasts begin their migrations, the myotomes become "innervated" by motor nerve fibers from the adjacent segments of the brain. They then migrate as a group taking with them their motor nerve fibers, sometimes following complex migration paths such those of the "hypoglossal cord" (Figure 2-18).

Those innervated by cranial nerves V, VII, IX and X follow simpler migration paths as they migrate into the cores of the branchial arches, positions once occupied by the lateral plate mesenchyme, which differentiated into the earliest vascular elements. After they have arrived in their "staging" areas, the myoblasts break up into groups of cells, each representing an individual muscle. As they then undergo their secondary migrations, each group takes with it the nerve fibers for that particular muscle. It is only after they reach their final positions that they become invaded by the local mesenchyme, which forms the connective tissue components of the muscle. In the case of the hypoglossal musculature, most of the myoblasts remain in place to form the intrinsic muscles of the tongue. Their arrival and subsequent proliferation is indicated by the lateral lingual swellings and copula of Figure 2-10A.

3.4 SKELETAL AND CONNECTIVE TISSUE DEVELOPMENT

The interface between skeletal and connective tissues of crest and mesoderm is important for the consideration of the pathogenesis of a number of malformations of the head and neck. This interface is described in Figure 2-19. Technically, the onset of bone formation is considered to define the onset of fetal development. Some cartilages are already present, and the forerunner of tooth development, the **dental lamina**, has already formed. For reasons of continuity, further consideration of development of the skeletal system will be incorporated into the description of the fetal period, to be considered later.

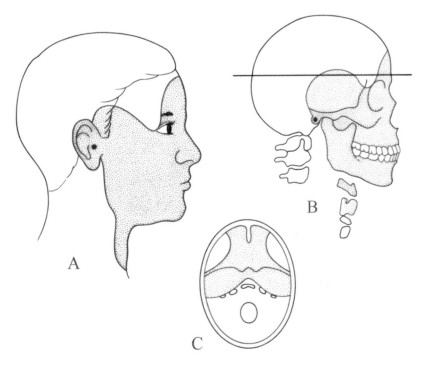

Figure 2-19: The approximate distribution (stipple) of connective (A) and skeletal (B) tissues of neural crest origin. The distribution of skeletal elements in the floor and walls of the cranial cavity (top of the skull removed) is indicated in (C).

3.5 OTHER TISSUES

Development of the pharyngeal glands and some of the general features of gland development were considered in the section dealing with pharyngeal development. Salivary glands develop as similar invaginations of the oral ectoderm. The anterior pituitary (adenohypophysis) is basically a gland also formed by an invagination of the oral ectoderm, which interacts with a portion of the undersurface of the brain, which forms the posterior pituitary (neurohypophysis). The lacrimal gland and duct form as a fold along the junction of the maxillary and lateral nasal processes. The skin and its appendages, such as facial hair, sweat and sebaceous glands, is usually considered to constitute a tissue. Aspects relevant to craniofacial malformations will be considered below.

4. MOLECULAR REGULATION OF NORMAL (AND ABNORMAL) EMBRYONIC DEVELOPMENT

4.1 HISTORICAL PERSPECTIVE

The experimental basis for most aspects of development (e.g., cell migration, inductive interactions, etc.) was developed from studies of amphibian embryos with little or no understanding of the underlying molecular mechanisms. A system for provision of the nutrients necessary for development that is largely unique to amphibian embryos made them particularly useful for developmental studies.

Nutrients, in the form of yolk platelets, are stored in the relatively gigantic fertilized egg, which divides into progressively smaller cells, each with its own supply of nutrients. There is no need for an outside source of nutrients, such as the yolks of avian and reptilian eggs (or their equivalent in fish embryos) or the placenta in mammals. The amphibian system required very large embryos whose tissues were easily manipulated for transplantation or culture in simple salt solution. Horstadius summarized the results of the amphibian studies in 1950, as did Holtfreter and Hamburger in 1955. Unfortunately, this unique nutrient supply system resulted in plump, relatively featureless embryos, not at all like the embryos illustrated in Figure 2-1. This appears to be the primary reason for the slow acceptance of the amphibian results by investigators working with higher vertebrate embryos.

It was not until the introduction of more sophisticated cell marking procedures, such as those using tritiated thymidine and the quail chromatin marker, that it was possible to extend the findings to higher vertebrates (see reviews by Johnston and Bronsky, 1995, 2002; LeDouarin and Kalcheim, 1992), and that the findings from amphibian embryos were widely accepted. Other techniques useful for the study of small embryos included other autoradiographic, histochemical, immunohistochemical and biochemical procedures, such as gel electrophoresis, as well as much more sophisticated techniques for cell and tissue culture.

Such technical advances; along with advances in molecular genetics (especially the extension of studies on the development of the fruit fly, Drosophila) have provided the basis for understanding molecular mechanisms underlying such developmental phenomena as induction, "fields" and segmentation. Investigators using cell culture began to identify "**growth factors**" that would stimulate cell proliferation, while teratologists studied alterations in development caused by other naturally occurring molecules such as retinoic acid (from the vitamin A family), corticosteroids and thyroxin.

When vertebrate embryos such as those of the chick and the mouse were examined for evidence of such molecules and the presence of gene products similar to those involved in Drosophila development, the basis for the molecular mechanisms involved in development was quickly established. The primary technique utilized was the identification of messenger RNA for the different molecules by radiolabeling their anti-sense DNA, which complexes with the appropriate RNA and can be demonstrated by autoradiography (see Figure 2-20).

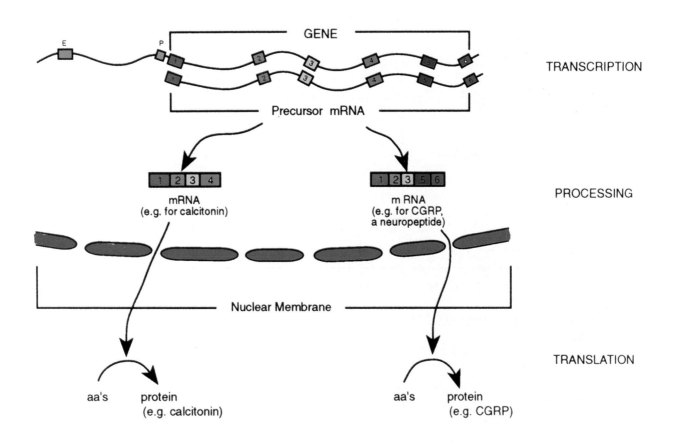

Figure 2-20: Gene transcription, processing and translation.

4.2 TISSUE INTERACTIONS

As noted earlier, cell movements and morphogenetic movements bring cells and tissues into close apposition with other cell populations. Interactions are mediated through the secretion of signaling molecules ("paracrine" factors), which diffuse over short distances to adjacent cells and alter the activity of "target" genes in these cells.

There are two principle mechanisms by which the signaling factors alter genes and these are illustrated in Figure 2-21. Much of evolutionary diversity arises through the duplication of genes and modification of the duplicated genes to serve similar or quite different functions. For example, there is a whole family of fibroblast growth factors (e.g., FGF1, FGF2, etc.). Also, their receptors are duplicated and modified (FGFR3, FGFR4, etc). The fact that the duplicated genes may have different receptors is illustrated by a mutation in FGFR3 that causes the common achondroplastic dwarfism (a defect in cartilage growth); while mutations in FGFR2 cause premature closure of craniofacial sutures, such as in Crouzon's syndrome.

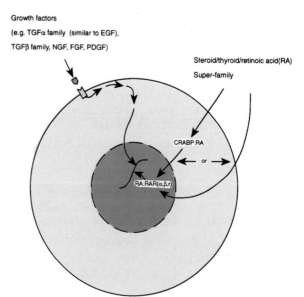

Figure 2-21: Most signaling factors, including the growth factors indicated, are water soluble and cannot get through the lipid layer of the cell membrane, necessitating a complex system of cell surface receptors and intracellular molecules in order to alter gene function. The steroids thyroxin and retinoic acid are insoluble and must be transported by carrier proteins.

These examples illustrate the divergent function of these receptors.

Figure 2-22 illustrates signaling factors and target genes functioning at different stages of development. This illustration is an oversimplification in that duplication and subsequent modification has resulted in sometimes very large families of signaling molecules such as the FGFs, which may have rather different functions at different stages of development. To a lesser extent, the same is true for the target genes.

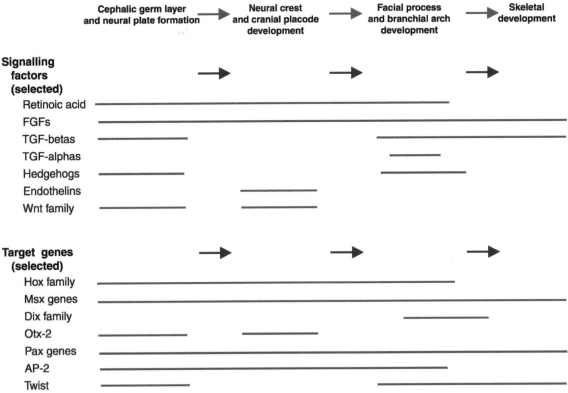

Figure 2-22: Indicates the periods of embryonic development during which different signaling molecules and target genes are active. The figure is somewhat of an oversimplification in that different members of a family of signaling molecules (e.g., different FGFs) may function at different times and these functions may be quite different. For example, FGF8 functions in growth promotion in the facial processes and limb buds, while other FGFs have the opposite effect in cartilage development, stimulating prechondroblasts to differentiate post-mitotic chondroblasts, thereby slowing cartilage growth.

4.3 DEVELOPMENT OF THE ANTERIOR NEURAL PLATE AND FOREBRAIN AND THEIR RELATIONSHIPS TO THE DEVELOPING FACE

From both evolutionary and developmental perspectives, there are two major divisions of the head. The hindbrain and visceral arches are more primitive than the forebrain and upper face. The forebrain and upper face are virtually absent in the sub-vertebrate chordates and the most primitive vertebrates (cyclostomes, such as the lamprey). The crest cells which migrate into the upper face are continuous with the mandibular arch crest and appear to be similarly programmed genetically but modified by the evolutionarily new forebrain and eye so that they do not form mandibular structures. The hindbrain develops as a series of segmental neuromeres that appear to be under the same type of developmental control in the most primitive vertebrates, the pre-vertebrate chordates and even invertebrates such as the fruit fly, Drosophila.

The neural crest cells themselves have much the same genetic activity as the neuromeres from which they are derived, and this will determine how they will react to the inductive influences of the endoderm and other tissues they encounter during and at the end of their migrations. The prechordal plate is essentially an extension of the notochord (Figure 2-2F and Figure 2-7B). As with the notochord, it is involved in bilateralization of the neural plate, an inductive interaction in which the notochord and prechordal plate alter the development of the overlying neural plate so that it separates structures such as the developing eye fields (Figure 2-2F) into two bilateral structures. Many years ago it was shown that experimental removal of the prechordal plate in amphibian embryos led to failure of separation of the eye fields and a large median eye similar to the case of human cyclopia illustrated in Figure 2-23D.

Cyclopia is considered to be a member of the holoprosencephaly ("single cavity fore-brain") series of malformations, in which underdevelopment of the forebrain leads to reduced sizes of the of the forebrain ventricles, sometimes to the point where only a single small midline ventricle remains. It has recently been determined that the inter-action between the prechordal plate and overlying neural plate is mediated by the production of a signaling molecule ("sonic hedgehog", Shh), found in Drosophila. It is produced by the prechordal plate and diffuses into the overlying neural plate, there-by altering its differentiation. Cyclopia can be produced by "knocking out" (rendering non-functional) the gene, or by interfering with its synthesis, which appears to be the mechanism by which veratrim alkaloids from a range plant produce cyclopia in sheep.

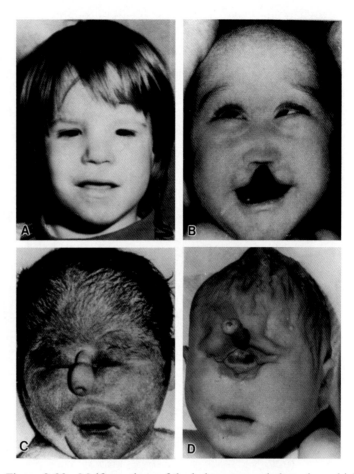

Figure 2-23: Malformations of the holoprosencephaly series, which is a grouping of somewhat loosely related malformations, where underdevelopment of the forebrain results in a tendency to form a "single cavity forebrain". Although rare, the best understood is cyclopia (D), which results from defects in signaling interaction between the prechordal plate (Figure 2-2F) and the overlying neural plate. Arhinencephaly (B, literally, "no nose") usually results from trisomy 13 or trisomy 19. The mildest form illustrated is the fetal alcohol syndrome (FAS). The tube-like structures in (C) and (D) are attempts to make a nose from a single midline olfactory placode trapped above the eye(s). From Johnston and Bronsky, 2002.

The other holoprosencephalies illustrated in Figure 2-23 probably resulted from somewhat different developmental alterations. Although the eyes are reduced in size, they remain bilateral, even in the most severely affected cases. The fetal alcohol syndrome (FAS, Figure 2-23A) is considered to be at the mild end of the spectrum. From a mouse model in which pregnant mice were given high (binge level) oral doses of ethanol at the time of germ layer development (about 16th post-fertilization day in the human), face (and brain) malformations very similar to the FAS occurred (Figure 2-24). The ethanol appears to have major effects on mesoderm formation and, although its effects on development of the neural plate are more severe in the midline, they are more diffuse than in the animal models for cyclopia noted above. This may account for the reduction in eye size seen in the non-cyclopia holo-prosencephalies. The nasal placodes, which are derived from the anterior neural plate, come to lie pro-gressively closer to the midline in more severely affected cases (Figure 2-25). Contact of the placodes as seen in Figure 2-25C results in a malformation similar to arhinencephaly (Figure 2-23B) in the mouse, but effects this severe are apparently not compatible with survival in the human, where they are usually associated with abnormalities in a chromosome (e.g., trisomies 13 and 19).

Somewhat related malformations are the otocephalies (Figure 2-26). In the milder cases (Figure 2-26A), the absence of the philtrum in the upper lip is similar to that found in the fetal alcohol syndrome (Figure 2-24A). In the otocephalies, the primary defect, at least in an animal model, appears to be in the mesoderm. In this model, a C57Bl mouse with defective gene function, the first cells to undergo cell death in the more mildly affected embryos are the cells in the mesodermal cores of the visceral arches. As noted above, these cells normally undergo cell death after they have vascularized the surrounding neural crest mesenchyme, but the timing is off, and the apparently initially normal crest cells die secondarily to the lack of vascular supply and the mandible sloughs to give a malformation similar to Figure 2-26A. The more severe malformation illustrated in Figure 2-26B presumably results from more severe mesodermal cell death.

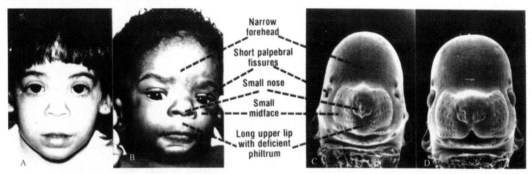

Figure 2-24: Children and a mouse model for FAS. Similarities between the facial structures in the affected mouse fetus and an FAS child are illustrated in (B) and (C).

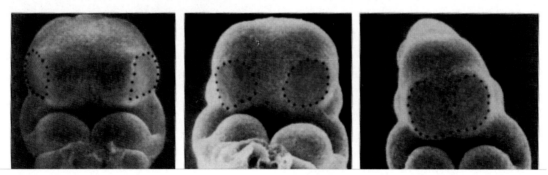

Figure 2-25: Scanning electron micrographs from a control mouse embryo (A) and mouse embryos (B) and (C) taken from a mother treated with ethanol at the time of germ layer formation. The degree of separation between the olfactory placodes to placodes situated closer to the midline, which is apparently the degree of separation sufficient to decrease the size of the premaxilla by an amount sufficient to cause the FAS. Contact of the placodes is apparently not compatible with survival in the human but produces malformation similar to the arhinencephaly illustrated in Figure 2-23B. From Sulik (1984).

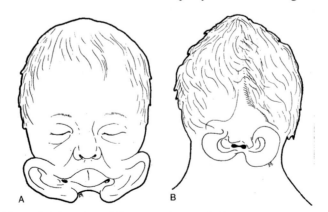

Figure 2-26: In the milder case of otocephaly (A), the mandible and associated structures are absent. In the more severe form illustrated, little more of the face than the ears are present, hence the name otocephaly (ear head).

4.4 NORMAL AND ABNORMAL MECHANISMS OF NEURAL CREST AND GANGLIONIC PLACODE DEVELOPMENT

Figure 2-7 summarizes some of the features of the vertebrate segmental plan for the embryonic head and neck. Much of the recent work on head segmentation in vertebrates is based on genetic studies of Drosophila. The chromosomal segment containing the Hox genes, which control head segmentation in Drosphila, has been duplicated on four mammalian chromosomes (Figure 2-27).

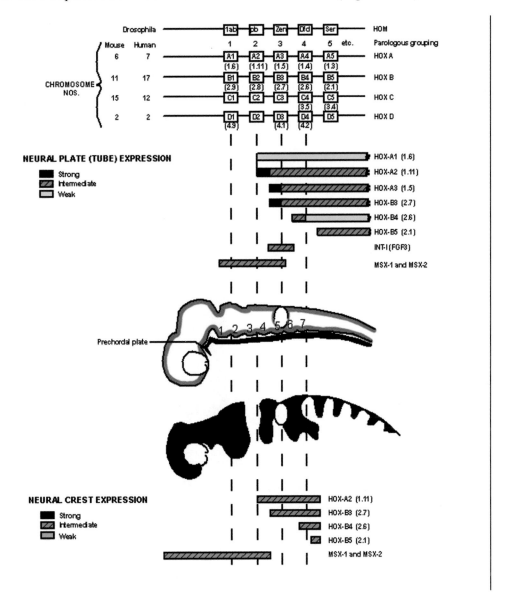

Figure 2-27: Control of segmentation in vertebrate embryos is apparently similar to that seen in Drosophila. The homeotic genes of Drosophila are replicated and modified on four different chromosomes in the mouse and human, each of the genes in the same head-to-tail sequence. Messenger RNA for the genes is progressively added beginning with Hox-A1 and Hox-A2 in rhombomere 4, which continue to be present as the messenger RNA of more Hox genes is added. The developmental significance of this "cascade" is described in the text.

As noted earlier, duplication with subsequent modification of genetic function appears to be a common strategy in evolution. It permits duplicated genes to adopt altered function without disturbing a critical developmental function of the parent gene. Gene activity in embryos can be monitored by the presence of messenger RNA produced by the genes.

Such studies show that as one proceeds from the more rostral to more caudal neuromeres, new genes are activated, while the originally active genes continue to produce their messenger RNA (Figure 2-27). For example, when the Hox-A2 gene is activated in the second (hyoid) arch crest cells, other Hox genes active in the first (mandibular) arch continue to produce their messenger RNA. If the Hox-A2 gene is experimentally "knocked out" in mouse embryos, the hyoid arch cells do not have the genetic information they require in order to respond appropriately to the inducing tissues of the hyoid arch and form, instead, another mandible.

These observations explain, at least in part, the results of classical studies in experimental embryology. For example, first arch crest cells used to replace second arch crest cells migrate normally into the second arch, but respond to local inducers by producing another mandible rather than hyoid arch skeletal elements. Also, when trunk crest cells are used to replace head crest cells, they migrate normally into the branchial arches but are unable to produce any skeletal elements. Forebrain crest cells, when used to replace first arch crest cells, respond to the first arch environment by producing a mandible, suggesting that they are basically first arch crest cells that are normally modified by the forebrain and/or eye with which they come into contact.

Newborns with the Retinoic Acid Syndrome (RAS), Figure 2-28A) first appeared after the introduction of the drug Accutane (13-cis-retinoic acid). This drug is very effective in the treatment of severe cystic acne and has gained wide acceptance. In spite of warnings that the drug was a known teratogen (as are other retinoids, including vitamin A), and was not to be not to be taken during pregnancy, accidental exposures have produced an unexpectedly large number of severe malformations such as that illustrated in Figure 2-28A.

This is apparently because of the decreased capacity of humans to metabolize an equally teratogenic

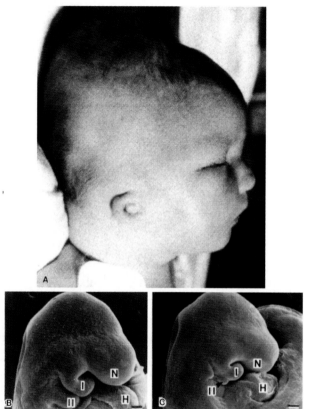

Figure 2-28: Child with retinoic acid syndrome (RAS), which results from the accidental administration of 13-cis retinoic acid, a drug used for the treatment of severe cystic acne. In addition to the deformities of the external ear resulting from major effects on the hyoid arch (B, C), there are usually many associated malformations, including those of the cardiovascular system and pharyngeal glands, which are life-threatening. There are also sometimes severe brain malformations, particularly of the cerebellum. (From Webster, et al., 1986).

metabolite of the drug, which builds up to high levels in the blood stream (Webster, et al., 1984). In an animal model for this malformation, Accutane administered before and during the migration of neural crest cells resulted in malformations virtually identical to those of the RAS (Figure 2-28A). Retinoids slow proliferation of embryonic cells and may also interfere with their migrations. In the animal model, large numbers of crest cells die both before and during their migrations, and migrating crest cells show excessive numbers of blebs on their surfaces.

The cell death is particularly pronounced for hyoid arch crest cells and results in virtual absence of the hyoid arch (Figure 2-28B,C). The gap in the sheet of crest cells between the mandibular and hyoid crest in normal development (Figure 2-7) results from normal ("programmed") death of crest cells in that portion of the neural folds, and Accutane broadens this area of cell death. While deficiencies in the mandibular crest cells can be made up by more anterior cells, this is not possible for hyoid crest, which is separated by the above-noted gap anteriorly and the developing ear posteriorly (Figure 2-7).

The longitudinal septum of the cono-truncal portion of the developing heart (Figure 2-17) is derived from crest cells, and failure of crest cell migration into this structure apparently leads to the associated abnormalities of the great vessels (arch of the aorta and pulmonary artery), which are normally formed by splitting of the cono-truncus through its septum. These vascular abnormalities and deficiencies of the thymus glands (whose mesenchyme is crest-derived) are usually fatal for RAS infants.

Considerable interest is being taken in the DiGeorge syndrome, partly because of its close similarity to the RAS, and partly because of the finding that it is caused by a deletion in chromosome 22. A similar deletion was found in patients with the velo-cardio-facial syndrome, which is basically the DiGeorge syndrome without the pharyngeal gland defects. Also, similar malformations can be caused through a very wide spectrum of experimental manipulations, all of them involving the neural crest in one way or another.

In a classic series of studies conducted by Kirby and associates, they first showed that the neural crest is responsible for the formation of the cono-truncal septum noted above, and that extirpations of post-otic hindbrain neural crest in the chick resulted in cardiovascular and pharyngeal gland defects similar to those found in the RAS, DiGeorge and other syndromes. Most recently, studies of mouse models for the deletion and knockouts of individual genes in the deleted region have shown that the deletion or just the knockout of one of its genes, a gene transcribing a transcription factor (Tbx), results in the cardiovascular defects (but not the pharyngeal gland defects). The primary effect seems to be on a subpopulation of crest cells that forms the smooth cells of the aortic arch vessels, fouling up the changes in the fourth arch vessels related to shut-down on one side and formation of the arch of the aorta on the other.

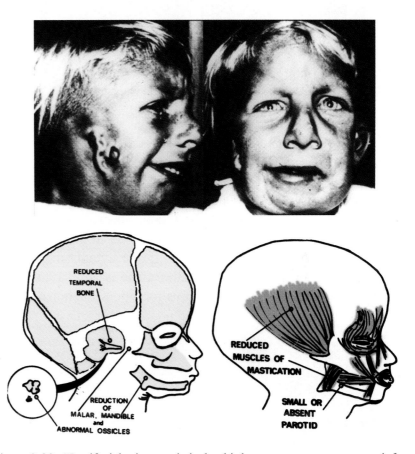

Figure 2-29: Hemifacial microsomia is the third most common severe craniofacial malformation after cleft lip with or without cleft palate and cleft palate only. It shares some of the characteristics of the RAS. The external and middle ear defects are similar but mostly unilateral. It has high incidence of similar cardiovascular malformations, but pharyngeal gland deficiencies have not been reported. There appears to be little or no effect on brain development.

While the developmental origins of **hemifacial microsomia** (Figure 2-29) are unknown, the frequently associated great vessel defects and similar ear defects suggest somewhat similar crest cell involvement.

Again, there appear to be no pharyngeal gland defects. Although usually unilateral, the defects may be bilateral, especially in more severely affected cases.

Administration of Accutane at a later stage results in massive cell death in and around the distal portions of the trigeminal ganglion. Placodal cells are migrating into the ganglion at the stage of administration. Again, this may be related to enhancement of cell death, which occurs normally when neurons which have failed to make peripheral connections degenerate. Treatment at this time produces malformations that are uncannily similar to those of the Treacher Collins syndrome (Figure 2-30), which, however, is caused by a single dominant gene.

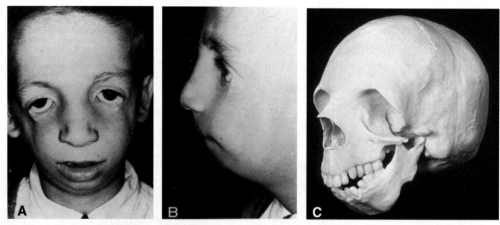

Figure 2-30: Treacher Collins Syndrome. In this syndrome, there are also similar but usually less severe defects of the external and middle ears. There is a high incidence of cleft palate, but little in the way of other malformations.

The cell death appears to overwhelm other cells in the area so that structures other than the ganglion are affected. These include the zygomatic bone and the proximal portion of the mandible. The high incidence of clefts of the soft palate may be related to deficiencies of the proximal portion of the maxillary process. Recently, a gene (TCOF-1) has been identified for the Treacher Collins syndrome. Unlike most genes involved in malformations, its product, treacle, is not a regulatory molecule but one that is broadly distributed and primarily involved in the organization of nucleoli and, possibly, in the transport of materials from the nucleus to the cytoplasm. Unlike the RA Treacher Collins model described above (which produced malformations similar to those of human Treacher Collins syndrome), a transgenic mouse hemizygous for a non-functional TCOF-1 gene demonstrated severe malformations that appear to have resulted not only from massive cell death in prospective ganglionic placodes, but also in many crest and other cells.

4.5 MECHANISMS INVOLVED IN NORMAL AND ABNORMAL PRIMARY PALATE AND SECONDARY PALATE DEVELOPMENT

The inductive interactions between the crest cells migrating into the upper face have been studied very little. Transplantation of these cells prior to their migration to the first arch region shows that they are capable of forming first arch skeletal elements, suggesting that they are somehow modified to form skeletal and connective tissues appropriate to the upper face when they migrate to that region. Evidence concerning the mechanisms involved in normal primary palate formation is slowly accumulating. Proliferation of mesenchymal cells in the facial processes is maintained at a relatively high rate, and epithelial-mesenchymal interactions are required.

There is some evidence that the high proliferation rate at least partly results from the action of growth factors (Figures 2-21 an 2-22). Experimental combinations of epithelia and mesenchyme in culture have shown that mesenchyme from the facial processes or branchial arches requires combination with epithelia in order to survive and proliferate, but that fibroblast growth factor (FGF) can replace the epithelia. This suggests the possibility that the epithelia may be producing this factor. *In situ* hybridization studies have shown that the distribution of FGF-8 and Ssh in the epithelia of the developing facial processes (and the branchial arches) is remarkably well defined (Figure 2-31), suggesting that these structures are being regulated, at least in part, by these molecules. Retinoic acid, msx and other regulatory molecules apparently also play major roles.

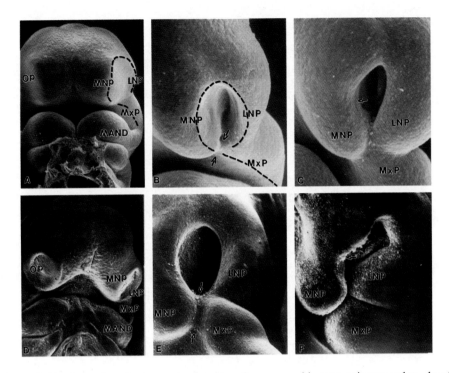

Figure 2-31: Scanning electron micrographs of mouse and human primary palate development, with broken lines added to summarize the findings of numerous studies showing the approximate locations of FGF-8 and Shh.

Clefts of the lip and/or palate (Figures 2-32 2-33 and 2-34) are by far the most common of the severe facial malformations. Like other common malformations, and other common diseases, most appear to have multifactorial etiology. It requires multiple predisposing factors to cause the malformation in each case. Any factors increasing the probability that facial processes will fail to contact and fuse would be considered to be predisposing factors. Examples of genetic factors include the more medial direction of medial nasal process growth and failure of epithelial seam differentiation in genetically predisposed mouse strains, and the presence of an unusual growth factor variant (TGF-alpha in Figures 2-21 and 2-22), which might interfere with epithelial fusion in human **cleft lip** and/or palate cases. Environmental factors appear to include cigarette smoking, which interferes with ATP formation, and the anti-epileptic drug Dilantin. ATP is the immediate energy source for all cells, and its reduction could affect many developmental phenomena, including cell division and morphogenetic movements. There is experimental evidence that interference with tongue removal may lead to cleft palate, and that large tongue size may contribute to cleft palate formation in humans. While there is a clear separation of cleft lip with or without cleft palate and isolated cleft palate in humans (see Figure 2-34), many of the predisposing factors noted affect both.

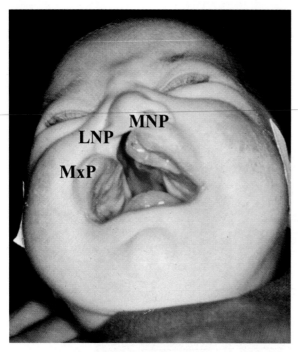

Figure 2-32: Unilateral cleft lip and palate.

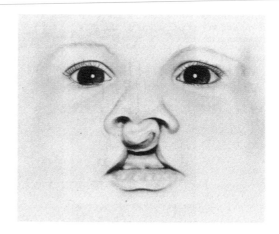

Figure 2-33: Bilateral cleft lip and palate. Structures in the midline are philtral portion of the lip (prolabium) and the premaxillary segment of the maxilla.

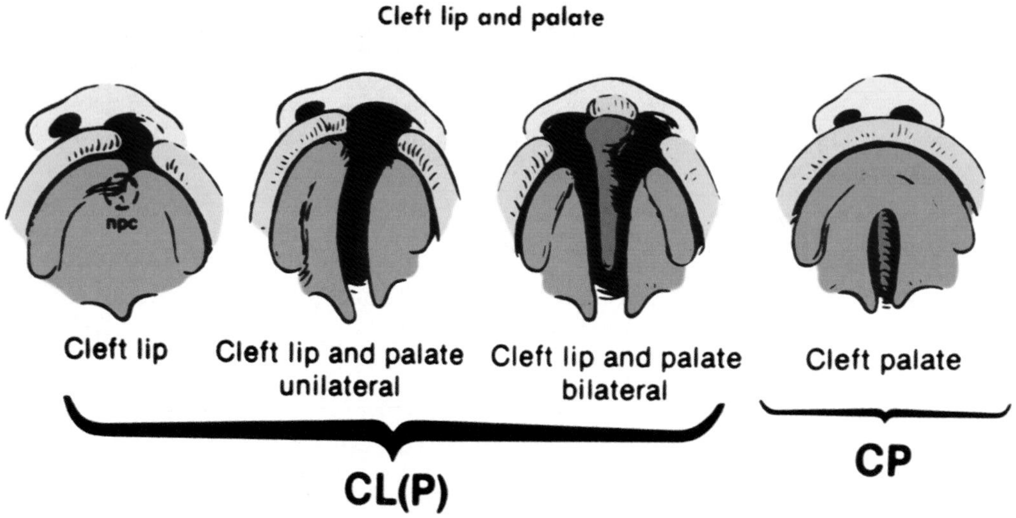

Cleft lip and palate

Cleft lip   Cleft lip and palate   Cleft lip and palate   Cleft palate
              unilateral   bilateral

CL(P)   CP

Figure 2-34: Diagrams of the complete forms of clefts of the lip and/or palate. The brackets indicate that clefts of the lip with or without cleft palate (CL(P)) are etiologically different than clefts of the palate without the cleft lip (CP).

The fusion and merging of the facial processes constitute "developmental weak points", which are subject to many genetic and environmental factors leading to abnormal development. The medial nasal processes are initially widely separated, and their failure to merge completely results in clefts of the nose as illustrated in Figure 2-35. In more severe cases, almost the entire upper face is cleft, and in these cases the brain is also affected with abnormalities in the corpus callosum, which connects the two cerebral hemispheres. Many of the less common forms of facial clefts such as the cleft jaw (Figure 2-36) may be instructive in understanding both normal development and the alterations leading to more common malformations.

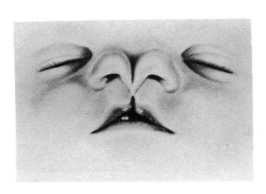

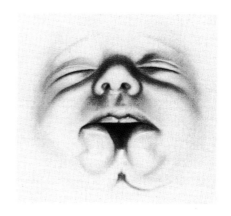

Figure 2-35: Rare median cleft of the nose and upper lip

Figure 2-36: Median cleft of the mandible and lower lip is even less common than medial clefts of the lip and nose.

5. FETAL DEVELOPMENT

The completion of embryonic development and the onset of fetal development are signaled by the completion of the secondary palate and the beginning of bone formation. These events occur at about the 55th to 60th day, or about the end of the first trimester. They are rather arbitrary landmarks. While growth and maturation are more predominant, many embryonic phenomena are still occurring, such as the migrations and differentiation of neuroblasts, which continue well on into postnatal life.

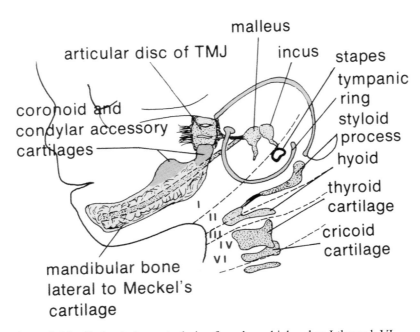

Figure 2-37: Skeletal elements derive from branchial arches I through VI.

Figure 2-37 illustrates the relation between the initial cartilaginous elements and the branchial arches (Roman numerals). The developing mandible envelops the distal portion of Meckel's cartilage. The development of the temporo-mandibular joint is complex (Figure 2-38). The condyles first form as independent cartilages lateral to Meckel's cartilage (Figure 2-38B) and are later enveloped by the developing ramus of the mandible (Figure 2-38B, C).

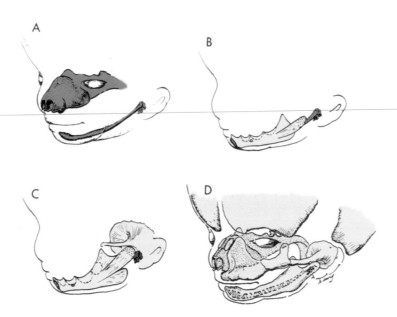

Figure 2-38: (A) Development of the cartilaginous nasal capsule and Meckel's cartilage at about 9 weeks. (B) By about 16 weeks, mandibular bone is enveloping Meckel's cartilage and the developing condyle is fusing with the mandibular bone. (C) At about 24 weeks, the condyle is articulating with the temporal bone. (D) The facial skeleton at about 30 weeks.

The initial skeletal element of the nose is the cartilaginous nasal septum (Figure 2-38A). Most of the capsule undergoes endochondral ossification. The majority of the mid-face skeleton is, however, formed by intramembranous ossification. The **cranial base** is formed by endochondral ossification. Portions of the cranial base remain cartilaginous to form the spheno-ethmoidal and spheno-occipital synchondroses, which function as growth centers.

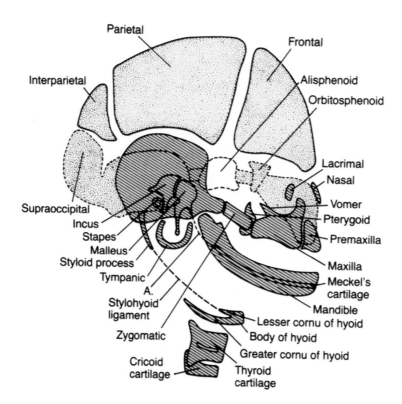

Figure 2-39: In this schematic drawing, the branchial arch bones are obliquely hatched, as are other facial bones. The bones of the cranial vault and the nasal septum are stippled.

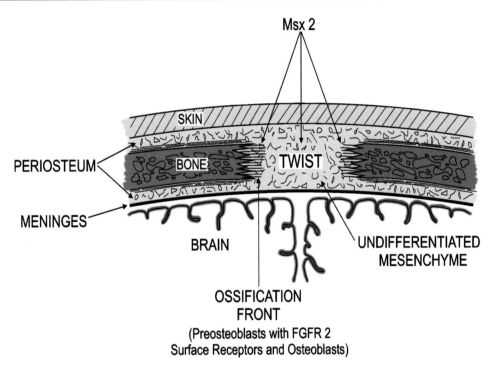

Figure 2-40: Distribution of some of the regulatory molecules involved in suture development. The interparietal suture is illustrated. From Johnston and Bronsky, 2002.

The relations between the branchial arch skeletal elements to those of the mid-face cranial base are schematically presented in Figure 2-39. Reference has already been made to the dominant role of neural crest cells in the formation of skeletal and connective tissues in the facial region. In Figure 2-19, the distribution of dermal and subcutaneous tissue, as well as the distribution of skeletal tissues of neural crest or mesodermal origin is illustrated. The mechanisms involved in suture development are illustrated in Figure 2-40. A principle regulatory gene is TWIST. Experimentally, the twist protein has been shown to function by binding to fibroblast growth factors (FGFs), which keeps them from complexing with FGF receptors on the surfaces of pre-osteoblast mesenchymal cells. Since the FGF/FGFR complex is needed for differentiation into the post-mitotic state, the twist protein keeps the preosteoblasts proliferating and enhances suture growth. Msx also stimulates osteoblast differentiation.There are a number of craniofacial malformations related to defects in skeletal development.

Very similar genetic defects cause two well-known defects, the common achondroplastic dwarf and Crouzon's syndrome. In both malformations, the genetic defects are in the cell surface fibroblast growth factor receptors (Figure 2-21). Defects in the TWIST protein and in Msx cause other types of premature suture closure (synostosis).

5. SUGGESTED READINGS

Avery, JK. Prenatal facial growth. In Moyers, RE (ed.) Handbook of Orthodontics, 4th Ed., Year Book Medical Pub.(2000)

Avery, JK. Essentials of Oral Histology and Embryology, 2nd Ed., CV Mosby, St. Louis 2000.

Dunhamel, B (1966) Morphogenese Pathologique. Paris. Masson et Cie.

Gorlin RJ, Cohen MM, Hennekam RCM. Syndromes of the Head and Neck, 4th Ed., Oxford University Press, Oxford, England 2001.

Greene RM, Weston WM. Craniofacial embryology. In: Master of Surgery. Cohen M, editor. Little, Brown and Co. 1996, pp 459-470.

Johnston, MC. Embryology of the head and neck. In: Plastic Surgery. McCarthy J, ed., WB Saunders, Philadelphia, 1990.

Johnston, MC. Understanding Human Development, In: Human Malformations and Related Anomalies, Stevenson RE, Hall JG, Goodman RM, Eds. Oxford University Press, New York and Oxford,1993, pp 30-64.

Johnston MC, and Bronsky PT. Craniofacial Embryogenesis: abnormal developmental mechanisms. In: Understanding Craniofacial Anomalies: The Etiopathogenesis of Craniosynostosis and Facial Clefting. Mooney MP and Siegel MI (eds.) Wiley-Liss. New York 2002.

Johnston MC, Hassel JR and Brown KS. The embryology of cleft lip and palate. Clin. Plast. Surg. 1975;2:195-203.

Johnston MC and Hazelton RB. Embryonic origins of facial structures related to oral sensory and motor function. In: Oral Sensory Perception, The Mouth of the Infant. Bosma JF, Ed., Charles C. Thomas, Springfield, IL 1972.

Johnston MC and Sulik KK. Embryology of the head and neck. In: Pediatric Plastic Surgery. Serafin NG and Georgeaide ND, eds. CV Mosby, St. Louis 1984.

Millicovsky G, Ambrose LJH, Johnston MC. Developmental alterations associated with spontaneous cleft lip and palate in CL/FR mice. Am J Anat 1982;164:29-44.

Noden DM. Vertebrate craniofacial development: The relation between ontogenetic process and morphological outcome. Brain Behav Evol 1991a;38: 190-.

Poswillo D. The pathogenesis of the first and second branchial arch syndrome. Oral Surg 1973;35:302-328.

Ross RB, Johnston MC. Cleft Lip and Palate. Williams & Wilkins, Baltimore 1972.

Sadler TW. Langman's Medical Embryology. 7th Ed. Williams & Wilkins, Baltimore 2000.

Sulik KK. Critical Periods for Alcohol Teratogenesis in Mice, with Special Reference to the Gastrulation Stage of Embryogenesis. Ciba Foundation Symposium no. 105, Pitman Books, Ltd., London 1984.

Sulik KK. Critical Periods for Alcohol Teratogenesis in Mice, with Special Reference to the Gastrulation Stage of Embryogenesis. Ciba Foundation Symposium no. 105, Pitman Books, Ltd., London 1984.

Sulik KK, Johnston MC. Embryonic origin of holoprosencephaly: interrelationship of the developing brain and face. Scanning Electron Micr 1982;1:309-322.

Sulik KK, Johnston MC, Webb MA. Fetal alcohol syndrome: Embryogenesis in a mouse model. Science 1981;214:936-938.

Taysi K, Tinaztepe K. Trisomy D and the cyclops malformation. Am J Dis Child 1972;124:170.

Waterman RE and Meller SM Normal facial development in the human embryo. In: Textbook of Oral Biology. Shaw et al. (Eds). WB Saunders Co., Philadelphia 1973.

Waterman RE, Meller SM. Alterations in the epithelial surface of human palatal shelves prior to and during fusion: A scanning electron microscopic study. Anat Rec 1974;180:111-135.

Webster WS, Johnston MC, Lammer EJ, Sulik KK. Isotretinoin embryopathy and the cranial neural crest: An in vivo and in vitro study. J Craniofac Genet Dev Biol 1986;6:211-222.

CHAPTER 3

Postnatal Craniofacial Development

Malcom C. Johnston

James K. Avery

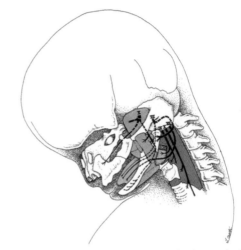

Figure 3-1: Illustration of nerve-muscle interrelations to emphasize the importance of understanding paths followed by cranial nerves as they follow the migrations of myoblasts innervated by cranial nerves V (blue), IX, X (green) and XII (yellow).

1. INTRODUCTION

This chapter will be divided into two major sections. First the development of the structural components will be considered, followed by physiological development. Clinical relevance will be considered, although much of these correlations will be left to later chapters.

2. STRUCTURAL DEVELOPMENT

2.1. THE RELATION OF STRUCTURE TO EARLY PRENATAL DEVELOPMENT:

As noted in Chapter 2, the development of muscle and nerve is, from the earliest stages, closely interrelated. The sometimes complex anatomies of the motor nerves and muscles they innervate (Figures 3-1 and 3-2) are closely related to their embryonic development and is best understood in this context.

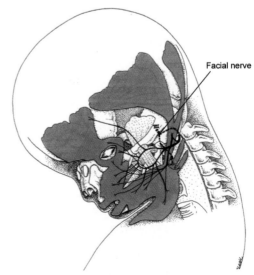

Figure 3-2: Illustration detailing the muscles innervated by cranial nerve VII.

The **myoblasts** arise from the myotomes of

somites that are directly apposed to the neural tube (Figures 2-2H and 3-3), so that neurites from motor neurons in the tube directly encounter the myotomes as they leave the tube. During their primary migrations (Figure 2-18), the myoblasts move as solid masses ("cords"), taking the neurites with them. Once they have reached their primary staging areas (e.g., in the cores of the branchial arches), most of the myoblasts migrate as individual cells, taking with them branches of the motor nerves.

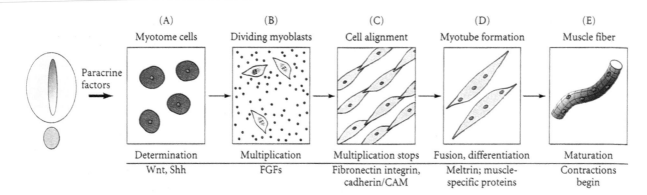

Figure 3-3: Differentiation of muscle cells as learned from *in vitro* studies. After fusion of the cells in an end-to-end pattern, nuclei become post-mitotic. While they are initially in the center of the myotube, they eventually come to lie under the cell surface. From Wolpert, et al., 1998.

Branches of the cranial nerves, which have mixed sensory and motor functions, innervate the craniofacial muscles. Myoblasts derived from the core "muscle" plates of the mandibular arch are innervated by the mandibular branch of the Vth cranial nerve and form the contractile components of the "jaw" muscles (Figure 3-1), while those derived from the hyoid (2nd) arch are innervated by the facial (VIIth cranial) nerve and provide the contractile components of the muscles of facial expression (Figure 3-2). The myoblasts derived from the 3rd arch contribute only to the stylohyoid muscle, which is innervated by the primarily sensory glossopharyngeal (IXth cranial) nerve.

The pharyngeal constrictors, as well as the muscles of the larynx and most of the muscles of the soft palate, receive their myoblasts from the 4th arch and are innervated by branches of the vagal (Xth cranial) nerve (Figure 3-1). Intrinsic and extrinsic muscles of the tongue are derived from the hypoglossal cord and are innervated by the hypoglossal (XIIth cranial) nerve (Figure 3-1). The extrinsic ocular muscle myoblasts have origins similar to the branchial arch musculature. In addition, this group of myoblasts also forms the contractile components of the levator palbebrae superioris, which is innervated by the oculomotor (IIIrd cranial) nerve, and which is involved in elevation of the upper eyelid. It is the only muscle of facial expression that is innervated by the facial nerve. Other "peculiarities" based on evolutionary and developmental considerations are described below.

During embryonic development, the vagal nerve is closely associated with the fourth aortic blood vessel, which persists on the right side to form the arch of the aorta. The laryngeal branch of the vagus, which provides motor innervation to the muscles of the larynx, gets caught behind the developing aorta and is dragged caudally by the aorta as it descends into the thorax. Hence the name, "right recurrent laryngeal nerve". The XIIth cranial nerve sweeps caudally (Figure 3-1) because the myoblasts of the hypoglossal cord migrate behind the **pharyngeal arches** and forward in the floor of the developing pharynx. Also, during the complex evolution of the soft palate, most of its myoblasts are derived from the fourth arch and are, consequently, innervated by the Xth cranial nerve (Figure 3-1), which also innervates other pharyngeal constrictors and, as noted above, the laryngeal muscles. A muscle primarily related to the middle ear (the tensor palatii, which is derived from the first arch and is innervated by the Vth cranial nerve) was drafted to stabilize the soft palate from above (Figure 3-1) in order to assist in the very complex movements involved in human swallowing and speech. The tensor palatii is also involved in regulating the opening of the middle ear **Eustachian tube** and a related muscle, the tensor tympani, is also innervated by Vth nerve. The involvement of the first and second arches in the evolution of the middle ear and **temporomandibular joint** (TMJ) were discussed in Chapter 2.

2.2. DIFFERENTIATION OF MUSCLE CELLS

Once they have reached their definitive locations, the myoblasts begin to fuse together to form **myotubes** (Figures 3-3C and D). At first the nuclei are lined up in the center of the myotube (Figure 3-3D), but later they migrate to the periphery of the cell (Figure 3-3E). These multinucleated muscle cells are usually termed muscle fibers. Each **muscle fiber** (cell) extends throughout the length of muscle, and a branch of an **axon** of an individual neuron serves each muscle fiber (Figure 3-4). The neuron and the muscle fibers it innervates are termed the "**motor unit**". The fibers of one motor unit are interspersed among the fibers of others and may cover an area several millimeters wide (Figure 3-4). When the neuron fires, all its innervated muscle fibers contract simultaneously and the total force (tension) exerted is a summation of the forces exerted by the individual motor units (Figures 3-4 and 3-5). The number of muscle fibers per unit depends on the intricacies of movements controlled by the muscle. For example, in muscles sub-serving the vocal cords of the larynx the number of fibers per neuron is about 5:1, while in the masseter muscle it is about 40:1.

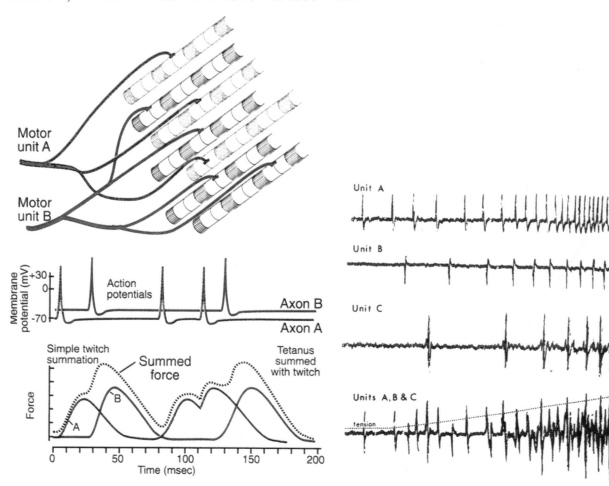

Figure 3-4: Summation of motor units. The morphological relations of two motor units are shown above and action potentials and twitches are shown below. From Rhoades and Pflanzer, 1992.

Figure 3-5: Diagrammatic representation of the action potentials of individual motor units (A, B, C) and the summation of their activities, as seen in an electromyographic recording.

Characteristic of all skeletal (and cardiac) muscle fibers are the **actin-myosin** arrays, which have a longitudinal periodicity, giving the muscle its striated appearance (Figures 3-3 and 3-6 through 3-8). Larger **myosin** filaments are interspersed between the finer **actin** filaments (Figure 3-4), and a sliding interaction between them gives the muscle its contractility. Primarily, the banding results from the more darkly staining myosin bands (Figures 3-3 and 3-6). Dispersal of the action potential from the neuromuscular **synapse** throughout the **muscle fiber** is greatly enhanced by a series of microtubules, termed T-tubules, and the **sarcoplasmic reticulum** (Figure 3-8).

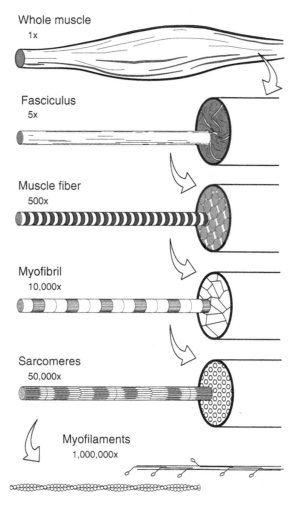

Figure 3-6: Levels of complexity in the organization of skeletal muscle. The approximate amount of magnification required to visualize each level of structure is indicated. From Rhoades and Pflanzer, 1992.

The actin-myosin arrays may be found in some muscle fibers very early in development, even before the secondary migrations occur, such as in the muscle plates in the branchial arches. Presumably these cells remain at or near their current position. Many prospective myoblasts remain unfused and they, presumably, are involved in the secondary migrations.

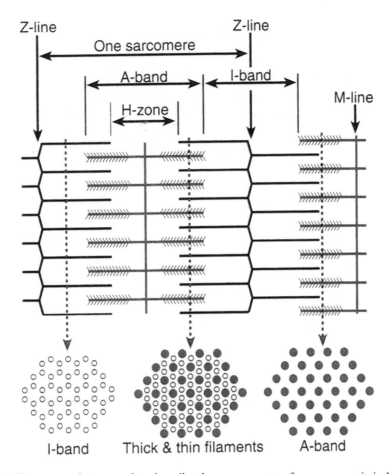

Figure 3-7: The nomenclature used to describe the components of a sarcomere is indicated above and their arrangement in cross-section below. From Rhoades and Pflanzer, 1992.

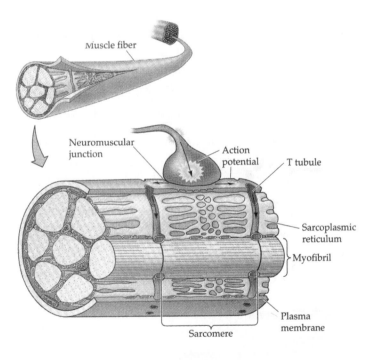

Figure 3-8: A schematic drawing of the three-dimensional relations of bundles of myofilaments to the **sarcoplasmic reticulum** and T-tubules, which transport the action potential from the neuromuscular junction. (Purves, et al., Life: The Science of Biology, 1997).

Muscle fibers differentiate into two main groups of cells: **muscle spindles ("intrafusal" fibers)** that are specialized to monitor stretch in the muscle, and the **extrafusal fibers** that give the muscle its power (Figure 3-7 and 3-8). The contractile **extrafusal fibers** show several overlapping characteristics that are related to the function of the muscle. In Type II fibers, the **actin**-myosin interaction (and hence the speed of contraction) is enhanced by the presence of **myosin ATPase**, which can be demonstrated in fibers histochemically as darkly staining substance, while fibers staining lightly for the enzyme are designated Type I (Figure 3-9). While muscle spindles contract to some extent, the contractions are basically concerned with increasing the muscle spindle's sensitivity to the degree of stretching in the muscle. In the craniofacial region, the sensory neurons of the trigeminal nerve are located in the brainstem (mesencephalic nucleus), in contrast to the trunk region, where they are located in the spinal ganglia. The spindles receive relatively small alpha efferent motor fibers whose cell bodies are located in the motor nucleus, as are the cell bodies of the motor neurons that innervate the extrafusal fibers. Other endings sensitive to stretch are the **Golgi tendon organs** (Figure 3-10), found in the tendons of the muscle. Similar stretch-sensitive endings are found in the temporomandibular joint. Of all the skeletal voluntary muscles, only the muscles of facial expression do not have muscle spindles. They insert primarily in the skin, and appear to rely on Golgi tendon organs and other sensory endings to monitor stretch.

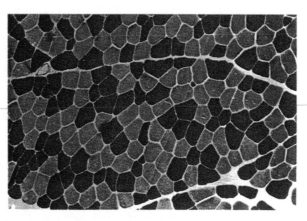

Figure 3-9: Cross-section of a muscle illustrating two major fiber types differentiated by their ATPase staining. ATP is the major source of energy, and higher levels of ATPase (more darkly staining cells) permit rapid contraction. From Rhingquist, 1973.

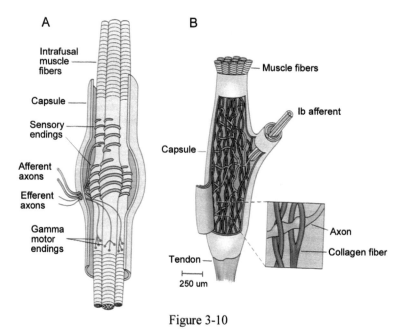

Figure 3-10

Figure 3-10: Two types of sensory endings for monitoring stretch in a muscle. The muscle spindle illustrated in (A) is modified **muscle fiber** very sensitive to the amount of stretch in the muscle while the **Golgi tendon organs** illustrated in (B) are less sensitive and more involved in protective reflexes. From Kandel, et al., 2000.

On the other hand, fatigue resistance, as is required in muscle involved in postural activity, requires a sustained energy supply, which is provided by the presence of mitochondria (Figure 3-9) and an adequate blood supply. These characteristics are found in Type I fibers as well as in Type IIA fibers, which also have myosin ATPase and are both fast and fatigue resistant. Type IIB fibers have only myosin-ATPase, and are fast but not fatigue resistant. Type IIB fibers are preponderant in the biceps muscle while the masseter muscle, which has both postural and rapid contraction functions, has a mixture of Type I and small Type IIB fibers.

2.3 HOW MUSCLES GROW

Since the nuclei of the multi-nucleated muscle fiber (Figures 3-3D and E) are post-mitotic and the fiber extends from one end of the muscle to the other (Figure 3-4), growth of the fiber lengthwise depends on the recruitment of cells in the vicinity. These cells are closely apposed to the surface of the fiber and form the **sarcolemma**. Although Moss and Leblond (1956) discovered this phenomenon years ago, many of the details have only recently been described. These nuclei are added primarily at the ends of the fiber.

In addition, new (secondary) muscle fibers are added during the growth period through the fusion of residual myoblasts. They are histologically indistinguishable from the primary fibers, but when the primary fibers are labeled with BUDR in the prenatal period, it has been demonstrated (Zhang and McLennan, 1999) that in muscle atrophy, as occurs following section of the motor nerve, the primary fibers maintain their nuclei, while secondary fibers lose theirs, beginning at their distal end. (Sort of like "last hired, first fired"!)

During muscle hypertrophy, as following exercise, the muscle increases its size through the addition of **actin** and myosin filaments, usually without addition of nuclei. In the adult, muscle fibers are added only with extreme levels of exercise. Tendons and other muscle attachments contribute little to growth, although they are capable of adjusting following major surgical procedures, such as those involved in lengthening of the mandible. There is a major change during growth in that muscles, during much of the growth period, insert into the periosteum, but eventually these insertions become surrounded by bone. There are numerous other structural changes in nerve and muscle during postnatal development, but these are best postponed following some further description of functional changes.

2.4 SYNCHONDROSES AND ARTICULATIONS OF THE **CRANIAL BASE** AND FACE

Growth Sites In The Cranial Base

The discussion of the period from birth to adulthood should include some discussion of articulations of the cranial base and face, since they make important contributions to growth in the cranial-facial area. One of the functions of the cranial base is as a buffer zone between the face, brain and palatal region. Early growth of the basicranium takes place by growth of the sphenoethmoidal and the sphenooccipital synchondroses.

These two synchondroses of the cranial base originate in cartilage during early prenatal life, as seen in Figure 3-11A. This cartilage is transformed into bone by endochondral bone development to develop the bony cranial base, as seen in Figure 3-11B.

Gradually, this cartilage structure develops into bone by endochondral development. Between the ethmoid, sphenoid and midline, cartilaginous sutures develop to provide for the lengthening of the cranial base. The chondocranium initially supports the base of the brain. As the brain expands during childhood, cranial sutural expansion responds in compensating growth. It is interesting that the articulations of the midline exist initially between cartilages that became bone by endochondral bone formation and, as long as the cartilage articulation exists, the bordering bone can grow and expand.

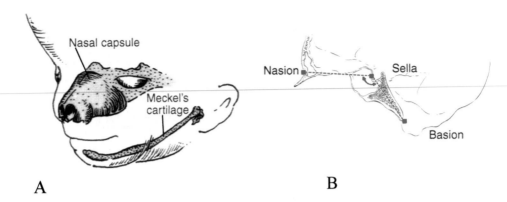

Figure 3-11: Part A.) Diagram of the prenatal nasal capsule that forms to support the sense organs of the nose and ears and the floor of the brain. This develops into the ethmoid and sphenoid bones in postnatal life. Part B.) Landmarks of the cranial base angle used to determine the angulation of this support base.

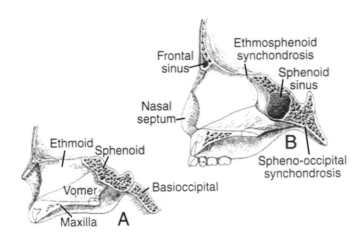

Figure 3-12: The face increases in height and length as the midline vomer, ethmoid, sphenoid and basioccipital bones grow and enlarge the cranial base.

In addition to the ethmoid and sphenoid there are other midline bones aiding in the anterior and ventral growth, and one of these is the **vomer** bone. Observe how the face grows in height as these bones grow during childhood to adulthood. A comparison of the relationship in a lateral view of the vomer and the ethmoid, sphenoid and basioccipital bones is seen in Figure 3-12. The originally cartilaginous chondocranium of the embryo and fetus is now changed in the adult into a midline made up of the nasal septum that maintains cartilage on its anterior parts, the bony ethmoid with its spreading lesser and greater wings, the sphenoid housing the **sella turcica**, the temporal spreading laterally and the occipital spreading posterior to the foramen magnum, around which these bones have developed. The vomer bone is a midline bone that grows beneath the ethmoid bone, which supports the nasal cavities. In (Figure 3-12A) we note the appearance of the basicranium in the newborn and how these bones grow to appear (Figure 3-12B) in the adult.

The **synchondrosis** is an interesting type of junction between bones. First it functions as an attachment to the two opposing bone fronts so that stability is maintained. Second, it functions as a means for growth of the bones bordering the sutures. Third, the cartilages are strong and provide stability of the cranial base. In the center of the synchondrosis is a resting zone where new cartilage cells arise and gradually migrate peripherally, where they increase in size and then divide in the periphery of the synchondrosis. New cartilage is then formed by this means, then calcifies and degenerates, providing space for bone to replace the cartilage along the surface of the bony front. This diagram and histologic view of a synchondrosis is seen in Figure 3-13.

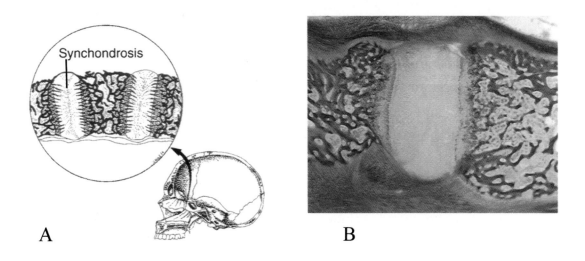

Figure 3-13: A.) Diagram of the location of the cartilage synchondrosis of the cranial base. B.) Appearance microscopically of the synchondrosis. New cartilage is formed along the periphery of the synchondrosis, which calcifies, disintegrates and new bone replaces it on the adjacent fronts.

The cranial base is a stable area and the sychondroses provide for a very important area of growth underlying the brain. In this way, they function in a manner similar to the epiphyseal plates of long bones. The cranial base and the nasal septum are very short in achondroplasia, as are the long bones. Achondroplasia is a deficit in cartilage growth caused by an abnormal FGFR-2 receptor.

The Facial Sutures

As the face grows during childhood the craniofacial sutures allow for enlargement of the brain and face. At birth, the sutures and fontanels between the bones of the skull allow the frontal, parietal and occipital bone to expand. Fontanels are connective-tissue-covered areas of the brain that are located superiorly, medially and laterally, as seen in Figure 3-14. At birth the premaxillary, maxillary, zygomatic and pterygoid sutures each contribute by allowing the adjacent bones to grow and contribute to the face. These facial sutures serve two functions: one in which they provide a means for the opposing bones to grow, and secondly to unite the bones of the face as they attach to the margins of the interfacing bones. During growth there is constant addition of bony increments along the margins of these junctions.

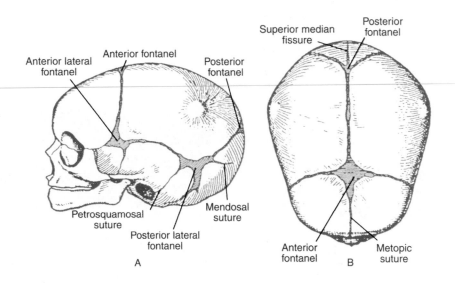

Figure 3-14: The appearance of the cranium at birth. The fontanels are located along the median suture and laterally at the corners of the parietal bones.

Sutures are the means by which growth can occur between these bones. Facial sutures are active during the growth of the head and face. The metopic or interfrontal suture closes at the end of the first year. The paired frontal bones then become unified. The coronal, sagittal and lambdoidal sutures fuse between 20 and 40 years. The spheno-temporal, the occipito-mastoid and squamous sutures may not fuse until age 70. By 10 years of age the skull is 95% complete, whereas the facial skeleton has achieved only 65% of its growth. The face increases 8 to 10 times its volume from birth, while the brain increases only 4 to 5 times its volume.

The second function of the facial suture is a means of uniting and articulating these bones. Facial sutures are composed of connective tissue that separates the opposing surfaces of the facial bones. These **collagen** fibers in their periphery are embedded in the adjacent bony face, and thus tie the bones together with a firm connective tissue bond. The central zone of loose connective tissue is where blood vessels, nerves and nerve endings as well as where osteogenic cells are located. These formative cells will gradually migrate to the periphery of the suture and facilitate new bone growth on the surfaces of the bones bordering the suture.

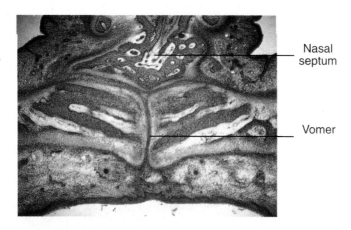

Figure 3-15. This is a cross section view of the face showing the midpalatine suture and the overlying vomer. These sutures allow an increase in size of the face postnatally.

The upper face grows by a complex pattern. As the nasal septum grows in the midline, the vomer grows below it, and the palate has a suture that provides growth in the midline. This arrangement is seen in Figure 3-15. Facial sutures are simple sutures, and an example of the simple suture is seen in Figure 3-16.

Sutural growth will result in enlarging facial bones to maintain a separation and are so positioned to cause the face to move forward and downward. There are four facial sutures, and they are named for the bones they interpose. They are the frontomaxillary, zygomaticomaxillary, zygomaticotemporal and the pterygopalatine. A comparison of the skull and the sutures of the newborn and the adult skull and its sutures indicate the relative size increase of each of the facial bones. Although the sutures maintain a similar relationship, there has been a great deal of growth of each of the bones bordering these sutures (Figure 3-16).

Where the craniofacial sutures are syndesmotic or made up of connective tissue, some are structurally different. The nasal suture is known as a simple suture in which the advancing bony fronts are separated by an outer layer, known as the fibrous capsular layer, in which fibers are embedded in the adjacent bony fronts and terminate at their other ends in the central zone of the suture. The attachment of the adjacent bony fronts by the capsular fibers provides for the integrity of the bony complex. The connective tissue suture thus serves as a hinge, which allows the interfacing bones to maintain a positional relationship as the bones grow.

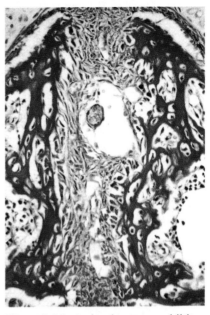

Figure 3-16. A simple suture exhibits collagen bundles in the outer layer, which penetrate into the adjacent bony fronts. In the central or intermediate zone blood vessels can be seen.

Sutures have the ability to bend during the addition of the lamina of bone along the surface of the opposing bony plates. Each of the sutures of the face function in different ways as their positions in the face dictate their direction of growth. Anteriorly, the nasal bone suture is a simple suture and contributes to the lateral growth of the nose. An example of this type of suture is seen in Figure 3-16. Other sutures of the face are simple sutures, although each has different effects on the growth of the face. Because of its horizontal position, the frontomaxillary suture contributes to downward growth of the maxillary bone. The zygomaticomaxillary and the zygomaticotemporal sutures contribute to anterior growth of the face. The relative position of these sutures can be seen in Figures 3-17 and 3-18.

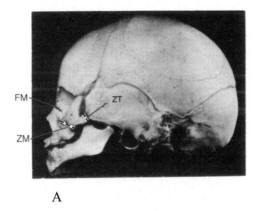

A

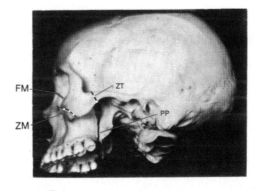

B

Figure 3-17: Sutures of the developing newborn face. FM: Frontomaxillary, ZM: Zygomaticomaxillary and ZT: Zygomaticotemporal.

Figure 3-18: Sutures in the adult face. Compare the location to that of the newborn. FM: Frontomaxillary, ZM: Zygomaticomaxillary and ZT: Zygomaticotemporal.

There are three types of syndesmotic sutures: the squamosal, the serrated, and the simple suture. The simple suture has been described earlier. The squamosal is characterized by an overlap of parallel surfaces of the opposing bones, which are located at an angle to the bones' surfaces. An example of two bones attached to a squamosal suture is the parietal and temporal bones on the sides of the face. The interface of the squamosal suture has collagen fibers with vascular channels present in the center of the suture, and penetrating fibers that attach to the opposing bony fronts. Many of these fibers in the suture are positioned in the long axis of the opposing bony plates. An example of this type of suture is shown in Figure 3-19. The third type of suture is the serrated or interdigitating type suture. This type of suture exists between the cranial bones and is designed to provide a maximum interface between the opposing bones. The function of this suture is to join the bones together with dense **collagen fiber** bundles. An example of this type of suture is seen in Figure 3-20.

In contrast to the synchondroses, which may provide a propulsive force separating bones as they do in the epiphyseal plates, sutural growth is generally considered too passive, with soft tissue growth providing the force separating the bones. This is most clearly demonstrated in the cranium, where growth of the brain provides the force separating the cranial vault bones. The importance of sutural growth is demonstrated by early closure (synostosis) as discussed in Chapter 2 and illustrated in Figure 2-40. If the cranial vault bones are not separated surgically, brain growth is inhibited and the downward force on the roofs of the orbital cavities causes the eyes to protrude (exophthalmos). In Crouzon's syndrome, the genetic defect is in the FGFR-2 receptor (see Chapter 2). The facial sutures also close prematurely, inhibiting midfacial growth. The midfacial deformity can, at least partly, be corrected by surgery.

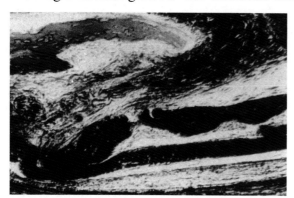

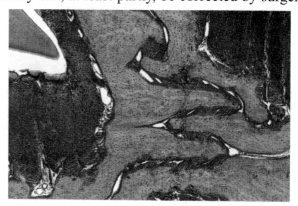

Figure 3-19: A squamous suture in the early stage of development prior to thickening of the overlapping bony plates. Note the presence of the longitudinally positioned fiber bundles.

Figure 3-20: This is a serrated cranial suture. Observe the interdigitating bony fronts and the dense fiber bundles between the interfaces. These sutures provide an interlocking to prevent movement between these bones of the skull except during growth.

3. FUNCTIONAL DEVELOPMENT

Functional development begins long before birth. Synapses, such as those illustrated in Figure 3-21, are set up during the embryonic period. Closure of the **secondary palate** and the onset of bone formation are often considered to signal the end of the embryonic period, but already the embryo is capable of opening and closing its mouth (e.g., Humphrey, 1965), a movement which appears to be necessary for withdrawal of the tongue from between the palatal shelves so that they may elevate. Complex functions such as swallowing are well developed in the fetal period. Fetuses have been observed sucking their thumbs well before birth.

During postnatal development from infancy through adulthood, there are many changes in such functional activities as the maintenance of posture, sucking and swallowing, speech and mastication. Many of them are related to the development of the dentition. Prior to tooth eruption, the tongue fills the space between the gum pads contacting the lips and cheeks along its outer edge. The eruption of the teeth alters many functions, such as the mechanism of swallowing, and enhances the development of speech. These complex functions will be dealt with later, after a consideration of some basic mechanisms such as the development of reflexes.

3.1 DEVELOPMENT OF **REFLEXES**

Many reflexes are established by the beginning of the fetal period in order to support the complex movements noted above. These are, of course, unlearned or spontaneous **reflexes**. Many of the reflexes established during postnatal development are learned, such as those involved in complex movements such as speech and walking. Some reflexes are abnormal, such as tongue thrusting, which frequently causes open bites. Consequently, the ability to modify such reflexes is of considerable interest in orthodontic treatment.

3.1.1. Simple Reflexes

Many simple reflexes are protective in nature. The jaw-closing **reflex** is easily demonstrable. The neuromuscular components are illustrated in Figure 3-21. If one attempts to forcibly depress the mandible, the jaw closing muscles immediately resist the movement. This is accomplished by the muscle spindle, which, in response to stretching, sends an impulse into the central nervous system through the mesencephalic nucleus, where the neuronal cell bodies are located, and from there to the motor nucleus to synapse with the neuronal cell body of the Vth motor neuron, from which an impulse travels back to the mandibular elevators causing them to contract and resist the depressing force. If a hard object is encountered when masticating food, sensory endings primarily in the periodontal ligaments send impulses to the central nervous system to depress the motor neurons, thereby protecting the teeth and periodontal structures. Painful stimuli from the periodontal ligament and TMJ have similar protective effects.

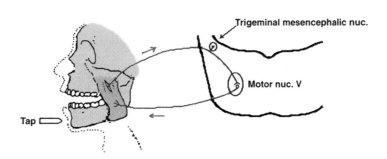

Figure 3-21: The gamma efferent loop in jaw closing muscles. From Junge, 1998

3.1.2. Complex Reflexes

3.1.2.1. Postural Activity of Nerve and Muscle

The mandibular and hyoid bones are best considered as floaters whose position is determined by the muscles to which they are attached (Figure 3-22). In the upright position, the mandibular elevators and the supra- and infra-hyoid muscles keep them in place, together with contributions from the tongue, cheeks and other muscle groups. The elevators and supra-hyoids counteract the effects of gravity. The cranium and face are balanced on top of the vertebral column. The bulk of the cranium and all of the face are in front the vertebral column, and the pull of gravity on these structures must be counteracted by postural activity of the posterior cervical muscles (Figure 3-22). The specialization of different **muscle fibers** for different muscle functions has already been considered. Muscles involved in postural activity are necessarily fatigue-resistant and are richly supplied with capillaries and Type I and Type IIA fibers that contain high concentrations of mitochondria.

There are numerous alterations in function that have major effects on the developing dentition. Perhaps the most severe are those caused by habitual mouth breathing, which is usually caused by obstruction of the airway, most commonly by nasal cavities that are too narrow. In order to provide an oral airway, the tongue and consequently the jaw must be carried in a lower position, which, over time, causes the mandibular angle to open, increasing the height of the lower face and the so-called long face syndrome. Another sequela of these alterations in posture is further narrowing of the maxilla related to the fact that the tongue no longer counteracts the inward pressure of the cheeks.

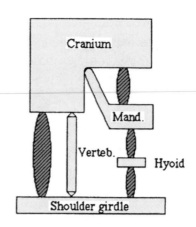

Figure 3-22: The cranium is balanced on the vertebral column by the posterior cervical muscles, counter-balanced by the mandibular elevators and the anterior neck musculature. From Sarnat, 1964.

Much more complex movements are involved in such functions as swallowing, speech and mastication, and these will now be described. The development of the dentition and the development of speech lead to many changes in functions of the orofacial musculature. These will be described separately in the sections below.

3.1.2.2. Swallowing

As noted earlier, one of the first of the complex **reflexes** to develop in the early fetal period is that involved in swallowing and sucking. The muscles and coordinating brain stem nuclei for each phase of swallowing are summarized in Figure 3-23. The electromyographic activity observed in many of these muscles as the bolus of food moves from the oral to the pharyngeal cavities and then into the pharynx and, finally, the stomach is illustrated in Figure 3-24.

MUSCLES OF DEGLUTITION

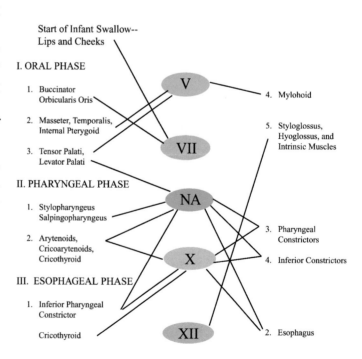

Figure 3-23: Schematic presentation of the muscles involved in swallowing and the brain stem nuclei involved in the coordination of their activity.

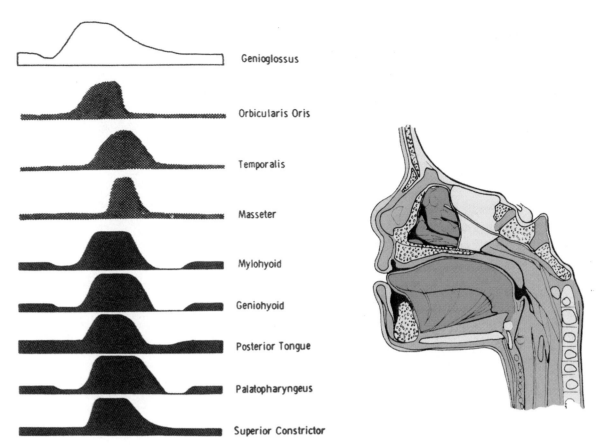

Genioglossus

Orbicularis Oris

Temporalis

Masseter

Mylohyoid

Geniohyoid

Posterior Tongue

Palatopharyngeus

Superior Constrictor

Figure 3-24: Pattern of activity of several muscles involved in a single swallow in the dog as determined by electromyographic activity. From Doty and Bosma, 1967.

Figure 3-25: In the newborn, the lack of dentition requires a different pattern of muscle activity in swallowing, as illustrated in Figure 3-26.

Prior to the development of the dentition the tongue extends to the lips and cheeks, filling the space between the **alveolar ridges** (Figure 3-25). In order to suck and swallow, the infant must maintain the seal between the tongue and the lips and cheeks. Contraction of the lip and cheek muscles can be demonstrated by electromyographic recordings (Figure 3-26). Following eruption of the teeth, activity of the cheek muscles is still necessary to clear any of the food bolus from the cheek vestibule, but from then on the seal is between the tongue and lingual surfaces of the teeth.

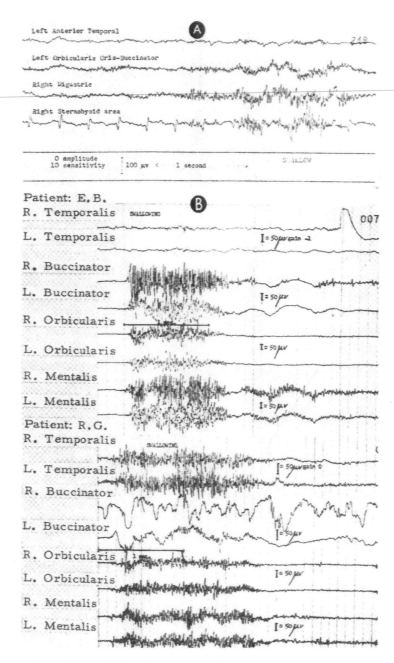

Figure 3-26: A.) Different swallowing patterns as demonstrated
by eletromyographs taken from different muscles in the infant, and
B.) following eruption of the dentition.

Tongue thrusting is a partial maintenance of the infantile swallowing pattern after the teeth have erupted. The tongue is thrust between the incisors and the anterior seal necessary for swallowing is made
between the tongue and lips (Figure 3-27), as it is in the infant. This abnormal pattern leads to an **anterior open bite**, which consists of failure of the incisors to make contact in the occlusal contact position
and an abnormal degree of protrusion of both upper and lower incisors.

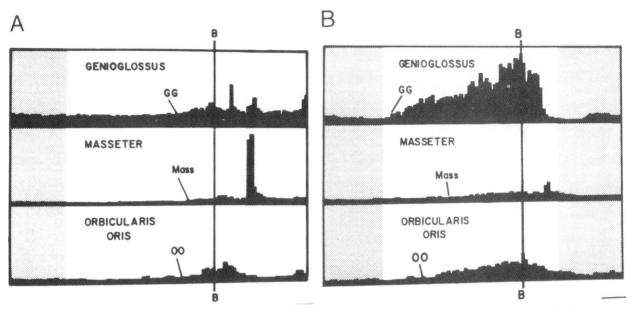

Figure 3-27: Histograms of electromyographic activity from normal and open bite patients. From Lowe and Johnston, 1979.

3.1.2.3. Mastication

Many of the muscles involved in postural activity also have other functions. For example, the masseter is involved in the relatively rapid movements of mastication and must be capable of rapid responses to avoid injuries to the teeth and the temporomandibular joint. The problem of occlusal interference has been noted above. Avoidance of premature contact as a learned (conditional) **reflex** is illustrated in Figure 3-28C. The presence of fairly large numbers of Type I fibers permits the masseter to carry out these functions. The masseter and other muscles involved in mastication also have numerous muscle spindles which help co-ordinate these movements and, together with sensory endings in the tendons, TMJ and periodontal tissues, in the protective functions.

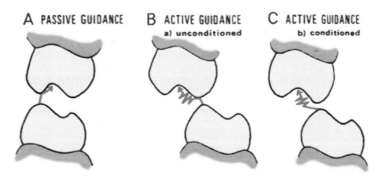

Figure 3-28: Active and passive occlusal guidance.

There is little doubt, however, that even minor occlusal interferences may at least temporarily alter postural muscle activity (Figure 3-28). Such changes were observed in one of this chapter's authors (MCJ) M.Sc.D. thesis in the electromyographic activity of the temporalis muscles in response to occlusal interferences in the mixed dentition caused by deciduous tooth exfoliation. These observations were later confirmed by more extensive studies.

The nature of the relationships between occlusion (and malocclusion) and facial growth has often been contentious. Except for the most severe malocclusions, it is now generally accepted that with modern soft diets, malocclusions do not have large effects on the ingestion of food. Also, it appears that normal occlusion is not necessary for normal facial growth. This has by no means always been the case. For many years, a prominent orthodontic program with a large following taught that normal occlusion was extremely important for normal facial growth, and used this argument to justify arch expansion without tooth extraction to relieve crowding, in the belief that the attainment of normal occlusion would stimulate bone growth to such an extent that the increased jaw size would be sufficient to accommodate all the teeth.

3.1.2.4. Speech

Speech is probably the most complicated of all complex reflexes. It was a major achievement in human evolution and involves precise coordination of many different systems, such as the neuromuscular systems already noted, as well as hearing. While the infant is capable of some aspects of speech, it is only with the eruption of teeth that many sounds are made possible. In particular, the articulation of consonants is greatly facilitated by the dentition, as illustrated in the conformations of oral structures in Figure 3-29. Vowels are less demanding.

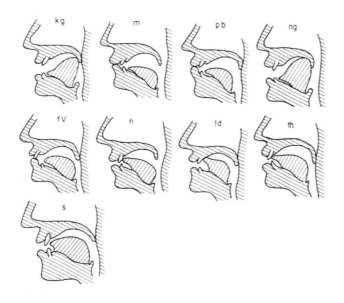

Figure 3-19

Figure 3-29: Articulation of consonant sounds is accomplished by a wide variety of tongue positions. From Jenkins, 1978.

The human shows remarkable abilities in overcoming severe abnormalities of physical structure in order to attain relative clarity of speech. One problem that is not easily overcome is **velopharyngeal insufficiency**, in which the inability to obtain a seal between the soft palate and the posterior wall of the pharynx prevents the accumulation of sufficient intraoral air pressure for the formation of plosive sounds and, consequently, results in nasal speech. This is a common problem in individuals with cleft palate where surgical closure may result in short soft palates, often with reduced mobility as in Figure 3-30A and D. Other neuromuscular defects (Figure 3-30C) or an excessively deep pharynx (Figure 3-30B) may further complicate the picture or cause velopharyngeal incompetence by themselves.

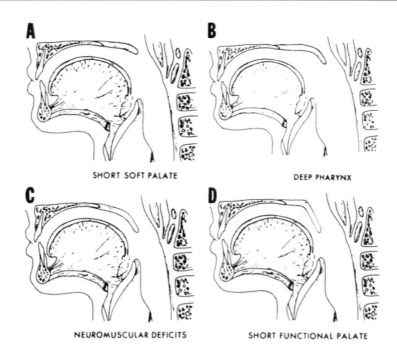

Figure 3-30: Velopharyngeal incompetency is a term used to describe the failure of the soft plate to contact the posterior pharyngeal wall during speech. It is responsible for the hypernasality of some individuals with clefts of the palate although, as indicated, it can result from a number of problems. From Warren, 1979.

4. SUGGESTED READINGS

Bazmajian, JV and De Luca CJ. Muscles Alive: Their Functions Revealed by Electromyography. 5th Ed., Williams and Wilkens, Baltimore 1985.

Bradley RM. Essentials of Oral Physiology. CV Mosby, St Louis 1995.

Carlson DS. Growth of the temporomandibular joint. In: Zarb GA, Carlsson GE, Sessle B, Mohl ND, editors. Temporomandibular joint. 2nd ed. Copenhagen: Munksgaard; 1994. p. 128-58.

Doty RW and Bosma JF. Effect of medullary lesions on coordination of deglutition. J Neurophysiology 1967;19:44-60.

5. Dubner R, Sessle BJ and Storey AT. The Neural Basis of Oral and Facial Function. Plenum, New York 1987.

Hinton RJ, Carlson DS. Effect of function on growth and remodeling of the temporomandibular joint. In: McNeil C, editor. Science and practice of occlusion. Chicago:Quintessence; 1997; pp 95-110.

Humphery T. The development of mouth opening and related reflexes involving the oral area of the human fetus. Ala J Med Sci 1968;5:126:127.

Jenkins GN. Physiology a Biochemistry of the Mouth. (4th ed) Blackwell, Oxford 1978.

Jonston LE (1985) New Vistas in Orthodontics. Lea and Febiger, Philadelphia

Junge D. Oral Sensorimotor Function. Medico Dental Media International, Pacific, Missouri 1998.

Kandel ER and Schwartz JH and Jessel TM (2000) Principles of Neuroscience. 4th ed. McGraw-Hill, New York

Lowe AA and Johnston LE. Tongue and jaw muscle activity in response to mandibular rotations in a sample of normal and anterior open bite subjects. Am J Orthodont 1979;1:345-351.

Miller AJ. Craniomandibular Muscles: Their Role in Function and Form. CRC Press, Boca Raton, FL 2000.

Moss FP and Leblond CP. Satellite cells as the source of nuclei in muscles of growing rats. Anat. Rec. 1971 170:721-435.

Moyers RE. The infantile swallow. Trans Eur Orthodont Soc 1964;40:180-187.

Opperman LA. Cranial sutures as intramembranous bone growth sites. Dev Dyn 2000;219:472-85.

Ringqvist M. Histochemical enzyme profiles of fibres in human masseter muscle with special regard to fibres with intermediate myofibrillar ATPase reaction. J Neurol Sci 1973;18:133-141.

Rhoades R and Pflanzer R. Medical Physiology. 2nd ed. Saunders, Ft. Worth, Texas 1992.

Sarnat BG. The Temporomandibular Joint. 2nd ed. Thomas, Springfield, IL 1964.

20. Storey AT (1988) Maturation of the orofacial musculature. In Moyers RE, Handbook of orthodontics, 4th ed. Yearbook medical publ., Inc. pp 73-94.

Warren DW. Aerodynamic studies of the airway: Implications for growth, breathing and speech. In MacNamara JA (ed.) Nasorespiratory function and Craniofacial growth Monograph, Center for Human Growth and Development, University of Michigan, 1979.

Wolpert LB, Beddington R, Brockes J, Jessel T, Lawernce P and Myerowitz E. Principles of Development. Current Biology Ltd., London 1998.

Zhang M and McClennon IS. The myotubal origin of rat muscle fibres affects the extent of tenotomy-induced atrophy. J Physiol 1999;519:197-202.

Purves, et al., Life: The Science of Biology. W.H. Freeman, 1998

CHAPTER 4

Growth of the Craniofacial Skeleton
Donald H. Enlow

1. INTRODUCTION

At birth, both the oral and nasal components of the face are proportionately small relative to the earlier and faster growing brain, neurocranium, and orbits. A prominent forehead overlies the yet diminutive midface and mandible. Although the facial airway is vertically short during early childhood, it is proportionate to small overall body and lung size. The tiny jaws are proportionate to early suckling and swallowing functions prior to the onset of later childhood masticatory actions.

Early in childhood, the transverse size of the face is notably broad relative to the short vertical dimension. The reason is that the basicranium is wide which, in turn, places articulations for the mandible and maxillae in their early, wide positions. Vertical facial growth later accelerates as precocious brain and neurocranial development declines, and definitive facial configuration takes form. Nasal capacity enlarges paced by continued growing body and lung size. Nasal expansion is produced by a descending relocation of the maxillary and mandibular arches, thereby lengthening the face vertically. The jaws also enlarge considerably as primary and secondary dentition comes into play, together with corresponding expansion of the musculature. Vertical facial size thus belatedly emerges into adult proportions as the breathing and chewing parts of the face progressively develop throughout childhood.

It is important to understand that the basicranium is a developmental template that establishes many structural features of the facial composite suspended from the cranial floor by sutures and condyles. The anterior endocranial fossae relate specifically to the nasomaxillary complex and set up the perimeter of the growth field within which the midface develops. The shape and dimensional proportions of the anterior endocranial fossae determine corresponding features of the nasal region just below it, and the palate is a direct configurational projection. A foreshortened but broad anterior basicranium establishes a like palate, whereas an elongate and narrow anterior basicranium sets up a correspondingly shaped and proportioned palatal arch. Palatal (and upper **alveolar arch**) placement is more protrusive, or less so, as determined by basicranial dimensions and degree of flexure.

In turn, the **apical base** of the maxillary dentition is established by the perimeter of the hard palate, and thus the configuration of the arch is a programmed four-level step-down from the anterior endocranial fossae and frontal lobes of the cerebrum.

The mandibular condyles and rami relate to the middle endocranial fossae and temporal cerebral lobes. This part of the basicranium establishes the proportions of the pharyngeal airway just below it, and the mandibular rami must grow and develop in a coordinated manner that matches the timing and constantly changing size of the middle basicranium and pharynx. These are all elaborately fine-tuned and sensitive developmental interrelationships.

Whereas the mandibular rami (and their component condyles: see below) relate to the middle cranial fossae and function to bridge the pharyngeal space, the size and shape of the mandibular bony and dental arches relate to the overlying maxillary arch, palate, and the anterior endocranial fossae. The vertical and anteroposterior positioning of the lower arch, however, is a key function of the developing rami.

A most significant biologic concept emerges from the conditions outlined in the previous paragraphs. That is, the actual developmental determinants, which program the size, shape and positioning of major facial parts, do not necessarily reside genetically within those regions themselves. Rather, their morphology and morphogenic patterns are, very often, developmental expressions of determining factors located outside of each region itself. This raises the fundamental question as to just what and where are the actual targets for clinical intervention intended to alter regional morphology and the growth process leading to it. It also calls into question the specific causes and sources of "rebound", since the original but continuing conditions that determine a given part's shape and size can reside in locations unaffected by the clinical procedure.

A good regional example of the situation just described is the incisor region ("premaxilla") of the maxillary complex. As seen above, the "genetics" that regulate its development are not wholly resident within its own tissues and cells, and changing childhood and ultimate adult sizes and shapes are designed largely elsewhere in the craniofacial complex. In addition, by far the greater amount of the premaxillary region's own growth movement is produced by other parts external to the region itself. Thus, if a clinician does not fully understand these basic morphogenic relationships, how can clinical rationale be understood since it "works with growth"?

A characteristic feature of the child's face is a retrusive mandible. The developmental reason is the differential nature of the precocious growth of the anterior endocranial fossae, which have completed most growth increases by about six years of age. Since this part of the basicranium is the platform from which the nasomaxillary complex is suspended by sutures, forward neurocranial enlargement carries the maxillae anteriorly with it. Condylar articulation of the mandible relates to a different, more posterior basicranial growth field with a different developmental timing (middle endocranial fossae). The result is a differential in the time of maxillary versus mandibular anterior displacements (see below) and a transient retrognathic condition.

Because variations in headform (dolichocephalic, **brachycephalic**, dinaric) are characterized by differences in anteroposterior and transverse basicranial proportions and flexure alignments, corresponding differences in facial patterns exist. Different facial types are known to respond differently to various clinical procedures, although a comprehensive catalogue has yet to be developed and compiled.

2. GROWTH, DEVELOPMENT AND MORPHOGENIC MOVEMENTS

2.1 DIFFERENTIAL GROWTH

Growth is a "differential" process, which means that different parts and regions undergo this complex process at different times, by different amounts, in different directions, and involve different but interrelated and interdependent functions. These factors are why the term "and development" properly accompanies the word "growth". Use of the word "growth" without elucidation can present an incomplete and misleading picture. The frequently used term "condylar growth" is a good example and actually encourages a serious oversimplification of complex, multifactorial developmental and clinical issues.

2.2 GROWTH MOVEMENTS

One of the most fundamental of all the important morphogenic concepts is the basic distinction between the two great types of growth movements. Most of the other concepts that follow are dependent on it, yet so often this distinction is bypassed in textbooks, lectures, journal reports and seminars involving facial development and effects of clinical appliances on the growth process.

2.1.1. Remodeling

Two distinct and quite different types of morphogenic movements occur for each and all craniofacial skeletal components (Figures 4-1 and 4-2).

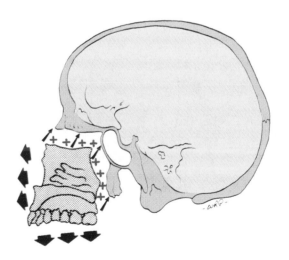

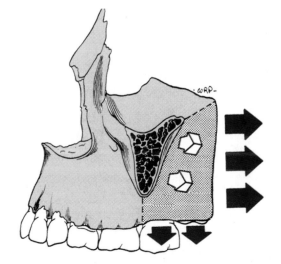

Figure 4-1: The entire nasomaxilla is displaced forward and downward by the enlarging soft tissues of the face and pharynx (large arrows). This separates the facial bones at their articulations, and the remodeling process (+) is activated at the same time which enlarges the bone into the places created by the displacement. (Adapted by Enlow, D., *Facial Growth*, 3rd Edition., W.B. Saunders, Pub., 1990)

Figure 4-2: The principle vector of maxillary arch lengthening is backward by remodeling at the maxillary tuberosity. (Adapted by Enlow, D., *Facial Growth*, 3rd Edition., W.B. Saunders, Pub., 1990)

They are, however, mutually serving and companion to each other. One of these, briefly described first, is produced by the coordinated mosaic of **remodeling** actions. These changes do not proceed, as often implied, primarily at special growth sites or centers. They take place on <u>all</u> inside and outside surfaces throughout all parts of any given bone. There are regional "fields" of osteogenic (osteoblastic and osteoclastic) activity that blanket all surfaces, the patterns of which are more or less characteristic for any given bone (Figures 4-3, 4-4, and 4-5).

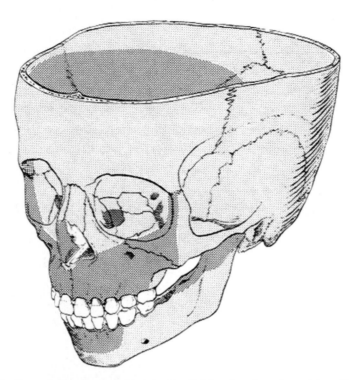

Figure 4-3: Remodeling is carried out by the fields of surface **deposition** (light areas) and **resorption** (dark areas) (Adapted from Enlow, D., T. Kuroda, and A. Lewis, Angle Orthod, 41:161 1971)

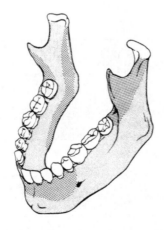
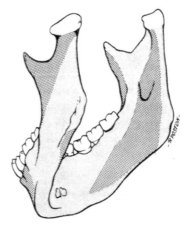

Figure 4-4: Remodeling fields of deposition (light areas) and resorption (dark areas) in the human mandible. Compare with 4-5, 4-6 and 4-8 (Adapted from Enlow, D., **Facial Growth**, 3rd Edition., W.B. Saunders, Pub., 1990)

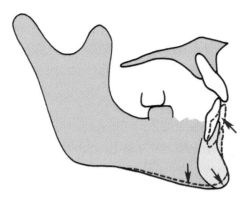

Figure 4-5: Fitting the mandibular anterior teeth to the maxillary arch involves alveolar remodeling adjustments. In this example, the lower teeth undergo retroclination into an overbite and overjet position involving surface resorption on the labial alveolar side. Deposition occurs on the mental protuberance. This combination produces the enlarging chin. There is much developmental variation in this part of the mandible. (Adapted from Enlow, D, *Facial Growth*, 3rd Edition., W.B. Saunders, Pub., 1990)

Remodeling is carried out by the various types of osteogenic connective tissues that occur on particular surfaces, including periosteum, endosteum, periodontal membranes, sutural membranes, condylar cartilages and synchondroses.

Several basic growth functions are carried out by the remodeling process, one of which is to provide overall enlargement. Many external surfaces are actually resorptive, and such locations have an endosteal side that is depository (Figures 4-5 and 4-6). To enlarge a given bone or some part of it, new bone is added onto whatever surface (inner or outer) faces the growth direction, with osteoclastic action on the contralateral side.

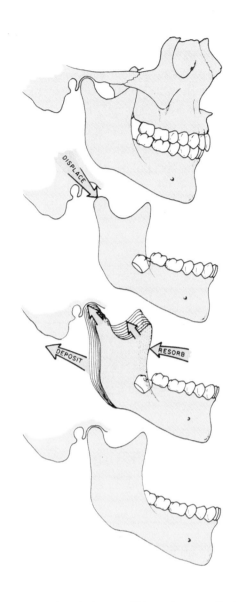

Figure 4-6: As the whole mandible undergoes displacement downward and forward, the ramus and condyle remodel in an opposite and backward direction. The extents of displacement and remodeling precisely compliment each other. (Adapted from Enlow, D., *Facial Growth*, 3rd Edition., W.B. Saunders, Pub., 1990)

For example, the oral side of the palate points inferiorly, and that bone surface is thus osteoblastic. The opposite nasal side is largely osteoclastic, and this combination moves the palate downward to contribute to nasal airway expansion (Figure 4-7). Variations in this combination, however, can produce configurational and rotational variations (see below), which is a second function of remodeling.

This is to establish the shape of a bone, and to progressively fine-tune it as development continues. In order to achieve both size and shape in the constantly changing child's craniofacial complex, the remodeling process produces successive relocations of its component parts (third function). This involves the remodeling movement, by means of osteogenic connective tissue actions, of all the parts progressively away from each other. Thus, to lengthen the corpus of the mandible, for example, the ramus is relocated posteriorly by periosteal, endosteal and condylar remodeling. This process also enlarges and reshapes the ramus itself at the same time. The area formerly occupied by the ramus is remodeled and converted into the elongating corpus at its distal end (Figure 4-6). Similarly, in order to enlarge the nasal chambers, the palate becomes relocated progressively in an inferior direction (Figure 4-7), and what was previously the palate becomes remodeled and converted into the expanding nasal region. (Note: The second type of growth movement, "**displacement**", is also involved, as described later.)

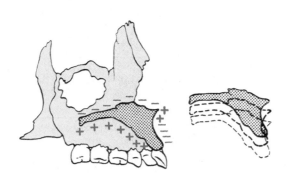

Figure 4-7: Palatal remodeling is produced by fields of resorption and deposition along the nasal and oral surfaces. (Adapted from Enlow, D., *Facial Growth*, 3rd Edition., W.B. Saunders, Pub., 1990)

A fourth major function of the remodeling process is to provide precision goodness of fit between a bone and its articulation(s) with other bones, and also its exacting fit with all of the attaching soft tissues. Consider the absolute perfection, with no tolerance whatsoever, of the **coronoid process** and its temporalis muscle; or a cranial nerve (moving as the whole head and brain grow) and its moving, precisely shaped and sized foramen; or a tooth root and its conforming socket. This ultimate matching and fitting is provided by reciprocal exchanges of **osteogenic**, **fibrogenic**, **cytogenic** and myogenic information among all of the multiple parts involved. Everything precisely fits because each bone is custom fitted to its contiguous tissues by turn-on and turn-off signals from those particular tissues. (Question: at what variable points does clinical intervention enter this cascade of events?)

A fifth function of remodeling is to provide ongoing adaptive adjustments of a bone to accommodate ever-changing intrinsic and extrinsic conditions and circumstances as they occur. All of the separate parts continue to function as each progressively grows, remodels, and develops.

It is noted that, although "remodeling" is often associated primarily with bone, the soft tissues themselves, including the osteogenic connective tissues, also have their own intrinsic growth and remodeling processes.

2.2.2. Displacement

The second major category of morphogenic growth movement is the process of **displacement** (also termed a **translatory movement**). This movement proceeds in concert with the remodeling (relocation) movements just described (Figure 4-6). Both must occur in conjunction with one another. Together, their combined movements are the movements of growth.

Displacement is the gross, *in toto* movement of a whole bone as it simultaneously undergoes relocation, shaping, sizing, and fitting by the companion remodeling process (Figures 4-1 and 4-6). Whole bones become carried apart (displaced) as all of the enclosing soft tissues grow and enlarge, thus separating bones at their articular junctions. Remember, soft tissues attach to the bones, directly or indirectly, by the anchoring fibers of Sharpey. Separations at the articular interfaces by this displacement process establish the "spaces" into which the bones remodel. Displacement determines the amount of linear elongation of a bone. Because bone-to-bone joints are the sites from which displacement movements proceed, they are noteworthy as the clinical targets for procedures attempting to either increase or to restrain the amount of movement or to alter the direction of movement.

3. CLINICAL SIGNIFICANCE OF DISPLACEMENT AND REMODELING INTERPLAY

Researchers have, historically, debated which of these two morphogenic movements is actually primary (first occurring) and which is a secondary sequel. That is, does remodeling cause a displacing push, or conversely, does displacement act as the pacesetting event, which subsequently activates remodeling? While this argument has been a great stimulus to research over the years, it is likely that the biology itself does not concern itself with any primary versus secondary confrontation. Rather, the two are complimentary, companion processes that proceed together in morphogenic coordination, one with the other, under the aegis of an intrinsic control system that is still somewhere beyond our full understanding.

To illustrate the importance of taking into account these two fundamental categories of growth movement, two examples are given. It is pointed out that past clinical research in facial development has not usually made a distinction between them. This is a shortcoming that has severely compromised research findings.

The first example, already mentioned briefly, involves the alveolar region in the incisor part of the maxilla, an area of frequent clinical attention. The extent to which "growth" in this premaxillary region is movement by remodeling versus displacement has almost never been considered or analyzed in clinical studies. A fingertip can be used for an analogy. Most of the fingertip's growth elongation away from the shoulder joint through the childhood years is by displacement as all of the intervening bones (humerus, radius, etc.) and their soft tissues progressively lengthen. Only a small fraction of the total extent of the fingertip's growth movement is a product of its own local remodeling. Similarly, most of the premaxillary growth movement is not a product of its own direct, intrinsic, local genetically determined remodeling within its own osteogenic matrix (Figure 4-1). Rather, by far the greater percentage of actual growth movement is produced 1.) in conjunction with all of the <u>other</u> regional ethmomaxillary areas above and behind as they all progressively enlarge, and 2.) by expansion of the **basicranium** and its soft tissues. Thus, where are the actual specific tissue targets for intervention into the growth control process as they relate to particular clinical objectives? Add to this consideration the factor of developmental "balance" described later.

A second example is the functional basis for how functional appliances actually operate. Briefly, the remodeling/displacement factor, as well as many other basic morphogenic concepts, again has been bypassed. Attention often still centers on such anachronisms as "condylar growth" (see below).

4. DEVELOPMENTAL ROTATIONS

4.1 REMODELING ROTATION

Rotations occurring during facial growth are an important consideration in understanding normal anatomic variations, etiology of malocclusions, and clinical interventions into the biologic process of facial development. However, the subject has become confused in the literature because of divergent systems for classifying them and the use of difficult to understand or inappropriate terminologies. Because all rotational growth movements are a natural product of one or the other of the two basic types of growth movement (remodeling and displacement), it seems a needless complication not to simply classify them as such, since that is just what they are. A "remodeling rotation" is produced by osteogenic connective tissues and involves osteoblastic and osteoclastic remodeling that alters the alignment relationship between parts in the same bone or between separate bones. A palatal rotation resulting from contrasting fields of deposition and resorption along its mesial-to-distal length on both the oral and nasal sides is one example. Another example is an alteration of the ramus-to-corpus alignment by remodeling of the growing ramus (Figure 4-8). This opens or closes the "**gonial angle**" to produce a ramus that is either more or less upright.

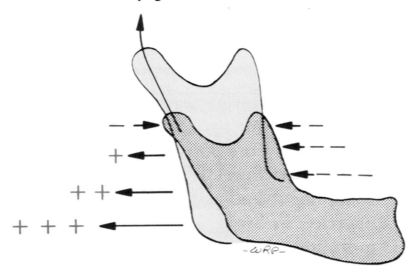

Figure 4-8: Variable fields of remodeling produce changes in the direction of the ramus development. In this example, the ramus is becoming more upright and the gonial angle is decreasing in order to accommodate the vertical enlargement of the nasomaxillary complex. (Adapted from Enlow, D., *Facial Growth*, 3rd Edition., W.B. Saunders, Pub., 1990)

4.2 DISPLACEMENT ROTATION

A "displacement rotation" is a realignment of a whole bone *in toto*, whether or not it is also remodeling at the same time. It is a result of mechanical force exerted on a bone from a source external to the bone itself. Thus, the palate can be rotated clockwise or counterclockwise because the whole maxilla can undergo rotations associated with differential extents of sutural growth or altered basicranial flexure. This occurs whether or not the palate is also "rotating" by its own osteogenic (periosteal-endosteal) remodeling at the same time. Similarly, a "displacement rotation" of the mandible takes place when the whole mandible realigns downward and backward or upward and forward in conjunction with either variable nasomaxillary vertical dimensions or variations in basicranial flexure or proportions. Frequently, a remodeling rotation can compensate for a displacement rotation. For example, brain and basicranial growth can lead to a middle cranial fossa rotation by displacement; but, a basicranial misfit with the mandible and maxilla can be precluded by an adjustive remodeling rotation of the ramus. (See Enlow and Hans, *Essentials of Facial Growth*, W. B. Saunders, Publishers, 1996, for further details and examples.)

It is pointed out that <u>combinations</u> of displacement and remodeling rotation are usually the rule, since if either one occurs, so must the other when involving articular junctions.

5. CONDYLAR FUNCTION

5.1 **CONDYLE** AS GROWTH CENTER

The clinical literature dealing with mandibular growth has tended to lag behind certain conceptual advances in recent years. Few researchers, familiar with the issues involved, still regard the condyle as a "growth center" responsible for a genetic blueprint that determines the course of mandibular development or which is a pacemaker for its remodeling and displacement processes. What essential growth functions, then, does the condyle indeed serve? Of course, it provides a pressure tolerant and compression resistant articular surface within a moveable joint. The condylar cartilage is also, as an endochondral "**growth cartilage**", a developmental equivalent to the traction-adapted periosteum elsewhere in the mandible. This means that the non-vascular condyle can provide for bone growth in a <u>pressure</u> situation, whereas intramembranous periosteal bone growth relates to tension conditions as in muscle and tendon attachments. Pressure relationships are not possible for highly vascular osteogenic tissues (periosteum, sutures) in which a low-threshold compressive force would close the sensitive capillary plexus.

Beyond this regional, mechanical articular developmental role, the condyle also participates in another, very significant growth function. This is far more noteworthy than its former presumed role as a "master growth center."

5.2 RAMUS-CONDYLE COMPOSITE

It is not <u>just</u> the condyle, however, but the <u>whole ramus</u> that performs this special developmental function. The particular condyle <u>and</u> ramus combination has been largely overlooked heretofore because the focus has been essentially on the condyle. It is the <u>whole</u> ramus, with its component condyle, that serves as the key regional adaptive structure responsible for properly placing the corpus and lower arch in functional position relative to the nasomaxillary complex above and middle cranial fossa behind. Because of architectonic complexities involved in the composite morphology of the whole craniofacial complex, a latitude of deviations is inevitable, but a "best fit" is achieved through developmental interplay among the ramus and the other principal cranial and facial parts. Herein lies the great functional significance of the whole ramus-condyle composite during facial growth. It provides for its own growth in such a way as to adapt to the multiple, variable, morphogenically changing conditions around it to give mandibular <u>arch</u> fitting, all the while functioning in attachments for the masticatory musculature.

The vertical development of the ramus must match the composite vertical lengthening of the nasal and oral parts of the midface and, at the same time, take into account changing vertical and horizontal basicranial growth and, further, the nature of flexure of the basicranium and its changes. Variations in headform type and resultant facial and basicranial configuration are also involved. Inadequate vertical ramus adjustive accommodation results in an open or deep bite. A tall order, indeed, for the ramus, but there is yet more.

At the same time all of the above developmental activities are underway, the anteroposterior breadth of the ramus must continuously growth-adapt to match the changing size of the **pharyngeal space**. The ramus bridges this space, which is size determined by the growing middle cranial fossae and temporal lobes of the cerebrum. Headform variations as well as geometric complexities and differences in the vertical and horizontal timing of nasal, oral, anterior cranial fossa, and middle cranial fossa development all come into play. Any significant ramus horizontal mismatch leads directly to mandibular arch **retrusion** or **protrusion**.

It is apparent that, for its developmental functions, the ramus is quite special. Yet, it has never been accorded the distinction it truly deserves in our teaching, anatomy textbooks, and understandings of etiologies of malocclusions, treatment theories, and how certain clinical treatment procedures actually work. All of the above, for example, underlie just how "functional regulators" operate. (See Figure 1-7 in Enlow, D. and M. Hans, *Essentials of Facial Growth*, W. B. Saunders, Publ., 1996.)

6. FUNCTION AND GROWTH INTERPLAY

6.1 FUNCTIONAL MATRIX

The question has often been asked, "Do you believe in the **Functional Matrix**?" A proper response, of course, can be "a form-function relationship is an old and respected principle in general biology." The problem is, then, why the Functional Matrix "theory" has not been successfully tested experimentally and thereby forthrightly either proven or discredited to everyone's satisfaction. To respond to this perplexing problem, which has bothered craniofacial theorists for over a generation, the following evaluation is presented.

If active parts of the mandible's **Functional Matrix** (masticatory muscles, for example) proceed to function, that is, to contract, the result is an upward and backward mechanical effect on the mandible. Yet, mandibular growth is described as forward and downward. Thus, there is a direct conflict that would seem to refute the Functional Matrix concept. Similarly, function of other Functional Matrix components, the facial musculature, has a backward and upward effect on the maxilla as well as mandible, thereby again conflicting with the conventional downward and forward facial growth tenet.

How can these troublesome hang-ups in growth theory be resolved? The answer parallels situations in many past research studies that have bypassed certain basic developmental principles, thus leading to dilemmas and fruitless outcomes.

Briefly, two important considerations were omitted in presenting the above problem, as they often have been in research attempts to "prove or disprove the Functional Matrix". First, basic distinction was not made between the **remodeling** movement of growth and the **displacement** movement. As emphasized before, this is essential, and unless done, proper growth interpretations are subject to confusion. The forward and downward "growth" referred to above actually represents composite displacement movements emanating from the basicranium as well as the ethmomaxillary and mandibular complex. Remodeling by osteogenic activity is the additional key aspect to be considered, but separately and unmerged into simplistic "growth". Enlargement, production of configuration, fitting, and all of the other essential functions of remodeling were simply ignored.

6.2 GROWTH ENLARGEMENT

The second basic omission is also a critical consideration. No basic distinction was made between function of the Functional Matrix (muscle contraction was the example given) and the growth and development of the tissue components comprising the Functional Matrix. Growth enlargement (separate from "function") of the masticatory muscles in length has a downward displacing effect on the mandible. Muscle enlargement in breadth has a mandibular protruding displacement effect. For the facial muscles, outward growth expansion (independent of their functional contractions), similarly, has an outward and downward carrying (displacing) effect on the maxilla as well as the mandible. While this is happening, function (contraction) signals the osteogenic tissues (periosteum and endosteum, condyles, sutures, etc.) to respond, thereby shaping and sizing the many regional parts of the lower and upper jaws to fit the very soft tissues and organs which generate the signals. Without distinguishing between function and growth, interrelated and physiologically inseparable as they actually are, meaningful interpretations of experiments are thus virtually impossible.

7. ARCHITECTONIC RELATIONSHIPS

7.1 BASICRANIUM AS A TEMPLATE

7.1.1. **Dolichocephalic** Headform

The term "**architectonic**" describes the dynamics involved in the reciprocal interrelationships that are ongoing among the many separate parts throughout the growing, functioning craniofacial composite.

There are two particular morphologic conditions that predispose such relationships and which underlie the establishment of an individual's facial form and pattern. One of these, as already mentioned, is the basicranium because it is the template for setting up the facial proportions and circumscribing the growth field within which the face develops. Thus, an elongate and narrow (**dolichocephalic**) headform relates to a corresponding facial configuration (leptoprosopic). The characteristic obtuse basicranial flexure and vertically long midface produce an inferoposterior alignment (displacement rotation) of the mandible with a resultant Class II tendency.

7.1.2. **Brachycephalic** Headform

Conversely, a rounded (**brachycephalic**) headform relates to a flatter, wider, and less retrognathic (**euryprosopic**) face. There is a much greater built-in tendency for an orthognathic profile or mandibular or **bimaxillary protrusion**. The dinaric headform has a long and narrow face, but because of its extreme basicranial flexure caused by the brachycephalization of the neurocranium, a lesser degree of mandibular **retrusion** than among dolichocephalics is usually seen. If a Class II exists in a dinaric individual, it is a different anatomic type because there are mandibular protrusive features mixed with the other regional facial features. Responses to clinical procedures are also different (See Enlow and Hans, *Essentials of Facial Growth*, W. B. Saunders, Publishers, 1996 and Chapter 7, Section 3 and Glossary).

Countless population variations and intermediate combinations of all these craniofacial typings exist. This is clinically significant because corresponding variations occur in the facial growth process. This means that a considerable range of sub-groupings also exists for Class I, II, and III malocclusions, and that responses to clinical procedures thereby vary in kind. Unfortunately, a comprehensive catalogue of such variations and their responses has yet to be worked out and compiled. This is because, simply, insufficient information presently exists to do so.

7.2 FACIAL AND PHARYNGEAL AIRWAY

Another architectonic relationship involved as a developmental determinant involves the facial and pharyngeal airway. This is of special significance because of direct involvement in the etiology of malocclusions and other dysplasias. In a real sense, the airway is a "keystone" within the face, structurally as well as developmentally. Any significant variation or any compromise of its shape and dimensions during development affects all contiguous facial parts. Mouth breathing and jaws-open swallowing, for example, require extensively different patterns of muscle functions which result in different signals to the osteogenic connective tissues of the nasal and mandibulomaxillary complex. This leads to different childhood growth patterns and divergent facial morphology. Growth has responded to achieve a revised state of balance, and the consequence is a balanced malocclusion.

8. MORPHOGENIC ADJUSTMENTS

As we have seen, facial growth is an ongoing, long-term process that constantly creates momentary imbalances produced by the growth changes themselves. As these changes proceed, however, growth also works toward composite balance. This requires interplays of continuous adjustments by the remodeling process. Growth changes and responses to growth changes among all the separate craniofacial parts ensure that 1.) everything more-or-less fits everything else (considering the multiple structural complexities involved), and that 2.) everything continues to function all the while.

8.1 NET COMPOSITE BALANCE

Growth thus functions as "nature's clinician." Because of architectural complexities, it is virtually impossible to achieve geometric perfection in overall structural assembly. Adjusting or balancing any one structural fitting would likely imbalance another, and so on. Net composite balance, thus, virtually always involves certain regional imbalances and certain malocclusion adjustments that have "corrected" what otherwise would have been a more severe malocclusion into one that is less so.

8.2 DEVELOPMENTAL ADJUSTMENT

A **leptoprosopic** facial type and **dolichocephalic** headform often have a Class II predisposition, and a **euryprosopic** has a greater Class III programmed tendency, as mentioned previously. During growth and development, however, the morphogenic process itself "compensates" to provide an aggregate anatomic balance to the extent possible in a given person, considering the limitless range of variations. Thus, childhood growth in most individuals converts such tendencies into a Class I or less severe Class II or III. Some of these intrinsic adjustments (not all) can be the same as utilized by clinicians in the design of certain treatment procedures.

A noteworthy example of a regional structure involved in developmental adjustment is the mandibular ramus, as mentioned briefly before. An infant that is "programmed" to become mandibular retrusive by virtue of an elongate basicranium, an obtuse basicranial flexure, a vertically long nasomaxillary region, a downward-backward mandibular "displacement rotation," and a closed ramus-corpus "remodeling rotation," can be subject to some measure of intrinsic correction by 1.) an anteroposterior broadening of the rami during growth to match the elongate middle cranial fossae and broad pharyngeal space; 2.) an upward drift of the anterior mandibular teeth to produce a dentoalveolar curve that closes what otherwise would have been an open bite; 3.) a vertical lengthening of the rami to match the vertically long nasal region; and 4.) an alteration in the ramus-to-corpus alignment ("gonial angle"), as seen in Figure 4-8.

8.3 PALATE

Another regional adjustive site is the palate. To enlarge the nasal chambers superior to it during development, the whole maxilla is displaced inferiorly, carrying the palate with it. The palate also remodels in a net downward direction. Why do both types of inferior growth movement occur? The reason is that the development of the basicranium as well as the maxilla and nasal region itself result in variable directions and amounts of maxillary "displacement rotations," carrying the palate with them. Leveling of the palate into functional position requires an adjustment by the remodeling process involving contrary depository and resorptive activities along the oral and nasal length of the palate. That is, the nasal/oral distribution of remodeling fields produces a "remodeling rotation" that corrects the "displacement rotation" by proper amount and direction.

8.4 LACRIMAL BONE

While virtually all regions and parts everywhere throughout the craniofacial composite are involved in some way and to some degree in give-and-take compensatory growth adjustments, another particular site is especially noteworthy, yet its special role has been all but unknown. This is the tiny flake of a bone, the lacrimal. Receiving little attention in textbooks and no special praise at all by anatomy teachers, this diminutive element provides a basic growth function so essential that virtually all normal neurocranial and facial development among all mammals depends expressly and specifically on it. This is why the **lacrimal bone** has survived as a separate little unit during evolution, whereas massive fusions and consolidations have occurred among the other cranial elements.

The lacrimal bone is an island surrounded by osteogenic sutural connective tissue. It is pivotally situated as a key hub among the constellation of major bones including the maxilla, ethmoid, frontal, and sphenoid. All of those great bones and their soft tissues are growing, remodeling, and displacing in a complex of different directions, at different times, and by different amounts involving different functions. The adjustive capacity of the lacrimal bone's sutural system operates strategically in the midst of actions shared by the multiple happenings around it. This provides the essential developmental buffer, which allows the divergent growth changes and the "sliding" of bones along their sutural margins to proceed. Without this, these differential morphogenic events would not be possible; everything would simply coalesce into a premature gridlock. This praiseworthy lacrimal function offers research opportunity to help better understand dysplasias such as **Crouzon's**, **Apert's**, **hypertelorism**, and similar growth-arrested conditions. Whether cause or effect, the lacrimal is certain to be involved in some basic way.

9. PERIODONTAL CONNECTIVE TISSUE

9.1 PERIODONTAL MEMBRANE

A component of the craniofacial composite that carries out morphogenic functions important to the clinician, yet which often has not been highlighted, is the **periodontal membrane**. It is referred to here as membrane rather than ligament because its developmental role extends far beyond just fibrous attachment, as connoted by the term ligament.

Consider the remarkable coordination involved in the symphony of actions that carry out ordinary intrinsic tooth movement, as well as clinically manipulated movements that utilize the same intrinsic growth process (See Chapter 8).

9.2 REMODELING MOVEMENTS

A tooth is moved by the pulling action of the periodontal collagenous fibers on the leading side (for example, by contractions of attached myofibroblasts in the periodontal membrane). As the tooth moves, the periodontal connective tissue itself, including its fibers, multiple cell types, and glycoprotein matrix also undergoes movement by the membrane's own remodeling process. As the periodontal membrane remodels and moves ahead of the tooth it is pulling, the **alveolar bone** on this leading side is removed by the membrane's **osteoclasts** and by amounts that <u>exactly</u> equal 1.) the distance the tooth is being displaced, 2.) the direction the tooth is being moved, 3.) the timing of these same events, and 4.) in the same directions, amounts, and timing of the periodontal remodeling movements. Then, on the trailing side of the tooth, the same **alveolar bone** and periodontal movements involving bone deposition proceed <u>in concert</u> by amounts, directions, and timing all equal and in <u>precise</u> coordination. There is no latitude for any differences whatsoever. The precision and the tolerances are exact with no margin of error at all. Even a minute differential in any of these events would shortly lead to either an **ankylosis** or a tooth-alveolar loosening. All of this is a most wondrous control and developmental system.

A tooth does not have an intrinsic capacity for its own mobility. While bone can be moved by the process of osteogenic remodeling, a tooth must be moved by some force external to it (displacement). For both bone and tooth, these growth movements are subject to manipulation by substituting extrinsic (clinical) control that replaces in part the intrinsic regulation of the morphogenic process. The factor of "architectonic balance" then comes into play, as outlined next.

10. ARCHITECTONIC BALANCE

It has been emphasized that clinical procedures intervene into the growth regulation system but utilize the same actual biology involved in ordinary development. Directions, amounts, or timing can be revised by altering in controlled ways the control factors that determine the course of growth. However, it has also been emphasized that growth works toward transient states of "balance" even as growth itself continuously creates regional imbalances. Clinical procedures also, of course, cause developmental and architectonic imbalances, and herein lay significant clinical problems because many possible contingencies exist. In brief, if the original conditions that caused some regional imbalance (such as basicranial proportions) were not altered by a given clinical treatment, the result can activate the growth process returning it to the original course of development. This, then, effectively erases the clinical results. The outcome, of course, is known as relapse, or rebound, but is actually "growth working toward a state of balance." However, the situation is multifactorial with many perplexing possibilities. For example, if growth could be accurately predicted, very early treatment could then allow many subsequent years of "normal" growth which could achieve revised states of clinically altered balance. For continued examples of these complicated problems, see Figure 1-1 in Enlow and Hans, *Essentials of Facial Growth*, W. B. Saunders, Publisher, 1996.

11. REGIONAL GROWTH SUMMARY

Beginning arbitrarily with the bony maxillary arch, the a.) remodeling and b.) displacement of each major craniofacial region is separately explained in Figures 4-9 to 4-25. This series illustrates the basic principle that the development of all facial and basicranial parts is necessarily interdependent in order to achieve precise fitting and necessary functional interrelationships. As each region is briefly described, the question is then asked for each region as to "what other region(s) must undergo comparable growth changes in order to ensure such fitting and uninterrupted function?" The series then proceeds to those part-to-counterpart regions in turn. All such regional growth processes proceed simultaneously.

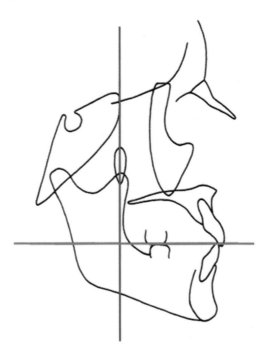

Figure 4-9: Two reference lines are shown. The horizontal line is the functional occlusal plane, and the vertical line extends from the interface between the anterior endocranial fossa and the middle endocranial fossa. Note that the former is the roof precisely overlying the facial airway and the whole nasomaxillary complex, and the latter is the roof for the pharyngeal space. (From Enlow, D., and R. Moyers, Growth and Architecture of the Face, J.A.D.A., 82:763, 1971.)

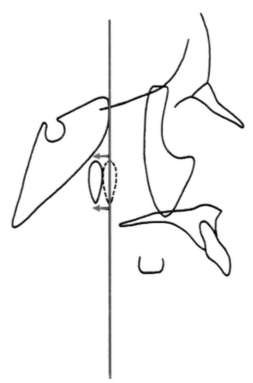

Figure 4-10: To achieve anteroposterior lengthening of the maxillary arch, the maxillary tuberosity remodels posteriorly, as revealed by its radiographic landmark, the pterygomaxillary fissure (PTM).

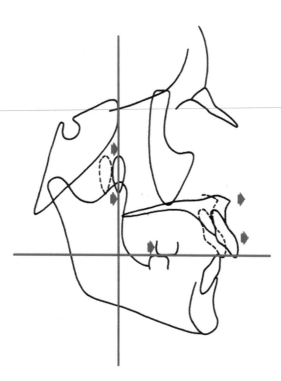

Figure 4-11: The maxillary tuberosity does not, of course, actually invade the space of the facial airway because the posterior remodeling (previous Figure) is accompanied simultaneously by anterior diplacement of the entire nasomaxillary complex by an equal magnitude. Note PTM is "returned" to the vertical reference line, from which it never actually departed.

Note that the premaxillary (incisor) region has become thrust protrusively even though the actual remodeling process itself occurred in the region of the tuberosity.

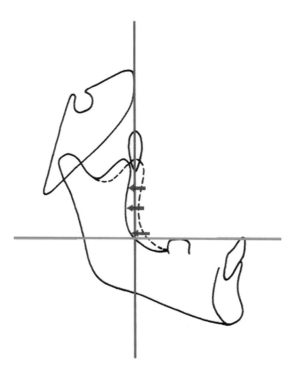

Figure 4-12: What must now "balance" the changes just described? The mandibular corpus must undergo comparable counterpart growth changes. To achieve corpus anteroposterior lengthening, the ramus must be moved posteriorly by remodeling. This stage shows the anterior border undergoing resorptive removal.

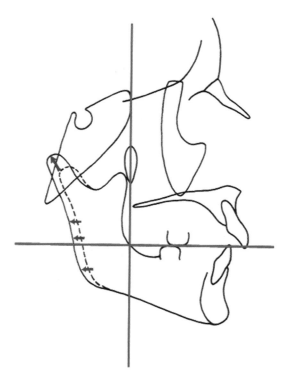

Figure 4-13: An equal amount of bone deposition is simultaneously added along the posterior border of the ramus. The magnitude of posterior ramus remodeling now equals that of the maxilla.

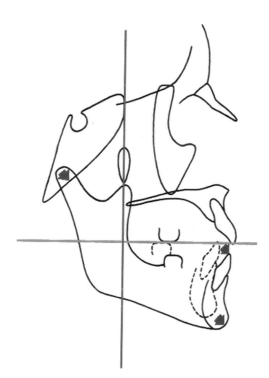

Figure 4-14: The entire mandible becomes displaced anteriorly by an amount that equals maxillary anterior displacment. Note that a vertical "separation" occurs between the maxillary and mandibular arches. Note also that a Class I molar relationship has been returned.

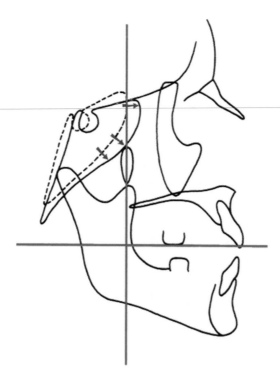

Figure 4-15: In conjunction with growth of the temporal lobes of the cerebrum, each middle endocranial fossa (right and left sides) enlarges by remodeling.

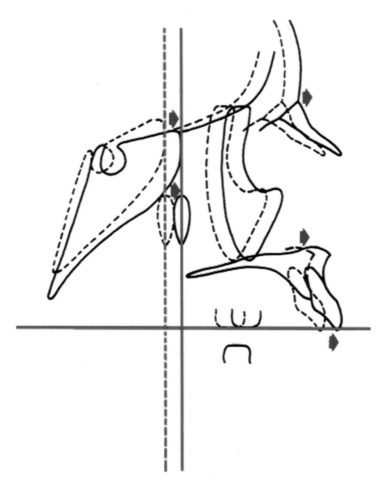

Figure 4-16: Growth of the middle endocranial fossae is accompanied by a protrusive displacement of the entire nasomaxillary complex suspended from the anterior endocranial fossae. This enlarges the underlying pharyngeal space.

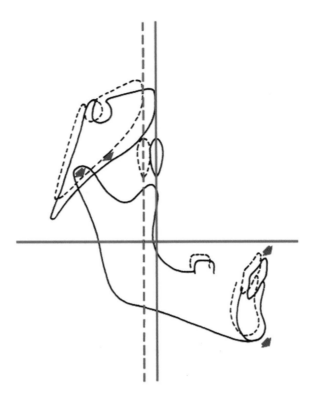

Figure 4-17: The mandible is also protrusively displaced, although the extent is much less than that for the nasomaxillary complex since the TMJ lies behind most of the protrusive growth of the middle endocranial fossae.

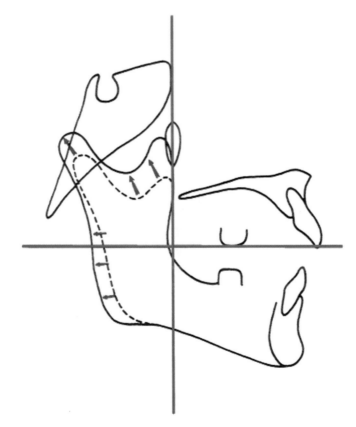

Figure 4-18: The anteroposterior breadth of the ramus must now enlarge to match the enlargement of the middle endocranial fossae. Since the ramus bridges the pharyngeal space created by the latter, the middle fossae and the right and left rami are development "counterparts."

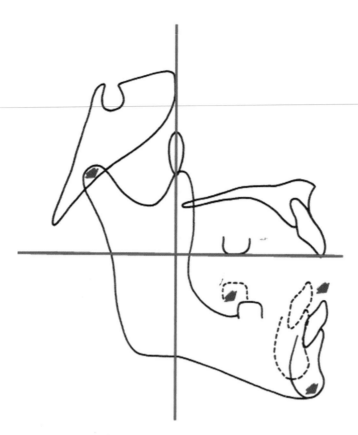

Figure 4-19: The entire mandible is displaced anteroinferiorly. Note that the occlusion becomes further separated, although a Class I anteroposterior relationship has again been restored.

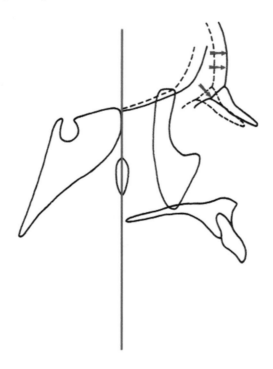

Figure 4-20: As the frontal cerebral lobes expand, the anterior endocranial fossae enlarge by remodeling and displacement to match. This continues until about the fifth or sixth year of childhood. Corresponding counterpart nasal airway expansion was seen in Figures 4-1 and 4-2, which continues for several years beyond anterior fossa enlargement. This results in the development of the frontal sinuses as the external frontal table separates from the internal table affixed to the brain.

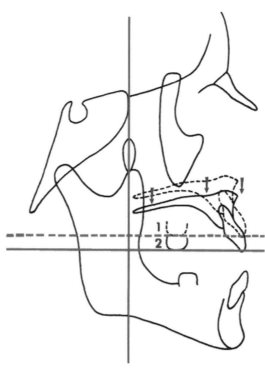

Figure 4-21: The entire nasomaxillary complex enlarges and becomes shaped by remodeling. The palate and **alveolar arch**, seen here, relocate inferiorly from 1 to 2 and, as it does so, levels any maxillary rotations caused by displacement (during regional changes in Figures 4-16 and 4-22). As the alveolar sockets remodel downward, each maxillary tooth <u>drifts</u> inferiorly with each of them. Note that this identifies the process of <u>vertical drift of teeth</u>, an important orthodontic factor that must be understood as an addition to the already well-known mesial drift. This is the considerable vertical movement of each tooth that the clinician "works with," yet the process is virtually unknown to many orthodontists. This fundamental growth process is NOT simply "eruption" or "**extrusion**."

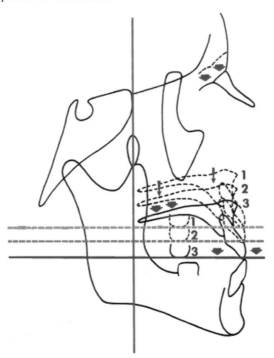

Figure 4-22: The entire nasomaxillary complex becomes displaced inferiorly from level 2 to level 3. As the ethmomaxillary complex undergoes displacement movement, all of the circumaxillary sutures become separated as sutural bone deposits simultaneously occur. Note that sutural osteogenesis does not "push" the bones apart, but rather, facial soft tissue growth expansion pulls on the attachment fibers anchored to the bone. This is the locomotor force producing displacement. Similarly, the displacement of the mandible is produced largely by the same process, rather than by "condylar growth," which is an old but incorrect notion.

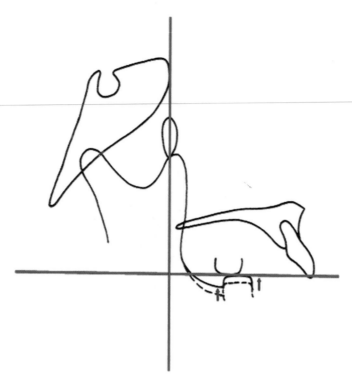

Figure 4-23: The mandibular teeth simultaneously drift superiorly into occlusion. If an anterior open bite is developing, a dentoalveolar curve of Spee often forms as a dental compensation to close the bite. (See Enlow and Hans, *Essentials of Facial Growth*, Saunders, Publisher, 1996.)

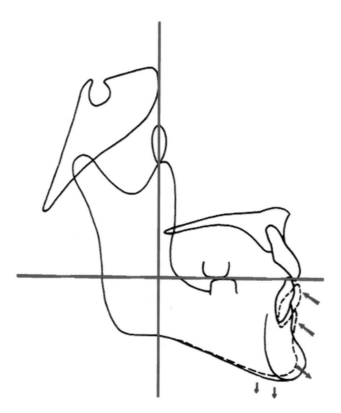

Figure 4-24: Bone deposition at the mental protuberance together with backward dental drift and alveolar remodeling produces the gradually enlarging chin over a many-year period.

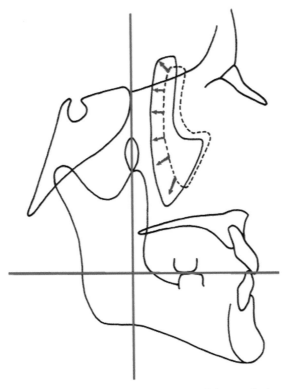

Figure 4-25: The malar protuberance and lateral orbital rim together remodel posteriorly so long as the **dental arch** increases in anteroposterior length, and then ceases.

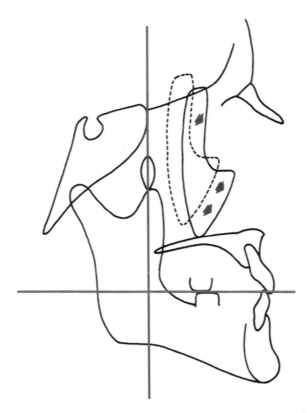

Figure 4-26: As the cheekbone and orbital rim remodel posteriorly, they become displaced anteriorly along with the whole maxillary complex. Note that the first molar retains its position aligned with the **<u>key ridge</u>**. The remodeling process enlarges and expands all of the complex maxillary contours, depressions, and elevations. The entire child's face undergoes a growth rotation in which the upper face becomes more prominent as the facial airway expands while the cheekbones and lateral orbital rims remodel retrusively.

Acknowledgement: This chapter was modified from Enlow, Chapter 2, in Kieferorthopadie, by G. P. F. Schmuth and A. D. Vardimon, Thieme Verlag Stuttgart, 1994.

Enlow and Hans, Essentials of Facial Growth, W. B. Saunders, Publishers, 1996

Enlow, D., Facial Growth, 3rd Edition., W.B. Saunders, Pub., 1990

Adapted from Enlow, D., T. Kuroda, and A. Lewis, Angle Orthod, 41:161 1971

CHAPTER 5

Development of the Dentition and Occlusion

James Mah
John Grubb
Robyn Silberstein
Michael L. Riolo

"When one looks closely at the processes of development, one observes order without minute **precision**, order within which there is flexibility and scope for revision and recovery from the unexpected."

David Poswillo, Mechanisms and Pathogenesis of Malformations, 1976.

1. ODONTOGENESIS

The development of teeth is a complex, highly coordinated process with remarkably consistent results. In spite of a long developmental time period and diverse **genetic**, **epigenetic** and **environmental** influences, there appears to be a beautiful redundancy in the regulation of odontogenesis. There are endless questions related to many of the major events seen from early tooth bud primordium to the expression of a definitely shaped crown. What are the factors that regulate migration of **neural crest cells** into developing branchial arches, initiate dental organ formation at the right time and place, and regulate the development of predictable size and shape of teeth? As practicing dentists and orthodontists we have always suspected a genetic component to tooth development and dental **anomalies**. Recent studies have strongly supported a role for specific genes in many aspects of dental development. There are several excellent and detailed reviews on the molecular control and mechanisms of tooth development. Currently, scientific goals are set for biologic tooth structure repair and whole tooth regeneration.

1.1 SUMMARY OF EARLY TOOTH FORMATION

There is extensive histologic and morphologic evidence of early tooth development (Figure 5-1). A reconstruction model is described from serial histologic sections of embryos and extracted teeth/jaws of fetal material. The origins of tissues that induce tooth formation are neural crest cells. This ectomesenchyme arises from the neural folds and migrates down the sides of the head along pathways underneath the skin. Interaction between oral epithelium and underlying mesenchymal tissue begins the histodifferentiation of teeth. The **dental lamina**, a thickening of the oral epithelium, grows into the underlying **mesenchyme** of the first branchial arch forming the epithelial buds. Development proceeds through the bud, cap and bell stages, which are named according to the characteristic epithelial shape. The oral mesenchymal cells around the bud form the dental papilla, which later give rise to the tooth pulp and odontoblasts. The oral epithelium gives rise to the enamel organ and, eventually, the ameloblasts (Figure 5-2).

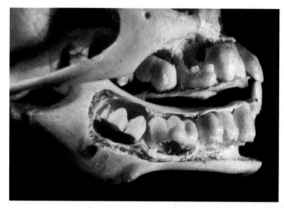

Figure 5-1: Early Tooth Formation. The lateral view of an 8 month old skull with the buccal plate removed to show the formation of the primary dentition.

The development of primary teeth begins in the embryonic stage at 4 weeks as epithelial thickenings at the lateral margins of the stomatodeum (the primordium of dental lamina). Total time for development of the primary teeth is between 2-4 years. In the maxillary arch there are basically four separate areas of odontogenic epithelial thickenings before week 5, but after that a broad band forms. The mandibular arch has two epithelial thickenings that extend almost to the midline. By day 37 both maxillary and mandibular arches show a contiguous plate of epithelium. This just follows **fusion** of the facial processes at day 35 or week 5. A successful fusion of the frontonasal and maxillary processes is an important **factor** in the formation of the continuous dental lamina. Consequently, when fusion is incomplete, as is the case with **primary palate clefting**, there is a higher incidence of abnormalities and/or **anodontia** in the premaxillary region (See Figure 6-5).

By day 39, the first sign of the dental papilla are seen as mesenchymal condensations surrounding the localized odontogenic epithelial swellings. Sixteen primary dental organs are observed as swellings or buds, each quadrant containing a central incisor, lateral incisor, cuspid and first molar. Approximately 2-3 weeks later condensations develop for the second primary molars. The permanent incisors, canines and premolars arise sequentially from the **lingual** aspects of the enamel organs from the fourth through ninth month in utero. Total time for development of the permanent dentition is approximately 18 years and begins in the early fetal stage. The permanent molars develop from a proliferation of the posterior aspects of the immediately anterior tooth. Thus, the dental lamina of the permanent first molar arises from the primary second molar at 4 months in utero.

By the 6th embryonic week, day 41, a cap-like formation or depression is seen in the epithelial swelling. The swelling is still broadly attached to the epithelial thickening at this point. Once the rim of the swelling becomes concave and begins enclosing the mesenchymal tissue of the dental papilla the outer enamel epithelium and inner enamel epithelium differentiate. All three structures of the tooth germ are present in the cap stage: the enamel organ, the dental papilla and the dental follicle. The four cell types present are the outer enamel epithelium (OEE), the inner enamel epithelium (IEE), the stratum intermedium (SI), which are the cells adjacent to the IEE towards the OEE, and the stellate reticulum (SR), which are the cells that fill the area between the OEE and IEE. The two areas of active cell proliferation, the cervical loop (where the OEE and IEE meet), and the **enamel knot** (the center of the enamel organ) is the organizing center.

The bell stage, week 10, demonstrates: 1.) deepening of the epithelial invagination; 2.) wider stellate reticular network; 3.) disappearance of the enamel knot; 4.) emergence of the enamel cord; and 5.) a more organized dental papilla and dental follicle; 6.) formation of the dentin matrix and deposition of the first dentin; and 7.) formation of the enamal matrix and calcification of enamel. Dentin (preceded by predentin) is first deposited by odontoblasts in the region of the incisal edges and cusp tips, then proceeds toward the cervical loop. There is a strong reciprocal influence of odontoblastic activity upon enamel formation. The predentin signals the internal epithelial cells to differentiate into ameloblasts and deposit the enamel matrix.

The late bell stage signals the onset of mineralization and establishment of crown shape and root development. Hertwig's sheath, derived from the fusion of the inner and outer enamel epithelia, establishes the dentino-enamel junction of the root and continues to form the pattern of the root(s). It organizes the odontoblasts and likely the periodontium. Hertwig's sheath and the dental lamina are resorbed.

The epithelial enamel organ ultimately produces the enamel, the dental papilla (a mesenchyme derivative) will form the dentin and pulp and the dental follicle (also a mesenchymal derivative) will form the the **cementum**, periodontal ligament (PDL), and **alveolar bone**. While tooth formation is a continuous process and there is some variability in timing, it follows a very predictable sequence of events.

Primary Teeth	Tooth Germ Begins Development	Mineralization	Eruption
Incisors	1 month in utero	4 months in utero	6 months post natal
Cuspids	1 month in utero	4 months in utero	18 months post natal
Molars	2 months	5 months in utero	12, 24 months post natal

Permanent Dentition	Tooth Germ Begins Development	Mineralization	Eruption
Incisors	4 months in utero	4 months post natal	6 years
Cuspids	4 months in utero	4 months post natal	9-13 years
Premolars	9 months in utero	2-3 years	11 years
First Molars	5 months in utero	birth	6 years
Second Molars	1 year	2-3 years	11-13 years
Third Molars	4 years	7-10 years	17-20 years

Table 5-1: Approximate tooth germ development, mineralization and eruption times of the primary and permanent dentitions.*

* Modified from Nery EB, Oka SW. Developmental Stages of the Human Dentition. In Clinical Dysmorphology of Oral-Facial Structures.

1.2 EPITHELIAL/MESENCHYMAL INTERACTIONS

There are a series of complex interactions between epithelium and mesenchyme that control the clearly defined sequence of events responsible for generating the tooth. Recombination experiments provide valuable information into the instructive and permissive aspects of the epithelial-mesenchymal relationship. Epithelium and mesenchyme of developing teeth are experimentally separated using matrix digesting enzymes and gentle mechanical **force**. When separated, both will proliferate but no tooth forms. Prior to the bud stage of development the potential to induce tooth **morphogenesis** resides in the epithelium. However, the epithelium can only specify tooth development in mesenchyme that is neural crest derived. Further, premigratory neural crest cells and early oral epithelium would only proceed to tooth development if first branchial arch epithelium was incorporated, as opposed to second branchial arch epithelium. This suggests that the epithelium provides an instructional role that may be locally controlled. After the bud stage, this inductive potential switches to the mesenchyme of neural crest origin. This includes dictating tooth structure, shape and details of enamel deposition. If the dental papilla is isolated and placed in isolation with epithelial lining from the vestibular sulcus, or even non-oral epithelium, it will form a fully developed crown. The dental papilla even has the ability to alter the previous history of the enamel organ epithelium. Molar dental papilla can direct the incisor enamel organ epithelium to reorganize into a molar enamel organ. This is typical of embryonic tissues only. As the fetus matures, responsiveness of the epithelium becomes more restricted and **ectopic** tooth inductions do not occur. When isolated dental papilla and enamel organ epithelium are recombined, a total reorganization of the epithelium takes place. The epithelium loses its complex dental structure, reverts back to a simple surface epithelium and begins new dental development. Even small patches of epithelial cells, permitted to reestablish contact with dental stroma, will resume tooth morphogenesis. This potential for tooth morphogenesis is apparently maintained for long periods of time in the epithelium. These data suggest that trauma must be severe and prolonged to abolish all traces of the dentition. Clinically, this is supported by the rarity of complete **anodontia** reported in the literature.

1.3 GENETICS AND PATTERNING

Currently there is considerable interest in understanding mechanisms that control initial tooth germ positioning in the developing embryo as well as the patterning. The pattern of the dentition is distinctly species-specific and thus strictly genetically controlled. Different types of teeth are positioned predictably along the **dental arch**; incisors, canines, premolars and molars. **Transpositions** are rarely seen (1% or less of the population), and when they do occur it usually involves teeth at the border of a series, such as canines. Further, molars essentially never develop at the front of the mouth.

Several theories have been proposed which address where and how certain teeth form. The Field Theory (Butler) suggests that teeth can be divided into three morphologic fields, the incisors, canines and premolars/molars. The "key" tooth is the most stable, i.e., the central, canine and first molar. The most distal teeth of each field are the most variable and the local environment controls the individual shapes. Clayton observed that the most posterior tooth of a series was missing most frequently and he hypothesized that these were "vestigial organs". However, there are clinical examples of congenitally missing first premolars or first molars when the second premolars or second molars are present. Svinhufvud, et al., suggested an anatomic model whereby certain embryonic regions are more susceptible to epigenetic influences and are "fragile" sites. For example, the union between the lateral maxillary and medial nasal processes is the region where missing and misshaped lateral incisors occur.

A more purely genetic role for missing teeth is the Clonal Model (Osborn). This suggests that the tooth primordia are prespecified and each migrating cell population is equipped with the necessary information to produce the different teeth. Sharpe elaborated on this theory that at very early stages of development, before initiation of tooth formation, the genes that are expressed in specific areas encode specific teeth, i.e., patterning genes. A number of different **homeobox genes** have been identified as candidate genes for possibly controlling neural crest prespecification such as Msx, Dlx and Pax genes.

Homeobox genes are a large group of genes that code for transcription factors responsible for regulating the expression of downstream target genes. They are highly conserved. They were originally discovered in the Drosophila specifying segment identity as homeotic genes. Homeotic genes feature co-linearity; i.e., spatial arrangement along a chromosome in the same order as the pattern of expression in the anteroposterior axis. The equivalents of the insect homeotic genes are the Hox genes in vertebrates. In mice and man there are 38 homeobox genes.

Msx and Dlx are expressed in first branchial arch mesenchyme in an interactive multiphasic pattern (i.e., temporally, spatially, and interactively). Msx-1 and Msx-2 are expressed in murine primitive streak mesoderm, neural crest cells and later stage embryos principally in areas where epithelial and mesenchymal inductive interactions occur. Prior to the initiation of odontogenesis Msx-1 and Msx-2 show specific fields of expression in the first branchial arch.

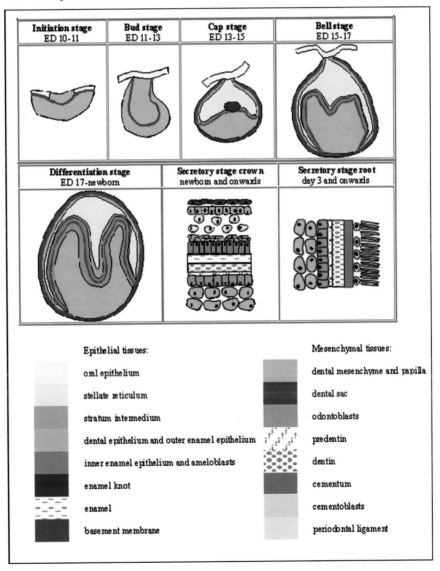

Figure 5-2: Web Site* for Gene Expression in Tooth. ED refers to embryonic days of mouse development. Developmental Biology Programme of the University of Helsinki, 1996. * http://bite-it.helsinki.fi

One of the most direct ways of assessing the importance of a particular gene in a developmental process is by altering the expression of that gene in a transgenic (i.e., genetically altered and defined) mouse embryo. Disruption of Msx-1 as seen in a **null mutation,** or lack of the gene, results in a complete absence of incisors and severely retarded molars. Msx-2 deficient mice show late defects (cuspal morphogenesis and root formation). Msx-1 and Msx-2 knockouts, double mutants, demonstrate arrests in early dental lamina and early bud formation. Therefore, both genes control inductive signals at distinct stages. Dlx-1 and Dlx-2 expression is found in the mesenchyme of future molar teeth. Null mutations of the Dlx genes results in the complete absence of maxillary molars.

There is evidence for the expression of a number of transcription factors, signaling molecules, growth factor receptors and extracellular matrix molecules in the mesenchyme of the first branchial arch. The expression of Pax9 has been shown to mark the mesenchymal regions at the prospective sites of all teeth prior to the morphological evidence. Pax9 deficient mice lack all teeth in addition to other developmental defects.

Bone Morphogenic Protein (**BMP**), the active component of osteoinductive extracts derived from bone, is also involved in signaling functions that mediate tissue interactions during development and are expressed in dental epithelium of early tooth morphogenesis. Of the fibroblast growth factor (FGF) genes known, seven are expressed in the developing tooth. Both BMP and FGF stimulate the expression of Msx1. There is evidence for the interaction of FGF and BMP in the regulation of early organ development both in a proliferation of cells as well as apoptosis, thus contributing to the differential cell proliferation seen in the enamel knot resulting in crown/cusp shapes. The most current and detailed review of molecular expression throughout odontogenesis can be found at the web site http://bite-it.helsinki.fi (Figure 5-2).

1.4 CLINICAL IMPLICATIONS

In order to identify genes involved in human tooth development and the mechanisms contributing to the defects, families with non-syndromal autosomal dominant tooth **agenesis** have been studied. **Oligodontia** (the absence of six or more permanent teeth) and **hypodontia** (the absence of less than six permanent teeth) have been studied with results indicating there is very likely **genetic heterogeneity**. There is compelling evidence for a point mutation in the Msx-1 gene on chromosome 4 contributing to missing premolars and third molars (familial tooth agenesis, FTA). A single arginine to proline amino acid missense mutation in the Msx-1 homeodomain has been identified (further study suggests the missense gene is non-functional, a haploinsufficiency). However, mutations in Msx1 and Msx2 have been excluded as a factor in familial hypodontia in a Finnish population missing lateral incisors. There is also evidence that a frameshift mutation occurs in a family with congenitally missing molars. DNA samples of the affected family members revealed an extra nucleic acid on the Pax9 gene on chromosome 14. The affected family members, each generation and both males and females, present different patterns of missing teeth. This would suggest an autosomal dominant pattern of transmission with **variable expressivity**.

In summary, **phenotypic variation** in missing teeth is noted between and within families. It is evident that multiple genes are involved in the etiology of missing teeth. Further, this would support a complex role or connection between genetic defects, the many transcription factors expressed during development (epigenetic factors) and individual variation.

2. MATURATION OF THE DENTITION

2.1 PRIMARY TOOTH RESORPTION AND THE PERMANENT TOOTH ERUPTION

Resorption of the primary tooth root is normally associated with eruption of the successor. **Osteoclasts** at the leading edge of the **eruption** follicle work to clear a path through the overlying bone and primary tooth, if present. This process seems to be well orchestrated with eruption and generally does not damage the adjacent teeth. Occasionally, if an erupting tooth is out of position with its eruption follicle contacting adjacent teeth, resorption of permanent tooth roots can occur. Primary tooth resorption can also occur in the absence of the successor, albeit at a much slower rate and less predictably. Additionally, traumatic events such as inflammation and trauma can hasten this process, while attachment of dental appliances such as splints and space maintainers to a primary tooth can delay resorption of its roots.

The two most significant events in the development of permanent teeth are initiation of calcification and the process of eruption. Most of our knowledge regarding these events has been obtained from serial radiographs. Common practice of evaluating calcification and eruption is also by radiographic means using a panoramic view. Calcification has been described by Nolla in ten stages, beginning from the presence of **tooth crypt** to completion of the root apex. However, these stages are

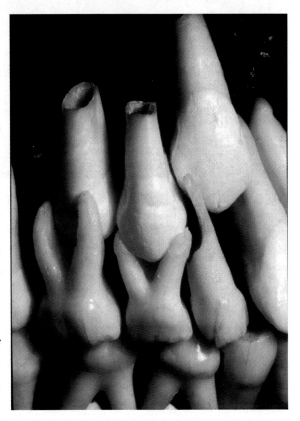

Figure 5-3: Primary Tooth Resorption and Permanent Tooth Eruption. A photograph of the 6 year old dentition. Notice the resorption of the primary roots as the permanent teeth erupt.

at times somewhat difficult to discriminate, and in practice are more practically described as a fraction of crown or root formation, such as ½ crown formed or ¾ root formed. There is great variability in calcification and eruption of the permanent teeth, much like that observed with sexual maturity and other growth indicators. There is some variability between the sexes as well, with girls generally slightly ahead of boys during the early calcification stages and girls well ahead of boys by 10 years of age. Racial variations and impact of socioeconomic status have been reported as well, although these data are not definitive.

2.1.1. Eruption

Teeth begin to erupt only after crown formation is complete; however, there is poor correlation between stage of root formation and rate of eruption. **Eruption** is a developmental phenomenon that moves a tooth from its crypt position through the alveolar process, in a path that is not always straight, into the oral cavity and into **occlusion** with its antagonist. This complex phenomenon involves a number of concerted biologic actions that are closely regulated. Simultaneous actions of elongation of the permanent tooth root, resorption of the primary tooth, increase in alveolar height and movement of the permanent tooth in the correct path through bone occur (Figure 5-4).

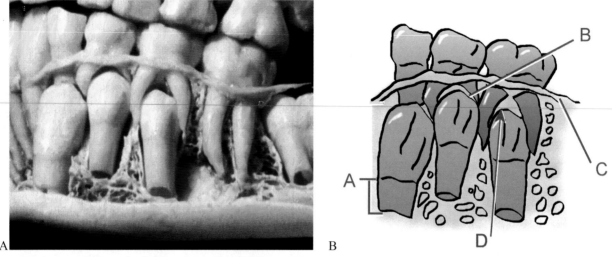

Figure 5-4A and B: Eruption of the Permanent Teeth. A.) The buccal plate has been removed from the mandible to show the developing permanent teeth. B.) The four simultaneous actions of eruption are shown: (A) elongation of the permanent tooth root; (B) resorption of the primary tooth roots; (C) increase in alveolar height and (D) movement of the permanent tooth in the correct path through bone.

Each of these actions is a phenomenon in itself, and despite the many studies on each of these events, they remain for the most part poorly understood. Abnormalities in any of these or related events can cause **impactions**, delayed eruption, **ectopic eruption** and a number of problems that lead to **malocclusion**. Additionally, despite the abundance of theories on eruption, none are proven and the phenomenon of eruption remains a mystery. Procedures for predicting emergence of a permanent tooth in the mouth are described in Chapter 16.

2.1.2. Variability of Eruption

Many recent studies on calcification, sequence and timing of eruption have focused on genetics, as these events seem to be largely genetically determined. Related to this, studies have shown that peoples of European descent generally erupt their teeth later than American blacks and American Indians. However, the precise role(s) of genes in the fundamental processes of calcification and eruption remain unknown.

> **Clinical Tip!**
> If a primary tooth is extracted after its successor has begun to erupt, the permanent tooth will erupt sooner. However, if the primary tooth is extracted prior to eruptive movements of the successor, eruption of the permanent tooth will be delayed.

Other factors that may influence eruption are socioeconomic status, nutrition, and mechanical disturbances. Although these factors are not as significant as genetics, they can influence eruption and, accordingly, should be taken into account in the evaluation of patients. In-depth study of the impact of economic status shows that tooth emergence in North American blacks and whites living at the poverty level tends to be delayed. Nutrition may also play a role, but only seems to be manifested at the extremes of nutritional variation. Mechanical disturbances may work to either hasten or delay eruption. Conditions such as periapical lesions, pulpitis, and pulpomy of a primary molar will hasten the eruption of the successor premolar. Similarly, if the primary tooth is extracted after the successor has begun eruptive movements, the permanent tooth will erupt sooner. However, if the primary tooth is extracted prior to eruptive movements of the successor, generally prior to root formation, eruption of the permanent tooth will be delayed. This delay is attributed to reformation of the alveolar process atop the successor, making eruption slower and more difficult. Trauma may cause intrusion or subluxation of the primary incisors resulting in disturbances of mineralization of the permanent incisors, and occasionally may even intrude the permanent incisors and/or halt eruption. In these instances, treatment during root formation may improve normal root development of the permanent incisor. Generally, traumatized primary teeth need to be reviewed periodically by the clinician to identify conditions that may interfere with eruption of the permanent successor.

2.1.3. Sequence of Eruption

Of the variable features of eruption, such as timing and sexual differences, the most clinically significant variable is the sequence or pattern of eruption.

First, the sequence of calcification is not indicative of the sequence of eruption into the mouth. Likely, the factors regulating eruption are not the same as those regulating calcification. Although there is wide variability of sequence of eruption into the mouth, the sequences, using the Palmer notation system, 6-1-2-4-3-5-7 and 6-1-2-4-5-3-7 occur almost 50% of the time in the maxilla, whereas the sequence (6-1)-2-3-4-5-7 and (6-1)-2-4-3-5-7 occur almost 40% of the time in the **mandible** (Figures 5-5, 5-6, 5-7). Note that these figures' sequences do not occur all the time (Figure 5-8); considerable variation is possible (Figures 5-9, 5-10). In fact, the time of clinical evaluation is important. For example, since incisors erupt at a faster rate than molars, it is possible that the molar began erupting first but at the time of evaluation the incisor has passed it by, creating the appearance that it had erupted first!

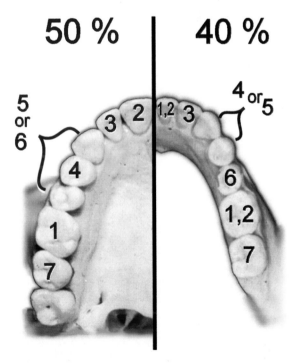

Average Eruption Sequence of Permanent Teeth

Figure 5-5: The most common eruption sequences for the maxillary (left) and the mandibular (right) arches are shown. This maxillary sequence is found in about 50 percent of the population, while the mandibular sequence is found about 40 percent of the time.

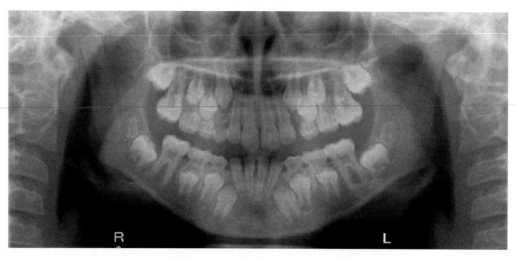

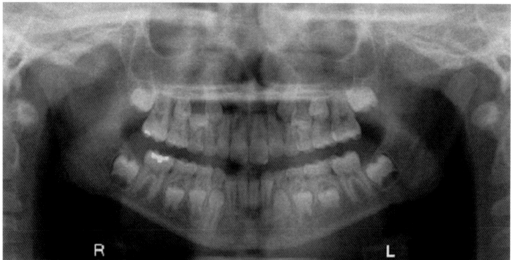

Figures 5-6 and 5-7: Panoramic radiographs showing common eruption sequences of 4-5-3 in the maxilla (top and bottom radiographs) and 4-5-3 (top) and 3-4-5 (bottom) in the mandible.

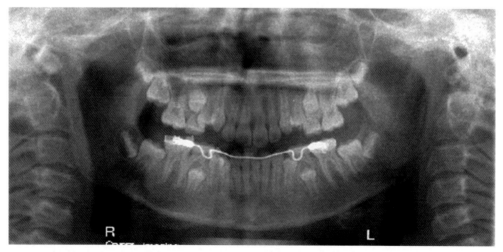

Figure 5-8: Panoramic radiograph showing eruption sequences of 4-3-7-5 on the left side of the maxilla, 3-4-7-5 on the right side and 3-4-7-5 on both sides in the mandible. Note the mandibular bilateral space maintainer in place to prevent mesial movement of the first permanent molars.

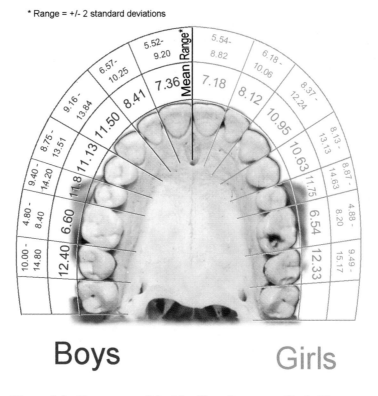

Figure 5-9: Emergence of the Maxillary Permanent Teeth. The mean times and +/- 2 standard deviations (late and early) of the emergence of the maxillary permanent teeth.

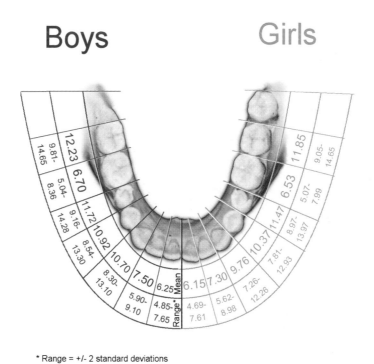

Figure 5-10: Emergence of the Mandibular Permanent Teeth. The mean times and +/- 2 standard deviations (late and early) of the emergence of the mandibular permanent teeth.

Although there seems to be no clinical significance attributed to either a 6-1 or a 1-6 sequence, the emergence of the second molar ahead of the cuspids or the premolars will likely result in shortened **arch perimeter** creating a **space deficiency** (Figure 5-8). Fortunately, the most common sequences of eruption are favorable for maintaining **arch length** during the **transitional dentition**. Clinicians involved in **serial extraction** treatments (more details on serial extraction in Chapter 17) favor an eruption sequence of 6-1-2-4-3-5-7 in the maxilla and (6-1)-2-4-3-5-7 in the mandible to allow for ease of extraction of the four first premolars as they emerge prior to the cuspids or second premolars (Figure 5-11).

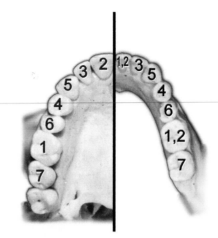

Prefered Eruption Sequence of Permanent Teeth

Figure 5-11: The preferred maxillary (left) and mandibular (right) permanent tooth eruption sequence for serial extraction and space management treatment.

2.1.4. Ectopic Eruption

Teeth erupting away from their normal positions are considered to be ectopic. This is distinctly different from impacted teeth, which are unable to erupt because of impedance, such as bone on the **anterior border of the ramus** above an erupting third molar. The most common ectopic teeth are the maxillary first permanent molars (Figure 5-12) and the maxillary cuspid, followed by the mandibular cuspid, maxillary second premolar, other premolars, and maxillary lateral incisors. Ectopic teeth occur significantly more often in girls than boys.

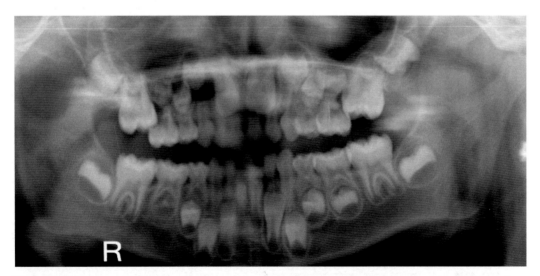

Figure 5-12: Panoramic radiograph showing ectopic eruption of maxillary first permanent molars and resorption of the distal root of the second primary molar.

Ectopic eruption of the maxillary first permanent molar occurs in approximately 3% of North American children and is associated with: 1.) large primary and permanent teeth, 2.) decreased maxillary **arch circumference**, 3.) posterior positioning of the maxilla, and 4.) atypical angle of eruption of the first molar. Treatment is best begun early in dental development in order to utilize the natural forces of eruption. Surgical uncovering and possible repositioning are often performed. More information on treatment of ectopic eruption can be found in chapters 13, 16, 17 and 20.

2.1.5. Factors Involved in Tooth Position During Eruption

Tooth eruption can be described in four stages: 1.) pre-eruptive, 2.) intra-alveolar, 3.) intra-oral, and 4.) occlusal (Table 5-2).

Stage of Eruption	Factors influencing tooth position
Pre-eruptive	Genetic determinants
Intra-alveolar	Presence/absence of adjacent teeth Rate of resorption of primary teeth Early loss of primary teeth Localized pathology Factors affecting growth of alveolus
Intra-oral	Lip, cheek, tongue muscles Extraneous objects (fingers, pencils, etc.) Spaces left by caries or extractions
Occlusal	Opposing tooth Muscles of mastication

Table 5-2: The Four Stages of Tooth Eruption and Factors Influencing Their Position

During each stage different factors may act upon the tooth to influence its position. In the pre-eruptive stage, the tooth position is thought to be genetically determined. In the subsequent stages, tooth position is influenced by a number of physical and mechanical factors. During the intra-alveolar stage, tooth position is also affected by the presence or absence of adjacent teeth, rate of resorption of the primary teeth, early loss of primary teeth, localized pathology, and any factors that affect the growth of the alveolus. During the intra-oral stage, when the tooth has entered into the oral cavity, forces from the lip, cheek, tongue or even extraneous objects such as fingers and pencils may work to change the tooth's position. Additionally, the tooth may **drift** into space created by caries or missing adjacent teeth (Figure 5-13). In the occlusal stage of tooth eruption, a complex system of forces determines the tooth's position. The upward forces of eruption and alveolar growth are countered by apically directed occlusal forces. At the same time, the muscles of **mastication** exert an influence through the interdigitation of the cusp tips.

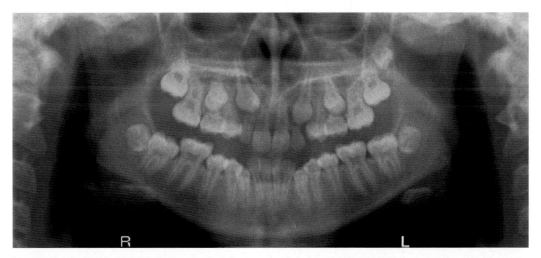

Figure 5-13: Panoramic radiograph showing premature loss of the maxillary primary cuspids and mesial drifting of the posterior teeth into the cuspid space, leaving little or no space for the permanent cuspids. Note also that the upper left permanent cuspid is abnormally positioned on the root of the permanent lateral incisor and has resorbed a significant portion of its root.

Another factor in determining tooth positions is the "**anterior component of force**" which is created by the forces of mastication (Figure 5-14). These forces are dissipated by the periodontal ligament to the surrounding **alveolar bone** and are mostly resisted in an occlusal-gingival direction. However, due to the slight mesial angulation of permanent teeth, a horizontal force vector is created in response to chewing forces. This mesially directed force is transmitted through the contact points of the teeth and is known as the "anterior component of force". This force is the result of both the axial inclinations of permanent teeth and the direction in which the occlusal forces are applied. Both are variable, and the latter depends on skeletal and muscle relationships.

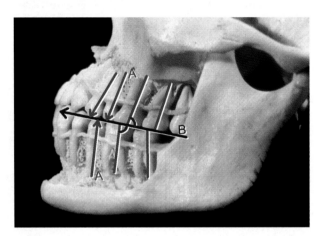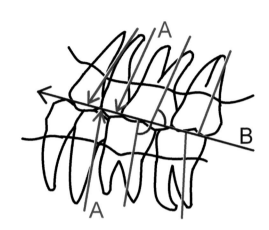

Figure 5-14: The Anterior Component of Force. The slight mesial angulation of the permanent teeth (A) direct chewing forces in an anterior direction (B).

It is important to distinguish between the anterior component of force and mesial drifting tendency, as the two are often confused. The former, as described above, is the result of muscle forces acting through the **intercuspation** of occlusal forces, while **mesial drift tendency** is an inherent disposition of teeth to drift mesially even before they are in occlusion.

3. DEVELOPMENT OF THE PRIMARY OCCLUSION

3.1 MINERALIZATION

Initiation of mineralization of the primary teeth is generally in the sequence of central incisors (14 weeks), first molars (15.5 weeks), lateral incisors (16 weeks), canines (17 weeks), and second molars (18 weeks); however, this sequence is not maintained throughout development, as the primary teeth develop at different rates. Suffice to say that primary teeth begin calcifying at 14 to 19 weeks. Mineralizing cusp tips continue to grow until they coalesce and form a complete tooth crown. As root formation occurs, the teeth erupt toward the occlusion. Both sequences of crown formation and eruption occur with biologic variations that include developmental variability, bilateral asymmetry, and sexual dimorphism.

3.2 ERUPTION

The typical sequence of eruption (Figure 5-15) is not of great clinical significance unless severe deviations occur. Indeed, significant variation, especially of the first and second primary molars, seems to exist without incident.

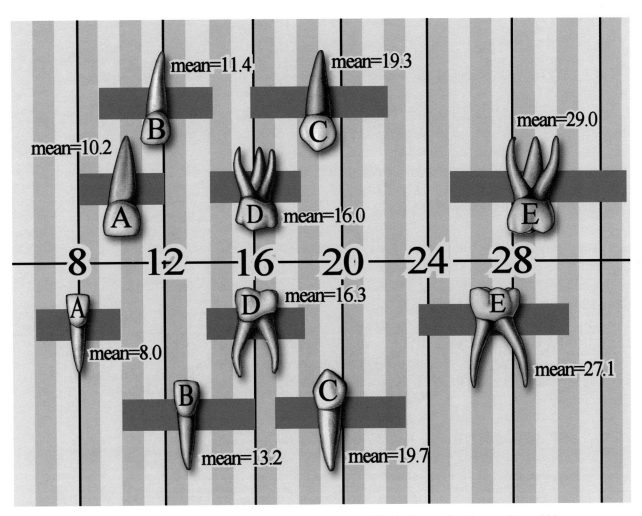

Figure 5-15: The Sequence of Primary Tooth Eruption. Centerline indicates time in months and blue rectangle indicates the standard deviation.

Of particular note, especially from a parent's perspective, a significant time in an infant's growth and development is the period of "teething". Parents report infant signs and symptoms such as vomiting, fever, diarrhea, and excessive crying. However there is disagreement among dentists, physicians and other professionals on the correlation of "teething" and systemic disturbances such as rhinorrhea, irritability, and diarrhea. The **diagnosis** of "teething" should be used with caution and not used freely, as serious unrelated problems such as upper respiratory infection, febrile convulsions, wheezing bronchitis, and infantile eczema can be overlooked.

3.3 PRIMARY DENTAL ARCH FORM

During formation and eruption of the primary teeth, the alveolar process develops vertically and horizontally. All the while, the **orofacial** musculature functions to influence the **arch form**. For example, habits such as persistent sucking can lead to significantly increased overjet. Most primary arches are ovoid in shape and display less variation than permanent arches. Early on in development, the tongue seems to play an important role in shaping of the dental arches, as the primary dentition is formed around it. This role is lessened with the establishment of occlusal reflexes and the change in lip activity from nursing to eruption of the incisors. The anterior regions of the dental arches increase in size slightly from birth to 12 months, with only very little subsequent increases thereafter. Posterior arch dimensions seem to increase more than those of the anterior, and are associated with eruption of the posterior teeth. The palatal vault width increases mostly from birth to 12 months and remains unchanged for the first 2 years.

3.4 PRIMARY DENTAL OCCLUSION

The most clinically significant aspect of the primary occlusion is the "flush terminal plane" relationship of the distal aspect of the primary second molars (Figure 5-21). This is the result of the second mandibular molar having a wider mesiodistal dimension than the second maxillary molar, and the occlusal relationship of the mandibular cusps articulating just ahead of the corresponding maxillary cusps. In the primary molars, the mesiolingual cusp of the maxillary second molar occludes in the central fossa of the mandibular second molar. The incisors are vertical with minimal **overjet** and **overbite**. When the terminal plane is straight, the first permanent molars are guided into an initial end-to-end relationship, considered normal for Caucasians in North America. Cultures with coarse diets have cuspal wear that removes cuspal interferences and allows a more forward position of the mandibular arch, leading to a more edge-to-edge incisal relationship and a distinct mesial step terminal relationship.

> **Clinical Tip!**
> A normal primary dentition should have:
>
> 1.) Spaced anterior teeth
> 2.) Primate spaces
> 3.) Straight/Mesial step terminal plane
> 4.) Near vertical relationship of anterior teeth
> 5.) Ovoid arch forms

4. DEVELOPMENT OF THE PERMANENT OCCLUSION

4.1 THE TRANSITIONAL DENTITION PERIOD

That period during which both primary and permanent teeth are present in the mouth is known as the mixed or transitional dentition period (Figure 5-16 and Figure 5-17). The permanent teeth that replace primary teeth are known as **successional teeth** (e.g., incisors, cuspids, premolars), while those permanent teeth that erupt posterior to the primary teeth are known as **accessional teeth**.

During the **mixed dentition** period, the pattern and sequence of eruption is intimately related to growth of the jaws. The mixed dentition period is characterized by two clinically significant events: 1.) utilization of arch perimeter and 2.) adaptive changes in occlusal relationships.

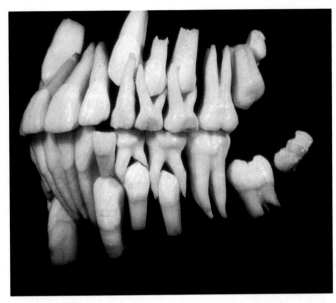

Figure 5-16: Mixed Dentition Period. A photograph of teeth during the mixed dentition period.

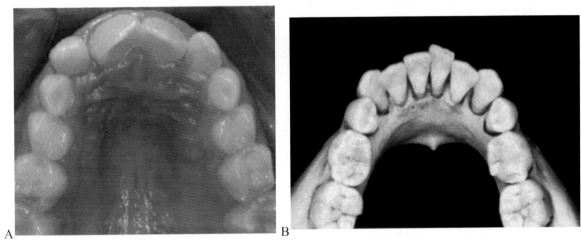

A   B

Figure 5-17: Two photographs showing misalignment and crowding of the permanent incisors. A.) Maxillary B.) Mandibular

4.1.1. Uses of the Dental Arch Perimeter

The dental arch perimeter is generally used for three events:

a.) Alignment of the permanent incisors, as they typically arrive crowded.
b.) Space for the cuspids and premolars.
c.) Adjustment of the molar occlusion. The permanent first molars typically erupt in an end-to-end relationship and must change to a Class I relationship for normal occlusion.

To accommodate the much larger permanent incisors, coordinated mechanisms occur to allow for this successful transition: 1.) the **arch width** slightly increases, 2.) the interdental spacing in the primary dentition is utilized, 3.) the permanent incisors tip **labially**, and 4.) the primary cuspids are moved distally (Figure 5-18). Despite these mechanisms there is still a slight space shortage and minor crowding that is not relieved until the primary cuspids are lost.

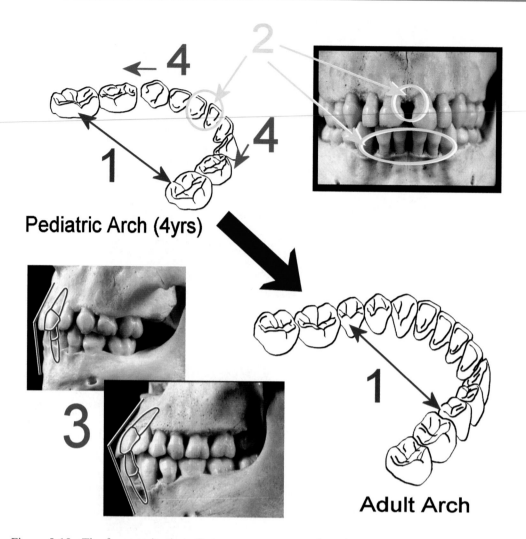

Figure 5-18: The four mechanisms that occur to accommodate the eruption of the larger permanent incisors: 1.) arch width increases; 2.) interdental spacing of the primary dentition is utilized; 3.) the permanent incisors tip more labially than the primary incisors and 4.) the primary cuspids move distally.

Since some posterior space is utilized for the incisors, available space for cuspid and premolar eruption and molar adjustment decreases. The cuspid and premolars erupt into the normally excessive (Figure 5-19). The **"E" space** specifically refers to the difference between the mesial-distal width of the larger primary second premolar and the permanent second premolar (Figure 5-20). If molar adjustment or **late mesial shift** is to occur there must be remaining space mesial to the permanent first molars. In practice, we see great variability and deviation from the ideal utilization of arch perimeter and late mesial shifts.

To restate the events, there is a mean negative value for anterior space as the permanent teeth are much larger, even if the interdental spacing and other mechanisms are accounted for. There is a mean positive value for space in the posterior since the combined widths of the c+d+e exceed the combined widths of the 3+4+5. However, the total is the important clinical consideration. The method of utilization of is the key factor in the transitional dentition.

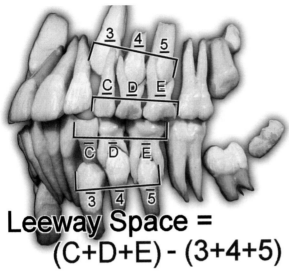

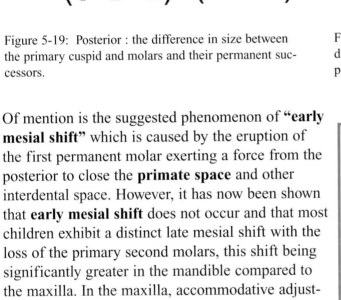

Leeway Space =
(C+D+E) - (3+4+5)

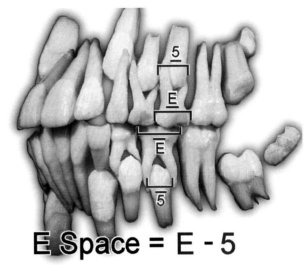

E Space = E - 5

Figure 5-19: Posterior : the difference in size between the primary cuspid and molars and their permanent successors.

Figure 5-20: "E" Space: the difference in mesial-distal dimension between the primary second molar and the permanent second premolar.

Of mention is the suggested phenomenon of **"early mesial shift"** which is caused by the eruption of the first permanent molar exerting a force from the posterior to close the **primate space** and other interdental space. However, it has now been shown that **early mesial shift** does not occur and that most children exhibit a distinct late mesial shift with the loss of the primary second molars, this shift being significantly greater in the mandible compared to the maxilla. In the maxilla, accommodative adjustments occur as in the mandible, but the matter is not as critical because the maxillary incisors procline more and the maxillary perimeter does not display the same tendency to shorten as in the mandible. Additionally, it is relatively easier to alter maxillary dimensions during treatment.

> **Early Mesial Shift**
> Closure of the primate and other interdental spaces from the posterior by erupting forces of the first permanent molar. This theory has, for the most part, been shown not to occur.
>
> **Late Mesial Shift**
> Mesial shift of the permanent first molar into the normally excessive posterior following eruption of the permanent cuspid and the premolars.

4.1.2. Changes in Occlusal Relationships in the Mixed Dentition

The flush terminal plane of the primary dentition allows for an end-to-end relationship of the first permanent molars. A Class I molar relationship is established through: 1.) late mesial shift after loss of the primary second molar, 2.) greater forward growth of the mandible relative to the maxilla, or 3.) a combination of both mechanisms, which is the most likely situation. **Cephalometric** studies show the dominance of skeletal patterns of growth over dental mechanisms of adjustment. A distal step in the primary dentition reflects a likely skeletal imbalance and will most likely result in a Class II molar relationship in the permanent dentition (Figure 5-22). The two most common paths are from a flush terminal plane to Class I (Figure 5-21) and from a mesial step to Class I occlusion (Figure 5-23).

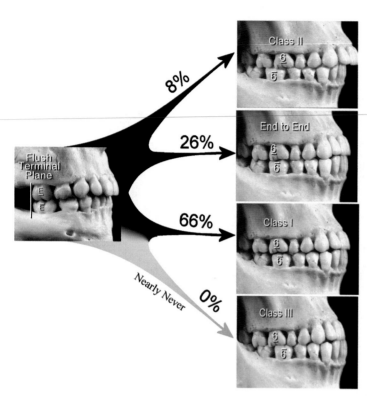

Figure 5-21: Approximate percentages of patients starting from a flush terminal plane relationship that end up in a Class I, Class II, Class III or end-to-end relationship.

Of particular clinical relevance are the factors that induce a flush terminal plane to follow something other than the normal path to a Class I or end-to-end relationship. For example, if a child with a flush terminal plane also has a mild Class II skeletal pattern and/or insufficient arch perimeter to allow for late mesial shift of the first permanent molars, an end-to-end (Figure 5-21) or Class II molar relationship (Figure 5-22) will result at the end of the mixed dentition period, depending on the severity of the factors involved. The most favorable situation is to achieve a Class I molar relationship prior to loss of the second primary molars, leaving sufficient arch perimeter for alignment of teeth without using any for molar adjustment (Figure 5-23). It is important to put the relative magnitude of skeletal and dental factors of the occlusal changes in perspective. In mild skeletal disharmonies, with large s, dental adjustments can be overcome with timely orthodontic intervention, but the amount of dental adjustment alone is simply insufficient to achieve a Class I molar relationship with a severe Class II skeletal pattern.

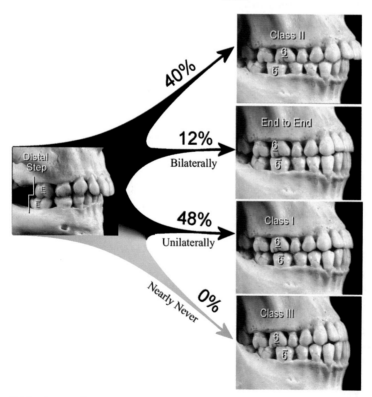

Figure 5-22: Approximate percentages of patients starting from a distal step relationship that end up in a Class I, Class II, Class III or end-to-end relationship.

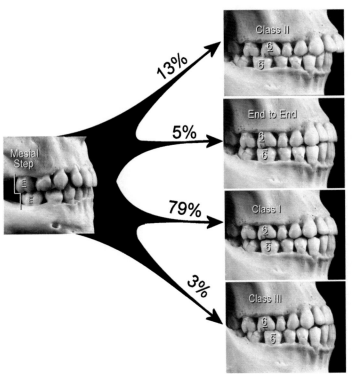

Figure 5-23: The percentage of patients starting from a mesial step relationship that end up in a Class I, Class II, Class III or end-to-end relationship.

Although a certain degree of predictability exists, one should also be aware of the great variation in the paths and not be fooled into assuming a precise path will be followed. It is not known why some patterns change and some remain constant or homeostatic, such as the Class II, end-to-end, or the Class I (Figures 5-21 through 5-23) relationships from the primary to the permanent dentitions. Knowledge of skeletal change offers some predictability of future occlusal relationships, but does not offer certainty and should be interpreted with caution, particularly in borderline situations. The only recourse for the clinician is to study and follow the patient closely to determine which path of occlusal change emerges and decide if intervention is necessary. Remember that the path of change is the result of both dental changes and, to a much larger extent, skeletal changes.

4.2 DIMENSIONAL CHANGES IN THE DENTAL ARCHES

To begin a discussion on dental arches, we must clarify the respective measurements of: 1.) the dental arch, the combined mesial-distal widths of the teeth, 2.) the dimensions of the **alveolar bone**/arch in which the roots reside, and 3.) dimensions of the mandible or maxilla proper, also known as the **basal bone** (Figure 5-24). During growth these values change in different fashions and will be dealt with in different sections of this book. Tooth sizes and growth of the bones of the craniofacial complex are dealt with in other chapters. In the following discussion we will deal primarily with growth changes of the dental arches.

The usual arch dimensions measured are: 1.) widths at the canines, primary molars (premolars), and first permanent molars, 2.) length (or depth), and 3.) circumference (Figure 5-25, 5-26). These measurements will be dealt with separately for purposes of simplicity and because they change somewhat independently of one another.

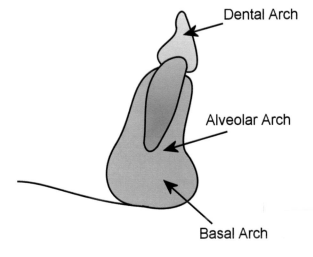

Figure 5-24: An illustration showing the difference between the dental arch (the combined mesial-distal widths of the teeth), the **alveolar arch** (the dimension of the alveolar bone, in which the roots reside), and the **basal arch** (the dimension of the maxilla and mandible proper).

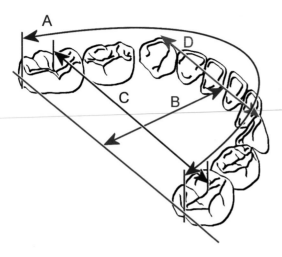

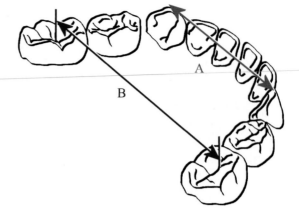

Figure 5-25: The three commonly used arch dimensions: (D) arch width, between the canines and (C) between primary second molars. The width between permanent first molars is also used; (B) arch length, or depth; and (A) arch circumference.

Figure 5-26. Arch width is measured between the primary canines (A), and the primary second molars or the permanent first molars (B).

4.2.1. Width

Key aspects relevant to width changes in the dental arches:

1.) Increases in dental arch width are almost totally related to alveolar process growth. At this time in craniofacial development there is little skeletal growth contribution in the maxilla and none in the mandible.

2.) The magnitude and manner of changes in dental arch width are significantly different between the maxilla and the mandible. Dental arch width increases correlate highly with vertical alveolar process growth, whose direction is quite different between the two arches. Maxillary alveolar processes diverge while the mandibular alveolar processes are more upright and parallel. As a result the maxillary width increases are much greater, and, of important clinical significance, the maxillary width can be more easily altered in treatment.

3.) Increases in dental arch width are more closely related to the events of dental development than to overall skeletal growth or chronological age.

In the mandible, the **intercanine width** increase is very slight, and most of this increase is the result of distal tipping of the primary canines into the primate space (Figure 5-27), since the mandibular incisors are not normally moved labially through time. No significant changes in arch width occur thereafter. In the maxilla, recall that the maxillary processes diverge, forming the palatal walls. The width increases tend to be timed more with periods of vertical alveolar growth, that is, during active eruption of teeth. Additionally, the maxillary permanent canines are placed further distally in the arch compared to the primary and erupt pointing mesially and labially. Hence, these events are important factors in widening and changing the shape of the maxillary dental arch. In this arch, there are also notable sex-related differences in the increase of maxillary intercanine width which are not as evident in the mandible (5.5 and 3 mm of sexual dimorphism, respectively).

Maxillary premolar width increases reflect the general widening of the arch coincident with vertical alveolar growth and is significantly greater than in the mandible.

In the mandible, width increases in the premolar region occur because the center of the premolar crowns are positioned further buccally than the centers of the crowns of the wider primary molars. When these measurements are taken at the buccal cusps, the increase in width is much less. The crowns of the first molars usually erupt in a lingually-tipped position and generally upright by the time of second molar eruption. As the first molars erupt, there is a sub-

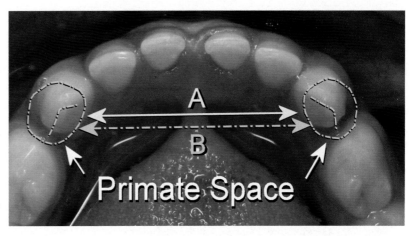

Figure 5-27: The canine to canine arch width of the mandible is affected by the primary canines tipping into the space between the canines and the primary molars, known as the primate space. This movement causes a slight increase in the arch width, as is shown by lines A and B in the figure above. Notice that the distance after the canine movement (B) is greater than the distance before the movement (A).

sequent increase in intermolar arch width, but this change is due to relative positions, rather than to an increase in size of the mandibular arch. Furthermore, some intermolar arch width is lost as both first molars move forward at the time of late mesial shift and assume a narrower distance along the convergent dental arch.

In summary, regarding the different mechanisms of width increase in the maxillary and mandibular arches: it is important to remember that the only postnatal mechanism for widening the basal bone of the mandible is that of deposition on the lateral borders of the corpus mandibularis. Such deposition only occurs in small amounts and is insufficient in helping the clinician interested in widening the mandibular dental arch. In contrast, the maxilla widens with vertical growth due to the divergent alveolar processes and, therefore, greater width increase is seen and more can be procured during treatment. Additionally, the mid-palatal suture can be split open during "rapid palatal expansion" to gain relatively large amounts of width.

4.2.2. Length or Depth

Dental **arch length** (or, more properly, **arch depth**) is measured at the midline from a point midway between the central incisors to a **tangent** touching the distal surfaces of the second primary molars or second premolars (Figure 5-28). Although measured and reported, it does not have the same clinical significance as **arch circumference**, and any changes in arch length are crudely associated with changes in arch perimeter. Occasionally, one-half the circumference is referred to as "arch length".

4.2.3. Circumference or Perimeter

The most important dental arch dimension is arch circumference or perimeter, which is measured from the distal surface of the second primary molar (or mesial surface of the first permanent molar) around the arch over the contact points and incisal edges in a smoothed curve to the contralateral point (Figure 5-29).

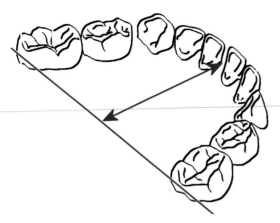

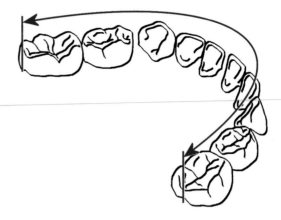

Figure 5-28: Arch depth is measured at the midline from a point midway between the central incisors to a tangent touching the distal surfaces of the second primary molars or second premolars.

Figure 5-29: The arch circumference, or perimeter, is measured from the distal surface of the second primary molar (or mesial surface of the first permanent molar) around the arch over the contact points and incisal edges in a smoothed curve to the contralateral point.

Prior to dental eruption, anatomic landmarks along the gum pads may be used to measure **arch circumference**. Using these methods along with dental measurements, it has been determined that the greatest incremental increases occur during the first two years of life and continues to increase until 13 years in the maxillary arch and 8 years in the mandibular arch. Then significant decreases occur in both arches mesial to the permanent first molars.

Mandibular arch circumference is reduced during the transitional and early adolescent dentition and is the result of several mechanisms: 1.) the late mesial shift of the first permanent molars as the "" is preempted, 2.) the mesial drifting tendency of the posterior teeth throughout life, 3.) slight amounts of interproximal wear of the teeth, 4.) the lingual positioning of the incisors as a result of the differential mandibulomaxillary growth, and 5.) the original tipped positions of the incisors and molars. The last point, in particular where incisors are tipped lingually and molars are tipped mesially, may shorten the available arch perimeter markedly as a function of the skeletal pattern, steepness of the occlusal plane, and vertical alveolar growth.

There is great variability in perimeter dimensions at various ages, and there are important sexual differences. The arch perimeter in females is particularly vulnerable to severe losses during the transitional and adolescent dentitions. Of particular clinical note is that moderate and severe caries and early loss of primary molars may dramatically increase the amount of arch perimeter loss. For details on the relationship between arch perimeter loss and malocclusion, see Chapter 7 on Etiology of Malocclusion.

The role of the mandibular third molar in crowding of the incisors is an often-discussed and researched topic. Despite the abundant literature on this relationship, no comprehensive and convincing studies on causation exist to date and the topic remains controversial. Some clinicians strongly feel that the third molars are responsible for anterior crowding and recommend their prophylactic removal during their early development, before they can disrupt the arch alignment or ruin orthodontic treatment results. The best clinical guides on this problem are still largely subjective, despite some ingenious efforts to predict the role of the third molar in "pushing" the other teeth forward.

In summary, the mandibular arch perimeter shows great variability in its continuing loss during normal development. This variation is due to differences in skeletal pattern, sex (female arches shorten more), and caries experience. This underscores the clinical importance of monitoring this dimension and preserving it during critical periods of development, for it is a dimension whose losses are difficult to recover.

Maxillary arch perimeter, in contrast, typically increases slightly. The very marked difference in angulation of the maxillary permanent incisors, as compared with the primary (Figure 5-30), and the greater increases in width likely account for the greater tendency to preserve arch perimeter, even though the permanent molars drift mesially in development. In the second and third decades of life, significant decreases in maxillary and mandibular arch perimeter occur, particularly in females. However, there is great variability as some individuals show decreases while others show increases.

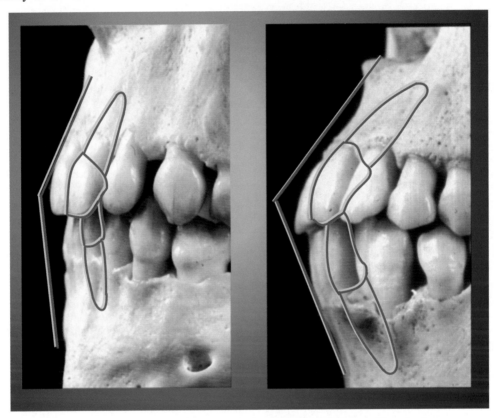

Figure 5-30: This figure shows the increased angulation of the maxillary incisors (right) as compared to the mandibular incisors (left).

4.2.4. Dimensional Changes During Orthodontic Therapy

An important fact is that it is much easier to increase dental arch width and length in the maxilla than it is in the mandible. It is relatively simple to increase the maxillary dental arch width and length, difficult to increase and retain the mandibular dental arch width, and difficult to move mandibular molars distally to significantly increase arch perimeter.

4.3 OVERJET AND OVERBITE

Overbite (the vertical overlap of the incisors) and overjet (the horizontal overlap) undergo significant changes during the primary and transitional dentitions (Figure 5-31). During the primary dentition, the overbite normally decreases slightly and the overjet is often at or near zero. From the early mixed dentition to the completion of the permanent occlusion, the average overbite increases slightly and then decreases; however, there is great variability in this behavior. Overbite is correlated to a number of vertical facial dimensions, such as **ramus** height, whereas overjet is a reflection of the anteroposterior skeletal relationship. Overjet may also be influenced by abnormal lip and tongue function as well as digit habits. During the growth of severe Class II and Class III malocclusions, the overbite and overjet must adapt to the abnormal skeletal relationships and thus behave differently than that just described.

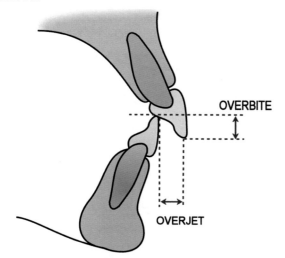

Figure 5-31. Overjet and Overbite. Overbite is the measurement (in millimeters or as a percentage overlap) of vertical overlap between the maxillary and mandibular incisors, while overjet is the measurement (in millimeters) of horizontal overlap of the incisors.

5. Suggested Reading

Early Odontogenesis

Avery JK. Essentials of oral histology and embryology a clinical approach. Mosby Inc. St. Louis; 2000.

Avery JK. Oral development and histology. Thieme. New York. 2001.

Ferguson MWJ. The dentition through life. In: Elderton RJ, editor. The Dentition and Dental Care. Oxford: Heinemann Medical Books;1990:1-29p.

Johnston MC, Listgarten M. Observations on the migration interactions and early differention of orofacial tissues. In: Slavkin HC, Bavetta LA, editors. Developmental Aspects of Oral Biology. New York: Academic Press;1972; pp 278-287.

Nery EB, Oka SW. Developmental stages of the human dentition. In: Melnick M, Shields ED, Burzynski NJ, editors. Clinical Dysmorphology of Oral-Facial Structures. Littleton: John Wright, PSG Inc ;1982:pp 401-438.

Osborn JW, Ten Cate AR. Advanced Dental Histology. Bristol: John Wright & Sons Ltd., 1976.

Piesco NP, Avery JK. Development of Teeth: Crown Formation. In: Avery JK editor. Oral Development and Histology. New York: Thieme, 1994: 70-93.

Poswillo D. Mechanisms and Pathogenesis of Malformations. British Medical Bulletin 1976; 32:59-64.

Kollar EJ. Epithelial-Mesenchymal Interactions in the Control of Tooth Shape and Size. In: Melnick M, Shields ED, Burzynski NJ, editors. Clinical Dysmorphology of Oral-Facial Structures. Littleton: John Wright, PSG Inc., 1982: 439-446.

Mina M, Kollar EJ. The induction of odontogenesis in non dental mesenchyme combined with early murine mandibular arch epithelium. Archives of Oral Biology 1987; 32: 123-127.

Thesleff I, Vaahatokari A, Kettunen P, Aberg T.Epithelial-Mesenchymal Signaling during Tooth Development. Connective Tissue Research 1995; 32:9-15.

Cobourne MT. The Genetic Control of Early Odontogenesis. British Journal of Orthodontics 1999; 26:21-28.

Ignelzi MA et al. Genetically engineered mice: tools to understand craniofacial development. Crit Rev Oral Biol Med 1995; 6:181-201.

McGinnis W. A conserved DNA sequence in homeotic genes of the Drosophila antennapedia and bithorax complexes. Nature 1984; 308:428-433.

Osborn JW. Morphogenetic gradients: fields versus clones. In: Butler PM and Joysey KA, editors. Development, Function and Evolution of Teeth. New York: Academic Press, 1978: 171-201.

Peters H, Balling R. Teeth where and how to make them. Trends in Genetics 1999; 15(2):59-65.

Peters H et al. Pax-9-deficient mice lack pharyngeal pouch derivatives and teeth and exhibit craniofacial and limb abnormalities. Genes Dev 1998; 12:2735-2747.

Qiu M et al. Role of the Dlx homeobox genes in proximodistal patterning of the branchial arches: mutations of Dlx-1, Dlx-2 and Dlx-1 and -2. Archives of Developmental Biology 1997; s185:165-184.

Satokata I, Maas R. Msx-1 deficient mice exhibit cleft palate and abnormalities of craniofacial and tooth development. Nature Genetics 1994; 6:348-356.

Sharpe PT. Homeobox genes and orofacial development. Connective Tissue Research 1995; 32:17-25.

Teixeira C. New horizons in understanding early tooth development. Clin Orthod Res 1999; 2:171-174.

Tucker AS, Sharpe PT. Molecular Genetics of Tooth Morphogenesis and Patterning: The Right Shape in the Right Place. J Dent Res 1999; 78(4):826-834.

Nieminen P et al. Gene defect in hypodontia: exclusion of MSX-1 and MSX-2 as candidate genes. Human Genetics 1995; 96:305-308.

Stockton DW et al. Mutation of Pax-9 is associated with oligodontia. Nature Genetics 2000; 24(1): 18-19.

van den Boogard M, Dorland M, Beemer F, Ploos van Amstel H. Msx-1 mutation is associated with orofacial clefting and tooth agenesis in humans. Nature Genet 2000; 24: 342-343.

Vastardis H: The genetics of human tooth agenesis: New discoveries for understanding dental anomalies. Am J Orthod Dentofacial Orthop 2000; 117:650-656.

Vastardis H, Karimbux N, Gutha S, Seidman J, Seidman C. A human Msx-1 homeodomain missense mutation causes selective tooth agenesis. Nat Genet 1996; 13: 417-421.

Maturation of the Dentition

Nolla CM: The development of the permanent teeth. J Dent Child 1960; 27: 254-266.

Melcher AH, Beertsen W. The physiology of tooth eruption. In: McNamara JA Jr, editor. The Biology of Occlusal Development, monograph 7. Craniofacial Growth Series. Ann Arbor Michigan, Center for Human Growth and Development, University of Michigan, 1977, pp 1-23.

Moorees CFA. Dentition of the Growing Child. Cambridge, Massachusetts, Harvard University Press, 1959.

Wise GE. Cell and molecular biology of tooth eruption. In: Biological Mechanisms of Tooth Eruption, Resorption and Replacement by Implants. Davidovitch Z and Mah J, editors.Harvard Society for the Advancement of Orthodontics, EBSCO Media, Birmingham, Alabama, 1998, pp 1-8.

Gaethofs M, Verdonck A, Carels C, de Zegher F: Delayed dental age in boys with constitutionally delayed puberty. Eur J Orthod 1999; 21:711-715.

Nanda SK. The developmental basis of Occlusion and Malocclusion. Chicago, Quintessence, 1982.

Van der Linden FPGM (ed). Transition of the Human Dentition. Monograph 13. Craniofacial Growth Series. Ann Arbor Michigan, Center for Human Growth and Development, University of Michigan, 1982.

Becker A, Chaushu S: Dental age in maxillary canine ectopia. Am J Orthod Dentofacial Orthop 2000; 117:657-662.

BeGole EA, Fox DL, Sadowsky C: Analysis of change in arch form with premolar expansion. Am J Orthod Dentofacial Orthop 1998; 113:307-315.

Valmaseda-Castellón E, De-la-Rosa-Gay C, Gay-Escoda C: Eruption disturbances of the first and second permanent molars: Results of treatment in 43 cases. Am J Orthod Dentofacial Orthop 1999; 116:651-658.

Baccetti T: Tooth rotation associated with aplasia of nonadjacent teeth. Angle Orthod 1998; 68(5):471-474.

Tschill P, Bacon W, Sonko A: Malocclusion in the deciduous dentition of Caucasian children. Eur J Orthod 1997; 19:361-367.

Development of the Primary Occlusion

Leighton BC. Eruption of deciduous teeth. Dental Practitioner. 1968: 200:836-842.

Development of the Permanent Occlusion

Baumrind S, Bravo LA, Ben-Bassat Y, Curry S, Korn EL: Lower molar and incisor displacement associated with mandibular remodeling. Angle Orthod 1997; 67(2):93-102.

Bishara SE, Jakobsen JR, Treder J, Nowak A: Arch length changes from 6 weeks to 45 years. Angle Orthod 1998; 68(1):69-74.

Bondevik O: Changes in occlusion between 23 and 34 years. Angle Orthod 1998; 68(1):75-80.

Brin I, Zwilling-Sellam O, Harari D, Koyoumdjisky-Kaye E, Ben-Bassat Y: Does a secular trend exist in the distribution of occlusal patterns? Angle Orthod 1998; 68(1):81-84.

Hunter WS, Smith BRW. Development of mandibular spacing-crowding from nine to sixteen years of age. J Can Dent Assoc 1972; 38:178-185.

Lindsten R, Ögaard B, Larsson E: Difference in dental lateral arch length between 9-year-olds born in the 1960s and the 1980s. Am J Orthod Dentofacial Orthop 2000; 117:663-668.

Moyers RE, Wainright R. Skeletal contributions to occlusal development. In: McNamara JA Jr, editor. The Biology of Occlusal Development, monograph 7. Craniofacial Growth Series. Ann Arbor Michigan, Center for Human Growth and Development, University of Michigan, 1977, pp 89-111.

Van der Linden FPGM. Facial Growth and Facial Orthopedics. Chicago, Quintessence, 1986.

Watanabe E, Demirjian A, Buschang P: Longitudinal post-eruptive mandibular tooth movements of males and females. Eur J Ortho 1999; 21:459-468.

Weiland FJ, Jonke E, Bantleon HP: Secular trends in malocclusion in Austrian men. Eur J Orthod 1997; 19:355-359.

Section II
Foundations for Orthodontics

This section deals with descriptive terminology, the classification and origin of malocclusion, the role of force and tissue response, tissue engineering, and clinical epidemiology.

Chapters:

CHAPTER 6

Introduction to Classification and Terminology

Joseph Damone II

1. INTRODUCTION

Classification of malocclusion should not be confused with the etiology. **Classification** is the morphologic description of the dental, skeletal, and soft tissue deviations from the norm while **etiology** deals with the cause. The morphologic approach to classification has prevailed because dental occlusions are defined by a set of morphologic conditions and there are very few individuals with malocclusions in whom etiological factors can be found. However, known etiologic factors must be considered in deciding the type, intensity, and duration of treatment that is to be provided to the patient.

Dentists must have an understanding of the terms that are used when describing an orthodontic problem in order to have a meaningful dialogue with other professionals. Without this knowledge of the terminology, each individual will have difficulty understanding the problem list that leads to a diagnosis, treatment objectives, and treatment plan for the orthodontic patient. Over the course of time, orthodontists have developed a system of classifying malocclusions by creating a glossary of terms that everyone understands and uses when communicating with other dental professionals.

Classifying malocclusions is the recognition of the morphologic deviation from a quantitative and qualitative norm. Attempts have been made to arrange the malocclusions according to groups having a recognized pattern of morphological defects or malformations that are not currently considered to constitute a syndrome or anomaly and, although helpful, there are major deficiencies with these attempts. Take for example the malocclusion that is classified as a Class II, Division I. The characteristics associated with this term represents only two areas of deviation. These are the first molar occlusal relationship and the maxillary anterior tooth inclinations. Therefore, one does not know any of the other characteristics that may be found within this category of malocclusion. You can begin to see, there is no simple description that will allow individuals to understand the myriad of problems that can be present in a malocclusion. The diversity that exists in the orthodontic population does not lend itself to simply classify a malocclusion with a few descriptive words, but must present a detailed description of the patient's problems. So when we speak of classifying a malocclusion, we are really describing the characteristics or the morphology that deviates from the norm. This type of description will allow the presentation of a clear picture to other professionals so they will be able to immediately understand a patient's orthodontic problem.

2. ORIENTATION PLANES

To begin to understand what we need to communicate, it is necessary to establish a plane of reference. Since individuals are three dimensional, there are three orientation planes that we use to aid in establishing a problem list. The **median plane, e.g., midsagittal plane** (Figure 6-1) is an imaginary plane that passes longitudinally through the middle of the head and divides it into right and left halves. This plane is used to describe anterior-posterior relationships and is referred to as the **sagittal plane**. The **frontal plane (coronal plane)** (Figure 6-2) is an imaginary plane that passes longitudinally through the body perpendicular to the median plane dividing the head into the back and front. This plane is used to describe superior-inferior relationships and is referred to as the vertical plane. The **transverse plane (horizontal plane)** (Figure 6-3) is an imaginary plane that passes through the head at right angles to the median and frontal plane dividing the head into upper and lower halves. This plane is used to describe right to left relationships. (See Glossary for varieties of plane definitions).

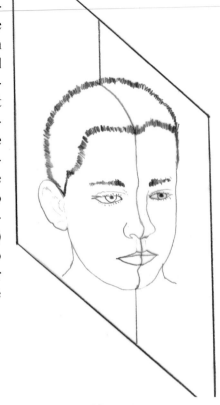

Figure 6-1

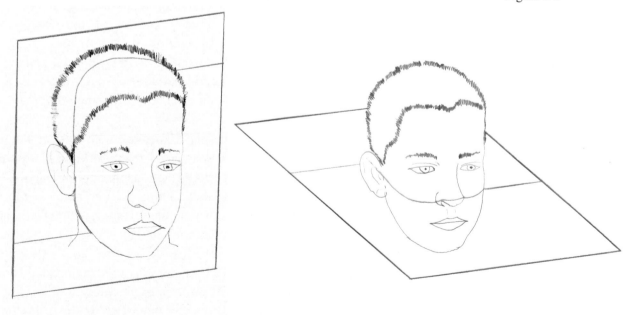

Figure 6-2

Figure 6-3

Along each orientation plane, there may be associated dental, skeletal, and soft tissue deviations. Since the objective of orthodontic treatment result is to create a balance between the dental, skeletal, and soft tissue patterns, a problem list is established for each of the orientation planes to include the hard and soft tissue patterns. The **global reference framework** of three mutually perpendicular, intersecting planes are used as a reference for measurements within the dentofacial complex. The clinician objective is to determine if there are any dentofacial deformities characterized by disharmonies of size, form and function. Utilizing these planes gives us a starting point from which to begin to characterize the orthodontic problem list.

3. SOFT TISSUE RELATIONSHIPS

It is the stature and face that we see first when we meet any individual. The soft tissue relationships of the nose, lips, and chin, are important when the final treatment objectives are reached for the patient. Therefore, we should begin to note the deviant characteristics of the soft tissues as they relate to the orientation planes before we ever begin the examination of the oral cavity.

Anthropologists use **craniometry**, which is the direct measurement of the head and dry skull, to arrive at the **cranial index** to classify the different head shapes found in the human population. The **cranial index** is the relationship established by the measurement of the length of the cranium from the forehead to the back of the skull as compared with the width of the head between the ears. Brachycephalic, **Mesocephalic**, and **Dolicocephalic** are the anthropometric terms that describe the three major categories of head shapes. Orthodontists have adopted these terms to aid in the case description and, since these are anatomical descriptions, there is no one type of malocclusion associated with them.

Brachycephalic (Euryprosopic) (Figure 6-4) is an individual that has a larger than average cranial width and usually presents with a broad square head shape and a low mandibular plane angle.

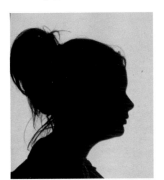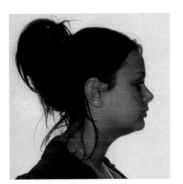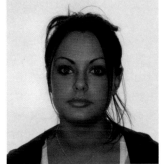

Figure 6-4

Dolicocephalic (Leptoprosopic) (Figure 6-5) is an individual that has a narrower cranial width and usually presents with a long narrow head shape and high mandibular plane angle.

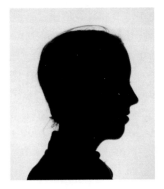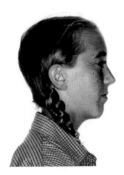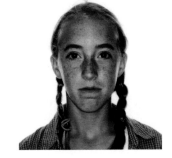

Figure 6-5

Mesocephalic (Mesoprosopic) (Figure 6-6) is an individual that falls between the brachycephalic and dolicocephalic pattern and has an average cranial width whose facial features appear well balanced in all of the orientation planes.

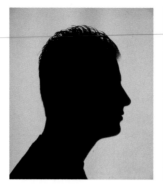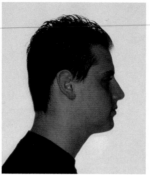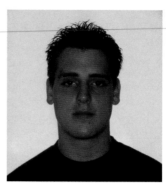

Figure 6-6

Brachyfacial and **Dolicofacial** are terms that combine the anthropologic term with the usually associated facial characteristics that one would find in these individuals. **Brachyfacial** is an individual that is characterized by a broad square face with a strong chin, flat lip posture, low **mandibular plane** and a straight profile. Dolicofacial is an individual that is characterized by a long, narrow face with a high mandibular plane angle, convex profile, poor chin development and an anterior-posterior face height imbalance.

3.1 FRONTAL FACIAL VIEW

Since we greet and talk with the patient from the front, this would be a good starting point for the beginning of our examination. This is called the frontal view and gives us the opportunity to determine the presence or absence of any facial asymmetries as determined by the midfacial plane. **Facial asymmetry** is a reduction of similarity or proportion between the right and left sides of the face or the craniofacial skeleton. It is important to note asymmetries because they may be associated with syndromes that influence the skeletal development. When a syndrome is diagnosed, it will make the case more difficult and can compromise the treatment result. Other asymmetries may be due to dental deviations and/or skeletal deviations. Therefore, diagnosing the morphologic deviation of the asymmetry is important because that would influence the treatment objectives and the **mechanotherapy** necessary to correct the problem.

The midline is a central reference line of a structure from which symmetry can be determined between the right and left side. The interpupillary line is the line connecting the pupils of the eyes and is used as a reference plane when evaluating facial asymmetry. The midline of the face is called the **facial midline** and is considered to be a line drawn perpendicular to the interpupillary line from **glabella** to the tip of the nose, passing the midpoint of the philtrum of the upper lip, and the midline of the chin. The **maxillary dental midline** is determined by drawing a line perpendicular to the maxillary occlusal plane through the proximal contacts of the central incisors and noting its relationship to the philtrum of the upper lip. The **mandibular dental midline** is determined by drawing a line from the proximal contacts of the central incisors perpendicular to the mandibular occlusal plane and noting its relationship with the facial midline, the maxillary dental midline, and the midline of the chin.

The lip posture and **lip line** are soft tissue patterns that provide us with the information about the musculo-skeletal pattern as influenced by the bones and the anterior tooth position. The lip line (Figure 6-7) is the amount of tooth and/or gingival tissue that is exposed at rest while the **smile line** (Figure 6-8) is the amount of tooth and/or gingival tissue that is exposed upon smiling.

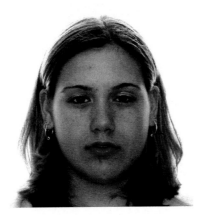

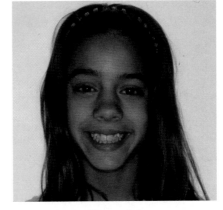

Figure 6-7   Figure 6-8

Lip incompetence (Figure 6-9) is the inability of the patient to have the lips contacting in the **rest position** without showing any muscular strain.

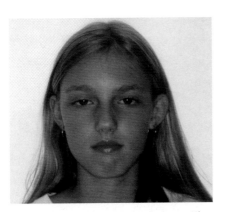

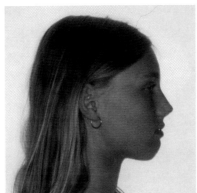

Figure 6-9

These characteristics must be included in a problem list because they play a role in determining the treatment objectives as well as the mechanics needed to improve or correct a gummy smile produced by a dental or skeletal protrusion.

3.2 PROFILE FACIAL VIEW

This view is necessary to evaluate the nose, lip, chin, and facial convexity. There are many variations to the profile and its characteristics do not necessarily relate to the occlusion of the teeth. The three profile types are convex (Figure 6-10), straight (Figure 6-11), and concave (Figure 6-12).

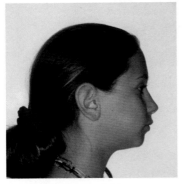

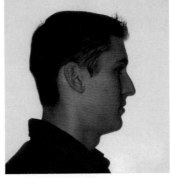

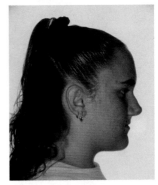

Figure 6-10   Figure 6-11   Figure 6-12

The profile determination is made by mentally drawing a line on the soft tissue from Glabella to Subnasale and then to **Pogonion** along the midsagittal plane (Figure 6-15A).

These profile types can be found in faces that present with an anterior or posterior **divergency**. The divergency of the face can be determined by mentally drawing a line from Glabella to Pogonion and observing its relationship to the **Frankfort plane**. If this line is approximately 90 degrees to the Frankfort plane, this individual is considered to have an orthognathic (straight) face (Figure 6-13) with no divergency.

If this line is less than 90 degrees, this individual is considered to have a **retrognathic** (posterior divergent) **face** (Figure 6-14) and, if the angle is greater than 90 degrees, this individual is considered to have a **prognathic** (anterior divergent) **face** (Figure 6-15B).

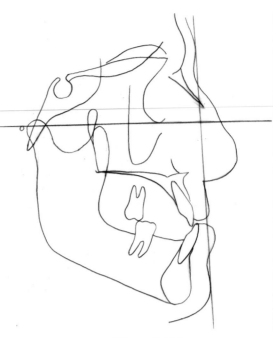

Figure 6-15A

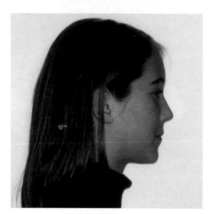

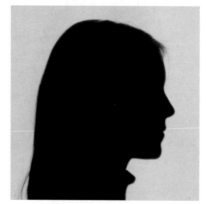

Figure 6-13

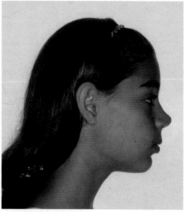

Figure 6-14

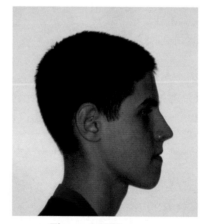

Figure 6-15B

4. DENTAL RELATIONSHIPS

To perform a through dental evaluation, the intraoral examination must be followed by the study model evaluation, and together they allow the dentist to create a detailed problem list. One should develop a sequence that is routinely followed so that no possible problem is overlooked during the evaluation process. The **arch form**, which is the shape of an individual **dental arch**, is examined first to look for malposed teeth and other related problems such as **supernumerary teeth**, malformed teeth, missing teeth and diastemas. Supernumerary teeth are extra teeth usually malformed and erupting ectopically. **Ectopic** is the term used to describe a condition in which a tooth develops or erupts into an abnormal position and **anodontia** is used to describe congenitally missing teeth. A **diastema** is a space between two teeth in the dental arch. However, this term generally refers to the space found between the maxillary central incisors even though the more accurate term would be a maxillary midline diastema.

The individual is asked to bite and the occlusion is examined for any sagittal relationship deviations. The terms to describe the malposed teeth are given to them by their relation with the line of occlusion and the facial midline plane. The terms used to describe the malposed teeth are their position as they relate to the orientation planes.

There are several positions that malposed teeth can adopt that were termed by Edward Angle as a malocclusion. However, Lischer suggested that the suffix version be used instead of the term occlusion when describing malposed teeth. Lischer used the word malocclusion to represent the malrelation of the arches. For example, a Class II, division I malocclusion describes an abnormal sagittal dental relationship. The following terms are used to describe the position of malposed teeth within the arch.

1.) **Mesioversion** is the term used to describe a tooth that is in the arch form but located nearer the midline of the face than it would normally be found.
2.) **Distoversion** is the term used to describe a tooth that is in the arch form but located farther from the midline of the face than it would normally be found.
3.) **Labioversion** is the term used to describe an incisor or canine that is outside the arch form and is located toward the lips.
4.) **Buccoversion** is a posterior tooth that is outside the arch form and located toward the cheek.
5.) **Linguoversion** is the term used to describe a tooth that is inside the arch form and located toward the tongue.
6.) **Infraversion** is the term used to describe a tooth that has not erupted to the occlusal plane.
7.) **Supraversion** is the term used to describe a tooth that is over-erupted.
8.) **Torsiversion** is the term used to describe a tooth that is rotated on its axis.
9.) **Transversion (Transposition)** is present when the teeth are in the wrong sequential order. An example of this is present when the maxillary first premolar assumes the position of the canine and the canine assumes the position of the premolar.

It is important to understand the meaning of each term because there are various combinations of these terms that might apply to a single tooth. For example, a tooth might be in a mesio-bucco-torsi-infraversion. Looking at this description one can see there are no conflicting terms. However, a tooth that is described as being in a bucco-linguoversion is represented by conflicting terms since a tooth cannot be buccal and lingual at the same time.

4.1 MAXILLARY AND MANDIBULAR DENTAL ARCHES

The arch form varies within each facial type and is noted for future reference in order to maintain continuity of the arch form during treatment. There are many variations that can be found in the arch form of the orthodontic patient population. However, they fall into three general categories: square, elliptical, and tapering. The type of arch form found in an individual usually follows the facial type. For example, a brachyfacial patient will usually have a broad, square arch form.

A decision to treat a case with tooth extraction is dependent upon the results of a dental arch space analysis. The **arch length**, also known as **arch perimeter**, is determined by measuring from the mesial surface of one molar to the mesial surface of the contralateral molar along the arch form presented by the teeth. This gives us a measurement that is known as **available space**. Measuring the mesio-distal dimension of the individual teeth from molar to molar gives us a measurement that is known as **required space**. The difference between the available space and required space is called an **arch length discrepancy** that could exhibit a deficiency (crowding) or excess (spacing). The arch length discrepancy is influenced by the individual tooth sizes. If there is a disproportionate relationship between the sums of the mesiodistal measurement of the maxillary teeth and the mandibular teeth, there is a **tooth size discrepancy.** This discrepancy can be further analyzed to determine if it is a posterior, middle, or anterior tooth size discrepancy. There are instances when one would measure only the mandibular anterior teeth to arrive at an **irregularity index**. The irregularity index is determined by measuring the linear displacement of the anatomic contact points of each mandibular incisor from the respective points of the adjacent teeth and the sum of these displacements represents the relative degree of anterior irregularity.

Arch width is the measurement taken across the arch as measured between contralateral teeth. The **intercanine width** is the measurement taken across the arch between the canines. The **intermolar width** is the measurement taken across the arch between the first molars. These measurements are used as a guide when fabricating arch wires in order to maintain the arch form during treatment.

4.2 SAGITTAL DENTAL RELATIONSHIPS

It was Edward H. Angle who published the first classification of malocclusion in 1890. This was a giant step forward because it subdivided major types of malocclusions and included the first clear and simple definition of normal occlusion in the natural dentition. He believed that the maxillary first molar was the key to the occlusion because it was always in the physiologically correct position with the skull and the variability that is presented comes from the mandible. The classifications were based on the relationship of the mesiobuccal cusp of the maxillary first molar and the buccal grove of the mandibular first molar. If this molar relationship exists, then it would follow that the teeth would align on a smooth curve that would result in a normal occlusion (Figure 6-16).

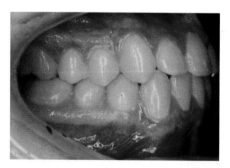 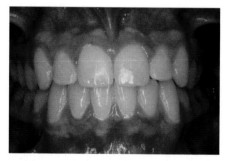

Figure 6-16

This postulation has held up over time as long as there were no other problems dealing with tooth size discrepancies and/or skeletal deviations.

The **Angle classification** describes three types of occlusion; however, if we consider his normal occlusion model, he actually has described four types of occlusion.

Class I malocclusion: A malocclusion where there is a normal molar relationship but the arch form is not correct due to factors relating to tooth position, dentoalveolar positions, and other causes (Figure 6-17). For example, there may be crowding, cross bites, and other morphologic deviations.

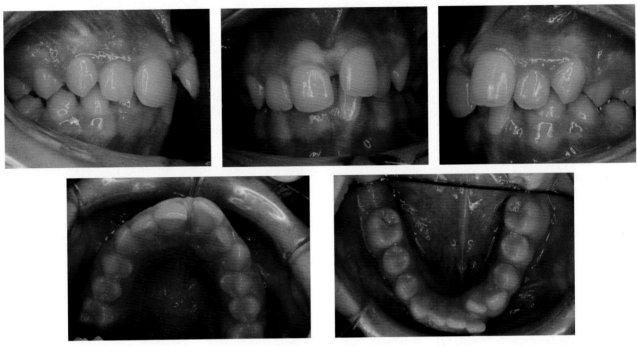

Figure 6-17

Class II malocclusion: A malocclusion where the molar relationship shows the buccal groove of the mandibular molar distally positioned when in occlusion with the mesiobuccal cusp of the upper molar (Figure 6-18). Within this classification there are variations to the maxillary anterior tooth inclinations that will determine the type of **Division** classification given to this malocclusion.

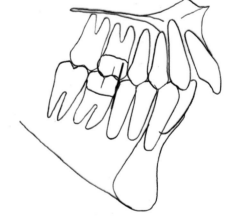

    1.) Division I: A Class II malocclusion where the maxillary anterior teeth are proclined and there is a large overjet (Figure 6-19).

Figure 6-18

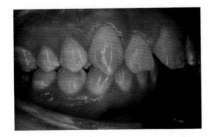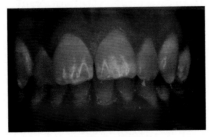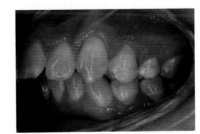

Figure 6-19

Proclination is the labial tipping of the anterior teeth.

2.) Division II: A Class II malocclusion where the maxillary anterior teeth are retroclined and there is a deep overbite (Figure 6-20). **Retroinclination** is lingual tipping of the anterior teeth.

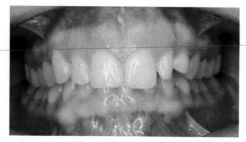 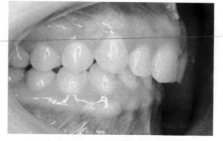

Figure 6-20   Figure 6-21

Associated with the Division II type of malocclusion there can be described three types of maxillary anterior tooth arrangement.

    a.) Type A: The four maxillary anterior incisors are retroclined and do not show any crowding (Figure 6-21).

    b.) Type B: The maxillary central incisors are retroclined and the lateral incisors are proclined (Figure 6-22).

    c.) Type C: The four maxillary incisors are retroclined without crowding with the canines positioned labially (Figure 6-23).

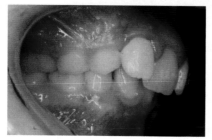 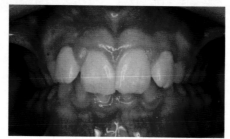 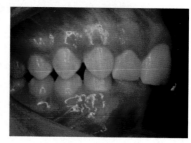

Figure 6-22   Figure 6-23

Class III malocclusion: A malocclusion where the molar relationship shows the buccal groove of the mandibular first molar mesially positioned to the mesiobuccal cusp of the maxillary first molar when the teeth are in occlusion, as in Figure 6-24 drawing. The photos in Figure 6-24 illustrate a Class III dental relationship where there is premature incisal contact leading to an anterior bite shift (a pseudo Class III).

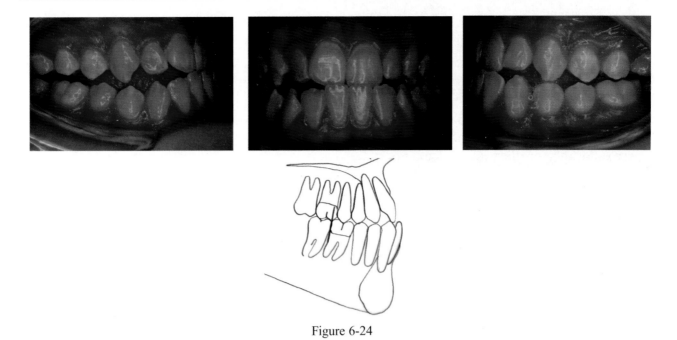

Figure 6-24

Even though these classifications are used throughout dentistry, we must remember that they do not describe the total picture.

Having determined the molar classification, we must now evaluate the anterior teeth and note the problems associated with their position. **Overjet** is the term used to describe the distance between the labial surface of the mandibular incisors and the incisal edge of the maxillary incisors. This is usually measured along the occlusal plane and is determined by the most anteriorly positioned incisors. **Crossbite** is a malrelation between the maxillary and mandibular teeth when they occlude with the antagonistic tooth in an opposite relationship to normal. It can involve one or more teeth and may be present in the anterior and/or the posterior teeth. When the maxillary central incisor is occluding with the lingual of the mandibular central incisor this is termed an **anterior crossbite** (Figure 6-24 center photo). To establish the problem arch, one would evaluate the arches to determine which arch form is deviant. If the maxillary **arch form** is skewed and there is an anterior tooth positioned palatally to the mandible, it is termed a maxillary anterior **palatal crossbite**. If the mandibular arch form is skewed, then it will be a mandibular anterior labial crossbite. Knowing where the deviation lies will allow for the proper planning to correct the crossbite.

4.3 TRANSVERSE DENTAL RELATIONSHIPS

When examining the transverse orientation plane, one is looking at the inclinations of the posterior teeth in both arches and the occlusion of the teeth. Posterior crossbites can be due to the malposition of the teeth and/or the skeleton and evaluating the intercanine and intermolar widths in the transverse plane will aid in determining which arch is malaligned. A **posterior crossbite** is present when the posterior teeth occlude in an abnormal buccolingual relation with the antagonistic teeth. There can be varying degrees of severity to the crossbite and they can be described as a unilateral or bilateral posterior crossbite. Careful examination of the dental crossbite is essential for determining the offending units because it will lead to the proper diagnosis and treatment. Looking at the inclinations of the teeth and determining if there are occlusal interferences will help to determine if there is a shifting of the mandible to the right or left and establish if the crossbite is unilateral or bilateral. The frontal **headfilm** should be evaluated to determine if there is an associated skeletal component to the deviation. The following terms are used to describe crossbites:

A **functional crossbite** is caused by an occlusal interference that requires the mandible to shift either anteriorly and/or laterally in order to achieve maximum occlusion.

A **buccal crossbite** is due to the buccal displacement of the affected tooth or teeth as it relates to the antagonistic tooth or teeth in the posterior segments of the arch.

A **lingual crossbite** is due to the lingual displacement of the mandibular affected tooth or teeth as it relates to the antagonistic tooth or teeth.

A **palatal crossbite** is due to the palatal displacement of the maxillary affected tooth or teeth as it relates to the antagonistic tooth or teeth.

A **complete crossbite** is found when all the teeth in one arch are positioned either inside or outside to the all the teeth in the opposing arch.

A **complete mandibular buccal crossbite** is present when all the mandibular teeth are buccally positioned to all the maxillary teeth if the mandibular arch is wide and a **complete maxillary buccal crossbite** when the maxillary arch is wide.

A **complete mandibular lingual crossbite** is present when all the mandibular teeth are lingually positioned to the maxillary teeth due to a narrower mandibular arch than the maxillary arch. A **complete maxillary palatal crossbite** is present when all the maxillary teeth are palatal to the mandibular arch due to the narrower maxillary arch. Both could be referred to as a scissors bite.

A **scissors-bite** is present when one or more of the adjacent posterior teeth are either positioned completely buccally or lingually to the antagonistic teeth and exhibit a vertical overlap.

4.4 VERTICAL DENTAL RELATIONSHIPS

The maxillary and mandibular vertical relationships can be associated with environmental factors, and/or skeletal deviations, and anklyosis of individual teeth or groups of teeth. **Anklyosis** is a fusion of two bones where they articulate and occur in the dentition when there is a fusion between the teeth and **alveolar bone**. Anklyosed teeth do not erupt with the vertical growth of the patient and are seen in the infraversion position.

An **overbite (positive overbite)** is determined by the amount of overlap of the mandibular anterior teeth by the maxillary anterior teeth and is measured perpendicular to the occlusal plane. The amount of overbite can be measured in millimeters or percentages of the overlap of the mandibular incisors by the maxillary incisors.

An **open bite (negative overbite)** is present when there is no vertical overlap of the maxillary and mandibular anterior teeth **(anterior open bite)** or no contact between the maxillary and mandibular posterior teeth **(posterior open bite)**. To effectively treat an open bite, one must determine if it is the result of an environmental factor or a skeletal deviation or both.

5. SKELETAL PATTERN

The skeletal pattern is examined by viewing the lateral and frontal cephalometric radiographs. The patient is placed in a **cephalometer** (cephalostat) which positions the head for the taking of a standardized head film. The standardized head films are used to evaluate the treatment response of the dentition and skeleton by comparing the pre-treatment tracing and post-treatment tracing.

Each radiograph is traced by hand or digitized using cephalometric points to create linear and angular measurements that are used to determine the hard and soft tissue deviations. There are approximately ten cephalometric analyses in use today. A **cephalometric analysis** is the process by which one evaluates the relationship between the soft tissue, teeth, and skeleton. Each presents a different set of values for the purpose of arriving at a diagnosis for an orthodontic problem. Analyses are named after the individual who described them in the literature and each focuses on the angles and measurements that were thought to give the most meaningful information that could be used to arrive at a diagnosis. There are some areas of overlap between each analysis and some enhance the diagnostic capabilities of others.

These analyses use cephalometric landmarks to draw the planes and record the various measurements for comparing the norms or standards established for the different races. There have been described 27 hard tissue landmarks, 15 soft tissue landmarks and 21 skeletal planes. Using the transverse, sagittal, and vertical orientation planes on the head films, a problem list is developed and integrated with other data to arrive at a diagnosis. There will be some terms that can be used in more than one orientation plane but the author has chosen to list them in one area to eliminate repetition.

5.1 LATERAL CEPHALOMETRIC RADIOGRAPH

The lateral cephalogram gives the orthodontist a sagittal view of the skeletal, dental, and soft tissue relationships. The deviations are considered to be measured along the midsagittal plane of the radiograph and represents a two-dimensional picture of a three-dimensional individual at the moment of the radiographic film's exposure.

Hyperdivergent and **hypodivergent skeletal pattern**s are morphological deviations from the norm and each requires a customized treatment regime. These deviant skeletal patterns were determined by relating them to the cephalometric norms. A **hyperdivergent skeletal pattern** (Figure 6-25) is one in which there is an excessive divergence of the skeletal planes. This type of individual is characterized by having a posterior divergent facial pattern with a steep mandibular plane angle, an anterior lower face height that is long with an open bite tendency, lip incompetence, and an often-associated Class II malocclusion. Other terms that have been given this pattern are the "High Angle" patient, "Vertical" patient, Long Face Syndrome, and Hyperdivergent Face.

A hypodivergent skeletal pattern (Figure 6-26) is one in which the skeletal planes are more parallel to each other. This type of patient is characterized by having an orthognathic facial pattern with a low mandibular plane angle, short lower anterior face height, and an often-associated Class II, Division II malocclusion. Other terms that have been given to this pattern are the "Low Angle" patient, "Horizontal" patient, and Hypodivergent Face.

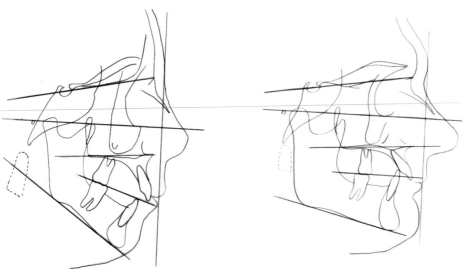

Figure 6-25   Figure 6-26

The deviations as well as the normal relationships (Figure 6-27 through Figure 6-31) that exist between the maxilla, mandible and the **cranial base** will also be evaluated with this radiograph.

Prognathism and **retrognathism** are the terms used to describe the position of the maxilla or mandible as it relates to the cranial base of the skull. The **cranial base** is the endochondral bone that forms the antero-inferior aspect of the brain case. Because the bones of the cranial base stop growing at a relatively early age, they are often used in the superimposition of serial cephalogram tracings as a reference structure to assess the growth of the jaws and/or mechanotherapy results.

Prognathism is a skeletal protrusion and retrognathism is a skeletal **retrusion**. Protrusion and retrusion are the terms used more frequently to represent these skeletal relationships as well as the position of the teeth as they relate to the maxillary and mandibular **basal bone**.

Bimaxillary prognathism (protrusion) (Figure 6-28) is present when both jaws protrude forward of the normal limits of the face.

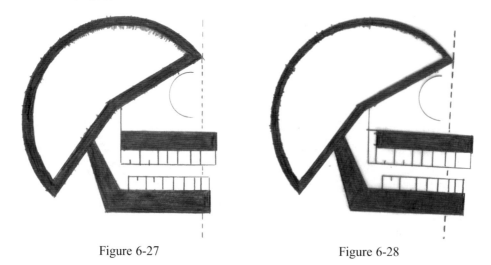

Figure 6-27   Figure 6-28

Maxillary prognathism (protrusion) is present when the upper jaw protrudes forward of the normal limits of the face.

Mandibular prognathism (protrusion) is present when the lower jaw protrudes forward of the normal limits of the face.

Bimaxillary dentoalveolar protrusion (prognathism) (Figure 6-29) is present when the anterior teeth of both jaws are positioned forward of the normal limits of the basal bone.

Maxillary dentoalveolar protrusion (prognathism) is present when the upper anterior teeth are positioned forward of the normal limits of the basal bone.

Mandibular dentoalveolar protrusion (prognathism) is present when the lower anterior teeth are positioned forward of the normal limits of the basal bone.

Bimaxillary retrognathism (retrusion) (Figure 6-30) is present when both jaws are posterior to the normal limits of the face.

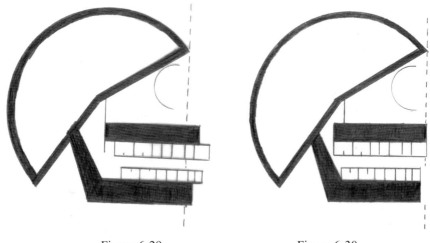

Figure 6-29   Figure 6-30

Maxillary retrognathism (retrusion) is present when the upper jaw is posterior to the normal limits of the face.

Mandibular retrognathism (retrusion) is present when the lower jaw is posterior to the normal limits of the face.

Bimaxillary dentoalveolar retrusion (retrognathism) (Figure 6-31) is present when the anterior teeth of both jaws are posterior to the normal limits of the basal bone.

Maxillary dentoalveolar retrusion (retrognathism) is present when the anterior teeth of the upper jaw are posterior to the normal limits of the basal bone.

Mandibular dentoalveolar retrusion (retrognathism) is present when the anterior teeth of the lower jaw are posterior to the normal limits of the basal bone.

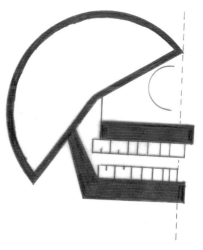

Figure 6-31

When a Class II or Class III malocclusion is present in a patient, it would be beneficial to know if it is a dental or a skeletal malocclusion. The angular and linear measurements that are obtained by using cephalometric analyses would give us the information needed to make that determination and treatment plan the correction.

5.2 P-A (FRONTAL) CEPHALOMETRIC RADIOGRAPH

The P-A cephalometric radiograph gives the orthodontist a transverse view of the skull. The head film is traced to evaluate the angular and linear measurements of the transverse dental and skeletal relationships. Ricketts has developed a detailed analysis that is useful for determining the various skeletal and dental patterns and it can assist the orthodontist in determining the maxillary bony width and aid in estimating the amount of expansion needed to correct a skeletal constriction. It would be beneficial for you to refer to the textbook **Orthodontic Diagnosis and Planning,** by R.M. Ricketts, et. al., that is referenced in the reading list to see a detailed description of the analysis and the interpretation of the results.

6. SUMMARY

A case description or classification is very difficult to present with just a few descriptive terms. There have been attempts to classify malocclusions in this manner, but the morphological variations found in the patient population will not allow this to become a reality. One must establish a routine during the evaluation of an orthodontic problem in order to look at all the different relationships between the hard and soft tissues. The morphologic variations that deviate from the norm will be the classification or description for an individual. These variations will be used to arrive at a diagnosis that leads to the development of the treatment objectives, treatment plan, and finally to the mechanotherapy necessary to resolve the problems and arrive at a balanced final result.

7. SUGGESTED READINGS

Diagnostic Data

Ackerman JL, Profitt WR. The Characteristics of malocclusion: a modern approach to classification and diagnosis. Am J Orthod. 1969; 56:443-454.

Angle EH. Classification of malocclusion. Dental Cosmos. 1899; 41:248-364, 350-357

Angle EH. The latest and best in orthodontic mechanisms. Dental Cosmos. 1928; 70:1143-1158

American Association of Orthodontists. Glossary of Dentofacial Orthopedic Terms, American Association of Orthodontists. Saint Louis, 1993.

Brin I, Weinberer T, Ben-Chorin E. Classification of occlusion reconsidered. Eur J Ortho. 1999; 21:169-174.

Dadkalogiannakis J. Glossary of Orthodontic Terms. Quintessence Publishing Co. Inc., Berlin, 2000.

Dawson PE. Evaluation, Diagnosis, and Treatment of Occlusal Problems. 2nd Edition. The C.V. Mosby Co., Saint Louis, 1989; Chapter 1.

Du SQ, Rinchuse DJ, Zullo TG, Reliability of three methods of occlusion classification. Am J Ortho Dentofacial Ortho. 1998; 113:463-470.

Farkas LG, Munro IR. Anthropometric Facial Proportions in Medicine. Charles C Thomas. Springfield, Ill. 1987.

Goodman RM, Gorlin RJ. The Face in Genetic Disorders. The C.V. Mosby Co., Saint Louis, 1970.

Graber TM. Orthodontic Principles and Practice. 2nd Edition. W.B. Saunders Co., Philadelphia, 1969.

Graber TM, Vanarsdall RL. Orthodontics – Current Principles and Techniques. 2nd Edition. Mosby Year Book Inc., Philadelphia, 1985.

Gravely JF, Johnson DB. Angle's classification of malocclusion: An assessment of Reliability. Br J Ortho. 1964; 1:79-86.

Grewe JM, Hagan DV. Malocclusion indices: a comparative evaluation. Am J Ortho. 1972; 61:286-294.

CHAPTER 7

Etiology of Malocclusion

Anne-Marie Bollen

1. INTRODUCTION

A **malocclusion** is a deviation from the desired form of occlusion as described in Chapter 5. While the word "malocclusion" specifically refers to the teeth, general usage also extends to surrounding tissues such as the bones and muscles of the jaws and face. A malocclusion, or deviation from the functionally and anatomically correct occlusion, like all other deviations from "normal" in biology, results from an interaction between **heredity** and **environment**. The interplay of external influences with the genetic blueprint or **genotype** of the individual results in an observed **phenotype**. The relative contributions of the genetic and environmental influences differ for different components of the phenotype.

Very little is known about the details of the **inheritance** for the many components that affect the occlusion. The head and face of vertebrates is a modular structure to which a wide range of cell lineages contribute (Chapter 2). Its development is dependent on a sequence of highly coordinated events such as cell migration, fusion of epithelia, cell polarization, cell signaling and specific extracellular matrix secretion. These events are precisely coordinated in spatio-temporal sense. This complexity makes the craniofacial complex sensitive to genetic mutation or environmental **teratogens**. One-third of all major birth defects involves the head and face. The complexity of its development also makes it difficult to sort out the role and influence of specific genes in the final morphology of the various craniofacial components.

Even less is known about the effects of the environment and how some genetic traits predispose subjects to greater influences from the environment. It is often difficult, if not impossible, to separate a hereditary from an environmental etiology. Any attempt to categorize etiologic factors is purely arbitrary. The craniofacial complex is continuously adapting to the environment within its genetic disposition.

A malocclusion is not a disease. A malocclusion is a symptom (or the end result) of disturbances in one or more of the components that influence the occlusion. The occlusion (the way the teeth fit together) results from an interaction between several components: the dentition, the facial skeleton, the **orofacial** musculature and other factors. A deviation in one or more of these components or sites may result in a malocclusion. The etiology of deviations in these sites, as discussed earlier, is a result of the interaction between genetics and environmental factors. Since the true etiology is not known, it has become customary to view deviations in either the dentition, the craniofacial skeleton or orofacial musculature as etiologies of the malocclusion. For example, a short mandible can "cause" a Class II malocclusion. The use of a deviation itself as an "etiology" bypasses the need to identify the true causes (genetic and environmental) that resulted in this deviation. This categorization into **etiologic sites** also has the advantage that it fits well with our regimen of diagnosis and treatment planning, where we tend to evaluate each site separately. Deviations in etiologic sites can lead to malocclusions, but **compensatory changes** in other sites may result in an acceptable occlusion. The remainder of this chapter will provide more detail about the contributions of each of the etiologic sites to malocclusions. Where possible, information is provided regarding the genetic and environmental causes for these deviations.

<u>Rationale:</u>

Why would one want to determine the etiology of a malocclusion? The rationale is that knowing what caused a problem may lead to strategies and treatments to correct and/or prevent specific malocclusions. To correct a malocclusion, ideally one needs to eliminate the cause of the problem. The true cause is a combination of genetic and **epigenetic** factors. However, since our knowledge of the contribution of these factors is scant, traditionally the "etiology" of malocclusions has been restricted to the diagnosis of deviations of "etiologic sites" (dentition, skeletal, neuromuscular and other factors). Also, eliminating the true etiology may not always be possible, especially for problems with a mainly genetic etiology (for example, missing teeth). In contrast, it is currently possible to correct most deviations of etiologic sites. However, with the boundaries of genetic manipulation forever pushing ahead, the future may yet bring us some unknown treatment possibilities.

We also tend to diagnose deviations from the normal separately for each of the etiologic sites. The available diagnostic tools to evaluate the various etiologic sites are discussed in Section III (Chapters 11-16). The resulting diagnosis will then lead to a treatment plan (Section III and IV, Chapters 16-21), aimed at correcting the malocclusion by eliminating its "etiology" (usually the problems diagnosed in each etiologic site) if possible.

2. ETIOLOGIC SITES THAT CAN CONTRIBUTE TO MALOCCLUSIONS

As explained above, due to our scant knowledge of the genetic and/or environmental etiologies of a malocclusion, it has been customary to approach the etiology of a malocclusion in terms of deviations from the normal in one or more of etiologic sites. Several etiologic sites can contribute to a malocclusion: the dentition, the craniofacial skeleton, and the orofacial musculature. In addition, there are some habits (which are not really sites) that can give rise to malocclusions. The "normal" or ideal condition of all aspects of each etiologic site have been determined from measurements on large groups of subjects who are without a malocclusion.

For each site the most common deviations leading to a malocclusion are listed. Deviations in each of the sites are the result of an interaction between heredity and environmental influences. Environmental effects include trauma, habits and disease (including malnutrition) as well as feedback and interaction between other etiologic sites. Deviations from the normal in any etiologic site may be a cause of a malocclusion or a secondary adaptation to a deviation in another site.

2.1 DENTITION

Examination and diagnosis of the dentition are discussed in Chapter 11. Several aspects of the dentition are under genetic control: calcification and tooth formation, eruption, tooth size and shape, and number of teeth. In the past few years, several genes have been identified that play a role during tooth development: **homeobox genes**, pax genes, HMG-box genes, zinc-finger genes and others. The precise mode of transmission is yet unclear for most of these (also see Chapter 14 on Dental **Dysmorphogenesis**). The following dental aspects can result in a malocclusion: number of teeth, size of teeth, eruption of teeth (location/direction and amount), and the health of the periodontal tissues.

2.1.1. Number of Teeth

-Supernumerary teeth
-Congenitally missing teeth
-Lost teeth (primary and permanent)

The inheritance of the number of teeth is autosomal dominant with variable penetrance. Therefore, the congenital absence of a certain tooth is often associated with **agenesis** and/or reduction in size of other teeth. While the number of teeth is inherited at birth, environmental conditions can lead to tooth loss, which may also result in a malocclusion.

2.1.1.1. Supernumerary Teeth

This condition is genetically determined. No precise information is available about the inheritance pattern, but there are indications that the presence of **supernumerary teeth** is linked to some skeletal dysplasias (for example, cleidocranial dysplasia). Supernumerary teeth are mostly located in the anterior maxillary region. They can be morphologically amorphous composites of dentin and enamel (usually conically shaped) or normally shaped duplicates of other teeth (Figure 7-1). Their location determines the extent to which they cause malocclusions. An impacted supernumerary tooth often is found accidentally on a radiograph and may not interfere with dental alignment or function. On the other hand, a fully erupted supernumerary will cause crowding since space for this extra tooth is seldom available (Figure 7-1) and there may be interference with occlusion.

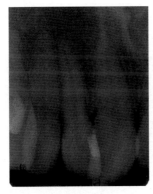 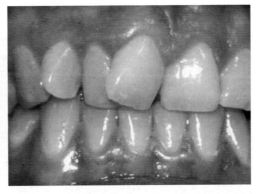

Figure 7-1: Supernumerary maxillary right lateral incisor. The presence of this extra full-sized tooth has resulted in crowding. Note the similar appearance of both lateral incisors.

2.1.1.2. Congenitally Missing Teeth: Hypodontia and Tooth Agenesis.

This condition is inherited as an autosomal-dominant, autosomal-recessive, or X-linked trait. The permanent teeth are more frequently affected than the primary teeth. The most common congenitally missing teeth are the third molars (20% in European and North American populations), second premolars (3.4%), and lateral incisors (2.2%). Missing teeth may result in problems other than esthetics. For example, absent mandibular second bicuspids can lead to retained mandibular primary second molars, which often become **ankylosed**. There are indications that congenitally absent lateral incisors are linked to peg lateral incisors on the opposite side as well as impacted cuspids (Figure 7-2).

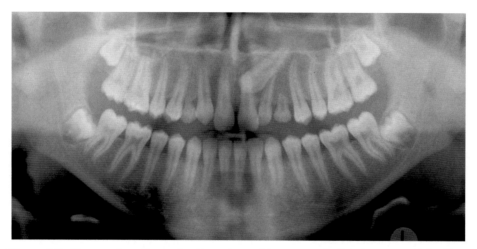

Figure 7-2: Panoramic radiograph of a patient with a congenitally absent maxillary right lateral incisor, a maxillary left peg lateral incisor, and a palatally impacted cuspid.

2.1.1.3. Lost Teeth (Primary and Permanent)

Early loss of primary teeth may be caused by extraction (for caries or other pathology; or in an attempt to "correct crowding") or trauma. Early loss of primary teeth may result in movement of the remaining teeth and eventually block out unerupted permanent teeth. Before extracting any primary tooth the effects of this removal on the space availability for the permanent dentition needs to be evaluated. The best space maintainer for an unerupted permanent tooth is the overlying primary tooth (Figure 7-3). Permanent teeth are lost due to caries, periodontal disease or trauma. This may result in tipping of neighboring teeth and/or **extrusion** of the opposing teeth. These changes may cause functional interferences.

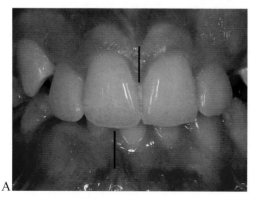 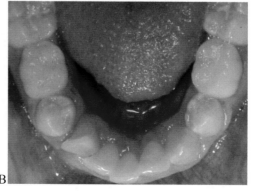

Figure 7-3: Unilateral extraction of the mandibular right primary cuspid has resulted in a midline shift. A.) Note the discrepancy between the upper and lower midlines and B.) the lack of space available for eruption of the mandibular permanent right cuspid.

2.1.2. Size of Teeth

The teeth are housed in the **alveolar bone**, which is positioned on the mandibular or the maxillary **basal bone**. The size of the bone base and the size of the teeth are both genetically determined. The linkage of the inheritance is unknown, but it is clear that a genetic blueprint for large teeth does not always coincide with genetically programmed large jaws. The obvious result of this mismatch is crowding of the dentition (Figure 7-4). Similarly, one can have teeth that are proportionally smaller than the space available in the jawbone. This results in spacing between the teeth. For most malocclusions involving crowding and/or spacing, it is unclear whether the primary etiology is the size of the jaws or the size of the teeth.

One other situation involving tooth size can lead to a malocclusion. This is when the size of the maxillary teeth is not in proportion to the size of the mandibular teeth. The result of this mismatch (the so-called Bolton discrepancy) may be visible as an undesirable overbite/overjet or as spacing/crowding (Figure 7-5).

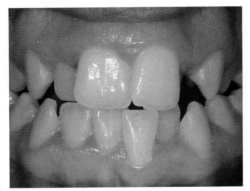
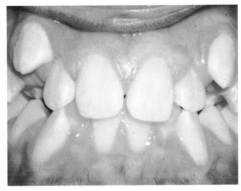

Figure 7-4: Discrepancy between tooth size and jaw bone. When the teeth are larger than the space available in the jaws the result is crowding (A and B). When teeth are blocked out of the dental arch this may result in a crossbite A.) or a scissors bite (reverse crossbite).

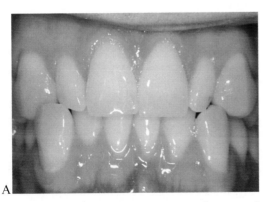
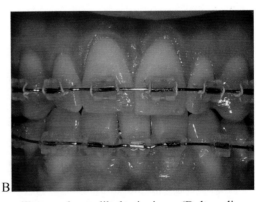

Figure 7-5: Tooth size discrepancy between the maxillary and mandibular incisors (Bolton discrepancy). A.) Note the smaller-sized maxillary lateral incisors. The mandibular cuspids are buccally displaced and in crossbite. B.) Same patient during treatment. One lower incisor was extracted. Note elimination of lower crowding and the crossbite. A desirable anterior occlusion and alignment is obtained despite the removal of one lower incisor.

2.1.3. Eruption of Teeth: Location/Direction and Amount

The ectopic development of a tooth may lead to the eruption of that tooth in a less than ideal position. This may lead to esthetic problems or functional interferences. Under some circumstances ectopically developing teeth do not erupt at all and become impacted (most notorious are maxillary cuspids). Also, the amount (too much or too little) of eruption of otherwise well-positioned teeth may give rise to malocclusions. The most common deviations in location and direction of dental position/eruption and the amount of eruption, are listed below.

Development/Eruption in the Wrong Place or Direction

While ectopic development is of multifactorial etiology, there is a genetic component which is linked to other dental inherited traits. For example: almost half of the patients with palatally positioned maxillary cuspids have anomalous or missing lateral incisors (Figure 7-2, Figure 7-7). Sometimes displaced teeth are a reflection of insufficient space availability. The teeth most affected are those erupting last in the arch (maxillary cuspids and mandibular second bicuspids). Depending on the tooth type, eruption in an undesirable place may have different consequences. For example, the palatal eruption of maxillary incisors may lead to a premature contact and a functional shift resulting in a crossbite (Figure 7-6). Mesial eruption of maxillary first molars may lead to premature loss of the primary second molars and loss of arch length. The buccal eruption of maxillary cuspids provides an undesirable esthetic alignment (vampire teeth, Figure 7-4B), however this eruption pattern may be more a result of deficient space in the arch than of an incorrect location of the developing tooth or a deviation in its eruption path.

When teeth switch places with neighboring teeth it is called a transposition (Figure 7-8). Transposition is an extreme type of **ectopic eruption** leading to a positional interchange of two adjacent teeth. Most common are maxillary transpositions (1 per 300 orthodontic patients), where a maxillary cuspid and first bicuspid transposition is most likely.

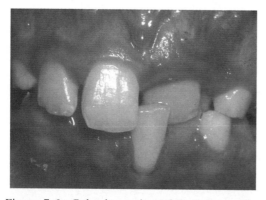 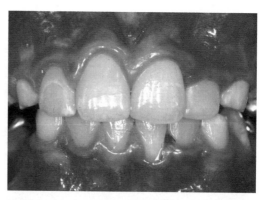

Figure 7-6: Palatal eruption of the left maxillary central incisor resulted in labial movement of the mandibular left lateral incisor. This tooth became periodontally involved: mobility and recession. The upper incisors were aligned (using upper molar **bands** and brackets on the upper four incisors). This resulted in spontaneous alignment of the displaced lower incisor with a decrease in its mobility.

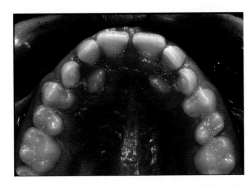

Figure 7-7: Palatal eruption of the maxillary cuspids. Also note the malformed left second bicuspid and a generalized reduction of the mesio-distal widths of the incisors. Dental malformations are often found in patients with palatal cuspid development, suggesting a genetic link between these traits.

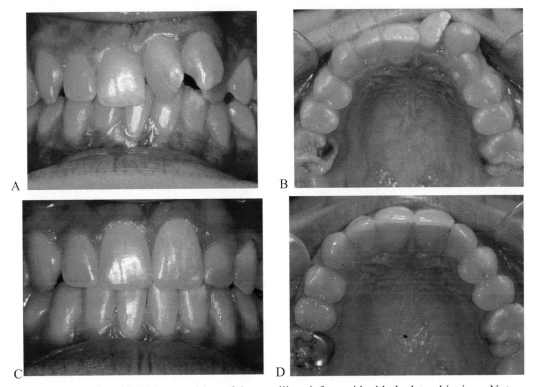

Figure 7-8: A.) and B.) Transposition of the maxillary left cuspid with the lateral incisor. Note the carious lesion on the upper first molar. This needs to be taken care of before the start of orthodontic treatment. C.) and D.) After orthodontic treatment which included extraction of the transposed cuspid. From the buccal the first bicuspid is indistinguishable from a cuspid.

Problems with amount of eruption

Deficient eruption results in teeth that do not reach the occlusal plane. This creates an open bite. Deficient eruption results in teeth that are only partially erupted in the oral cavity, or in teeth that fail to emerge in the oral cavity (failure of eruption, or impaction).

Deficient eruption is usually caused by environmental influences. Examples are deficient incisor eruption as a result of a digit habit (Figure 7-15), and deficient molar eruption as a result of altered tongue posture and/or function. Impaction is of multifactorial etiology. There is a genetic component, as well as localized interference with eruption (such as supernumeraries, odontomas, and cystic formations).

Most common are impacted maxillary cuspids (Figure 7-2), and third molars. The incidence of impacted maxillary cuspids is 1-3% in the United States and Europe. The prevalence of permanent first and second molar impaction is 0.06%.

Sometimes the periodontal ligament ceases to exist and bone fuses with cementum and dentin. A tooth affected as such becomes **ankylosed**. An ankylosed tooth is tightly stuck to the alveolar bone (osseo-integrated) and cannot move. Such teeth cannot erupt and therefore seem to become "submerged" compared to neighboring teeth. Primary teeth are more susceptible to **ankylosis** than permanent teeth.

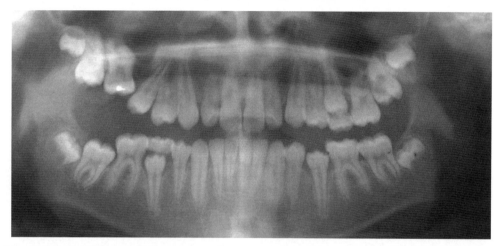

Figure 7-9: Deficient eruption of a maxillary right first molar. The tooth is completely submerged below the gingiva. However, at one time it was present in the oral cavity (note the occlusal filling) before continued normal eruption ceased. Note the effects on the position of the neighboring second bicuspid.

Increased eruption occurs when no opposing dentition is present. The absence of opposing teeth can be the result of extractions (due to severe caries or periodontal disease) or the result of a severe malocclusion. For example, in a Class II case where the mandibular incisors do not occlude with the maxillary incisors the mandibular incisors may extrude, leading to an increased **curve of Spee** in the lower arch. This in turn may result in an impinging anterior deep bite. Depending on where the lower incisors occlude with the palate, this may lead to loss of periodontal attachment palatal to the maxillary central incisors (Figure 7-10). Extrusion of teeth may also be the result of periodontal disease, where the decreased **anchorage** of the tooth in the alveolus leads to tooth migration and extrusion (Figure 7-11).

Generalized increased eruption of the dentition results in opening of the bite, a long lower face height and a divergent facial pattern. There are indications that in some individuals with low muscle tone the reduced masticatory forces allow greater eruption of the dentition. This combination of low muscle tone, increased dental eruption and skeletal open bite is often found together. It is unclear, however, which is cause and which is result: the reduced muscle tone, the increased dental eruption or the inherent skeletal growth pattern.

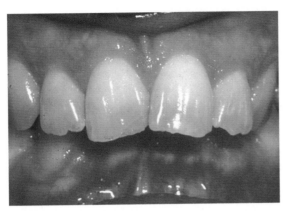
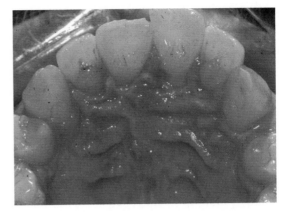

Figure 7-10: Loss of periodontal attachment palatal to the maxillary incisors due to over-erupted lower incisors (increased curve of Spee). Note the anterior deep bite (100%).

2.1.4. Periodontal Tissues

Teeth are held in the alveolar process by the periodontal ligament. Loss in this attachment apparatus can lead to movement of the involved teeth. While there seems to be some genetic predisposition to periodontal disease, certain environmental factors (such as smoking) certainly contribute. When the health of the periodontal tissues deteriorates, teeth will become more mobile. Migration of maxillary central incisors can lead to flaring, over-eruption, diastemas and rotations (Figure 7-11).

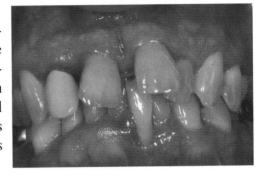

Figure 7-11: Loss of periodontal attachment has led to upper incisor flaring and over-eruption, as well as diastemas.

2.2 Facial skeleton

Examination and diagnosis are discussed in Chapter 11. Craniofacial morphology is a polygenic quantitative trait determined by genetic and environmental factors. Studies on twins and close relatives have shown the important role of the genetic background for the size and morphology of the facial skeleton. Family-line-twins studies have shown a strong genetic determination of the cranial base (shape and size), the palate (anterio-posterior and vertical position), the mandible (position and size), facial height and facial type. Growth pattern and timing of growth are, to a certain extent, genetically determined.

The genes have been mapped for some clinical malformation syndromes. One should realize that isolating genes responsible for severe developmental malformations does not necessarily point to the genes that play a role in the malocclusions we see in everyday practice. Most malocclusions are not the result of true malformations, but represent normal development with a less than "ideal" **outcome**. Such subtle variations in size, shape or direction of the skeleton cannot be studied with **knockout animal models** where entire genes are deleted, severely affecting the animal's craniofacial (and often postcranial) structures. In addition to the genetic contribution, other factors influence the phenotype. Even for the more severe craniofacial syndromes (such as **cleft palate**, **craniosynostosis**, Apert Syndrome), genetic mutations have been mapped to specific genes, but the way these mutations express themselves as the observed phenotype have not been completely resolved.

The potential influences of the environment on the craniofacial skeleton are well known. Prenatal trauma or fetal positioning can interfere with normal craniofacial growth. An example is inhibited or asymmetric mandibular growth due to intra-uterine pressure of an arm or leg against the face. Postnatal trauma and habits can have similar effects if they take place during growth. The ability of the craniofacial skeleton to adapt to environmental influences can be used to treat situations of less than ideal craniofacial growth. Pressure against bone reduces and/or redirects its growth. Clinical examples include **headgear** and chincup treatment. Tension across a patent (non-ossified) suture increases the distance between the two neighboring bones. If this space is then allowed to fill in with newly formed bone, the overall bone structure becomes larger than it would have been without this intervention. Clinical examples include rapid palatal expansion and facemask treatment. Changing the function of the craniofacial complex creates different pressures and tensions on the facial skeleton. This results in a variety of skeletal adaptations. Clinical examples include a diversity of functional appliances (for example the **activator** and bionator, the Herbst, and Frankel appliance), all of which change craniofacial morphology through a change in function.

The shape, size and position of the mandible and maxilla contribute most to malocclusions. When diagnosing the contribution of these bones to the malocclusion (a process called cephalometric analysis) each bone is evaluated individually and in relationship to the other skeletal components (See Chapter 15). The shape, size and position of the other skeletal components can aggravate or eliminate (compensate) the malocclusion.

1.) Maxilla. The maxilla can be excessive or deficient in all three planes of space. For example: a maxilla too long or positioned too far forward may result in a skeletal Class II malocclusion. A deficient maxilla in the anterio-posterior direction may lead to a skeletal Class III patient (Figure 7-12). A narrow maxilla (compared to the width of the mandible) results in a posterior cross-bite. When a maxilla is positioned too far vertically it may result in an **anterior open bite**.

2.) Mandible. The mandible can be excessive or deficient in all three planes of space. A mandible too long may result in a Class III malocclusion, a mandible too short in a Class II malocclusion. A mandible growing too vertically in a posterior direction may result in a Class II malocclusion and an anterior open bite (Figure 7-13).

3.) Other. The bony chin button is important in the esthetics of the lateral profile. A deficient chin prominence may aggravate the appearance of an already deficient mandible. A chin button that is too prominent may make an otherwise skeletal Class I pattern less attractive.

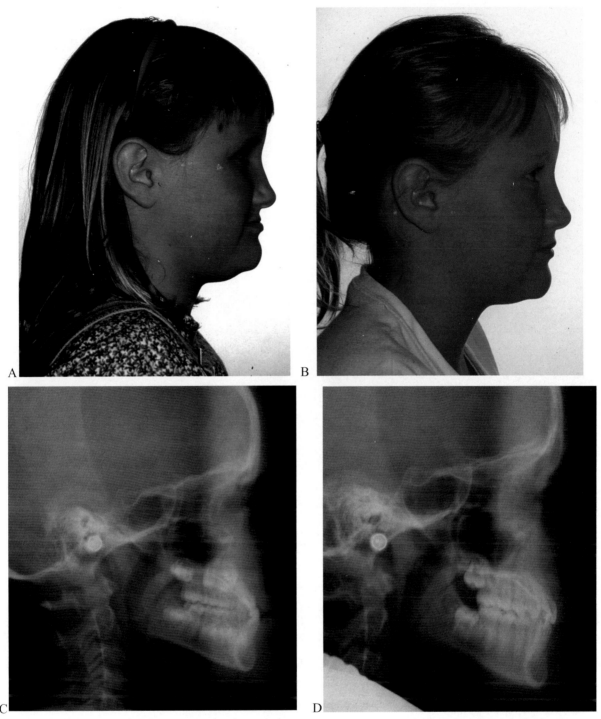

Figure 7-12: A.) A patient with a deficient maxilla in the anterio-posterior and vertical direction (age 7y 9m). B.) Facemask treatment brought the maxilla forward and down resulting in a more harmonious facial profile (age 8y 10 m). This treatment is based on the capacity of the craniofacial skeleton to adapt to external stimulae. C.) and D.) The lateral cephalograms of this patient before treatment and at age 10y 4m.

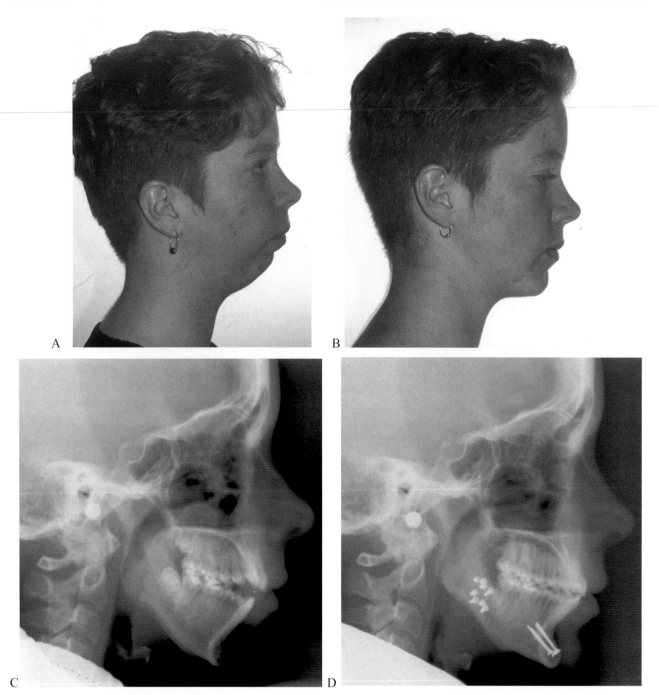

Figure 7-13: A.) and C.) A patient with an anterior open bite resulting from a posterior rotation of the mandible. The maxilla is in a good position. B.) and D.) Same patient after orthodontic treatment combined with orthognathic surgery. The mandible was rotated up, moved forward and a chin button added (genioplasty). Note the metal screws used to keep the bone segments in their new position after surgery.

2.3 OROFACIAL MUSCULATURE

Examination and diagnosis are discussed in Chapter 11. The muscles mainly involved are the muscles of mastication (5th cranial nerve), the facial muscles (7th cranial nerve) and the tongue. The neuromuscular system is partially determined by heredity. During development, however, myoblasts are secondary to developments in other tissues. Their development, migration, and orientation seem to be dictated by the changes in other craniofacial tissues such as bone. However in return, muscle activity directs and guides the development of several skeletal structures (such as the temporomandibular joint). While the genetic contribution to the neuromuscular system is clearly important, the environment plays at least an equal role in the development and patterning of the different muscles (Chapter 3). External factors such as pain and types of food ingested influence muscle contraction patterns. These feedback mechanisms rely on proprioceptors in the periodontal membrane and other sensory receptors. The jaw muscles exert a direct effect on the shape and size of certain facial skeletal components through their ligamentous insertions. An example is the effect on the **gonial angle** by the masseter. The craniofacial muscles also play an indirect role in the patterning and functioning of other structures such as the temporomandibular joint. This characteristic can be used to correct a malocclusion. For example, functional appliances to correct Class II malocclusions have been shown to cause changes in the facial musculature, the position of the mandible, and the location of the temporomandibular fossa.

Direct muscular activity on the teeth mainly comes from the tongue. The continued positioning and/or activity of the tongue to one area of the dentition can lead to tooth movement with a resulting malocclusion. Examples include an anterior open bite in response to an anterior **tongue thrust**, or a **posterior open bite** resulting from a posterior tongue position. There is indication tongue size may be under genetic control. Tongue thrusts may be genetically determined, or the result of avoiding the pharyngeal region (due to nasopharyngeal diseases such as tonsil hypertrophy), or as an adaptation to an open bite caused by a digit sucking habit.

Jaw muscular activity also has an indirect effect on the dentition and facial skeleton through the occlusion. It has been suggested that the decreased occlusal forces resulting from smaller and/or less active jaw muscles may result in greater continued dental eruption associated with skeletal open bite malocclusions. Increased muscle activity may lead to clenching and/or grinding. Under certain circumstances this activity may lead to severe dental wear and result in a malocclusion (Figure 7-14).

One should realize that it may not always be possible to determine the original cause of a malocclusion. The neuromuscular system (as well as other facial components such as teeth and skeleton) is very adaptive. The musculature continuously adapts to the external environment and changes in the orofacial area. For example, a habit such as thumb-sucking may inhibit eruption of the incisors, thus resulting in an anterior open bite. To seal off the oral cavity during swallowing, the tongue may be pushed forward during each swallow. If this abnormal tongue activity remains after the habit has been discontinued, normal incisor eruption may be prevented. Evaluation of a patient who has discontinued a digit habit but with an adaptive tongue thrust may lead to the conclusion that the tongue thrust is the initial etiology of the anterior open bite.

2.4 OTHER

A variety of habits can influence the teeth and jaws and result in a malocclusion. The most common is digit sucking. Thumbs and/or other fingers can exert strong forces that may result in malocclusions (Figure 7-15). The dentition is mostly affected (tooth eruption and position) but the skeleton can also be affected (narrow maxilla and a high palatal vault). As discussed earlier, there may be changes in neuromuscular activities as a secondary response to the changes directly caused by the habit, such as an anterior tongue thrust.

Soft tissue can also contribute to malocclusions. A large low-attached frenum can result in a midline diastema. The frenum (a large mucosal fold) may need to be removed to allow closure of the diastema. Scar tissue following surgery may restrict growth of the craniofacial complex. An example is the retruded maxilla following cleft lip repair.

The relationship between respiration and craniofacial morphology has been debated for many years.

Mouth breathing has been implicated as a cause of the long face syndrome (adenoid facies), a condition characterized by an increased anterior lower face height, steep mandibular plane angle and a constricted maxilla. While some studies have indicated some changes in craniofacial morphology after removal of the nasal obstruction and subsequent change from chronic mouth breathing to nose breathing, the data are inconclusive and most studies fail to find the relationship between facial morphology and respiratory mode. This is another example of our limited knowledge regarding the interaction between the genetically determined craniofacial growth pattern with exogenic influences (such as breathing pattern).

Diet has also been indicated as a cause of malocclusion. Some investigators have implicated bottle feeding to be less ideal than breast feeding. Also, a soft diet may lead to less inter-dental wear resulting in larger sized teeth and more crowding.

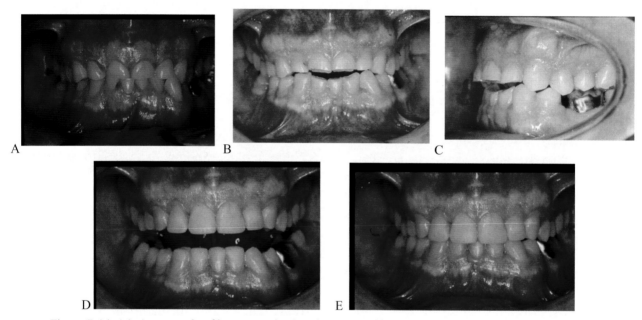

Figure 7-14: A.) An example of how extensive bruxism can result in a malocclusion. The maxillary incisors cannot be rebuilt due to the over-erupted upper and lower incisors and the end-to-end occlusion. B.) Orthodontic treatment of the upper and lower arches has intruded the incisors. B.) and C.) Frontal and left lateral view of open bite created after orthodontic treatment. D.) and E.): Temporary restorations to the anterior maxillary and mandibular teeth. Photos from Dr. Marissa Keesler.

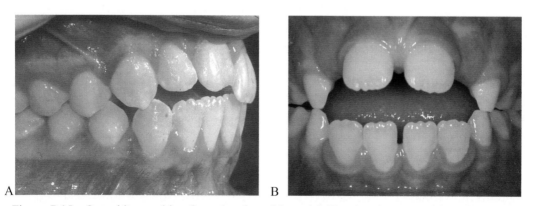

Figure 7-15: Open bite resulting from thumb sucking. A.) The thumb was positioned below the right lateral and central incisors. B.) The thumb was positioned in the anterior region. Note the constricted maxilla (end-to-end cuspid relationship). A narrow maxilla is commonly found in young, avid thumb suckers. This is an example of skeletal adaptation to external influences. For both patients note the retained mammelons on the lower incisors.

3. SUGGESTED READING

Introduction and Rationale

Hart TC, Marazita ML, Wright JT. The impact of molecular genetics on total health paradigms. Crit Rev Oral Biol Med 2000; 11:26-52.

Thorogood P (Ed) Embryos, genes and birth defects. John Wiley & Sons Ltd, Chichester, UK, 1998.

Etiologic Sites that Can Contribute to Malocclusion

Baccetti T. Tooth anomalies associated with failure of eruption of first and second permanent molars. Am J Orthod Dentofacial Orthop 2000;118:608-610.

Epstein CJ. The new dysmorphology: application of insights from basic developmental biology to the understanding of human birth defects. Proc Natl Acad Sci 1995;92:8566-8573.

Ferguson CA, Tucker AS, Sharpe PT. Temporospacial cell interactions regulating mandibular and maxillary arch patterning. Development 2000;127:403-412.

Garvey MT, Barry HJ, Blake M. Supernumerary teeth – an overview of classification, diagnosis and management. J Can Dent Assoc 1999;65:612-616.

Goldenberg M, Das P, Messersmith M, Stockton DW, Patel OI, D'Souza RN. Clinical, radiographic, and genetic evaluation of a novel form of autosomal-dominant oligodontia. J Dent Res 2000; 79:1469-1475.

Ho NC, Jia L, Driscoll CC, Gutter EM, Francomano CA. A skeletal gene database. J Bone Miner Res 2000;15:2095-2122.

Hu D, Helms JA. The role of sonic hedgehog in normal and abnormal craniofacial morphogenesis. Development 1999;126:4873-4884.

Hunter D, De Lange M, Snieder H, MacGregor AJ, Swaminathan R, Thakker RV, Spector TD. Genetic contribution to bone metabolism, calcium excretion, and vitamin D and parathyroid hormone regulation. J Bone Miner Res 2001; 16:371-378.

Kluemper GT, Vig PS, Vig KW. Nasorespiratory characteristics and craniofacial morphology. Eur J Orthod 1995;17:491-495.

Langberg BJ, Peck S. Tooth-size reduction associated with occurrence of palatal displacement of canines. Angle Orthod 2000;70:126-128.

Liu W, Wang H, Zhao S, Zhao W, Bai S, Zhao Y, Xu S, Wu C, Huang W, Chen Z, Feng G, He L. The novel gene locus for agenesis of permanent teeth (He-Zhao deficiency) maps to chromosome 10q11.2 J Dent Res 80:1716-1720, 2001.

Mundlos S. Cleidocranial dysplasia: clinical and molecular genetics. J Med Genet 1999;36:177-182.

Northway WM. Anteroposterior arch dimension changes in French Canadian children: a study of the effects of dental caries and premature extractions. Master's Thesis: Universite de Montreal. 1977.

Northway WM. Wainright R, Demirjian A. Effects of premature loss of deciduous molars. Angle Orthod. 1984;54:295-329.

Northway WM, Wainright R. D E Space - a realistic measure of changes in arch morphology: space loss due to unattended caries. J Dent Res 1980;59:1577-1580.

Northway WM. The not-so-harmless primary first molar extraction. JADA Dec 2000; 131:1711-1720.

Peck S, Peck L. Classification of maxillary tooth transpositions. Am J Orthod Dentofac Orthop 1995;107:505-517.

Pelsmaekers B, Loos R, Carels C, Derom C, Vlietinc R. The genetic contribution to dental maturation. J Dent Res 1997;76:1337-1340

Peter H, Balling R. Teeth. Where and how to make them. Trends Gen 1999;15:59-65.

Prece JW. The incidence of unerupted permanent teeth and related clinical cases. Oral Surg 1985;59:420-425.

Saunders SR, Popovich F, Thompson GW. A family study of craniofacial dimensions in the Burlington Growth Center sample. Am J Orthod 1980;78:394-403.

Scheiner MA, Sampson WJ. Supernumerary teeth: a review of the literature and four case reports. Aust. Dent J 1997; 42:160-165.

Shapira Y, Kuftinek MM. Maxillary tooth transpositions: characteristic features and accompanying dental anomalies. Am J Orthod Dentofacial Orthop 2001;119:127-134.

Taylor RW. Eruptive abnormalities in orthodontic treatment. Semin Orthod 1998;4:79-86.

Vastardis H. The genetics of human tooth agenesis: new discoveries for understanding dental anomalies. Am J Orthod Dentofacial Orthop 2000;117:650-656.

Whittington BR, Durward CS. Survey of anomalies in primary teeth and their correlation with the permanent dentition. N Z Dent J 1996; 92: 4-8.

Zhu JF, Marcushamer M, King DL, Henry RJ. Supernumerary and congenitally absent teeth: a literature review. J Clin Pediatr Dent 1996;20:87-95

CHAPTER 8

Force Systems and Tissue Response

Daman D. Thanik

Richard Kulbersh

James K. Avery

1. INTRODUCTION

Orthodontic tooth movement occurs from application of forces acting on the teeth. These forces could be produced by **orthodontic appliance** combinations such as wires, brackets, springs, loops, elastics, etc. or by the musculature that envelops the teeth such as lips, cheeks and the tongue. The teeth and their associated structures (cementum, **periodontal ligament** (PDL) fibers, **alveolar bone**) and gingival tissues respond to these forces with a complex biological reaction that results in the movement of teeth through **bone**. The teeth and the surrounding tissues, including the **gingiva,** collectively represent the periodontium (Figure 8-1).

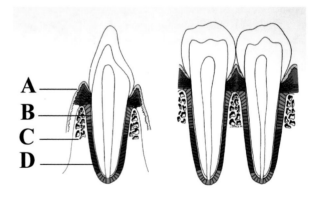

Figure 8-1: Diagrammatic view of periodontium (Latin *peri*: around; Greek *odous*: tooth). Mandibular Incisor (left view). The tooth is enclosed in the periodontium which consists of : A.) Gingiva covering the alveolar bone and the extra-alveolar cervical cementum, B.) cementum, C.) alveolar bone with marrow spaces, D.) periodontal ligament interposed between the bone and tooth cementum.

The cellular elements of the periodontium, regardless of how the forces are generated and applied to the teeth, respond solely to the stress and strain produced in their immediate environment.

The orthodontic medium to which physical forces are applied is biologic. This biologic medium is composed of three structures:
1.) Teeth
2.) Periodontal Ligament
3.) Alveolar Bone

2. TEETH

The teeth can be described as levers to which various combinations of forces can be applied by orthodontic appliances to produce specific types of tooth movement. The tooth is attached to the adjacent alveolar bone by means of the fiber apparatus of the PDL. PDL fibers also attach the tooth to the gingival tissues. The dentition consists of four types of teeth: incisors, cuspids, bicuspid and molars. The roots of these teeth are of different lengths and different morphologic configurations.

The smaller roots of teeth like mandibular incisors have a smaller root surface to alveolar bone ratio than, for instance, mandibular first molars. This consideration is of great significance in clinical orthodontics as the amount of PDL, and thus the **anchorage** value of a single tooth or group of teeth, is influenced by the root surface to alveolar bone ratio. Jarabak constructed a table of arbitrary anchorage values to provide a working guide for establishing comparative values for application of safe, effective force. If an arbitrary value of 1 was assigned to the smallest tooth, the mandibular central incisor, and 10 to the biggest tooth, the mandibular first molar, then the anchorage value with respect to root surface to bone surface ratio for each of the other teeth can be roughly visualized. In the maxillary arch, the first molars have the maximum anchorage value (9-10), followed by the cuspids and second molars (8-9), premolars (5-7), central incisors (4-5), and lateral incisors have the least (2-3). In the mandibular arch, the first molar has maximum anchorage value (10), followed by second molars (8-9), cuspids (7-8), each of the premolars (5-6), lateral incisors (2) and central incisors (1). These varied anchorage values can be combined to develop biologic resistance units to facilitate extensive movements of certain teeth while moving others only slightly.

In biologic terms, the term "**anchorage**" means the relative value of resistance offered by **bone**. Absolute resistance as found in hard substances like a rock or a large piece of metal is non-existent in alveolar bone. Thus, in clinical practice of orthodontics, anchorage means differential values of resistance existing between tooth units. The differing values of resistance offered by tooth units are due in part to both mechanical and physiologic factors. The determinant mechanical factor is the amount of collagenous fibers in the **periodontal ligament**. For example, teeth severely compromised by periodontal disease will have reduced amounts of collagenous fibers. The teeth with long or multiple roots have a PDL with more collagenous fibers than the teeth with smaller roots. The physiologic factor is dependent upon the ability of the alveolar bone to remodel and the PDL to repair and regenerate itself after an injury.

The anchorage values of alveolar bone vary in a wide range. It is influenced by age, hereditary factors, physiology of bone, diet, hormonal factors and general state of health. When the clinician is moving teeth by application of orthodontic forces, in fact he is changing the architecture of the alveolar bone, and in many instances even that of the **compact bone** of the labial and lingual plates.

It is important to understand that during the process of histologic remodeling of bone, the deposition of calcium occurs in two stages. During the first stage, osteon (**Haversian** system) is being built up to about 70-75% of what will be the final load of calcium stored by the osteon. The rest of the calcification of osteon proceeds at a very slow rate until finally completed. Animal experimentation utilizing radioactive tracers has shown that the dynamics of calcification is rapid at first, and substantially slows down as calcification approaches its terminal stage. This aspect has profound implications in planning of retention in orthodontic patients after the orthodontic appliances are removed. What is true for compact bone has been also confirmed for cancellous bone. Like compact bones, the trabeculae of cancellous bone are made up of varying layers of calcium. Engstrom and Engfled confirmed that the calcium content in the osteon is alternately high and low from one lamella to the next. Microradiographic studies clearly show this to be taking place in newly developing **bundle bone**. The differences in calcium content values become virtually nonexistent after the osteons are fully calcified.

3. GINGIVA AND PERIODONTAL LIGAMENT

It is a soft tissue structure, composed of connective tissue fibers, cellular elements, blood vessels, nerves, ground substance and interstitial fluid interspersed between the connective tissue and fiber bundles. Also present are the undifferentiated mesenchymal cells. The PDL fibers are mainly of the collagenous type and surround the root of the tooth. By means of its fiber apparatus, it attaches laterally to the surface of the tooth on one side and the bony socket wall on the other (Figure 8-2).

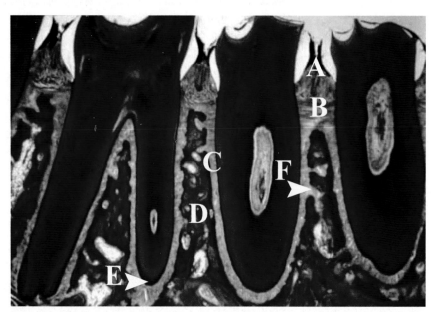

Figure 8-2: Histologic longitudinal section of the normal periodontium (buccal view). A.) interproximal gingival tissue; B.) transseptal fibers stretching from one tooth to the other over the septal bone; C.) intra-alveolar part of the periodontal ligament; D.) interdental bone with marrow spaces; E.) cementum (note variation in thickness of PDL on mesial–distal root surfaces versus apical region); F.) communicating channels between marrow spaces and PDL.

The PDL extends from the cemento-enamel junction to the apex of the root. It is approximately 0.3 mm to 0.4 mm wide. The width of the PDL is not uniform. It varies in different areas of the root surface of the tooth and in different tooth types. The average width of the periodontal ligament is wider in older persons than in younger ones, and two to three times wider in functioning teeth than non-functioning teeth. Functioning teeth are surrounded by dense **collagen fiber** bundles that correspond to the direction of **force**, whereas non-functioning teeth display poorly developed and poorly organized structure of the connective tissue that makes up the fiber bundle system of the PDL.

The **physiologic width of the PDL** can be defined as that width which it attains when the tooth is in function. **Biologic width is the width of the PDL** of a tooth that is not in function, for example, an impacted tooth or a tooth that has no occluding opponent. The physiologic width is greater than **biologic width**. The greatest width of the PDL is in the crestal and apical portions of the alveolar socket (Figure 8-2). The smallest width of the PDL is at the fulcrum of the root, which is generally located slightly below the middle of the root. The factors that influence the width of the PDL are: 1.) age, 2.) hormonal influences and 3.) the functional demands brought to bear on the teeth. The PDL is a richly vascularized and resilient tissue. It can have its structure, blood supply, nerve supply and function partially and totally destroyed, yet it has the capacity for almost complete repair and regeneration.

The periodontal ligament essentially fulfills four functions:
>   1.) Supportive function
>   2.) Formative function
>   3.) Nutritive function
>   4.) Sensory function.

3.1 SUPPORTIVE FUNCTION:

The supportive function of the PDL is performed by the collagenous fibers. Structurally the fibers are non-elastic. The slight elasticity in the fibers does not arise from their composition, but rather from the wavy configuration of their bundle-like arrangement. The main cellular elements (cell types), which produce collagen fibers, are called **fibroblasts**.

The fibers in the periodontium are divided into two groups: These fibers are called principal fibers and are arranged in distinct bundle groups.

>   - Extra-alveolar group of fibers (Gingival Group)
>   - Intra-alveolar group of fibers (Dentoalveolar Group)

The extra-alveolar fibers, as the name implies, are located outside of the bony socket, whereas intra-alveolar fibers line the inside of the alveolar socket, attaching the tooth to the **bone**. In both groups fibers extend from cementum into gingival tissues and from cementum to the **cribriform** plate of the **alveolar bone**.

3.1.1. Extra-Alveolar Group (Gingival Group)

The alveolar bone does not cover the whole of the root surface of the tooth. The margin of the alveolar bone follows the outline of the cemento-enamel junction and is located a short distance (approximately 1.5 to 2.0 mm apically) from this C-E junction, both on the labial and lingual sides of the tooth and interdentally. The crest (margin) of the bone on the labial and lingual sides is thus at a lower level than the crest at the interdental bone, called the bony septum. This area of the root surface, which is not covered by alveolar bone, affords the area of attachment to the extra-alveolar fibers of the PDL.

The principal fibers in the extra-alveolar group extend from cementum into the gingival tissues. (Figure 8-3)

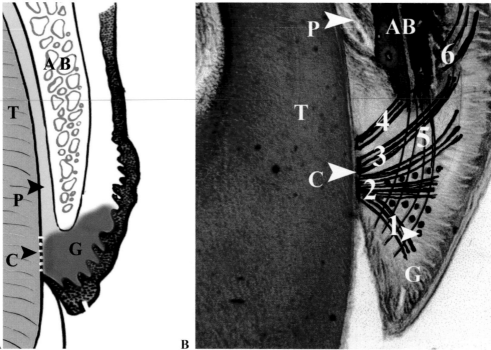

Figure 8-3: Diagrammatic representation of the histology of the gingiva. Frontal view, left maxillary canine. Part A: G: Gingival fibers; P: Periodontal fibers; C: Cementum—extra-alveolar cementum affords attachment to gingival group of fibers; AB: Alveolar Bone—showing buccal cortical plate and lamina dura next to PDL and trabecular bone between the two; T: Tooth root—surface covered with layers of cementum. The major portion of free marginal and attached gingiva is comprised of collagen fiber bundles (G). The periodontal ligament space (P) in an adult is 0.2–0.3 mm wide. Collagen fiber bundles are approximately 4 microns thick, occupying about 60% of the space. PDL fiber bundles traverse from cementum (C) to the alveolar bone (AB). Part B.: Extra-alveolar (dento-gingival) fiber bundles of left cuspid viewed in longitudinal section. Five of the gingival fiber groups (G) are shown. 1. Circular fibers appear as dots when cut in cross section. 2. Dento-gingival group fibers are the most superiorly placed, and their three sub-group fiber bundles extend from the cementum vertically and horizontally into free gingiva and apically into attached gingiva. 3. Dento-periosteal group fibers from the cementum extend apically after passing over the alveolar crest. 4. Dento-alveolar fibers extend from cementum in an apical direction and insert in the alveolar crest. Note that these fibers, along with dento-alveolar fibers of the intra-alveolar PDL fiber group, resist extrusion of teeth. 5. Alveolo-gingival fibers fan out into free and attached gingiva. Note the presence and location of periosteal–gingival group fibers (6).

Beside these, there are also fibers that extend from the tip of the bony crest into the gum tissues and into the cementum of the tooth. There are seven types of extra-alveolar groups of fibers. Four of the extra-alveolar group, namely, circular (circumferential), dentogingival, dentoperiosteal and transseptal, have direct implication in orthodontic tooth movement. They are named as follows: (Figure 8-3B)

3.1.1.1. Circular Fibers

3.1.1.2. Dentogingival Fiber Group

A.) Vertical Direction
B.) Horizontal Direction
C.) Apical Direction

3.1.1.3. Dento-Periosteal Fibers

3.1.1.4. Dento-Alveolar Fibers

3.1.1.5. Alveolo-Gingival Fibers

3.1.1.6. Transseptal Fibers

3.1.1.7. Interpapillary Fibers

The extra-alveolar group is divided in the following way (Figure 8-4).

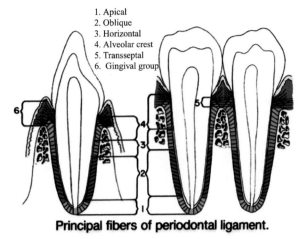

1. Apical
2. Oblique
3. Horizontal
4. Alveolar crest
5. Transseptal
6. Gingival group

Principal fibers of periodontal ligament.

Figure 8-4: Diagram of the orientation of periodontal ligament fibers of the extra-alveolar (dento-gingival) and intra-alveolar (dento-alveolar) PDL groups. They are: 1) apical group, 2) oblique group, 3) horizontal group, and 4) alveolar crest group. The level of attachment of fibers in #4 group to cementum is more incisal relative to the alveolar crest, and it has great clinical significance when attempting crown-lengthening procedures. Note: the inter-radicular group of fibers located between the roots of molar teeth is not shown in this diagram. The extra-alveolar group is indicated by #5, transseptal and #6, gingival groups. For detail of #6 group see Figure 8-3.

Starting from the incisal and looking toward the bony crest are the circular fibers, which encircle each tooth in the area of the **free gingiva**. Then there is the gingival fiber group, which consists of three sub-groups. The gingival fiber group also includes the circular fibers. The fibers in the three sub-groups of gingival fibers closest to C-E junction travel from the cementum in a generally vertical direction, ending in the free gingival margin after crossing through the fibers of the circular ligament.

The fibers in the second and third sub-group extend horizontally and slightly incisally and apically to the corium of the **attached gingiva**. The dento-periosteal fiber group, which is apical to the gingival fiber group, crosses over the crest of the **alveolar bone** and merges into the fibers of the buccal or lingual periosteum covering the alveolar bone. This arrangement of fibers resists the displacement of the gingiva. The major bulk of the free and attached gingival tissue is composed of dense, fibrous connective tissue. These fibers have also been called the gingival ligament. The dento-gingival group of fibers is the most superiorly placed fiber group and the most numerous, and is organized into thick **collagen** bundles. The dento-alveolar group of fibers extends from the cementum in an apical direction and inserts into the alveolar crest. This type of arrangement of fibers is instrumental in resisting **extrusion** of teeth.

The alveolo-gingival group of fibers (see Figure 8-3B) is attached to the alveolar crestal bone and extends into the **gingiva**, whereas the interpapillary ligament, as identified by Melcher, can be seen extending from the buccal papilla to the lingual papilla above the interdental septum, in the bucco-lingual plane. The significance of this is to resist the displacement of the gingiva during mastication.

The transseptal group of fibers is also part of the gingival group of fibers of the PDL. They can only be visualized in histologic sections in the mesio-distal plane since they do not extend into the gingival tissues. The fibers are organized into large bundles that run interproximally from the cementum of one tooth to the cementum of another tooth above the interdental septum (Figure 8-5).

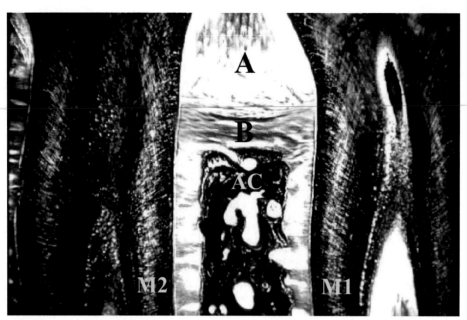

Figure 8-5: Fiber bundles viewed in mesiodistal section between two molar teeth, (M1, M2) above the crestal bone (AC). In interdental areas the transseptal fiber bundles (B) serve to stabilize the arch in mesiodistal dimension. They extend over the alveolar crest (AC) from cementum of one tooth to the other. The collagenous fiber bundles of transseptal fibers has been implicated in orthodontic rotational relapse, as well as in the loss of crestal bone related to aggressive intrusive move-ment of one tooth relative to another, tipping of teeth excessively mesially or distally incident to loss of adjacent teeth, and in orthodontic tooth movement.

Because they don't extend into the gingival tissues, they are termed accessory gingival fibers. The transseptal fibers are not seen in the bucco-lingual plane, whereas the circular (circumferential) fibers appear as dots or dark oval spots in the histologic sections. Thus the circular, free gingival and transseptal fibers are categorized as belonging to the extra-alveolar group of fibers. In histologic section, Atrinim & Hagerman has shown that the fibers of these groups all intermingle as part of a single mesh-work.

3.1.2. Intra-alveolar Group (Dento-alveolar group)

The intra-alveolar area extends from the crest of the **alveolar bone** to the apex of the root. Based on position and orientation of fibers, four relatively distinct fiber bundle groups in the PDL can be identi-fied in single-rooted teeth and five groups in multirooted teeth (Figure 8-6).

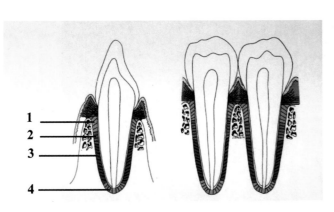
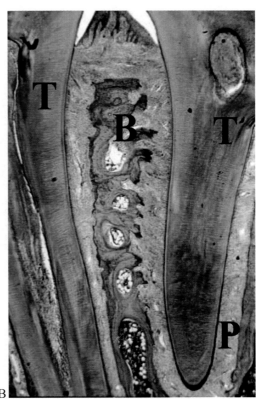

A   B

Figure 8-6 Orientation of periodontal fiber apparatus (intra-alveolar) of left central incisor and premolar (A) and molar teeth (B). Part A: (1) Alveolar crest group, (2) horizontal group, (3) oblique group, (4) apical group. The orientation of the fibers in relation to tooth and bone is indicated by their names. Most prevalent group is oblique group. Part B: Histologic longitudinal section of normal periodontium. (T) Tooth root covered with cementum, (P) Periodontal ligament, (B) Interdental septal bone

The fibers of the ligament are called the principal fibers, and they are named as follows: the alveolar crest group, the horizontal group, the oblique group and the apical group. As the name implies, the alveolar crest group extends from the extra-alveolar coronal area of the tooth to the alveolar crest (Figure 8-7A). This layer of fibers lies immediately below the transseptal fibers of the extra-alveolar group. The fibers in this group are not exactly horizontal. Cemental attachment of fibers is slightly incisal to the crestal attachment. Just like the apical group, they resist extrusion of the teeth. A short distance from the crest in the apical direction, the horizontal group is present (Figure 8-7B).

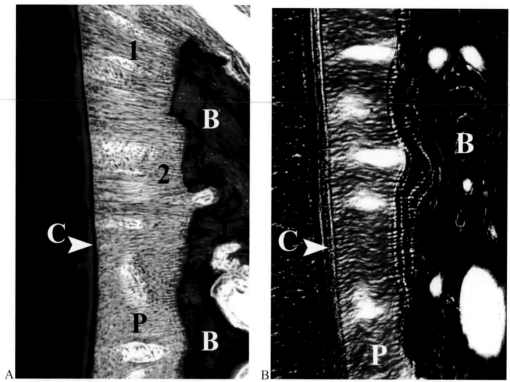

Figure 8-7: Histologic longitudinal section of periodontal ligament with interstitial spaces shown. Bone (B); cementum (C); PDL (P). Part A: **Alveolar crest fibers** (1) extending from alveolar crest obliquely upward toward extra-alveolar part of the tooth. Horizontal fiber group (2) travels perpendicularly from tooth to alveolar bone proper. Part B: Higher magnification of (A). Showing horizontal fiber bundles (2) running from cementum to bone. Sharpey's fibers can be seen embedding in bundle bone of the alveolar bone proper and into the incrementally layered cementum. Note the perpendicular orientation of fibers to bone and tooth surfaces. Haversian bone also clearly shown. White areas seen are interstitial spaces into which blood vessels and nerves run. The fibers attaching to the bone are thick fiber bundles, less numerous and widely spaced in comparison to the fibers and fiber bundles attaching to the cementum. Thus interstitial spaces (white areas) are wider and closer to the bone than cementum.

The fibers in this group (horizontal group) travel perpendicularly from the tooth to the alveolar bone. This horizontal orientation of the fibers resists tipping or horizontal movement of the teeth. Histologically, the fibers of the oblique group are most abundant and constitute two-thirds of the principal fiber apparatus of the PDL. The oblique fibers (Figure 8-8A) extend from root surface to the **bone**. The attachment to the root is more apical than to the alveolar bone. This arrangement of fibers suspends the tooth like a hammock, and plays an important role in resisting vertical intrusive forces encountered during masticatory function.

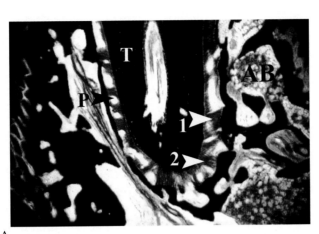
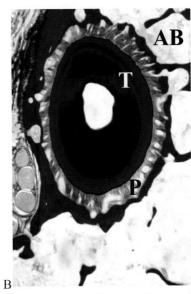

Figure 8-8: Longitudinal and cross sections of root showing the orientation of periodontal ligament fibers with interstitial spaces. Alveolar bone: (AB), PDL: (P), and Tooth: (T). At some places communication between PDL and bone marrow spaces can be seen. Part A: Oblique fiber group (1) extends from alveolar bone proper to a more apical location on the tooth. They constitute the bulk of PDL fibers. Apical fiber group (2) radiates apically from the tooth to the bone like a tent. This arrangement of fibers resists extrusion of the tooth and stabilizes the tooth against torsional stresses. Part B: Note variation in width of PDL, and interstitial spaces between fiber bundles. Blood vessels and nerve bundles run through these spaces vertically parallel and closer to the bone surface.

In the area of the root tip, the apical group of fibers extends from the root cementum to the bone and is arranged perpendicularly to the curved apex of the tooth (Figure 8-8B). The direction of these fibers functions in resisting vertical extrusive forces. The last, or fifth, group of fibers is the interradicular group. These are found between the roots of the multirooted teeth, such as molars and premolars. The principal fibers are arranged perpendicular to the alveolar bone and the root surface. These fibers resist lateral and vertical movements of the teeth.

To summarize, the extra-alveolar and intra-alveolar groups of principal fibers of PDL join the alveolar bone to the teeth and the teeth to each other, and forms a continuous unit that supports and unites the teeth. The continuity of the **dental arch**, in large measure, is dependent on the integrity of the gingival and periodontal fiber system. There is some controversy with respect to whether the fibers are continuous between the tooth and the bone or are made up of smaller lengths and spliced together. Some investigators have thought that some of the fibers of the PDL, especially human PDL fibers, were continuous from cementum to the cribriform plate of the alveolar process.

Sicher in 1923 investigated the phenomenon of tooth eruption of the rapidly erupting teeth of rats and guinea pigs and showed histologically that the principal bundle fibers are anchored both into the cementum of the tooth on one side and the **alveolar bone** on the other, and then run toward the middle of the periodontal ligament. This middle part is termed the intermediate zone, where the fibers are spliced or connected by short, intermediate plexus fibers of collagen and a collagenous cementing substance, both of which are the products of the fibroblastic cells. These intermediate fibers form a network of fibers running in all directions. Based on these observations, Sicher suggested that it was the intermediate zone or plexus where the adjustive processes take place primarily. Zwarych and Quigley in their study of mouse molar teeth have not been able to demonstrate the presence of the intermediate plexus. Their findings supported the concept that principal fibers were continuous from the cementum of the tooth to the alveolar bone. Sicher, in an effort to explain what occurs during tooth movement, reiterated his earlier stance that the intermediate zone, although quite narrow in man, does exist. If this zone is indeed present the following biological events can easily be explained. Small movements of teeth during masticatory function can be ascribed to the stretching and widening of the mesh-like arrangement of individual fibers in the intermediate plexus, because as such the individual fibers of collagen are non-elastic. Presence of an intermediate plexus means that the growth of the principal fibers would occur at the free end in the middle of the PDL. Under excessive pressure the intermediate zone would unravel, and intertwining fibers become unspliced, or torn apart, instead of the principal fibers being ripped apart from the alveolar bone or the tooth cementum.

3.2 FORMATIVE FUNCTION

At least five types of cells are present in the PDL space. Three of them are builders, one is a bone remover and one is a scavenger. The three builder cells are fibroblasts, **cementoblasts** and **osteoblasts**. The bone remover is the osteoclast, and the scavenger is the macrophage, or histiocyte. In addition to the above cells, there are also present undifferentiated mesenchymal cells in the interstices of the principal fibers of PDL and along the blood vessel walls. When given the proper stimulus the mesenchymal cells proliferate to become progenitor cells of fibroblasts, osteoblasts and cementoblasts. Scavenger cells and **osteoclasts** are brought into the PDL space through the blood circulation from the hematopoetic system (bone marrow).

3.2.1. Fibroblasts and Periodontal Ligament

The periodontal ligament, like all connective tissues, has two basic constituents – cells and the extracellular substance. The cells found in the periodontal ligaments are fibroblasts, cementoblasts, osteoblasts, osteoclasts, cementoclasts, and also undifferentiated mesenchymal cells. The extracellular substance is made up of two components – the fibers, which are primarily collagen, and the ground substance. The ground substance fills the interstices between the fibrils, the cells, the blood vessels and nerves. The ground substance provides the pathway between blood vessels and cells through which all metabolite regulatory substances and cellular waste products must pass.

Though the bulk of the **periodontal ligament** is made up of fibrous connective tissue, it is very cellular and vascular. The fibroblasts, osteoblasts and cementoblasts originate from undifferentiated mesenchymal cells, whereas osteoclasts and macrophages possibly have hematogenous origin. The normal rate of proliferation of fibroblasts and also of osteoblasts and cementoblasts in mature periodontium is relatively low. However after stimulation, there is a ten to fifteen fold increase in the periodontal ligament fibroblast cell population. This increase may occur primarily by division of cells positioned perivascularly within the PDL. It is presently uncertain whether the cells have a common progenitor or stem cell, or if each cell has its specific progenitor cell.   The fibroblasts of the periodontal ligament synthesize collagen fibrils and the extracellular substance, and are also responsible for its destruction and subsequent removal under normal physiologic conditions. This function continues throughout life. The vascular network supplies all the nutrients and regulatory substances to the cells and removes the waste products. The fibroblasts have long processes and they communicate with other fibroblasts, which give them their stellate appearance.

The fibroblasts are responsible for the production of **collagen**. They are derived from ectomesodermal tissues. They contain a nucleus, a rich network of endoplasmic reticulum, a well-developed Golgi apparatus and abundant mitochondria. The precollagen polypeptide chains, which aggregate into tropocollagen molecules, are synthesized in the granular endoplasmic reticulum. The group of ribosomes called polyribosomes, rather than individual ribosomes, is involved in the process of protein synthesis. The tropocollagen proteins are secreted from the cisternae of the granular endoplasmic reticulum, and are exocytosed into the extracellular space in the soluble form, where they later aggregate into collagen fibrils. The mechanisms, which control its aggregation in close vicinity to the cell membrane, are unknown. Electron microscope studies of PDL fibroblasts show the presence of microfilaments and microtubules that are usually credited with the locomotion of cells. The capacity of fibroblasts to move within the PDL depends on several inherent attributes that these cells possess. 1.) They are capable of synthesizing and degrading collagen. In addition to the enzymatic activity of collagenase, recent electron microscopic and histochemical studies suggest that they also are capable of directing phagocytosis. 2.) In vitro studies suggest that the fibroblasts can tie and untie their connection to the collagen substratum on which they move. 3.) Fibroblasts are interconnected to each other by cellular processes. Individual fibroblasts can connect, disconnect and reconnect with different fibroblasts as needed by means of these cellular processes.

The **resorption** of collagen is probably accomplished by hydrolysis of polypeptide chains of collagen macromolecules. It is believed that proteolytic enzymes, possibly collagenases, attack the fibers and reduce them into small fragments, then these fragments are phagocytized by phagocytic types of cells and digested intra-cellularly by their lysosomal enzymes. The cells implicated are: osteoclasts, fibroclasts, foreign body giant cell macrophages and blood vessel endothelial cells.

Collagen in the PDL is not an inert tissue. It is continuously resorbed and replaced during normal function, so that the amount resorbed and newly synthesized at a given time is equal. In normal adults, this active removal and replacement of collagen is referred to as collagen **turnover**.

By utilizing biochemical and radioactive tracer materials in experiments on rat skin, gingiva, PDL and alveolar bone, Sodek found that there is a very high rate of turnover of collagen in the periodontal ligament, and that the rate decreases with aging. Using skin collagen as a baseline tissue, it was found that mature alveolar bone collagen turns over approximately 2 ½ times faster, gingival collagen 3 times faster and PDL collagen 15 times faster than dermal collagen. This high turnover in the connective tissues of the periodontium, especially in that of PDL, indicates that they are very active and dynamic metabolically. Sodek has calculated the half-life of collagen in the PDL of rat molars to be about 1 day, that of gingiva about 5 days and that of skin about 15 days. Further discussion with respect to different types of **collagen** and in which other tissues they are found is presented in the section on osteoblast cells and **bone**.

The ground substance of the PDL tissue is characteristically comprised of protein polysaccharides, which are proteins combined with mucopolysaccharides. There are four mucopolysaccharides, which possess a very similar structure – hyaluronic acid and three chondroitin sulfates: A, B, and C. The principal mucopolysaccharides in connective tissues are chondroitin sulfate A and C and hyaluronic acid. The polysaccharide component is synthesized in the Golgi apparatus. The protein entity is assembled on the granular endoplasmic reticulum, and from there it travels to the Golgi apparatus where it becomes attached to mucopolysaccharides and then extruded into the extracellular space.

3.2.2. Cementoblasts and Cementum

The cementoblasts are highly specialized cells whose function is similar to that of the osteoblasts. They lie in close proximity to the surface of the cementum. The cementum is formed initially by **appositional growth**, like bone, by the **cementoblast**s, which deposit the organic matrix in layers (Figure 8-9).

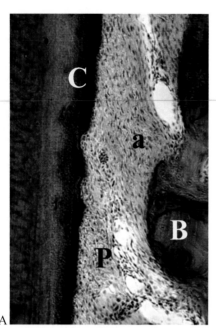
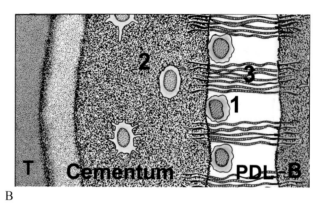

Figure 8-9. Histology of longitudinal section of root area showing attachment of PDL (P) principle fibers (a) to cementum (C), and bone (B). Part A: The surface of the cementum shows resorptive zones. The incremental line pattern of cementum (C) deposition is seen. PDL fiber bundles (a) (Sharpey's fibers) penetrate the newly laid down matrix. The sizes of the perforating bundles are smaller but greater in number in cementum than in alveolar bone. Part B: Diagrammatic representation of relationship of Sharpey's fibers in the newly laid cementum. Sharpey's fibers are small, thinner but greater in number in the cementum, whereas in the bundle bone of the alveolar bone proper they are longer, thicker and less numerous. Bundle bone (B); Tooth (T); Cementoblasts (1); Cementocytes (2) and Sharpey's fibers (3)

The **cementoblasts** may be associated with fibroblasts in the PDL and develop from the undifferentiated cells in the PDL. The collagen fibers being produced by fibroblasts in the PDL close to cementoblasts become embedded in the organic matrix as it is produced and deposited by cementoblasts. These are called Sharpey's fibers and remain almost totally unmineralized. The collagenous fibers in the organic matrix laid by cementoblasts, unlike Sharpey's fibers, are completely mineralized. The cementoblasts give rise to precementum, also called cementoid, in comparison to osteoblasts, which give rise to a prebone substance called osteoid. Cementoid is the non-mineralized organic matrix framework of the cementum. The cementoblasts in the newly developing cementum are in the recently laid uncalcified matrix, which lines the surface of the cementum. As the cementoid calcifies, some cementoblasts may get trapped in the calcifying matrix to become **cementocytes**. The fibers produced by **fibroblasts** in the PDL (Sharpey's fibers) get firmly attached to the cementum on one side and to the mineralizing bone of the **lamina dura** on the other. The fibers are oriented at right angles to the surfaces of the root and bone. The cementocytes exist in the lacunae and develop long cytoplasmic processes that radiate from the cell body and extend into the canaliculi. These processes communicate with other neighboring cementocytes via their processes. In contrast to this, the cementocytes in the deeper layers of cementum, closer to the dentin, exhibit few intracellular organelles and are in varying stages of degeneration. The cells in deeper layers become non-vital and empty lacunae appear.

The cementoblasts give rise to two kinds of cementum: 1.) cellular, and 2.) acellular (Figure 8-10).

The **cellular cementum** most often is seen in the apical third of the root, whereas the acellular cementum covers the remainder of the tooth. Cementum varies in thickness. It is thicker apically (150 microns to 200 microns) than it is cervically, where it is only 20 microns to 50 microns thick. It consists of approximately 50-55% organic matter and water and 45-50% mineral material. The mineral contents are in the form of hydroxyapatite crystals. Although cementum looks like bone morphologically, it is unlike bone physiologically. It contains no (1) blood vessels or nerves, (2) does not resorb as easily as bone and (3) contains no Haversian canals and does not appear to remodel. Throughout the lives of the teeth new cementum is continually being added to the old cementum, thus increasing its thickness. The continuous deposition of cementum at a relatively constant rate is a biologic characteristic of the tissue. Based on autoradiographic studies, the activity and mineralization rates of the cemental layers are slower than those of bone. The combination of constant cementum production, however slight it may be, and relatively slow mineralization may indicate that some cementoid is usually present on the outer surface of the cementum. Thus the continuous cementum deposition is essential to ensure the presence of resorption-resistant cementoid, which then could serve to provide and maintain the protection of the matured calcified cementum. The only time cementum is ever removed from teeth is when forces of high magnitude are placed against them, either in function or orthodontically—more so orthodontically than in function. Bone, on the other hand, is always in a state of flux; it is continually breaking down and remodeling.

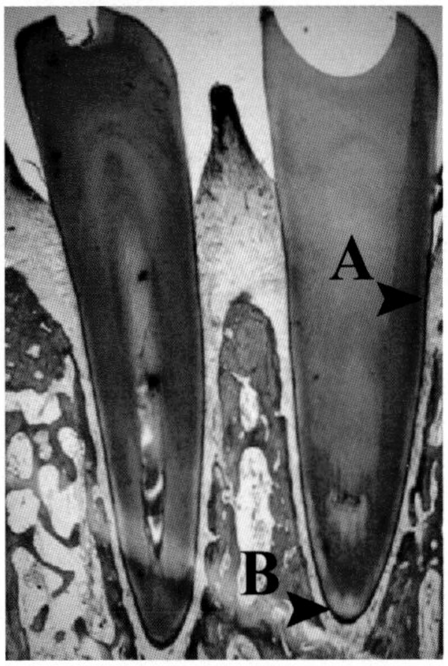

Figure 8-10: Longitudinal section of roots of teeth shows thickness of cementum. Note that cementum is thinnest in the root area closer to the **cemento-enamel junction** (A) and gradually increases in thickness at the apical region (B).

3.2.3. Bone Cells and Bone

Bone is a complex biologic system. Although bone is made up of dense tissue, at no time after its formation is it static. It is composed of three components: organic matrix, inorganic matter and water. The organic matrix component is made up of collagen fibers (95%), mucopolysaccharides (mostly chondroitin sulfate complex to protein) (4%), and other constituents including some reticular fibers (1%). Of the total bone mass, organic matrix component constitutes approximately 20%. The inorganic matter component constitutes about 70%, and the water component, approximately 10%. Morphologically, organic constituents in bone are indistinguishable from collagen and ground substance in other connective tissues. The inorganic matter (mineral content) is composed of calcium, phosphate, carbonate and citrate. The basic unit is made up of hydroxyapatite crystal ($Ca10$ $(Po4)6$ $(OH)2$), which is 35% calcium and has a definite lattice structure with a three-dimensional configuration.

As a general description, **bone** is a very dynamic tissue. Bone deposition during growth; remodeling during the process of development, internal structural transformation during its process of maturation and, in addition, the control of mineral homeostasis are all made possible by the cells of bone. There are three classes of bone cells that perform different functions. They are as follows:

- Osteoblasts – bone formation
- Osteocytes – bone maintenance
- Osteoclasts – bone resorption

These cells are probably one cell type, which changes appearance as it performs different functions. These cells mostly come from cells that have potential to form the cells of bone. These undifferentiated (precursor) mesenchymal cells of the PDL have the ability to proliferate and be converted into mature specialized connective tissue cells like osteoblasts and fibroblasts. The conversion from precursor mesenchymal cells in the PDL to mature specialized cells is brought about by at least two methods:

1.) Process of **differentiation**, meaning a permanent transformation of a precursor cell into a specific cell, or

2.) Process of modulation, meaning a temporary and reversible transition of one cell type into another specialized cell type; for example, osteoblasts transforming into osteoclasts.

Once the cells have differentiated into specialized cells, they lose their potential to proliferate. Therefore, mitotic activity occurs only in less-differentiated forms of mesenchymal cells. Precursor connective tissue cells that have the capacity to turn into cells with bone-forming potential are called mesenchymal cells in embryonic life. Mesenchymal cells in the postnatal period are not so distinct. The perivascular connective tissue cells and the reticular cells, for the most part, are present in the bone marrow and have the potential to transform into bone-forming cells, as they show a rapid rate of proliferative activity. These cells have been described as osteogenic cells, osteoprogenitor cells or pre-osteoblasts. The life cycle of the osteoblast is comparatively short, approximately two weeks. The osteoblasts are constantly being formed throughout life through the process of differentiation or modulation of precursor osteogenic cells, depending on the demand. As the osteoblasts retreat while laying down the organic bone matrix, many of them get embedded into their own secretions and become osteocytes.

3.2.3.1. Osteoblasts

This cell is responsible for the synthesis of the extracellular matrix of bone, i.e., the collagen and the ground substance of the bone (mucopolysaccharide–proteoglycan). According to Anderson, it may also be the initiator of the process of mineralization in the newly laid organic matrix of bone called osteoid. The osteoblasts are generally incapable of mitotic cell division and must arise by the process of modulation from precursor mesenchymal cells. They can probably also transform into other bone cells by the process of modulation, and into reticular cells by regressive modulation.

Morphologically, the osteoblast is columnar in shape and is characterized by the following organelles: a single nucleus, a very prominent rough endoplasmic reticulum indicative of active protein synthesis, a well-developed Golgi apparatus and a moderate number of mitochondria, all present in the cytoplasm of the cell, bound by the cell membrane. The cytoplasm of the mature osteoblasts contains a high content of ribonucleic acid (RNA). These morphologic features are suggestive of a cell very actively engaged in synthetic processes requiring large amounts of energy.

The osteoblasts are found in the deeper layer of the periosteum (close to the bone surface) and PDL (close to the **lamina dura**) and lie over the surface of the bone, around the trabeculae of the spongy bone, or lining the canals of the Haversian system including lacunae and canaliculi. The osteoblasts manufacture the collagen on the ribosomes, which are located along the endoplasmic reticulum. Collagen type 1 a straight-chain peptides of approximately 1000 amino acids are synthesized as intracellular precursors called a pro-α chain. By virtue of different amino acid sequences, two α-1 and one α-2 peptides unite in a triple helical structure called procollagen. The molecules of procollagen accumulate within the cisternae of the endoplasmic reticulum. From this site the procollagen molecules are transported to the Golgi apparatus, where they are presumably packaged into **transport vesicles**. Based on the observance of 680 A° periodicity, a characteristic feature of collagen fibrils found in these vesicles, it is suggested that the procollagen may aggregate here to form some **collagen fibers**, even before being secreted into extra-cellular space. But the major portion of the collagen fibrils are probably secreted out into the extra-cellular space in the form of procollagen, where final modification occurs with the stepwise conversion of procollagen to collagen molecules by the action of two specific procollagen peptidase enzymes. The free collagen molecules then assemble into their respective fibrils under the influence of cross-linking enzyme lysyl oxidase.

The collagen fibers produced by osteoblasts constitute the principal extra-cellular structural component of the bone, such as the organized fibrillar meshwork of collagen fibers and the unorganized amorphous ground substance. Each fiber is made up of smaller fibrils, which are composed of collagen molecules, which, in turn, are arranged in linear fashion. Collagen molecules are composed of three polypeptide chains known as α chains, coiled linearly into a triple helix. There are four distinct types of interstitial collagen molecules designated as Type I, Type I trimmer, Type II and Type III. **Type I collagen** is found predominantly in more rigid connective tissues such as bone, dentin and ligaments. Type II collagen is restricted to hyalin, elastic and fibrocartilage. **Type III collagen**, along with Type I trimmer, is found in more flexible connective tissues such as deeper layers of skin, vessel walls, PDL and the framework of many organs.

The collagen fibers of the bone produced by the osteoblasts are embedded in a ground substance, which is also synthesized by the osteoblasts. The ground substance consists of water, proteoglycan, hyaluronic acid and glycoproteins. Proteoglycan consists of a protein core with long side chains of chondroitin and keratin sulfate. They are often complexed with hyaluronic acid, and together they are known as the proteoglycan complex. Glycoproteins are molecules consisting of a protein core with short carbohydrate, or sugar, side chains. The relative amount of the above substances in the ground substance of the PDL is not known.

The actual mechanism by which the osteoblasts are stimulated to produce osteoid is not known, nor is the mechanism that determines the completion of matrix formation. Stimuli such as fracture healing and tension or pull on the margin of the bone produce osteoblastic activity.

3.2.3.2. Osteocytes

As the osteoblasts are producing new bone matrix they occasionally get surrounded by the matrix. The enclosed osteoblasts are now called osteocytes and reside in small holes called lacunae. In the lacunae the cell body is surrounded by non-mineralized lacunar material. The cells are connected to the blood vessels of the Haversian system by small tubes called canaliculi. The canaliculi are extravascular, their function presumably being to promote diffusion of tissue fluids required for maintenance of osteocytes and interstitial substance. The osteocyte has an oval nucleus of small size. In its cytoplasm there are few mitochondria and a small Golgi net. The endoplasmic reticulum is not prominent. These observations indicate a reduced protein synthetic function of the cell. Osteocytes can be easily identified by two characteristic features: (1) they reside within the calcified bone matrix chambers called lacunae and (2) they exhibit numerous cytoplasmic projections radiating from the cell body in all directions and extending into fine channels called canaliculi. By this arrangement, an extremely large area of the cell membrane-bone interface is obtained, which is crucial to the regulation of calcium concentration in the blood, the main function of the osteocyte. The other apparent function of the osteocyte is, by its cytoplasmic processes extended into the canaliculi, to maintain open pathways within the bone and to transport nutrient and materials from blood to bone and back. In a 3 mm section of certain bones there are 20,000 osteocytes and lacunae (Figure 8-16).

The life cycle of an osteocyte begins with its envelopment and ends with cell death. The normal life expectancy of an osteocyte is 25 years. In its beginning period, the cellular organelles still resemble and function like those of the osteoblasts. As the cell matures, the Golgi complex and its associated vesicles become more prominent, suggesting a rise in lysosomes to aid in the resorptive phenomenon. No mitosis has been observed to occur.

In a physiologic process called osteolysis, which is unique to osteocytes, mineral is withdrawn from and later returned to the calcified matrix surrounding the lacunae and canaliculi, thus providing calcium when needed to maintain the delicate control of the mineral homeostasis. During this process, the matrix is demineralized. If the process of osteolysis is prolonged, then several lacunae can become confluent, with the result that their osteocytes are freed. The fate of an osteocyte thus freed is unknown. It is postulated that it may revert to a new primitive cell and become part of the cell population of the marrow or become an osteoclast by the process of regressive modulation.

The last stage of the osteocyte's life is degenerative, characterized by vacuolization of its organelles, followed by death and degeneration. The death is generally brought about if the canaliculi become plugged and its nutrient supply is cut off. After death, the matrix surrounding the canaliculi becomes mineralized, whereas the lacuna is left empty.

3.2.3.3. Osteoclasts

The osteoclasts are multinucleated giant cells of mesodermal origin. This cell is most responsible for the resorptive aspect of bone remodeling. It is classically associated with erosion pits (resorbing bone) called Howship's lacunae resulting from a resorptive process called osteoclasis. The Howship's lacunae are cup-shaped depressions on the resorbing surface of hard tissue. Some researchers believe that the activity of the osteoclasts produces the lacunae. The osteoclast has the most fascinating life history.

The osteoclast cells can have multiple nuclei, ranging in number from two to one hundred. Depending upon the number of nuclei, the size of the cell increases to the extent that it can be the largest cell of the body. These nuclei resemble those of osteocytes and osteoblasts. The cytoplasm of the cell is often foamy and contains mitochondria and vacuoles, which are prominent. The mitochondria are more numerous per unit area than in the osteoblasts, indicating the potential energy requirement of the cell for its activity. The vacuoles are of big size and located near the brush border, and can be several microns in diameter.

One of the most distinguishing features of an osteoclast is the specialized cell membrane, found at the site of bone **resorption**, called the brush border. In tissue culture studies, the brush border extensions of the osteoclasts exhibit complex zones of infolding of the plasma membrane next to the resorbing matrix and shows active rough undulating motion. These foldings are in constant flux and are not true microvilli. These cytoplasmic extensions are only a fraction of a micron wide but several microns long. The spaces between these fingerlike projections or folds are tortuous and often show matrix debris between them when viewed under the electron microscope. The folds terminate as vesicles or vacuoles and apatite crystals are sometimes apparent in these vacuoles, brought into the cell by the process of pinocytosis. Based on the observations made in electron microscopic and histochemical studies, the **resorption** of hard tissue occurs in two phases. The extracellular phase involves the initial breakdown of a small area of hard tissue into partially dissolved fragments. In the intracellular phase, the osteoclast appears to ingest the breakdown products and complete the dissolution process. The process of bone resorption at the brush border probably entails both physical as well as enzymatic activities. Many lysosomes containing acid phosphotases are present in the cytoplasm close to the ruffled border of the cell. As the osteoclast attacks the hard tissue matrix with its lysosomal hydrolytic enzymes, the collagen fibrillar meshwork of bone is disrupted and exposed and crystals of inorganic salts are released. The freed crystals are taken into the cytoplasmic vacuoles of the osteoclast and are gradually digested within it. The disrupted fibrils are destroyed by the nearby fibroblast-clast cells, which are capable of both synthesis and degradation of collagen. One osteoclast can destroy, depending upon its size, the bone formed by 100-1,000 osteoblasts. Thus, for quite a large number of osteoblasts, there may only be one or two osteoclasts present.

The origin of the osteoclast is controversial and its fate is unknown. The osteoclast originates in the stroma of the undifferentiated mesenchymal precursor cells of the bone marrow and is brought as a preosteoclast into the PDL via blood circulation. The preosteoclasts are derived from circulating promonocyte derivatives. At times osteoclasts also arise by fusion of smaller cells, such as osteoblasts and osteocytes that are liberated from resorbing bone, or the fusion of spindle cells of macrophages. No mitotic figures are seen in the osteoclasts. Some researchers maintain that the lineage of the precursor cells of osteoclasts is the same as that of osteoblasts (i.e., mesenchymal cells).

The stimulus for PDL osteoclasis is possibly related to mechanical and metabolic inductive processes. Roberts and colleagues believe that since osteoclasts originate in the marrow, production of precursor cells of osteoclasts is under systemic and hematopoetic control. However, with mechanical loading, there is a mechanism for specific localization of osteoclastic resorption within the PDL. Mechanical induction is a specific response and occurs only in areas that have been modified or altered due to stress and strain and used by orthodontic forces. The mechanical stimulus for osteoclasis is probably related to electrical current – engendered in the bone by bending associated with mechanical stress. It is well known, based on many investigations, that bone deformation leads to the development of electric potential, presumably piezoelectric effect. How these electric signals are translated into many activities of osteoclasis has not been determined. Osteoclasts have very few specific bone-related metabolic hormone receptors. Calcitonin is the only osteoclast receptor that is directly related to calcium homeostasis or bone adaptation. In contrast, the osteoblasts have a whole host of bone-related receptors, such as parathyroid hormone (PTH), growth hormone (GH), estrogen, etc.

3.2.4. Scavenger Cells (Macrophages or Histiocytes)

Blood may be considered as a tissue consisting of free cells (corpuscles) and a fluid intercellular substance, or plasma. Genetically and structurally, blood is related to the connective tissues. The blood cells develop in the reticular connective tissues of the blood-forming organs and enter the bloodstream in a fully formed condition. The structural components of mammalian blood are not all true cells, and thus are often designated as the formed elements. They include red blood cells, the white blood cells (leukocytes) and the blood platelets. The red blood cells are limited to the bloodstream, whereas the white blood cells (leukocytes) function in the loose connective tissues and use the bloodstream merely as a vehicle of transportation.

In contrast to red blood cells, which contain hemoglobin and perform their function in the bloodstream, the white blood cells function in the connective tissue, where they have been described as wandering elements. They arise, function and die outside of the bloodstream. The bloodstream only acts as a place of temporary residence and a means of transportation from their place of origin to their destination in the connective tissues. The leukocytes possess a nucleus, thus are true cells. They show the capability of active amoeboid movement, by virtue of which they are capable of passing through the cell walls of the blood capillaries. The white blood cells can be divided into two groups:
1.) White blood cells (leukocytes), and 2.) non-granular form (agranulocyte) and granular form (granulocyte).

3.2.4.1.1. Non-granular form (agranulocytes):

Non-granular leukocytes include 1.) lymphocytes, which are small in size, and 2.) monocytes, which are of bigger size. These are comparatively undifferentiated and can reproduce by mitosis, not in the bloodstream itself, but may divide in the connective tissues, and in blood-forming organs.

3.2.4.1.1.1. Lymphocytes:

The lymphocytes of the normal circulation vary in size from 6-10 microns. They constitute about 20-25 % of the white blood cells. The lymphocytes of normal circulation are similar to the small lymphocytes of lymphoid organs. Large, immature lymphocytes are usually confined to blood-forming tissues, but may become abundant in the blood stream during certain pathological conditions such as lymphocytic leukemia. It is frequently very difficult to differentiate some of the medium sized lymphocytes from the small monocytes. This is easier to understand if one accepts the view that lymphocytes can differentiate into monocytes. The lymphocytes migrate through the walls of the capillaries and display marked motility in the connective tissue. Their function is not entirely clear, but it is believed that in the connective tissue they can develop into plasma cells and monocytes, and from monocytes into macrophages.

3.2.4.1.1.2. Monocytes (Large Mononucleated Leukocytes):

Monocytes are large cells, which constitute from 3-8 % of the leukocytes. They vary in size from 12-15 microns in diameter. Large monocytes are more active than small ones, but not as much as the neutrophil and eosinophil. The monocyte continually sends out and withdraws pseudopodia, and assumes an appearance somewhat like an octopus. In tissue culture, the monocyte can be made to enlarge and take on the appearance of, and with all the characteristics of, typical macrophages. In the body, they migrate readily through the capillary walls into the surrounding connective tissues, where they display their phagocytic characteristic. They develop into macrophages, which cannot be distinguished from the connective tissue histiocytes, and engulf not only fine particles, but also coarser masses, cells and cellular debris.

3.2.4.1.2. Granular form (granulocytes):

The granulocytes are characterized by the presence of specific types of granules in their cytoplasm and, according to the nature of this granulation, they are divided into 3 groups: neutrophilic, eosinophilic, and basophilic leukocytes. They are further characterized by the presence of many-lobed (polymorphous) nucleus, thus they are called polymorphonuclear neutrophil leukocytes. The granulocytes also differ from the non-granular leukocytes (lymphocytes and monocytes) in that they are more highly differentiated and cannot be reproduced by mitosis. The granulocytes give positive oxidase and peroxidase reactions due to the presence of a certain oxidizing enzyme.

The polymorphonuclear neutrophilic leukocytes (PMN) vary in size from 8-12 microns. They are the most numerous of white blood cells. They constitute about 60-70 % of the total white blood cells. The nucleus shows S- or horseshoe-shaped forms. The cytoplasm shows fine granules, which are neutrophilic. They are more active than any other blood cell. They advance by amoeboid movements, usually with the nucleus in the rear. After migration from the blood stream into the connective tissues, the neutrophils phagocytize bacteria and other small particles. Thus, they have also been called the microphages, or small eaters, in contrast to macrophages, or large eaters. They produce powerful proteolytic enzymes that act within the cell, as in the digestion of phagocytized bodies, or the enzymes are liberated and get outside the cell body. The neutrophils are attracted to devitalized tissue, bacteria or other foreign bodies by chemotaxis. The cells reach those places by amoeboid movements and they liberate the proteolytic enzymes, either by secretion, or, more commonly, by disintegration and rupture of the leukocytes themselves, which then become pus corpuscles. They are considered the first line of defense against invading organisms. The life span of various types of leukocytes is quite variable. Within the blood stream, the length of life for neutrophils is probably three days, and less than 24 hours for the lymphocytes. Senile and dead cells are removed in the spleen and liver by the process of phago-cytosis. Throughout their life there is an active proliferation of immature forms of blood cells to replace mature blood cells that are constantly being destroyed. The formed elements (red blood cells, white blood cells and blood platelets) of the blood are divided into two groups according to the location of their development in the adult. Agranulocytes (lymphocytes and monocytes) proliferate chiefly in the lymphoid tissues and are classified as lymphoid elements. Erythrocytes and granulocytes (neutrophils) normally develop in red bone marrow (myeloid tissue), and are classified as myeloid elements. Red bone marrow, like lymphoid tissue, is composed of a framework of stroma of delicate reticular connec-tive tissue in the meshes of which lie various kinds of cells. The majority of the free cells in red mar-row are immature, developmental stages of the granular leukocytes and erythrocytes. Red bone mar-row may also contain mature erythrocytes, granular leukocytes and a few lymphocytes and monocytes. Marrow is a soft tissue that occupies the medullary cavity of the long bones, the larger Haversian canals of the **compact bone**, and all the spaces between the trabeculae of spongy bone.

3.2.4.1.3. The Histiocytes or Macrophages

They are found in all loose connective tissues. The cells described as resting, wandering cells have been found to be identical with these histiocytes. The cells are irregular in shape with short and blunt cyto-plasmic processes. It is characterized by a small nucleus in comparison to the nucleus of the fibroblasts. The cytoplasm contains coarse granules and vacuoles. They take up trypan blue, colloidal carbon, etc. and store it in their vacuoles. They show active amoeboid movement and great phagocytic capacity under abnormal conditions, such as inflammation.

Macrophages or histiocytes are widely distributed throughout the body. Since they are present in loose connective tissue, therefore, they are present in all fascia. They also occur in the connective tissues of different organs, but the proportion of histiocyte to fibroblast varies considerably in the sinusoids of the liver, in the lymphoid organs and in the bone marrow. In the aggregate they form the "Macrophage System" or reticuloendothelial system.

3.3 NUTRITIVE FUNCTION

All periodontal tissues, but especially the PDL, have a rich blood supply. This is due not only to the high metabolism of the cell and fiber-rich tissue, but also to the mechanical and functional demands that are placed on the periodontium. Under normal physiologic conditions, occlusal forces are resisted by the PDL and the alveolar process and by means of tissue fluids and its shift within the PDL space, as well as by the circular and longitudinal blood vessels of the ligament. These blood vessels provide network functioning in "dampening" (shock absorbing effect, hydraulic pressure distribution, etc.) the change in shape of the ligament, which occurs when teeth are occluded. When mechanical forces are applied to the teeth, the root is pressed into the membrane on one side and the fibers of PDL are thus pressed against the bony wall of the alveolus, which in turn compresses the blood vessels in this area and necessitates a readjustment of the blood flow to prevent congestion. On the opposite side of the tooth root the fibers of the PDL are placed under tension. The blood vessels that are running between the fiber bundles are compressed and their lumen become flattened and narrow, thus reducing the blood flow.

When the mechanical **force** is light and applied reasonably and slowly, the vasomotor system takes care of this required modification in blood flow. It is well prepared to do so, because the same phenome-non occurs when the teeth are functioning during swallowing and mastication. Thus, within justifiable limits, there is absolutely no danger in applying pressure and tension to any of the teeth. On the other hand, when the force applied to the tooth is severe, the vasomotor nerves are paralyzed and the blood vessel walls injured, so that the lumen of some of the arteries and veins become greatly enlarged from loss of muscular tonus of the vessel walls, while other blood vessels are completely closed. These events bring about diapedesis of the blood elements and thrombosis and other degenerative changes appear in the structure of the tooth, PDL and **bone**.

The main arteries of the periodontal tissues and **alveolar bone** in the maxilla and mandible are the branches of the external carotid artery. In the maxilla these are: 1.) anterior and posterior alveolar arteries, 2.) infraorbital artery, and 3.) greater palatine artery that, in turn, are branches of the 3rd or pterygopalatine portion of the maxillary artery. In the mandible, the artery is the inferior alveolar artery with its mental, incisal and lingual branches, which is a branch of the first or mandibular portion of the maxillary artery, which in turn arises from the external carotid artery. In addition to buccal and facial arteries, the sublingual artery, the branch of lingual artery arising from external carotid, supplies the mucous membranes of the mouth and gums. The branches of the alveolar arteries of both maxilla and mandible pass occlusally in all directions into the PDL space, interdental bony septum, interradicular bony septum and gingival tissues.

The blood vessels circle the tooth and connect with others that run vertically from the tooth apex to the **gingiva**. These vessels are located in the PDL space nearer to wall of the alveolus than the cementum. As they pass upward through the wider interstitial spaces, which are closer to the bone surface, they receive branches from and give off branches to the bone of the alveolar wall. They end by anastamosing with blood vessels of the gingiva and help supply this tissue. When a cross section of a tooth root is viewed, the regularity of longitudinal vessels can be seen (Figure 8-11A). A longitudinal section through the periodontium clearly illustrates the communicating branches of the longitudinal plexus (Figure 8-11B).

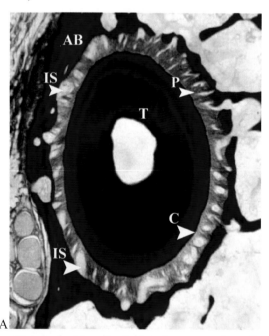 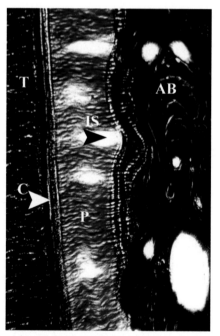

Figure 8-11: Histological longitudinal and cross-section of periodontal ligament illustrating vascular and neural supply pathways. Alveolar bone (AB), PDL (P), Tooth (T), Cementum (C), and Interstitial Space (IS). Part A: Note irregularity of the interstitial spaces (IS) between the PDL fiber bundles (P). At places communicating channels between alveolar bone (AB) and interstitial space (IS) can be seen. Part B: Interstitial spaces (IS) between the principal fiber bundles (P) through which ascending and descending blood vessels, nerve bundles and lymphatics run. Note the spaces are wider closer to the Alveolar Bone (AB).

3.3.1. Vascularity of the **Periodontal Ligament**

The anatomical assessment of the arrangement of the arterial system connected with PDL shows that this structure (PDL) is supplied by vessels that come from three sources:

1.) From the main arteries of the mandible and maxilla such as alveolar arteries, from the branches of which dental arteries enter the PDL space through the apical portion of the alveolus, before it enters the pulp canal.
2.) From vessels (interdental, interradicular) that enter through the perforations in the wall of the **alveolar bone proper** or lamina dura.
3.) From vessels that course through the gingival tissue near the area of junctional epithelium (Figure 8-12).

The vessels of the ligament form an elaborate anastamosing network, which provides the ligament with an interrelated chain of vessels. This network of blood vessels ends in coiled loops near the alveolar crest and in the apical areas. The elaborate and extensive arrangement of blood vessels in the PDL, and intercommunication between ligament vessels and septal bone and crestal bone vessels through the perforations in the alveolar bone proper can be visualized in histologic sections when tissues were perfused with India ink. Within the PDL the vascular network is especially dense, taking on the appearance and character of a thick woven basket. In view of this, therefore, ligament is highly vascular tissue, suggesting a need for a copious blood supply.

Not only does the copious supply of blood aid and assure safety during the active period of tooth movement, but it also offers a source of help after orthodontic movement is completed and the bone of the alveolar process is reconstructing itself. During the orthodontic retention period, the network of blood vessels assures the supply of essential building materials for reconstruction of PDL and bone tissues and also provides means of transport for elimination of waste products. The observations discussed above support the view that the formative and nutritive functions of the ligament constitute a critical aspect of ligament physiology.

3.3.2. Vascularity of Alveolar Bone

The (lamina dura), labial and lingual cortical plates with their **Haversian bone**, and the trabecular bone of the alveolar process are supplied by interdental and interradicular and other smaller subdivisions of the main arteries which supply the bone of the maxilla and mandible. Outer cortical plates are also supplied by periosteal arteries. Bone is highly vascular tissue. Arteries enter the cancellous or trabecular bone of the maxilla and mandible and the alveolar bone from all sides and

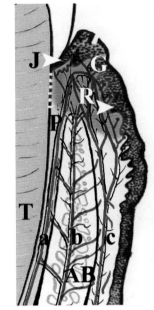

Figure 8-12: Diagrammatic representation of the blood supply and neural pathways of the periodontium: PDL (P), Gingival Tissue (G), Alveolar Bone (AB), Tooth (T), Junctional Epithelium (J), and Rete Ridges (R). Three sources of vascular and nerve supply are illustrated: Dental artery and nerve bundles (a) entering the PDL space (P) in the apical area, coursing toward the gingiva. In the PDL, they are located closer to the bone surface than cementum. Alveolar artery and nerves (b) run in the substance of the spongy bone toward the alveolar crest, and communicate with the PDL (P) and gingival tissue (G) through perforations in the lamina dura and alveolar bone (AB) in the crestal area. Periosteal blood vessels and nerves (c) run along the cortical surface of the alveolar bone (AB) and anastamose with the terminal blood vessels and nerves of the PDL (P). Note: The blood vessels (a, b, c) exhibit frequent anastamoses with each other. Adjacent to junctional epithelium (J), blood vessels form a dense plexus with numerous venules and in the area of the rete ridges, and capillary loops (R).

branches until they become oriented to the outline of the marrow spaces formed by the individual trabeculae.

3.3.3. Vascularity of Gingival Tissues

Gingival connective tissues are highly vascular. The blood vessels supplying this area have their origin in the structure of the periodontium, and extend into the lamina propria of the free gingival tissues. The first source of supply is from the branches of the periosteal vessels originating from the lingual, palatal, buccal and labial arteries. These vessels give off secondary branches along the labial and lingual surfaces of the **alveolar bone**, and can be readily seen through the stretched oral and vestibular mucosal tissues. The second source of supply is from the dental arteries that run vertically in the PDL compartment and exit in the area of junctional epithelium into the substance of free gingival tissues. The third source of gingival supply is from the interdental septal arteries, which exit into the periosteal side of the alveolar process through the perforations in the cortical plates and crestal bone of the alveolar bone. Both dental (PDL arteries) and interdental septal arteries are the branches of alveolar arteries that run in the maxilla and the mandible. These alveolar vessels anastamose with vessels from the periosteum to form the vascular bed of the gingiva. Observations made in young spider monkey PDL by Grant and Bernick (1972) observed that the septal vessels arborize to enter and anastamose with PDL vessels. In the transseptal region, a rich anastamosing plexus is formed by the branches of interdental septal vessels from the distal surface of one and mesial surface of the adjacent tooth, and also the crestal branches of the buccal and lingual gingival vessels. From this anastamosing plexus, arborizations arise and proceed into the lamina propria of the free gingiva to form terminal vascular loops. This arrangement of anastamosing vessels can be clearly seen in histologic sections, where gingival tissues have been perfused with injected India ink.

3.4 SENSORY FUNCTION

The nerve supply of the periodontium, which includes gingiva, cementum, PDL, and alveolus, is derived mainly from the trigeminal nerve, or the fifth cranial nerve. The teeth and their investing tissues in the maxilla and the mandible are supplied by the maxillary and mandibular branches of the fifth cranial nerve. These nerves, in general and with slight variations, have the same point of entrance and same distribution as the blood vessels. The most important afferent nerves for the alveolar process and the periodontium are:

A.) In the maxilla, the posterior superior alveolar, middle superior alveolar and anterior superior alveolar nerves, and the greater palatine nerve supplying the **gingiva**.

B.) In the mandible, the main source is the inferior alveolar nerve and its branches- dental, incisive and mental; and the buccal nerve supplying the mucosa and the gingiva.

3.4.1. Innervation of the **Periodontal Ligament**

The nerve supply of the PDL in both maxilla and mandible is derived from three sources:

A.) Nerve fiber bundles coming from the periapical area arise from the dental branches of the alveolar nerves and enter the PDL space along with the nerve trunk entering the pulp canal.
B.) Nerve fiber bundles branching from the interdental septal and interradicular septal nerves pass into the PDL space through opening in the walls of the or lamina dura.
C.) Terminal nerve fibers of the gingival nerves anastamose across the alveolar crest with the terminal branches of the PDL in the crestal area.

The majority of the nerve fibers supplying the PDL pass through foraminae in the base of the **alveolar bone** to enter the PDL space in the area of the root apex, while others enter in the lateral wall of the lamina dura. The nerve fibers entering the PDL in the apical area run coronally parallel to the root surface along with the blood vessels and encircle its root. These nerves are located in the middle compartment of the PDL, whereas blood vessels run closer to the bone surface in the outer compartment. The main nerve supply to the PDL is from the nerve fiber bundles that enter the PDL space through foraminae in the lateral wall of the alveolar socket. After entering the PDL space they divide and run apically and coronally and form plexuses with the nerves that run vertically from the tooth apex to the gingiva.

The nerve bundles in the PDL are both myelinated and unmyelinated and usually lie adjacent to the blood vessels running parallel to the long axis of the tooth. Based on the observations made by many researchers in the experimental animals, the PDL space can be conveniently divided into three parts. The part closer to the cementum (inner zone) about 30 %; the part closer to the alveolar bone (outer zone) 50 %; and the part in between the two (middle part) about 20 %. In longitudinal histological sections, small fiber bundles and blood vessels are located in the wider interstitial spaces that are present in the outer part of the ligament, whereas larger nerve trunks and small blood vessels traverse the ligament in the interstitial spaces between the principle fiber bundles in the middle zone.

PDL nerve endings have been studied in several animal species using histological and histochemical techniques. Kubota and Osanai (1977) showed, in the shrew, a higher density of free nerve endings in the apical part of the PDL, similar to the distribution of nerves. The nerve endings in the PDL are usually situated in the inner third of space close to the cementum and end in the PDL itself, while others describe free nerve endings in the **cementoblast** layers. Itoh, et al., (1981) showed nerve fibers terminating in the sub-cementoblastic and cementoblastic layers, some running parallel to the cementum. The free nerve endings contain neurotubules, neurofilaments and vesicles.

Three types of terminal nerve endings are found in the PDL which are free of a **myelin** sheath: a) one terminating in a spindle or knob-like swelling; b) forming loops or rings around the **collagen fiber** bundles of the principal fibers, and c) free nerve endings which are receptors of pain. Many nerve endings are receptors for proprioceptive stimuli. The proprioceptive endings allow accurate localization of the pressure in respect to its magnitude and direction. Proprioceptive reflexes are the first line of defense to protect the teeth from sudden overload by inhibiting muscular activity. Pain reflexes are the second defense mechanisms, which come into play when suddenly biting upon hard substances like a small stone or bone fragment, or when the teeth are subjected to very heavy loads.

Single myelinated and unmyelinated nerve fibers are also seen in the inner zone, which is also termed as the cemental zone. There, the terminal endings are in close relation to the fiber bundles and free endings are usually apparent between the fibers. It is suggested that they supply the mechano-receptor. The detection of forces applied to the teeth is attributable to the mechanical receptor in the periodontium, particularly those in the PDL. Pain can be evoked by direct stimulation of the PDL or by heavy pressure applied to a normal tooth. Since most of the nerves in the PDL arise from the interdental septal area, the proprioceptive and pain sensations are not impaired by removal of the apical parts of the ligament, as in apicoectomy, or by removal of the gingival portion, as in **gingivectomy**.

As elsewhere in the body, fibers from the sympathetic system, which are mostly unmyelinated, run parallel to the long axis of the tooth in close vicinity to the PDL blood vessels and may have a vasomotor function. The physiological effect of sympathetic autonomic activity in the PDL is upon regional blood flow. The sympathetic innervation to the PDL blood vessels can modulate the vascular blood pressure.

There is no experimental evidence that indicates the presence of parasympathetic innervation in the PDL.

4. **ALVEOLAR BONE**, GENERAL DESCRIPTION

Clinical orthodontics requires the movement of teeth through bone. The orthodontic appliances employed to move the teeth depend on the ability of the alveolar bone to permit such movement. Thus, a precise knowledge of osseous physiology is essential. Bone is a rigid form of connective tissue always organized into definite structure: the bones. Bone consists of cells, collagenous fibers and a viscid ground substance of mucopolysaccharide. The tissue specific cell type, the osteoblast, produces both phases of that tissue's organic matrix. These phases are (1) the organized fibrillar meshwork of **collagen fibers** and (2) the unorganized amorphous ground substance.

The organized fibrillar phase is almost, but not quite, completely formed by collagen. This is a polymerized protein that forms a little more than 90% of the dry weight of bone matrix. The morphology, chemical constitution and histologic characteristics of collagen have been previously discussed in this chapter. The general consensus is that the osteoblasts secrete the precursors of collagen into the surrounding ground substance, where the final polymerization into mature collagen takes place. In other words, collagen maturation is an extracellular event.

Ground substance, the unorganized amorphous ground substance synthesized by the osteoblasts, forming the unorganized phase of the organic matrix, is chiefly water. In addition, mucopolysaccharides are present in small but physiologically significant concentration. The most important of these substances are chondroitin sulfates A and C, kerato sulfate, and hyaluronate. Their total concentration is below 1% of the free dry weight.

Bone has mechanical, supporting and protective functions, which are served with conservation of mass and weight. It also serves as a storehouse for the calcium ion. The skeleton contains approximately 97% of the total body calcium. The bone is characterized by its hardness and by the presence of cells (osteocytes) with branching processes. The hardness is due to a complex mineral substance (hydroxyapatite) composed primarily of calcium, phosphate, carbonate and citrate plus several other trace elements. Though bone is hard, it is metabolically labile, plastic, and highly sensitive and reactive to mechanical stimuli. It is a highly organized vascular tissue and increases in size only by apposition of new bone on one of its free surfaces.

4.1. STRUCTURE OF THE ALVEOLAR PROCESS

The **alveolar bone** is that part of the maxilla and mandible that supports the roots of the teeth. The alveolar bone's development is a function of tooth development, and alveolar bone development occurs during root formation. The **basal bone** is that part of the jaws on which the alveolar process is situated. Histologically it is impossible to distinguish any difference between so-called basal bone and alveolar bone. The alveolar bone is made up of two components:

    A.) alveolar bone proper.
    B.) supporting bone. (Figure 8-13, 8-14)

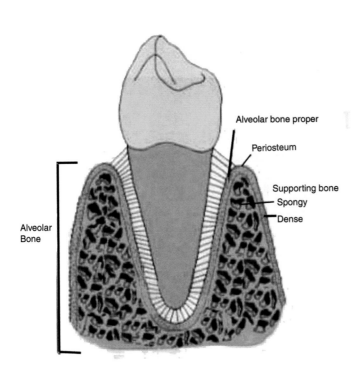

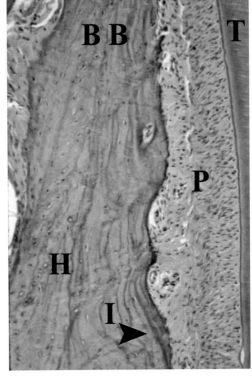

Figure 8-13: Diagrammatic view of the alveolar bone. Alveolar bone is divided into two parts: **Alveolar bone proper**: it is a specialized type of dense bone composed of bundle bone and Haversian bone. It appears radiopaque in radiographs and is, therefore, called the lamina dura. Bundle bone is so named because it is penetrated by PDL fibers. The supporting bone, as the name implies, supports the alveolar bone proper and is made up of both spongy and compact bone. Labial and lingual surfaces of the supporting bone, which are covered by periosteum, are made up of dense cortical plates, which are composed of bundle bone and Haversian bone. Note the level of the alveolar crest relative to the **cementoenamel junction**.

Figure 8-14. Histology of alveolar bone proper, longitudinal section. The following areas are identified: Tooth (T), PDL (P), Bundle bone (BB), Haversian Bone (H), Incremental layers (I).

4.1.1. The alveolar bone proper (Figure 8-14) is that bone which lines the socket and is also called lamina dura. It is a dense bone, the deep layer of which is Haversian bone. The superficial layer next to PDL gives attachment to the periodontal ligament fibers.

The **alveolar bone proper** (lamina dura) is perforated by many small foramina, which carry blood vessels, nerves and lymph vessels from the trabecular bone to the periodontal ligament. This is also called cribriform plate. The lamina dura is thicker during active tooth eruption and relatively thin during normal function. During tooth movement it is thicker on the tension side and less thick, or even absent, on the pressure side of the PDL. The coronal border of the alveolar bone is called the alveolar crest, which is located 1-1.5 mm below the cemento-enamel junction of the teeth.

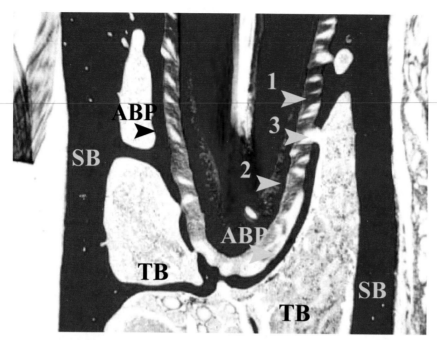

Figure 8-15: Histologic longitudinal section of a root shows alveolar bone proper and supporting bone. The alveolar bone proper (ABP), or the bony socket wall, is a modification of compact bone. It contains perforating fibers (Sharpey's). The fibers pierce the socket wall at right angles or slightly obliquely. The Sharpey's fibers in the cementum are also seen (2). The fiber bundle originating from bone (1) are much larger, widely spaced and less numerous than those inserting in cementum (2). Communicating channel between PDL and marrow spaces (3). Supporting Bone (SB) with Trabecular Bone (TB) between buccal and lingual cortical plates, and also between supporting bone, and alveolar bone proper (ABP).

4.1.2. Supporting Bone

The **supporting bone** (SB, Figure 8-15) includes the remainder of the alveolar bone, which is composed of **compact bone** plates that make up the labial, buccal and lingual cortical plates on the outer surface of the alveolar process, which is covered by periosteum. An intermediate layer of spongy bone, more appropriately called trabecular bone (TB), is present between the labial and lingual cortical plates and also between the cortical plates and lamina dura. Blood vessels, nerves, lymph vessels and adipose tissue fill the trabecular spaces.

4.2 CLASSIFICATION OF BONE TISSUE

Bone may be classified from its histologic characteristic as:

    A.) embryonic bone, or woven bone
    B.) compact bone, cortical bone, or lamellar bone:
            i. Haversian system; osteonal bone
            ii. Bundle bone
    C.) Spongy or trabecular bone

4.2.1. Embryonic bone—

Embryonic bone is also referred to at times as woven bone. Its structure is highly variable, disorganized, poorly mineralized and weak. This is made up of irregular, delicate bars and lamellae of bone, which form a small meshed network. The lamellae and bars are arranged without regular order or particular direction. This type of arrangement suggests that there has been no functional stress upon the bone. This type of bone is found normally during healing of fractures or extraction wounds, and only later is replaced by mature bone. As the name suggests, this immature, coarse fibrillar bone is characterized by the greater number, size and irregular arrangement of the osteocytes and irregular course of its fibrils. Per unit volume of bone there are greater numbers of cells and a reduced volume of calcified intercellular substance (ground substance). This structural arrangement makes this immature bone more radiolucent than mature bone. This explains why bony **callus** cannot be seen in radiograms at a time when histologic examination of the fracture reveals a well-developed union between the parts. Similarly, dental sockets of the extracted teeth appear to be empty at times when it is almost filled with immature bone. There is a lag period of 2-3 weeks between the visibility in the radiographs and actual bone formation. The woven bone does serve a critical initial role in the wound healing process by rapidly filling the gap between osseous fragments, providing continuity and strength for fractures and osteotomy segments. During orthodontic tooth movement, the first bone formed is woven type, which later on either gets converted into compact bone or remodeled into lamellar or Haversian bone. The understanding of this aspect of bone maturational processes has an important clinical implication with respect to orthodontic retention and postoperative follow-up of orthognathic surgical patients. In the steady states condition this bone is not found and readily disappears.

4.2.2. **Compact Bone**

This has also been described as cortical bone, or composite bone, which is composed of lamellar bone, Haversian bone, or osteonal bone and bundle bone (Figure 8-16). Compact bone or cortical bone of long bones is sandwiched between periosteum and endosteum, and can increase in size or **drift** in the same direction by appropriate bone apposition or bone **resorption**. These activities are responsible for external transformation. Internal transformation of compact or cortical bone involves the development of the Haversian system. The cortical bone is an osseous tissue which is formed by deposition of lamellar bone, the name given to layers of bone within the fibrillar framework of the woven bone, which is formed first. Roberts and coworkers described this as cancellous compassion. This type of bone, which is a resultant composite of woven and lamellar bone, is first formed in response to orthodontic **force**, and is also known as primary osteon. It is fairly strong bone and can sustain a normal functional load for a long period of time, but is ultimately remodeled into secondary osteon, or secondary spongiosa. The bones of adults are entirely of the remodeled variety, i.e., secondary osteon or secondary spongiosa. The cortical bone in the alveolar process is identical to bone elsewhere and is in a constant state of flux. The compact bone is dense and fairly solid **bone** tissue found as the outer layer of practically all bones and consists of three groups of osseous lamellae (Figure 8-16A):

1.) The circumferential lamellae
2.) The Haversian system of lamellae
3.) The interstitial lamellae.

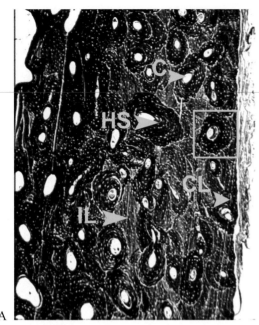

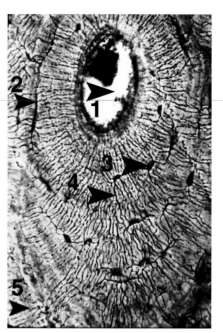

A   B

Figure 8-16: Histological cross sections of mature cortical bone showing: the Haversian System (A), and normal osteon (B). Part A: Haversian System (HS): Haversian canals (C); interstitial lamellae (IL); circumferential lamellae (CL). Multiple units of Haversian system are shown. Each unit is called an osteon, made up of central Haversian canal (C), surrounded by concentric layers of lamellae or lamellar bone. In each lamella, white dots represent empty spaces called lacunae (3) in which osteocytes reside. Part B: Haversian canal (1), lamellae (2), lacunae (3), canaliculi (4), interstitial lamellae (5). Higher magnification of A (boxed area). It shows single unit of Haversian system called an osteon. White circular area is Haversian canal (1), surrounded by multiple concentrically-arranged layers of bone lamella (2), black flattened spaces in the layers of lamellae, called lacunae (3), which contain bone cells—osteocytes—with their extended cellular processes (4) interconnecting the lacunae to each other in the same lamella and adjacent lamellae, and also to the central Haversian canal (1), are thin thread-like channels called canaliculi (4). Note: There are approx. 20,000 lacunae and osteocytes in three mm section of certain cortical bones. All the canals, lacunae and canaliculi are covered by a layer of osteogenic membranes, which are continuous with each other.

1.) The circumferential lamellae. These lamellae are composed of layers of dense bone built one upon another and arranged circumferentially around the shafts of long bones. It is this arrangement that gives them their name. The bone cells responsible for forming bone layers are osteoblasts. As the osteoblasts are producing new bone matrix, they occasionally get surrounded by their own matrix. The enclosed osteoblasts are now called osteocytes, and reside in small holes called lacunae. These trapped cells in the lacunae are connected to the blood supply of the Haversian system by small tubes called canaliculi, which are really lymph channels. The flat bones like those of the cranium also have surface lamellae that resemble the circumferential lamellae of long bones. They are found on both inner and outer surfaces of the bones.

2.) Haversian system. Traditionally, the Haversian system, or osteon, has been described as the basic unit of bone. Haversian systems consist of following components (Figure 8-16B):

The Haversian canal, which is a blood channel and has a direct connection with the larger central canal in the medullary cavity of the long bones. The Haversian canals also communicate with the external periosteal surface of the bone by means of other bony channels called Volkmann's canals. The Volkmann's canals penetrate cortical bone in an oblique direction, connecting with the Haversian system, thus providing vascular channels which carry blood vessels that come off from those of the periosteum and lymphatic passageways for metabolic exchange and carrying soluble signals such as hormones. Thus, it is seen that the blood supply of bone comes from vessels thesupply the periosteum, and these blood vessels give off branches that traverse the canals of Volkmann and then pour their contents into the Haversian canals, which in turn empty them in the large marrow cavity of the bone.

The lamellae are layers of bone arranged concentrically around each Haversian canal.

The lacunae, or small holes or spaces within the lamellae and between the lamellae contain osteocytes. Each osteocyte is linked to the neighboring osteocyte in the same lamella and to osteocytes in the adjacent lamellae through an intricate net of thread-like processes that traverse the canaliculi.

The canaliculi, or lymph channels, interconnect the lacunae to the Haversian canals and bring nourishment to the trapped bone cells, the osteocytes. The Haversian system, or osteon, runs more or less parallel to the long axis of the bone. It is an irregularly cylindrical, branching and anastamosing structure with thick walls and it has a narrow lumen, the Haversian canal. The canals are 22 to 110 microns in diameter, surrounded by four to twenty concentrically arranged lamellae of bone in a single system, each from 3 to 7 microns in thickness. The Haversian canals carry one or more, usually two, blood vessels. These are, for the most part, capillaries and post-capillary venules.

3.) The interstitial lamellae consist of layers of bone placed between the various Haversian systems, filling in the inner spaces and binding these systems together. In their structural composition are also formed lacunae and canaliculi and osteocytes.

The organizational network of osseous canals and channels described above enable cross-communication in terms of exchange of signaling molecules that may lead to bone cell activation among osteocytes and endosteal and periosteal lining osteoblasts, thus facilitating and promoting physiologic and functional responses.

Bundle bone: The bony areas of cortical or **compact bones**, which contain a great number of Sharpey's fibers, are given the name of bundle bone. The **alveolar bone proper** shows thick collagenous fiber bundles of PDL penetrating the bone surface and embedding into the substance of the bone. Bundle bone is a functional adaptation of the lamellar structure for attachment of tendons and ligament. In the case of teeth, the collagenous fiber bundles of the PDL, called Sharpey's fibers, insert themselves at right angles to the bone surface of the cribriform plate. Distinct layers of bundle bone are usually seen adjacent to the PDL.

4.2.3. Spongy Bone

It is also referred to as cancellous and trabecular bone. This type of bone tissue consists of a network of osseous matrix, the strands of which are called trabeculae. These trabeculae are made up of several layers of lamella, and enclosed within their membrane-lined walls are fairly large spaces that are filled with bone marrow. In the bone of the alveolar process, the sizes of the trabeculae are small in the crestal area and progressively become larger in the apical area. This has profound implications in planning an orthodontic force system to move teeth. In the buccal or lingual crestal area, heavy forces applied to teeth will not allow the undermining bone resorption, because the cortical plate of the outer surface more or less merges and fuses with the lamina dura. For physiologic tooth movement, a large trabecular pattern of spongy bone is essential.

4.3 NERVE SUPPLY OF BONE

The nerves of the periosteum are sensory, therefore this tissue is very sensitive. They also enter the marrow cavity, coursing along the nutrient arteries. Vasomotor nerves also follow the arteries, entering the cortical bone through Volkmann's canals. Innervation to the periodontium and especially to the PDL is discussed previously in the section on sensory function.

4.4 VASCULAR SUPPLY OF BONE

The marrow spaces in the spongy bone are well supplied by blood vessels. Blood vessels are also found in the Haversian canals and Volkmann's canals. Blood vessels in the Volkmann's canals connect the periosteal blood vessels with the medullary blood vessels. The blood supply of a bone comes from two sources. One source supplies the bone marrow, the trabecular part, and the other the compact bone, or the Haversian system. The vessels for each supply come from the periosteum and pass through Volkmann's canals to their destination. They intercommunicate with one another. The veins follow the course of the arteries. Vascularity of the periodontium is also discussed in the section on nutritive function.

5. TISSUE CHANGES WITH APPLICATION OF FORCE

Teeth move and change position during tooth formation and eruption. After teeth erupt into occlusion, they then erupt passively and may more gradually change position due to late growth changes or tooth wear. The periodontium responds to tooth movement, whether through physiologic forces or sustained mechanical force from orthodontic appliances. This is because the periodontium has a remarkable ability to be modified.

The tooth is said to be in control of its environment. The tooth's movement is mediated through the **periodontal ligament**, the cementum and the alveolar bone proper. These tissues reflect any response of the tooth's movement that causes pressure and tension on opposing sides of the root of the tooth. Pressure causes resorption of the bone and cementum on the pressure surface of the root as tension causes bone and cementum formation on the opposite, or tension, surface of the root. This response mechanism is observed in any case of tooth movement, whether is be physiologic **drift** or by mechanical means (Figure 8-17).

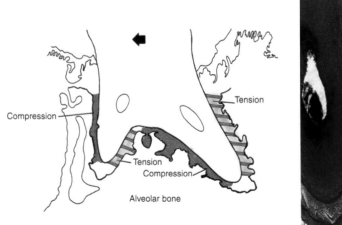
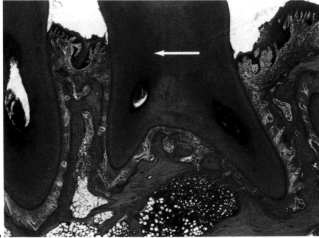

A   B

Figure 8-17A and B: Tooth movement to the left, with areas of compression and tension adjacent to the tooth's surface. A.) Zones of compression and tension in tooth movement, B.) tooth movement to the left (arrow).

Tooth movement is also more difficult to achieve in dense bony areas and more easily attainable in porous bony areas. Thus the mandibular teeth may be more difficult to move than most maxillary teeth.

5.1 ROTATION AND BODILY FORCES

As we learned from the previous description of the periodontium, the fibers of the periodontal ligament resist in a direction perpendicular to the tooth's surface during normal function. Thus the interstitial spaces are open and tissue fluid circulated freely through these spaces. Application of force, however, alters this condition, as in the case of rotational force.

In the case of a single-rooted tooth, force will take place along the entire root of the tooth, causing compression of the periodontium along the surfaces of both the tooth and the bone. On the opposite surface of the tooth and bone, tension will occur as the periodontal fibers become stretched between these two surfaces. Tension will lead to deposition of bone and of cementum on the tooth's root surface.

A more complex situation occurs in the rotation of a three-rooted tooth, such as a molar. Initially, again, the related periodontium shows periodontal fibers with open interstitial spaces. When force is applied in rotation of this tooth, the root periodontium shows compression along the advancing surface and tension along the trailing surface (Figure 8-18).

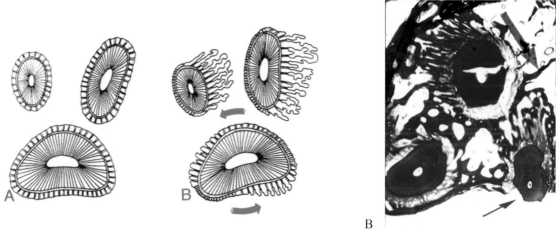

A   B

Figure 8-18A and B: A.) Diagram of normal periodontium around a three-rooted tooth. B.) Rotation of tooth results in bone loss ahead of advancing surfaces and bone and cementum deposition on trailing surfaces. In the early stages of rotation there is little change in the periodontal tissues. All of the roots do not move an equal amount. One root is the center of rotation while the other two appear to rotate about this axis. Also, most roots are oval rather than round, and this complicates tooth movement. Thus we see more bone deposition adjacent to two roots than the third.

5.2 EXTRUSIVE AND INTRUSIVE FORCES

These forces attain very different results and must be applied with care. The periodontal fibers are in tension, especially in the alveolar crest and fundic regions of the socket. Light extrusive forces are most effective in developing bone lining the alveolar socket. This type of **force** enables compensatory bone to grow in the entire socket area.

Intrusive force causes relaxation of the free and attached gingival fibers and loss of bone throughout the socket. Good results are more difficult to obtain with intrusive forces than with tipping or rotation (Figure 8-19).

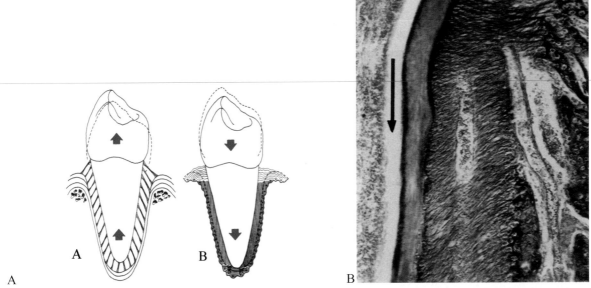

Figure 8-19A and B: Part A: Extrusion of a tooth (A) causing tension over the entire socket. Intrusion of tooth (B), causing resorption over the entire surface of the alveolar bone. Part B: Histology of intrusive movement. Note the loss of bone and cementum.

5.3 TIPPING AND BODILY MOVEMENT

Tipping a tooth results in resorption of bone and possibly tooth surface at the apical zone of the root, as well as in the alveolar crest area on the opposite side of the tooth. Also, as happens with other directional forces, a zone of deposition occurs on the sides of the tooth opposite the **resorption**. The results of this force are different for a short-rooted than a long-rooted tooth.

In the short-rooted tooth with incomplete roots, there is more space for the tooth to be tipped than in the long, completed root. In the latter case, there is strong resistance to tipping by the apical fibers and less periodontal space available, so **force** maintenance of longer duration is needed. This is seen in Figure 8-20. The center of rotation, or fulcrum, is noted by the small circles on the root surface.

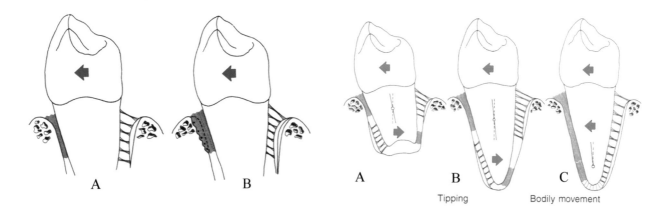

Figure 8-20A: In purple: results of tipping type of tooth movement. (A) early (B) late. In green: Change in point of rotation of tooth in young forming root (A), completed root, (B), and mature periodontium (C).

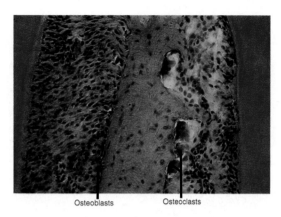

Figure 8-20B: Osteoblasts and osteoclasts in the bifurcation zone. Left- tension zone. Right-compression zone.

5.3.1. Force of Bodily Movement

This is a more complex movement than tipping, as the entire root surface of the tooth is being moved from point A to point B. This takes a greater force than tipping a tooth and will create resorption along the front in which the tooth is moved and tension along the entire surface that the tooth is being pulled away from. On the pressure front, resorptive sites appear along both the bone and the cemental surfaces, as well as changes in the periodontal tissue. The interstitial spaces in the pressure zone will exhibit decreased blood circulation and crushing of some of the fiber groups. This can be seen in Figure 8-21, where cell death appears in the peripheral alveolar bone where osteocytes have ceased function and will be lost as the bony front resorbs.

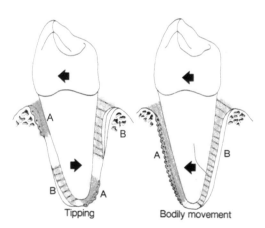

Figure 8-21A: Tipping movement compared with bodily movement. (A) represents the compression areas of the periodontal ligament and (B) represents the tension areas of the periodontal ligament. With the bodily movement such as depicted here, changes occur over the whole affected side of the periodontal ligament root surface.

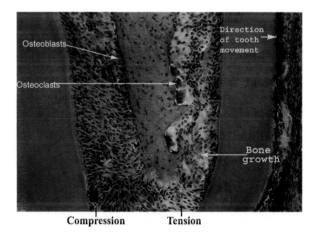

Figure 8-21B: Osteoblasts and osteoclasts in the bifurcation zone. Left- tension zone. Right-compression zone.

A great deal of activity still takes place along this front, as this is a necessary feature of the resorptive process. Cementum will not contact alveolar bone in this process but maintain periodontal fiber tissue along this front. Along the tension front, a different type of activity occurs as the fibers are under tension and the bone quickly activates; here bone is stimulated to begin formation.

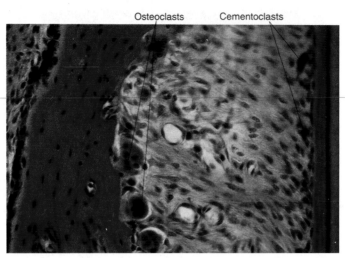

Figure 8-22: Tension along the opposite surface of a root that is undergoing **bodily movement**. Activity in the compression zone (late). Observe the osteoclasts on the bone and the resorption on the root surface.

The **perforating fibers** of the **periodontal ligament** are buried in the surface of the cementum and the alveolar bone. Application of tension on these fibers is the stimulus to cause activity of the hard tissues. Note the black staining, which indicates activity of oxidative enzymes in the cementoblasts that will, in turn, form cementum along the surface of the root. The presence of osteoclasts along the alveolar bone and cementum is indicative of the beginning of resorption of these hard tissues. To the left in Figure 8-22 is the surface of bone where bone deposition is occurring, indicated by the activity of osteoblasts at the site of the black stain.

5.3.2. Hyalinization Zones

Zones of **hyalinization** are caused by a force applied too greatly or too rapidly in tooth movement, resulting in a loss of blood supply in the ligament and adjacent alveolar bone. Compression has caused a cessation of blood flow in the area and may be seen histologically (Figure 8-23). Radiographically, the area will appear as a close apposition of the tooth and bone with a lack of change in bone density. Hyalinization causes the loss of cell activity and loss of fibrillar nature of the **collagen fibers** in the compression zone. The loss of cells and cell activity results in the lack of tooth movement temporarily. The most unfortunate effect of hyalinization is the possibility of **undermining resorption**. This is usually seen in the bone underlying the area of compression and hyalinization. The extent of damage due to undermining **resorption** is unpredictable and may result in extensive bone loss. In some cases there may be **root resorption** as well as undue bone resorption. Usually, when the compressed area of bone is resorbed the tooth movement then continues. It is said by some investigators that the change in bioelectric potential of the bone causes the onset of resorption. The importance of radiographic assessment cannot be over-stressed.

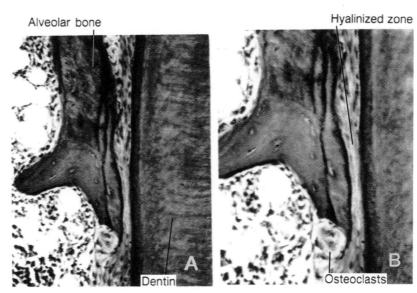

Figure 8-23: Zone of hyalinization of the periodontal ligament and zone of undermining resorption. Part A: compression and hyalinization of periodontal ligament caused by excessive tooth movement. Part B): higher magnification of (A) shows undermining resorption adjacent to the hyalinized zone.

5.4 STABILITY AND RELAPSE

The stability of teeth is due to the equilibrium they are in from the combined forces of chewing, swallowing, tongue and cheek movements. Tooth movement alters that equilibrium, and to regain that equilibrium the teeth depend on the new bone, ligament and cementum formation. New fiber and hard tissue formation and their maintenance is dependent on retention. Most clinical tooth movement produces a stable result; however, there are exceptions in which root loss or prolonged bone resorption may occur. Whereas bone loss and formation is usually a relatively rapid process, gingival fibers require a prolonged period of retention and may never fully remodel.

6. SUMMARY

The alveolar process is guided by intrinsic factors, the teeth, and extrinsic factors, the changes during the growth of the face. The bones supporting the teeth are made up of the fundic or **alveolar bone proper**, the compact, cortical plate and the cancellous bone that lies between the two. The periodontal ligament is made up of groups of fibers: the apical, oblique, horizontal, alveolar crest and interradicular groups. The dentogingival groups of fibers are made up of the free and attached gingival fibers, the circular and transseptal bundles. The periodontal ligament turns over collagen rapidly and has an active population of **fibroblasts** that both form and destroy collagen, and that is the reason that the ligament responds so well to treatment. Interstitial spaces separate collagen bundles and house blood vessels, nerves, nerve endings and lymphatics. Cementum is the hard tissue covering the root surface that functions as an attachment of the perforating fibers of the periodontal ligament. Cementum is the thinnest at the cervical region and thickest at the apical area of the tooth root.

A number of factors relate to the effects of force, such as the age and health of the patient as well as the amount of force, the length of time it is applied, and the direction and the point of application of the force. On the pressure front of the moving tooth, either resorption of **alveolar bone**, compression of the periodontal fibers and resorption of the cementum and possibly the root may occur. On the other hand, it was noted that undue compression might cause **hyalinization** of the ligament and bone and underlying resorption. There may be diminished width of the periodontal space from the 0.5 mm normal, although this distance will be restored in a short period of time. On the tension side of the tooth, the periodontal fiber bundles appear stretched, and gradually new bone plates appear as the tooth moves from this position. In all cases, the periodontal space is maintained and may increase slightly until bone and cementum deposition occurs. In most cases of clinical tooth movement there is produced a stable and successful clinical result.

7. SUGGESTED READING

Structural Organization of Periodontal Ligament

Berkovitz BKB and Moxham BJ. Tissue changes during tooth eruption. In: Teeth Vol. 6, Handbook of Microscopic Anatomy (Okesche A and Volbrath L, eds), 2nd edition, Springer-Verlag, Berlin 1989, pp 21-71,.

Berkovitz BKB. The structure of the periodontal ligament: an update. Eur J Orthod 1990;12:576.

Devlin H and Ferguson MWJ. Alveolar ridge resorption and mandibular atrophy. A review of the local and systemic factors. Br Dent J 1991;170:101-102.

Glimcher MJ Mechanism of collagen calcification: Role of collagen fibrils and collagen-phosphoprotein complexes in vitro and vivo. Anat Rec 1989;224:139-153.

Moxham BJ Studies on the mechanical properties of the periodontal ligament. In: Current Topics in Oral Biology (Lisney SJW and Mathews B, eds), University of Bristol Press, Bristol. 1985, pp 73-82,

Toms SR, et al. Nonlinear stress-strain behavior of periodontal ligament under orthodontic loading. Am J Orthod Dentofacial Orthop 2002;122:174-179.

Cells of Periodontal Ligaments

Avery, JK (Ed.). Oral Development and Histology. Thieme, New York. 2001, pp. 226-274.

Avery JK. Essentials of oral histology and embryology a clinical approach. Mosby. St. Louis, Missouri 2000.

Chambers TC Regulation of osteoclast development and function. In: Biology and Physiology of the Osteoclast. (Rifkin BR and Gay CV, eds), CRC Press, Boca Raton, Florida, 1991, pp 337-356.

Davidovitch Z, Nicolay OF, Ngan PW and Shanfeld JL. Neurotransmitters, cytokines and the control of alveolar bone remodeling in orthodontics. Dent Clin North Am 1988;32:411-435.

Holtrop ME Light and electron microscopic structure of osteoclasts. In: Bone, volume 2: The Osteoclast (Hall BK, ed), CRC Press, Boca Raton, Florida, (1990b), pp 1-30.

McCulloch CAG and Bordin S Role of fibroblast subpopulations in periodontal physiology and pathology. J Periodont Res 1991;26:144-154.

McCulloch CAG, Nemeth E, Lowenberg B and Melcher AH Paravascular cells in endosteal spaces of alveolar bone contribute to periodontal ligament cell populations. Anat Rec 1987;219:233-242.

Melcher AH and Chan J (1981) Phagocytosis and digestion of collagen by gingival fibroblasts in vivo: a study of serial sections. J Ultrastruct Res 77, 1-36.

Roberts WE, Mozsary PG and Klingler E (1982) Nuclear size as a cell-kinetic marker for osteoblast differentiation. Am J Anat 165, 373-384.

Ten Cate A. Richard, Oral Histology, Development, Structure and Function, Chap. 13 Periodontium pp 253-288, St Louis, Mosby, 1998.

Vasculature of Periodontal Ligament

Barker JH. Lymphatic vessels in human alveolar bone. Lymphology 1982. 15, 1-13.

Berkovitz BKB The structure of the periodontal ligament: an update. Eur J Orthod 1990;12:51-76.

Tang MFP, Sims MR, Sampson WJ and Dreyer CW. Evidence for endothelial junctions acting as a fluid flux pathway in tensioned periodontal ligament. Arch Oral Biol 1993;38:273-276.

Innervation of Periodontal Ligament

Berkovitz BKB. The structure of the periodontal ligament: an update. Eur J Orthod 1990;12:51-76.

Byers. Dental sensory receptors. Int Rev Neurobiol 25, 39-94. Lambrichts I, Creemers J and van Steenberghe D (1992) Morphology of neural endings in the human periodontal ligament: an electron microscopic study. J Periodont Res 1984;27:191-196.

Nakamura TK, Hanai H and Nakamura M. Ultrastructure of encapsulated nerve terminals in human periodontal ligaments. Jpn J Oral Biol 1982;24:126-132.

Roberts WE, Goodwin WC Jr and Heiner SR. Cellular responses to orthodontic force. Dent Clin North Amer 1981;25:3-17.

Developmental Aspects and Force Movement on Teeth

Berkovitz BKB and Moxham BJ. The development of the periodontal ligament with special reference to collagen fibre ontogeny. J Biol Buccale 1990;18:227-236.

Davidovitch Z, Nicolay OF, Ngan PW and Shanfeld JL. Neurotransmitters, cytokines and the control of alveolar bone remodeling in orthodontics. Dent Clin North Am 1998;32:411-435.

Davidovitch Z. Tooth movement. Crit Rev Oral Biol Med 2, 411-450. Premolars following experimental tooth movement. Scand J Dent Res 1991;80:357-368.

Nicolay OF, Davidovitch Z, Shanfeld JL and Alley K. Substance P immunoreactivity in periodontal tissues during orthodontic tooth movement. Bone Miner 1990;11:19-29.

Roberts WE, Goodwin WC Jr and Heiner SR. Cellular responses to orthodontic force. Dent Clin North Amer 1981;25:3-17.

Rygh P, Bowling K, Hovlandsdal L and Williams S. Activation of the vascular system: a main mediator of periodontal fibre remodelling in orthodontic tooth movement. AM J Orthod 1986;89:453-468.

Ten Cate A Richard, Oral Histology, Development, Structure and Function, Chap 14, Physiologic Tooth Movement and: Eruption and Shedding. St Louis, Mosby, 1989, pp 289-314.

CHAPTER 9

Tissue Engineering in Orthodontics

William L. Murphy

David J. Mooney

1. INTRODUCTION

Novel strategies for replacing diseased or damaged tissue offer widespread potential in the field of dentistry. Oral diseases are extremely prevalent, in essence affecting most individuals at some point during his/her lifetime. Diseases such as periodontitis, caries, and oral cancer are common, and present significant treatment challenges to the dental field. In addition, there are major complications associated with current orthodontic treatment. **Root resorption**, **ankylosis**, periodontal damage, instability, and relapse are important concerns with no ideal treatment method. The use of metallic or non-degradable polymeric prostheses has been successful in many cases for oral tissue replacement; however, these materials are not ideal because they do not resorb over time. Prosthetic materials often necessitate a second surgical procedure for removal, and they typically do not integrate very well with the host tissue. Recently there has been a trend toward growth stimulation strategies and expansion approaches in lieu of tooth removal. In light of the importance of growth stimulation in both orthodontics and periodontology, the rapidly growing field of **tissue engineering** may be uniquely suited to providing novel orthodontic therapies.

Given the composition of the oral tissues, the contribution from the field of tissue engineering likely lies in regeneration of fibrous tissue associated with the periodontal ligament, and bony tissue associated with cementum, **alveolar bone**, and **maxillofacial** bones. Orthodontic difficulties such as ankylosis and **root resorption** can be principally attributed to periodontal disease or damage. More generally, damage and loss of the periodontal tissues is a problem observed in over 90% of people age 13 or older. Although many of these cases are caused by gingivitis, more advanced clinical periodontal detachment is also widespread. Progression of periodontal disease can result in deepening of the **gingival sulcus**, detachment of the periodontal ligament and resorption of alveolar bone. In addition to the difficulties related to periodontal tissue loss, there is also a tremendous need for bony tissues for replacement of oral and maxillofacial bones lost in treatment of skeletal malocclusion, congenital defects, or trauma. Orthodontic forces during development have a profound effect on bony tissues in the maxillofacial region because of the dynamic nature of bone modeling and remodeling. There are an estimated 16 million untreated cases of skeletal malocclusion in the United States, and 1.2 million of these cases are severe enough to be considered handicapped. Novel methods of engineering bone tissue may provide an exciting new tool for orthodontic treatment and **orthognathic surgery**.

The general objective of regenerative medicine is to spur the regenerative process while simultaneously suppressing the natural repair process (i.e., development of fibrous scar tissue). There are three pertinent cell types in regeneration of orthodontic and periodontal tissues. Alveolar bone can be regenerated by **osteoblasts**, bone-forming cells involved in the production, mineralization, modeling, and remodeling of bone tissue. Cementoblasts are involved in production of the cementum, the mineralized connective tissue that anchors **collagen** fibers of the periodontal ligament to the tooth and seals dentin tubules in the root. Periodontal ligament **fibroblasts** (PLFs) produce fibrous connective tissue and can be employed to regenerate a damaged or detached periodontal ligament (gingival fibroblasts and gingival epithelial cells also play a smaller role in the soft tissue repair process). In addition to **tissue regeneration**, a critical requirement in this process is the blockage of cell types that can hinder tissue regeneration, such as epithelial cells from the apical root sheath, and connective tissue cells not associated with the periodontal ligament. These cells are active in the tissue repair process, and their activity results in build-up of scar tissue in the defect region. Osteoblasts may also be considered a hindering cell type in situations in which ankylosis prevention is a primary goal. The predictable manipulation of each of the above cell types in the regenerative process is the goal of current orthodontic and periodontal tissue engineering research and clinical work. Integration of cementogenesis, osteogenesis, and development of periodontal ligament fibers amid the negative influence of tissue repair processes is a complex task that may benefit from the advantages of the developing field of tissue engineering.

Three general strategies have emerged for engineering of tissues. The first is a **conductive approach**, in which synthetic materials amenable to infiltration of specific cell types are implanted into a site of disease or damage. The materials provoke conduction of desired cell types while physically blocking conduction of unwanted cells associated with the tissue repair process, thus creating a pathway for selective cell infiltration. The second approach is an **inductive approach** that involves the inclusion of **bioactive factors** (e.g., **growth factors**) into the aforementioned synthetic construct. The factors are chosen to spur the infiltration of the appropriate cell types, and induce the formation of a specific type of tissue. The third approach is a **cell-based approach** in which synthetic constructs are seeded with cells *in vitro* prior to implantation. Each approach is described in some detail below with emphasis on bone regeneration, and recent results pertinent to oral tissue regeneration. Investigators are currently applying **conductive, inductive, and cell-based approaches** (or hybrids thereof) to virtually all tissue types.

It is important to recognize that problems relating to loss of tissue structure and function extend beyond the field of dentistry. Tissue loss and late stage organ failure are two of the most substantial health problems in the United States from both a financial and humanitarian standpoint. It has been estimated that half of the annual health care budget is spent on patients suffering from these conditions, an allocation in excess of $400 billion per year. At the present time the standard tissue replacement therapies are either direct transplantation from an **autologous** donor site or **allogenic transplantation**. Current therapies are severely limited by the amount of tissues available for transplantation, and demand for tissues significantly outweighs supply.

In addition to donor tissue shortage there are other complications associated with therapeutic transplantation. The use of autologous transplants avoids significant immune response and reduces the likelihood of immune rejection. However, **autologous transplantation** is non-ideal, as it requires multiple surgical procedures and thus multiple risk of infection, surgical complications, donor site morbidity, and potential tissue **resorption**. Concerns associated with **allogenic transplantation** include immune response in the recipient tissue and pathogen transfer. Furthermore, allogenic transplants have shown poor new tissue formation, particularly in the case of demineralized bone allografts. The critical limitations inherent in these therapies have prompted the development of tissue engineering strategies (Figure 9-1). Tissue engineering strategies have been applied to virtually all tissue types, and particularly significant progress has been made in the areas of skin, cartilage, and bone regeneration.

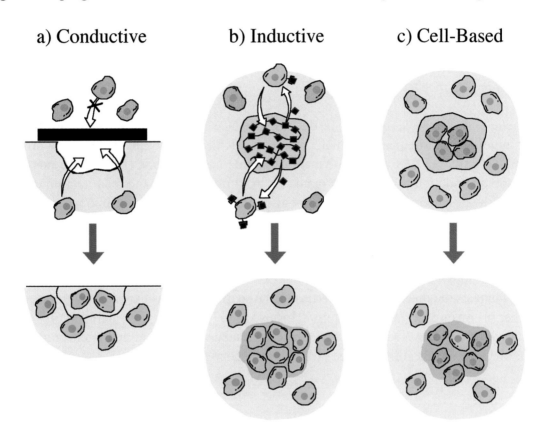

Figure 9-1: Schematic representation of the three general tissue engineering strategies: a.) conductive, b.) inductive, and c.) cell-based.

2. CONDUCTIVE APPROACH

A considerable challenge in the engineering of tissues lies in the ability to stimulate tissue regeneration by specific cell types while avoiding interference from cells associated with the tissue repair process. A method for alleviating the problem of non-selective cell conduction is to use synthetic polymer **scaffolds** as conduits to guide new tissue growth. Scaffolds can be designed to simultaneously conduct desired cell types and physically block conduction of undesired cell types, a strategy **termed guided** tissue regeneration **(GTR)**. The main principal underlying the GTR approach is that progenitor cells capable of tissue regeneration dwell in the healthy tissue adjacent to a defect and can conduct onto a synthetic construct without infiltration and interference of other cell types. In most cases, a natural or synthetic **degradable** construct is chosen so as to degrade and disappear in concert with new tissue development. This may result in formation of a natural tissue in the diseased or otherwise damaged area with no remnants of the **degradable scaffold**. The basic requirements of the system (along with the properties described below in "significant design challenges in tissue engineering") are **degradability** of the scaffold material over a controllable time scale, and selectivity of cell conduction.

2.1 DEGRADABLE MATERIALS

Although there has been widespread use of non-degradable materials as synthetic implants, they are limited as a material for regenerative therapy due to the necessity for multiple surgical procedures. A second procedure can hinder the process of new tissue formation. Procedures for replacement of natural tissue without remnants of the implant material call for the development of **degradable** scaffolds as conduits for cell migration and tissue formation. Several such materials, both natural and synthetic, have been considered as possible tissue engineering scaffolds. Among natural materials, formulations of bovine collagen have been studied most frequently, and have been successful in guiding osseous tissue regeneration while deterring the infiltration of interfering cells. The collagen constructs are chemotactic for fibroblasts, support cell growth, and show low cytotoxicity. Cross-linking of collagen molecules by means of chemical reagents such as glutaraldehyde and epoxides extends membrane degradation time and improves mechanical properties.

Several synthetic materials have proven to be **degradable** over a predictable and controllable time scale. The most commonly used **degradable** materials for GTR are composed of poly(α-hydroxy esters), specifically poly(lactide) (PLA) and copolymers of lactide and glycolide (PLG). It is possible to predictably tune the degradation time of these materials by simply varying the relative amounts of lactide and glycolide in the polymer. These materials are also attractive since they have long been approved by the Food and Drug Administration for use as surgical sutures. Recent modifications on the poly (α-hydroxy acid) materials make them more attractive for use in bone tissue regeneration. Both PLA and PLG materials have been mineralized to varying extents via a one step, room temperature process. Growth of a continuous mineral layer on the inner pore surfaces of the scaffolds (Figure 9-2) prior to implantation enhances the mechanical properties of the scaffolds, and is expected to enhance osteoconductivity. Other promising degradable materials for use as GTR membranes include Polyvinyl Alcohol (PVA), Polyethylene Glycol (PEG), Polyethylene Terephthalate (PET), and hydrogels composed of gelatin or low molecular weight formulations of the polysaccharide alginate.

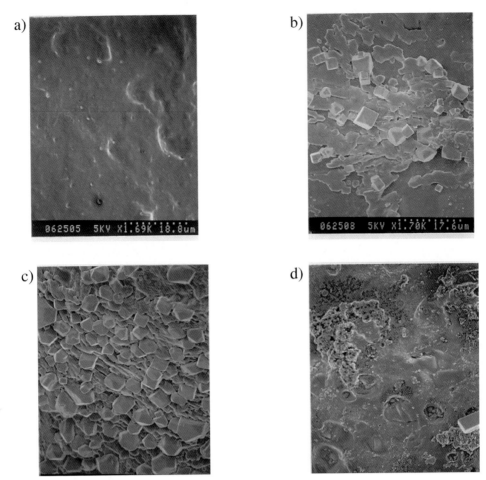

Figure 9-2: SEM micrographs of mineralized PLG scaffolds: Inner surface of a single pore of: a)A control scaffold prepared by solvent casting, particulate leaching process, not incubated in simulated body fluid (SBF); b)A scaffold incubated in SBF for 6 days displaying small mineral crystals growing on the polymer substrate; c)A scaffold incubated in SBF for 10 days displaying a large density of mineral crystals growing on the polymer substrate; d) A scaffold incubated in SBF for 16 days displaying a continuous mineral film grown on the polymer substrate (From: Murphy W.L., et. al., J. Biomed. Mater. Res. 2000;50:50-59.).

2.2 SELECTIVE CELL CONDUCTION

Selectivity of cell conduction can most easily be achieved by blocking cell migration across a polymer construct. Parameters that dictate a material's ability to block trans-construct cell migration are **total porosity**, pore size distribution, and interconnectedness of pore structure. The pore size of a material must be greater than approximately 10 microns to support cell infiltration and allow cell migration within a scaffold. As expected, the ability of cells to migrate within a scaffold increases with increasing pore size. One way of selectively conducting cells may involve creating a material with a continuous, interconnected pore structure on one side, and a non-porous surface on the opposite side via creative polymer processing. In this way, one can impel cells on one side of a construct to infiltrate while blocking cells on the opposite side that may interfere in tissue development. One may also be able to provide selectivity of cell conduction by varying the extent of mineral formation on opposite sides of a porous polymer scaffold. Mineralization would be a favorable technique in orthodontic bone regeneration applications, since the presence of a mineral layer generally enhances bony tissue ingrowth. **Degradable** materials that have been mineralized *in vitro* include phosphorylated chitosan, poly(ethylene terephthalate), poly (vinyl alchohol), poly (hydroxyethyl methacrylate), and the aforementioned poly (α-hydroxy acids).

2.3 THE STATE OF CONDUCTIVE APPROACHES IN DENTAL APPLICATIONS

Currently, the standard therapy for treatment of advanced periodontal disease involves the use of synthetic constructs (both **degradable** and non-degradable) as conduits for progenitor cells and barriers to infiltration of etiologic agents (e.g., bacteria). Researchers and clinicians in the dental field have attempted to use several materials to optimally meet design requirements. The most commonly used membrane for GTR is composed of expanded polytetrafluoroethylene (ePTFE) (Gore-Tex, W.L. Gore and Associates, Flagstaff, AZ, USA). This material has been relatively successful both in achieving periodontal attachment and in regenerating bone tissue, and it is chemically and biologically inert. However, ePTFE is not **degradable**, and therefore the use of the material requires a second surgical procedure for removal.

There has been significant progress in the use of **degradable GTR** materials composed of poly(α-hydroxy esters) in the periodontal field. A recent multicenter clinical study using two separate formulations of three-dimensional poly(lactic acid) (PLA) **GTR** membranes, Guidor (John O. Butler) and EpiGuide (THM Biomedical), shows that the materials provide a scaffold for tissue regeneration while causing no major infections, flap sloughing, adverse reaction, or delayed healing. The PLA materials also effectively prevent epithelial cells and gingival connective tissue from contacting the root surface, avoiding undesirable interference and development of scar tissue during oral tissue development. Guidor is a hydrophilic membrane formed from poly(lactic acid) and softened by a citric acid ester plasticizer for increased malleability, and EpiGuide is a hydrophilic membrane with a flexible open pore structure facilitating fluid infiltration and adherence to the surface of teeth. These materials show comparable results despite differences in mechanical properties, processing methods, and overall structure. A third, more recently developed PLA membrane system is Atrisorb (Atrix Laboratories, Inc.). This system consists of dissolved PLA in a carrier, N-methyl-2-pyrrolidone. The liquid form transforms into a pliable solid upon contact with aqueous solution, and thus can be readily molded into any desired structure. Successful clinical results have been reported using Atrisorb to regenerate the periodontal ligament and resorbed alveolar bone. A comparison of PLA membranes with non-resorbable ePTFE membranes shows no significant difference in vertical attachment level, horizontal attachment level, probing depth, and gingival margin location. Over the long term the **degradable** implants are favored, since they avoid a second surgical procedure and further patient trauma. Each of these materials could prove very useful in the prevention of alveolar bone resorption and ankylosis.

3. INDUCTIVE APPROACH

Recent tissue engineering approaches have been concerned with more accurately mimicking the processes of embryonic development and wound healing. Inductive approaches to engineering tissues are aimed at manipulating the process of tissue formation by controlled surface immobilization or delivery of **various bioactive factors** involved in developmental processes. Extracellular matrix molecules or small peptide sequences that promote cell adhesion and migration can be immobilized onto the surface of a tissue engineering scaffold to affect cellular organization during new tissue development. In addition, soluble signals such as polypeptide **growth factors** and plasmid DNA can be delivered locally from three-dimensional, porous scaffolds to exert a higher level of biochemical control over new tissue development. Inclusion of these pleiotropic macromolecules into tissue engineering constructs has implications for cellular control. **Inductive factors** can provide the means for manipulating cell proliferation, chemotaxis, **differentiation**, and matrix synthesis, and thus exhibit broad potential in regenerative medicine.

3.1 PEPTIDE/PROTEIN IMMOBILIZATION

An inductive tactic for selective cell conduction involves the immobilization of extracellular matrix (ECM) molecules or small peptide sequences on the surface of a synthetic construct. This approach takes advantage of the receptor-mediated selectivity of cell recognition. Proteins with ECM-derived amino acid sequences, or the ECM molecules themselves, can be used to bind specific cell types, leaving undesired cell types with no mechanism to adhere to the material surface. Control of cell adhesion, migration, and spatial distribution can be achieved via peptide immobilization or adsorbed protein layers on the surface of a membrane. Further uses of this approach are dependent on identification of adhesion sequences that exclusively bind certain cell types, a topic of extensive study in molecular cell biology. Potentially, this **inductive** method could be combined with physical blockage of unwanted cell migration to form a membrane with controlled pore structure and immobilized adhesion molecules, exerting a high level of control over cell migration.

3.2 FACTOR DELIVERY

Delivery of soluble signals (i.e., polypeptide growth factors, plasmid DNA) is a key aspect of new **inductive** methods to engineer tissues. Delivery of **bioactive factors** locally can induce cellular activity selectively, potentially stimulating tissue regeneration rather than tissue repair (i.e., scar tissue formation). Growth factors have been identified for several cell types and can potentially be exploited to induce regeneration of lost or damaged tissue. For example, vascular endothelial growth factor induces proliferation of vascular endothelial cells, and thus it may be very useful for inducing vascular tissue regeneration and vascular growth into regenerating tissues.

Although **bioactive factors** may be potent, their effects are typically transient, and inductive tissue engineering methods call for controllable, sustained, and localized delivery. Delivery systems must also maintain the **bioactivity** of the factors to be delivered, and processing techniques for delivery systems must guard against denaturation and degradation of proteins and nucleic acids. Many delivery systems take advantage of controlled **degradation** of synthetic polymer materials to release significant quantities of factor over an extended time scale. It is possible to tune polymer properties to manipulate the release profile over time, and thus precisely direct the regenerative process temporally. A recent study shows release of vascular endothelial growth factor (VEGF) from hydrogels composed of the polysaccharide alginate. The release is sustained at a constant rate (~5%/day) over a period of 14 days in culture (Figure 9-3). Additionally, the release from alginate hydrogels enhanced **bioactivity** when compared to VEGF added directly to the culture medium. The most commonly used materials for sustained drug delivery include PLG microspheres, and the aforementioned alginate hydrogels.

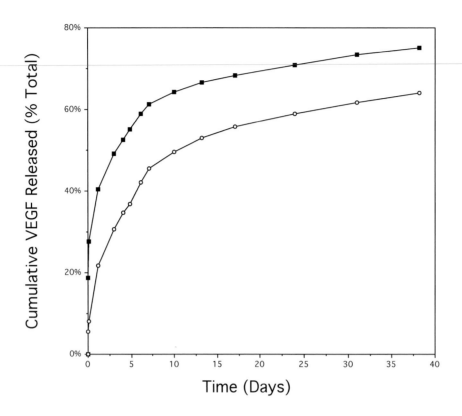

Figure 9-3: Cumulative release of VEGF from alginate hydrogel beads gelled in either 1.0M CaCl2 (o), or 0.1M CaCl2 (n) as a function of time (From: Peters, MC, et. al., J. Biomat. Sci.: Polym. Edn. 1998;9:1267-1278).

Specifically in orthodontic tissue engineering, many of the relevant **bioactive factors** have been identified for periodontal ligament fibroblasts (PLFs), gingival fibroblasts, and osteoblasts. Investigators have developed various delivery systems specifically for the delivery of platelet derived growth factor (PDGF) to periodontal tissues. PDGF is the most potent known factor in periodontal ligament regeneration, and has received the most attention from researchers. Transforming growth factor beta (TGF-b), PDGF, and basic fibroblast growth factor (bFGF) have shown strong chemotactic and mitogenic effects on PLFs, with the two latter factors also spurring matrix synthesis. Sustained delivery of bFGF has been accomplished from gelatin hydrogels and alginate hydrogels. TGF-b has also been released from alginate, along with methylcellulose gels, collagen, and PLG scaffolds. In each case cellular response was amplified when factors were delivered in a sustained and controlled manner when compared to the direct addition of factors both *in vivo* and *in vitro*.

The most potent known growth factors related to oral and maxillofacial bone regeneration are the class of peptides known as **bone morphogenetic proteins** (BMPs). The observation of the unique ability of demineralized bone matrix to induce bone tissue formation in extraskeletal sites led to the isolation and discovery of BMPs as inductive factors. Since their discovery, BMPs, have been delivered from several materials to induce formation of new bone tissue in a variety of skeletal and extraskeletal sites. BMP-delivery vehicles examined thus far include demineralized bone matrix, PLG, b-tricalcium phosphate, and hydroxyapatite. In each case, BMPs in conjunction with a natural or synthetic carrier material, *in vivo* induced dramatic increases in the amount and mechanical strength of bone regenerated when compared with the carrier materials alone. BMPs have also been delivered to the periodontium via a collagen matrix carrier and induced cementogenesis and development of a functional periodontal ligament.

Members of the BMP family have diverse effects on mitogenesis, differentiation, chemotaxis, and matrix synthesis of bone-forming cells, and many of the 13 BMP sequences cloned thus far have been analyzed in the context of bone **morphogenesis**.

The combination of BMP's with a carrier material is critical. BMP's injected directly into bone defects tend to diffuse away quickly and have a very limited **inductive** effect. Carrier materials not only curb diffusion of the factor away from the regeneration site, they also provide a substrate for conduction of osteogenic cells and promote **osteointegration**. It is important to note that surface characteristics and geometry of the substrate for tissue development are of critical importance in osteoinduction by BMPs. Given the appropriate carrier material, BMPs could prove to be an invaluable tool in orthodontic and periodontal treatment of alveolar bone resorption, replacement of lost teeth, and general reshaping of oral and maxillofacial bones.

3.3 TISSUE ENGINEERING SCAFFOLDS FOR INDUCTIVE FACTOR DELIVERY

A combination of **bioactive factor** delivery and **conductive tissue engineering approaches** may provide active control over the function of cells that migrate into a three-dimensional, porous scaffold. Although **guided tissue regeneration (GTR)** approaches have achieved success in regenerating tissues with minimal inflammatory response, greater control over cell-cell and cell-macromolecule interactions is desirable. Clinically used **GTR** scaffolds have several properties amenable to cell conduction, but they are passive, and in general they exercise a low level of biochemical control over new tissue formation. Recently, several investigators have developed schemes for inclusion of **bioactive factors** into natural and synthetic scaffolds to exert control over local tissue regeneration.

Ideally, one would like to controllably deliver **bioactive factors** directly from degradable, synthetic scaffolds for tissue regeneration. This scheme would allow for simultaneous induction of tissue formation, and conduction of progenitor cells onto the matrix. Inductive factors included into the scaffold material can be delivered in a sustained manner, which amplifies their inductive effects by controlling diffusion of the factor away from the regeneration site. Recent studies have shown sustained release of **bioactive factors** from sponges composed of PLG or collagen intended for use as tissue regeneration scaffolds. The scaffolds are over 93% porous (Figure 9-4), and are thus amenable to cell infiltration and tissue growth. The controlled release of VEGF has been accomplished from both mineralized and non-mineralized PLG scaffolds by incorporating the factor into a novel gas foaming process for production of the scaffold. The release from non-mineralized 75:25 PLG was sustained over 60+ days *in vitro*, and the VEGF retained over 90% of its **bioactivity**.

Although delivery of polypeptide growth factors is an attractive method for inductive tissue engineering, the direct alteration of cell function on the genetic level may have a more substantial effect. The localized delivery of DNA in tissue engineering is exciting because it offers the ability to recruit specific cells as bioreactors to produce inductive factors.

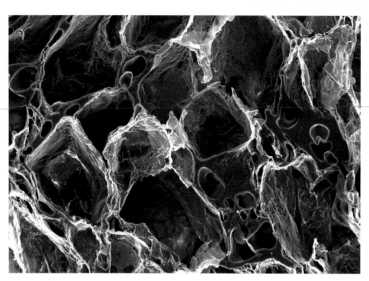

Figure 9-4: SEM micrograph of the cross section of a gas foamed/particulate leached 85:15 PLG scaffold (From: Murphy W.L., Gilhool K.A., Kohn D.H., Mooney D.J. In: Mineralization in Natural and Synthetic Biomaterials, Materials Research Society, Vol. 599. P. Li, P. Calvert, R.J. Levy, T. Kokubo, C.R. Schneid, Eds., 1999).

Inducing certain cells to act as micro-bioreactors may improve the **efficiency** and specificity of factor delivery, and exert a new level of control over cell activity during tissue development. The sustained release of DNA encoding for platelet derived growth factor (PDGF) has also been accomplished from the PLG sponges. Release was sustained for periods of up to a month *in vitro* (Figure 9-5), and the delivery led to the transfection of a large number of cells *in vivo*. Delivery of DNA enhanced extracellular matrix deposition and blood vessel formation *in vivo* exhibited the functional potential of the technique. Delivery of plasmid DNA encoding for bone morphogenetic protein-4 (BMP-4) has been accomplished from **collagen** sponges, and the localized delivery led to the formation of local bone foci similar to bone formed by BMP autoinduction.

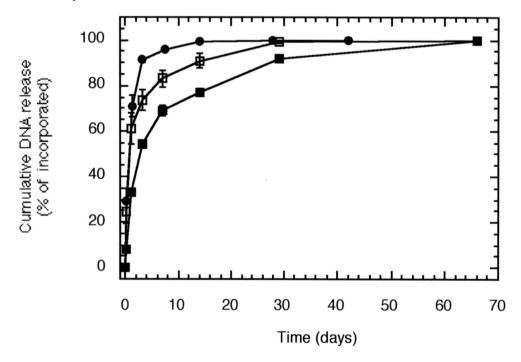

Figure 9-5: Cumulative release of plasmid DNA from 75:25 PLG with an inherent viscosity of 0.2 (l), 85:15 PLG with an inherent viscosity of 0.7 (o), and 75:25 PLG with an inherent viscosity of 0.7 (n) as a function of time (From: Shea, LD, et. al., Nature Biotechnology 1999;17:551-554).

4. CELL-BASED APPROACHES

Although **conductive and** inductive approach**es** have great potential, cell transplantation approaches are also currently being pursued due to key limitations in these approaches. Even if inductive factors are able to control cell migration and activity, the factors have not been identified for all cell types, and there may be cell types for which factors do not exist. Also, each approach relies on the postulate that progenitor cells reside in the tissue adjacent to a defect and will conduct onto a material construct *in vivo* when provided with an appropriate migratory environment. An intrinsic limitation is the inability to precisely predict and control which cell types conduct onto a construct and which biological factors are involved in the process of tissue development. A third limitation of inductive and conductive strategies is the time lapse between implantation of a scaffold and development of a tissue. In some applications a waiting period between implantation and tissue development is unacceptable, and it is desirable to have engineered tissues on hand for transplantation. Each of these limitations can potentially be addressed by directly transplanting the desired cell types to the deficient site.

Cell-based tissue engineering schemes involve seeding of cells onto a synthetic construct *in vitro* and subsequent transplantation of the construct. Using cell-based approaches, one can transplant cells directly with or without a material carrier, or allow cells to grow and form tissue for a period of time *in vitro* prior to implantation. In the latter approach, the culture environment can be controlled during the process of tissue development. An exciting advantage of *in vitro* tissue engineering is the possibility of treating a multitude of patients from a single biopsy, which may circumvent the problem of tissue and organ donor shortages (Figure 9-1).

One can potentially obtain the necessary cells for *in vitro* tissue development or cell transplantation via allogenic or autologous biopsy. **Allogenic cell sourcing** techniques are desirable because they involve minimal patient trauma; however, they also run the risk of tissue rejection and necessitate the use of immunosuppressant drugs. **Autologous cell sourcing** circumvents concerns about cell or tissue rejection, but requires multiple surgical procedures with a time lapse in between for cell expansion in culture.

Cell-based schemes have yet to be attempted in orthodontic or periodontal regenerative therapy. Several methods for **cell-based tissue engineering** of bone have been developed, and could prove useful in the regeneration of alveolar bone. Three dimensional culture systems have been developed for osteoblast-like cell lines and marrow stromal osteoblasts using PLG scaffolds. Osteoblast-like cells and rat calvarial osteoblasts follow their classic differentiation pathway within a three-dimensional, porous polymer scaffold, and the osteoblast-like cells are able to form a three-dimensional tissue with architecture similar to that of native bone after 12 weeks in culture. These scaffolds may eventually be used clinically to enhance bone regeneration by delivering progenitor cells to the wound site or by growing bone tissue in culture for transplantation.

5. MECHANICALLY-INDUCED BONE MORPHOGENESIS: DISTRACTION OSTEOGENESIS

One particular technique used to affect *de novo* formation of bone tissue, **distraction osteogenesis**, does not employ any sort of external scaffold system, bone graft, or inductive factor delivery and thus it does not precisely fall into any of the aforementioned tissue engineering schemes. In contrast to the aforementioned methods, which endeavor to spur the regenerative process while simultaneously suppressing the natural tissue repair process, this technique actually utilizes a natural tissue repair response to spur regeneration of bone tissue. The technique involves cortical fracture of a bone followed by gradual separation (distraction) of the two resulting bone ends. The basic concept relies on the initial formation of a temporary bone-like substance between and around the ends of a fractured bone, termed the temporary callus. Formation of the temporary callus is brought about by the presence of a copious blood supply carrying osteoprogenitor cells and inductive factors to direct the regenerative process. The temporary callus is then lengthened using an external fixative device to stretch the bone ends and the surrounding muscle and fascia apart. During the gradual stretching process the temporary **callus** begins to remodel into a definitive callus due to the resorptive activity of **osteoclasts** and the bone forming ability of osteoblasts in response to various mechanical forces. The gradual stretching process is followed by a consolidation period in which the newly formed bone matrix is mineralized and fully becomes the definitive callus, which can scarcely be distinguished from natural bone tissue. This process is effectively equivalent to the process that occurs upon pathological bone fracture. Distraction osteogenesis (also termed osteodistraction) is routinely used to treat long bone abnormalities, and has more recently been applied to the maxillofacial region since its inception by Guerrero in 1990.

Since the basic concept of osteodistraction is to advantageously manipulate a pathological process, there are critical variables to address in order to ensure optimal union between the fractured bone segments and avoid fibrous nonunion. The five significant objectives in the osteodistraction process are: 1. a "clean" fracture with optimal preservation of osteogenic tissue, 2. an adequate time lapse between fracture and **distraction** (latency period) to allow for temporary callus formation, 3. an optimal rate of **distraction** to allow for callus elongation, 4. stability of bone segments during **distraction**, and 5. an adequate time lapse between the end of distraction and the removal of the external distraction device to allow for mineralization of newly formed bone tissue (the "consolidation period"). Many techniques and external fixative devices have recently been developed to manipulate these variables. The simultaneous insertion of autologous bone grafts from the iliac crest is usually necessary and advisable for limb lengthening. Therefore, although in principal the process avoids the disadvantages of introducing a foreign material, grafting is generally necessary to augment *de novo* bone formation. Nevertheless, this process has proven to be eminently useful in limb lengthening, and may prove clinically useful in the treatment of craniofacial defects.

6. SIGNIFICANT DESIGN CHALLENGES IN TISSUE ENGINEERING

Although the above approaches offer contrasting methods and techniques for directing regeneration, there are certain requirements that pervade the field of tissue engineering. First, growing cells require a **degradable**, biocompatible, and mechanically stable substrate to support and encourage their growth, proliferation, differentiation, and function. Furthermore, as the tissue forms into a three-dimensional mass of appreciable volume the tissue absolutely requires a vascular supply, and in some cases neural infiltration. In addition to the basic survival concerns, cells must be provided with the appropriate signals if one is to exercise control over new tissue formation. As more complex formulations for engineering tissues are developed, spatial and temporal control over cell function at the level of specific cell types may become increasingly important. Such concerns may call for novel strategies for presentation of **bioactive factors** to cell populations.

6.1 BIODEGRADABILITY/BIOCOMPATIBILITY

Materials used as constructive scaffolds for tissue development must be **degradable** over a predictable and controllable time scale so that one can synchronize material clearance and natural tissue formation. This requirement is even more important in the context of recent **inductive** tissue engineering techniques in which material **degradation** is a major parameter determining factor delivery. The materials must also degrade into products that are physiologically acceptable and cause minimal inflammatory response in the body. Commonly used **GTR** materials such as expanded poly(tetrafluoroethylene) (ePTFE) fall short of these requirements, and thus require a second surgical procedure for removal. Given recent clinical evidence that degradable materials are as effective as ePTFE membranes at guiding tissue regeneration, the non-degradable materials are likely to be unacceptable for the next generation of **GTR** constructs for orthodontic and periodontal tissue engineering.

The factors determining a material's predictability and controllability of degradation include degradation mechanism (i.e., enzymatic, hydrolytic, etc.), molecular weight, inherent viscosity (I.V.), and polydispersity (molecular weight variability). Molecular weight and I.V. can be predictably varied in synthesis of many materials to imply control over degradation and ensure coincidence of regeneration and scaffold departure. A variety of biodegradable polymers and hydrogels have been employed as regenerative scaffolds. The most widely used materials are the poly (α-hydroxy acids), specifically PLA and PLG. They have a simple hydrolytic degradation mechanism and their products of degradation are natural metabolites (lactic and glycolic acid), and thus pose minimal threat of inflammatory response in the host tissue. Simply by varying the relative amounts of PLA and PGA present in a matrix formulation one can vary degradation time from days to several months, while also controlling the scaffold's mechanical properties.

6.2 ADEQUATE SURFACE AREA/VOLUME RATIO

Another key material requirement is a large surface area/volume ratio to support tissue development and facilitate nutrient transport. A highly porous material with a largely interconnected pore structure promotes cell activity by extending the substrate area for growth and proliferation while also allowing for mass transport. The interconnectedness of the pore structure expedites mass transport, which is absolutely essential in the region of a developing tissue with little or no vascular supply. An open pore structure is advantageous for the diffusion of nutrients and wastes to and from functioning cells. This requirement is especially important in a **degradable** system, since clearance of degradation products is also desirable.

Methods abound for producing PLA, PGA, and PLG materials with interconnected pores. Most methods are dependent on a phase transition, and require the use of organic solvents, which are undesirable due to the possibility of cytotoxic residual solvent from processing. Recently developed processing techniques use high pressure gas foaming of PLG sponges in combination with particulate leaching to produce an open-pore structure without cytotoxic residuals (Figure 9-4). One of the major advantages of the gas foaming process is the ability to include **bioactive factors** into polymer processing for production of inductive regeneration scaffolds.

6.3 MECHANICAL INTEGRITY

Cells exert contractile forces on their substrate material, potentially collapsing the structure of a three-dimensional scaffold and destroying the shape of the resulting tissue. Mechanical integrity of the scaffold material is necessary for resistance of contractile cellular forces during tissue growth. In addition, many tissue engineering scaffolds both *in vivo* and *in vitro* are subjected to externally applied mechanical forces that play a role in tissue development. Mechanical forces can be very important in the development of a tissue, and several *in vitro* tissue engineering strategies have been designed to apply external forces that mimic *in vivo* developmental conditions. Even on the single cell level, control over mechanical properties can determine the activity of cells on the surface of a construct, and mechanical signaling via the adhesion substrate may be a key factor in development of many types of tissue. Cells can be spurred to proliferate or differentiate depending on their mechanical interaction with a substrate material. Control over these cell surface interactions could be a major parameter in the design of scaffolds for controlled tissue regeneration. Some materials, such as PLG scaffolds and alginate hydrogels, can be processed so that their mechanical strength is controlled, potentially implying control over the shape of the final tissue product and the forces applied to cells within the material constructs. For example, it is possible to engineer smooth muscle tissue with a predefined structure by increasing the mechanical integrity of the scaffold material, and the development of engineered smooth muscle tissue can be regulated by externally applied mechanical forces. Control over tissue shape is quite important in cosmetic applications for aesthetic purposes, and is desirable in many tissue engineering applications, including orthodontic applications.

6.4 VASCULAR AND NEURAL INFILTRATION

Poor survival of most cell types post-implantation is a significant problem in cell-based tissue regeneration due to hypoxia of cells deep within a construct. Also, several tissue types require neural ingrowth to properly function (skeletal muscle, urological tissue, etc.). Developing tissues require a vascular supply for transport of nutrients and waste. Rapid vascularization has been a topic of intense study, and a variety of **angiogenic** factors have been identified. Recent studies have focused on the inclusion of inductive factors into tissue engineering scaffolds to spur **angiogenesis**. Although investigators have had some success in promoting rapid angiogenesis, several challenges remain. The angiogenic cascade involves the sequential action of several distinct **bioactive factors**, and rapid angiogenesis may require complex inductive factor delivery systems.

The challenges of vascular and neural infiltration highlight the advantage of a highly porous scaffold material. Open-pore structures (Figure 9-4) facilitate vascular and neural ingrowth and can promote the survival of a growing tissue. Although porous scaffolds may passively allow for tissue ingrowth, the process of tissue infiltration can potentially be improved and augmented using the previously described inductive tissue engineering methods.

7. FUTURE DIRECTIONS

Guided tissue regeneration has proven to be an apt method for regeneration of the oral tissues, specifically in periodontal applications. Although attempts with **degradable** and non-degradable materials have been relatively successful, a new level of spatial and temporal control over tissue development may offer a higher degree of success. The challenges to tissue regeneration mentioned above each apply specifically to orthodontic and periodontal tissue engineering. **Degradability** of the scaffold material has been shown to be beneficial when compared with non-degradable dental implants in periodontal applications, and biocompatibility is key to avoid immune responses and cytotoxicity. The maxillofacial region is subjected to significant mechanical stress, which highlights the importance of scaffold mechanical integrity in oral and maxillofacial applications. In addition, many of the oral and maxillofacial tissues are bulk tissues of appreciable volume (i.e., periodontal ligament, alveolar bone, cementum, etc.), and thus rapid **angiogenesis** may be a key requirement for oral tissue engineering scaffolds to ensure cell survival.

Future studies in the field of tissue engineering will likely focus on developing novel model systems to study the role of environmental cues in tissue development. An understanding of the factors that dictate tissue development will lead to design of novel scaffolding systems for tissue engineering. Elucidation of the effects of cellular spatial organization on tissue development may lead to the design of scaffolds with tightly controlled surface features to guide cell adhesion and migration. The localized, sustained, and temporally-controlled delivery of the appropriate soluble inductive factors promises to be a key component of novel inductive tissue engineering strategies. For engineering of hybrid tissues such as the interfacial region between the periodontal ligament and alveolar bone, co-transplantation of multiple cell types may be advantageous. Recent work has been aimed at expanding the field by combining **conductive, inductive, and cell-based approaches**. This may enhance the selectivity of cell migration, while also providing environments conducive to development of the desired tissue.

8. SUGGESTED READINGS

Principles of Tissue Engineering: Second Edition; Lanza, R.P., Langer, R., Vacanti, J., Eds. New York, NY.: Academic Press. 2000.

Langer R, Vacanti JP. Tissue Engineering. Science 1993:260:920-925.

Crane GM, Ishaug SL, Mikos AG. Tissue engineering of bone. Nature Medicine 1995;1:1322-1324.

Alberg, E., Hill, E.E., Mooney, D.J. Craniofacial tissue engineering. Critical Reviews in Oral Biology and Medicine 2001;12: 64-75.

Hermann JS, Buser D. Guided bone regeneration for dental implants. Current Opinion in Periodontology 1996;3:168-177.

Hubbell JA. Synthetic biodegradable polymers for tissue engineering and drug delivery. Current Opinion in Solid State Materials Science 1998;3:246-251.

Giannobile WV. Periodontal tissue engineering by growth factors. Bone 1996;19:23S-37S.

Ripamonti U, Reddi AH. Tissue engineering, morphogenesis, and regeneration of the periodontal tissues by bone morphogenetic proteins. Critical Reviews in Oral Biology and Medicine 1997;8:154-163.

Soskolne WA. Subgingival delivery of therapeutic agents in the treatment of periodontal diseases. Critical Reviews in Oral Biology and Medicine 1997;8:164-174.

Colton CK. Implantable biohybrid artificial organs. Cell Transplantation 1995;4:415-436.

Golub ES, Green DR. (Eds) In: Immunology a Synthesis, Chapter 37: Transplantation, 1991 p. 658-670.

Klagsbrun M, D'Amore PA. Regulators of angiogenesis. Annual Reviews in Physiology 1991;53:217-239.

CHAPTER 10

Clinical Epidemiology and Malocclusion

Burcu Bayirli

1. INTRODUCTION

Correct **diagnosis** is a crucial part of a patient's treatment. As a result of the diagnostic process, a clinician classifies the patient's target **disorder** (malocclusion). That classification determines the treatment that will follow based on knowledge that should be derived from research. Although personal experiences may be a guide to clinical decision making, clinicians' experiences are not enough for the clinician to be able to understand all the mechanisms that lead to a malocclusion and the correction of that malocclusion. Actually, these experiences may be misleading.

Clinical predictions from prior experiences and/or knowledge of the biology of malocclusion are **hypotheses** to be tested by research. It is very hard to predict the course of treatment in an individual patient, because there are genetic, physical, and psychosocial factors that affect the **outcomes** of a treatment. In orthodontics, for instance, the skeletal and dental manifestations of the patient's growth pattern, patient cooperation, and clinician's skill are some of the factors that influence the results of a particular treatment plan. In addition to these factors, the **biases** of the clinician may lead to **systematic errors** that would distort the clinical observations resulting in erroneous conclusions. Also, there is usually not a one to one relationship between an effect and its cause. Therefore, understanding the distribution and **determinants** of health and disease in groups (clinical epidemiology) is necessary for clinicians to determine the accuracy of clinical information.

Epidemiology enables clinicians to make accurate treatment decisions for their patients through development and application of valid and reliable clinical observation methods as well as best clinical evidence. For instance, patients receiving different treatments are observed and the characteristics of those patients with different treatment outcomes are identified. Systematic and **random errors** are minimized during these observations through application of epidemiological methods. Consequently, the characteristics that may lead to different treatment results are determined to isolate the treatment effects. Thus, it is important for clinicians and epidemiologists to collaborate with each other, because both fields have a lot of useful information to offer one another.

Unfortunately, in traditional clinical perspective, clinicians use their and other colleagues' prior experiences to diagnose and treat a patient. Clinicians have been hesitant to express a patient's probability of presence in various risk, diagnosis, or treatment categories. Instead, they are concerned with their individual patients. Therefore, one may say that the traditional clinical perspective does not support the exchange of information between epidemiology and clinical disciplines. This chapter will attempt to clarify why collaboration between epidemiology and clinical disciplines is essential starting with causal inference and multifactorial etiology.

2. CAUSAL INFERENCE AND MULTIFACTORIAL ETIOLOGY

Malocclusion is a developmental problem—a significant variation from the normal range of growth or morphology. Hereditary and environmental factors are important influences on development. It is unlikely that any part of the facial skeleton is solely determined by Mendelian genetics. Malocclusions are determined by a combination of hereditary and environmental factors.

To a large extent, genes may determine the size and shape of the bones and teeth, but the environmental forces act to change these characteristics. The hereditary and environmentally acquired traits become so interwoven that it is difficult to isolate the different pieces of the puzzle as demonstrated in the following example:

> "Both the right set of genes and the yellow corn diet are necessary to produce yellow shanks. A farmer with several strains of fowl who feeds them only yellow corn would consider yellow shanks to be a genetic condition, since only one strain would get yellow shanks, despite all strains getting the same diet. A different farmer who owned only the strain liable to get yellow shanks but who fed some of the birds yellow corn and others white corn would consider yellow shanks to be an environmentally determined condition because it depends on diet. In reality, yellow shanks is determined by both genes and environment; there is no reasonable way to allocate a portion of the causation to either genes or environment (Rothman and Greenland, 1998)."

Both the clinician and the scientist face the same challenging task of solving this complex puzzle.

2.1 GAME THEORY

Holland (1998) compares this endeavor to a game in which the scientist and/or clinician are one of the players and nature is his/her opponent. In a game, even if each player makes a plan at the outset, the course of the game is full of surprises for the players, because they are not aware of each other's strategies. In orthodontics, the scientist and/or clinician try to model the rules of facial growth to understand the development of malocclusion. The expression of genes in the offspring is a guide to how certain facial and occlusal characteristics are acquired. The **outcome** is still a surprise, because of the changing effects of the environment on facial growth.

Consequently, the scientific challenge lies in the ability to model the interactions of the genes with environmental influences (i.e., forces of the musculature). Holland says that one has to understand emergence (see the quotation below) to solve this scientific problem and understand nature's strategy:

> "A wondrous vine emerges when Jack plants the seed for his beanstalk, and it unfolds into a world of giants and magic harps. When we were children, Jack's miraculous beanstalk wasn't so far removed from the everyday miracles of fall colors and germinating seeds. Now that we're grown, seeds still fascinate us. Somehow these small capsules enclose specifications that produce structures as complicated and distinctive as a giant redwood, the common day's-eye (daisy), and a beanstalk. They are the very embodiment of emergence—much coming from little (Holland, 1998)."

In short, emergence is what one has to decipher to make causal inferences. Game theory and emergence leads us to the necessity of consideration of multifactorial etiology to achieve the scientific conquest.

2.2 IMPORTANCE OF MULTIFACTORIAL ETIOLOGY IN CAUSAL INFERENCE

In their discussion of "Causation and Causal Inference", Rothman and Greenland (1998) define the term "complete causal mechanism" as "a set of minimal conditions and events that inevitably produce disease or target disorder; 'minimal' implies that all of the conditions or events are necessary." This definition stresses the importance of considering the role of every etiological factor in the onset of a disorder.

For instance, one could hypothesize that mouthbreathing may cause crossbites in some people. One has to realize, however, mouthbreathing will not lead to crossbites in everyone. The challenge lies in the answer to this question: When does mouthbreathing cause crossbites? In other words, one has to know the other factors that act in accordance with mouthbreathing to cause crossbites. Assumption of a one-to-one relationship between mouthbreathing and crossbites would be naive. Actually, there are probably a number of different causal mechanisms—some sharing a few of the same etiological factors—that cause the same disorder, such as crossbite.

At the end of the 19th century, the perception of cause was very different than it is today. The reason for this difference is that the interest in causation started with the efforts to treat infectious diseases. The basic belief underlying Koch's postulates was that a disease has one particular cause. Although these postulates were a great contribution to medicine, they do not apply to chronic diseases (i.e., cancer) and/or various disorders (i.e., malocclusion). Even for an infectious disease that has specific bacteria that causes it, the assumption of a one-to-one relationship between this disease and the specific bacteria may be dubious. For example, there are behavioral factors that would determine the occurrence of an infectious disease. Unless certain behavioral factors exist, the mere presence of the bacteria may not always lead to the development of a specific infectious disease in an individual. Furthermore, the relationship of the factors among themselves results in different effects as well. When a treatment effect or a disorder has more than one cause, a change in one of the causes may have a substantial effect, for instance, on the treatment outcome.

As scientists and clinicians, we have to identify all these possible causal mechanisms to avoid being ignorant and, thus, unfair to patients. When only one component of a whole mechanism that produces a disease is known, equal risks are assigned to individuals with this one known cause and same treatment is carried out on all of them. Employment of the same treatment strategy on patients with similar occlusal manifestations, but different causal mechanisms may be the reason why a certain treatment works on most of the patients, but not all. Therefore, etiology of a disease should be included in the diagnosis. Etiologic classification becomes very important if one wants to include etiology in diagnosis. Unfortunately, in orthodontics, various malocclusions with different causes and prognoses are classified as the same type of malocclusion. **Angle classification** does not differentiate the causes of malocclusion types. Inconvenient classification schemes lead to problems both in diagnosis and treatment planning.

3. DIAGNOSIS

In diagnosis, clinical and radiographic data are interpreted to differentiate various clinical disorders with similar manifestations. Sackett and associates (1991) mention that social, psychological, and economic status of the patient should influence the diagnosis, because the treatment plan is finalized according to patient's concerns and wishes. These factors become even more important for orthodontic treatment in which the goal is to correct the target disorders of a malocclusion, some of which may be lacking any pathologic symptoms.

Unfortunately, patients and clinicians have different definitions for successful orthodontic treatment. A patient's definition of successful orthodontic treatment is based on their expectations from this treatment. Accordingly, clinicians and researchers need to understand these expectations and develop methods to measure them, so that patient expectations from treatment may be included as outcome measures in the studies of treatment effect. For example, **quality of life** and **utility** measures could be developed for orthodontics and incorporated into indices, scales, and rating systems to reflect patient values.

Many occlusal indices have been developed to measure malocclusion and determine treatment need. Most of these indices use professional judgment to derive their criteria. As a result, these indices do not address all the issues that are related to oral health, such as self-perception of oral health. Bader and Ismail (1999) recommend that dimensions important to the clinicians as well as to the patients should be included in the classification of oral health care outcomes.

Investigators who realize that esthetics have important psychosocial consequences have incorporated esthetics into their occusal indices, such as Dental Aesthetic Index (DAI) and the Index of Orthodontic Treatment Need (IOTN). Yet, Birkeland and associates (1996) claim that many occlusal traits are not represented in the esthetic component of IOTN. Also, neither of these indices are designed to be used in an African-American population. There are variations in the types of malocclusions and dental conditions observed among different races and ethnicities. The inclusion of these criteria above would enhance the **validity** of the indices and the data gathered through the application of these indices would provide information on the prevalence and severity of malocclusion. If standard valid and reliable as well as objective diagnostic criteria are developed, these indices could be used as outcome measures, too.

These valid and reliable criteria incorporated into the indices can also be used in diagnostic tests. Valid and reliable diagnostic tests may be very useful to the clinician during the diagnostic process. A valid test should have a high **sensitivity** and **specificity.** Sensitivity (Table 10-1) refers to the capability of the test to accurately determine those individuals with the disorder. Specificity (Table 10-1) refers to the capability of the test to accurately determine those individuals without the disorder. In an ideal world, all diagnostic tests should have a 100 % sensitivity and specificity; however, most of the tests are not able to correctly identify all the true positives and true negatives (Table 10-1). A false positive is an individual without the disorder identified as having the disorder; a false negative is an individual with the disorder identified as not having the disorder. Sensitivity and specificity address the following questions, respectively:

1.) What is the probability that the test result is positive, if the patient has the disorder?
2.) What is the probability that the test result is negative, if the patient does not have the disorder?

Table 10-1: Sensitivity, specificity, positive predictive value, and negative predictive value of a diagnostic test

Test result	True classification of patients	
	Disorder	No disorder
Positive	A=True positive	B=False positive
Negative	C=False negative	D=True negative

$$\text{Sensitivity} = \frac{A}{A+C}$$

$$\text{Specificity} = \frac{D}{B+D}$$

$$\text{Positive predictive value} = \frac{A}{A+B}$$

$$\text{Negative predictive value} = \frac{D}{C+D}$$

From a clinical point of view, one also needs to know the positive and negative predictive value of diagnostic tests (Table 10-1). Positive predictive value is the probability that the patient has the disease, if he/she tests positive for the test. In other words, what is the probability that the individual has the disorder, if the test result is positive? On the other hand, negative predictive value is the probability that the person does not have the disorder if the test result is negative. The above definitions relate to the validity of the diagnostic tests. One has to realize that reliability of the test is just as important. A test is reliable if its results can be reproduced.

Although valid and reliable tests assist the diagnosis, clinicians make their final diagnosis by applying their knowledge and experience. Thus, they have to be able to comprehend the scientific literature as well as have a thorough judgment. Obviously, diagnosis is a very subjective process; therefore, it is very hard to be absolutely certain of any diagnosis. Clinicians can only estimate the probability of a patient having a certain disorder. They seek evidence to support their hypothesis to establish the correct diagnosis. Sackett and colleagues (1991) claim that this approach to diagnosis leads to errors and is the opposite of the scientific approach. In scientific studies, investigators try to disprove a hypothesis. Correct approach to diagnosis is crucial, because after the diagnosis is completed the clinician selects the best treatment for the patient and errors during diagnosis would lead to an incorrect treatment decision.

4. TREATMENT DECISION

Sackett and associates (1991) discuss the steps to determine the best treatment for patients. First of all, treatment objectives are identified. Then, the clinician decides on the best treatment to achieve these treatment objectives. Finally, the ultimate treatment target is determined.

In orthodontics, the treatment objectives are identified to correct malocclusion through employment of specific treatments. One should know the effect of these treatments on the particular malocclusion and the prognosis of malocclusion. The functional and esthetic disadvantages of not receiving any treatment needs to be assessed. Relapse tendencies as well as their mechanisms should be identified. In addition, patient's social, psychological, and economic status as well as concerns must be addressed before the treatment objectives are finalized.

Before treatment starts, clear treatment targets are defined. Specific treatment mechanics to achieve the various treatment targets are determined. For example, Steiner determined incisor angulations to achieve an acceptable occlusion according to various degrees of ANB angle and called them Steiner compromises. Methods such as this one enable the clinician to quantify the treatment targets. Quantification makes these targets easier to observe and their achievement becomes easier to assess.

Furthermore, the patient needs to be involved in the process to achieve the treatment objectives and targets. This involvement increases patient compliance and treatment success. Accordingly, the clinician discusses the best therapy options with his/her specific patient to achieve the selected goals. Three methods are used to select a treatment approach as described by Sackett and colleagues in 1991: abdication, induction, and deduction.

"Abdication" is a method of treatment selection that reminds one of medieval times. Treatment is accepted on faith and suggestions of professors and/or colleagues. Actually, modern science emerged when abdication was left behind and inductivism began as scientists started to inquire about their observations.

In the method of "induction", observations are made to form inferences about natural events. In other words, an orthodontist observes patients in his/her practice. Then, he/she assumes that patients in the future will respond to a specific treatment the same way patients in the past did. Indeed, such observations are helpful, because they lead to formulation of new ideas and hypothesis testing. Unfortunately, clinicians are observing merely one event after another—mandibular growth is observed following the delivery of a functional appliance— and it would be premature to assume a causal connection between two events that take place one after another. As early philosophers pointed out, two events may be happening consecutively by pure chance. The problems with induction led philosophers and scientists to seek sounder methods for scientific reasoning.

The method of "deduction" was introduced as Karl Popper (1959) claimed that it is impossible to prove a hypothesis. On the other hand, consistent observations that do not agree with a hypothesis imply that the hypothesis is false. This approach respects induction only as a method to create new ideas and encourage hypothesis testing. The deductive approach led to today's hypothesis testing in scientific studies.

There are various study designs that employ the deductive approach. Sackett and colleagues (1991) as well as many other researchers advocate the "randomized clinical trial" as the gold standard. Treatment decision may be based on the results of randomized clinical trials if the clinician is using the strategy of deduction. Unfortunately, randomized clinical trials have not yet been carried out to answer most of the questions an orthodontist may have about various treatment strategies. Tulloch and associates (1990) indicated that only 76% of 50 studies that investigated the effectiveness of growth modification in the correction of Class II malocclusions had control groups, and that none of them had employed randomization in their study protocols. Similarly, in 1996 Harrison and colleagues assessed types of studies published in two orthodontic journals over a 5-year period and reported that only 2.8 % of the clinical articles were randomized clinical trials. The rest of the studies either had non-randomized controls or did not have any controls. It is appropriate to use the results of these other study designs as long as they follow valid scientific methods. Research should be conducted to develop methods to summarize the existing data for the best possible incorporation of this information into clinical practice. For instance, it would be helpful to develop methods to evaluate the non-randomized clinical trials. Still, randomized clinical trial is the gold standard, if it is ethical and feasible to conduct. One should never forget that some medical treatments that were thought to be effective as a result of the conclusions derived from weak study designs were later demonstrated to be ineffective in randomized clinical trials.

Lack of evidence with regard to the orthodontic treatment outcomes makes it challenging to determine the best treatment for each patient. Therefore, the clinician should be able to read the available literature critically and apply the best available evidence to his/her patients. As a result of the application of the best available evidence, treatments should be more beneficial and less harmful. In order to be able to critically evaluate the available evidence, one must be familiar with different types of study designs.

5. STUDY DESIGNS

5.1 CLINICAL TRIALS

In clinical trials, investigators compare specific treatments to receiving no treatment, as well as two or more treatments to each other by studying subjects randomly assigned to the various study groups. Investigators administer the treatment, and then measure the outcome of this treatment.

5.1.1. Treatment Selection

The various treatments or interventions that are being administered to the subjects and controls should be sufficiently different from each other so that a significant difference between the groups may be detected, if one exists at all. These treatments should be feasible to be applied in clinical practice. The treatment protocol must be clearly defined for **reproducibility**. Due to the high cost and time required to conduct clinical trials, these trials should be carried out on treatments that basic knowledge is already available from other types of studies.

5.1.2. Subject Selection

Assembly of the study cohort starts with defining inclusion and exclusion criteria. These criteria affect the **generalizability** of the results of the study, because the narrower the selection criteria are, the smaller the sample size gets. It is easier to have a sufficient sample size if there is a large patient pool to select the study participants from.

After these criteria are precisely defined an adequate sample size is calculated. In order to calculate the sample size, the magnitude of a clinically significant treatment effect needs to be estimated. If there are not conclusive data on the selected outcome or outcomes, there may be different opinions about a clinically significant treatment effect.

Afterward, subject recruitment starts. This process requires a lot of time, effort, and financial resources. In clinical trials, a run-in phase may be included before the recruited subjects are randomly assigned to the study groups. In the run-in phase, all subjects are given a placebo treatment. The purpose is to be able to identify the compliant subjects so that **bias** arising as a result of not being able to maintain the assigned groups is avoided. Then, only the compliant subjects are included in the clinical trial. For certain treatments or interventions, such as surgical procedures, however, inclusion of a run-in phase may not be possible. In such situations, the random allocation to study groups should be delayed until the compliant subjects are determined.

5.1.3. **Randomization**

Randomization means that all the subjects have an equal or a known chance of inclusion in any of the groups. As a result of randomization, factors that would distort the **association** should be evenly distributed among the groups. Still, demographic variables and known predictors of the outcome should be measured for each group and compared to each other to assure that the various groups are similar, at least with respect to these factors. At times, chance variation leads to dissimilar groups and, therefore, bias. In that case, these factors must be controlled in the analysis. To further avoid any bias, blinded studies are carried out if possible.

5.1.4. **Blinding**

Various biases may be introduced into a study when the researcher and/or clinician as well as the patient is aware of the treatment assignment. In some randomized clinical trials, it may be possible to blind the researchers and the study participants. Researchers should be blinded at three points during the trial: treatment assignment, treatment administration, and the measurement or determination of the treatment outcome. Double-blind studies are the ones in which neither the patient nor the researcher know the treatment assignment. Sometimes only the study participants can be blinded. Unfortunately, blinding is not possible with certain treatments or interventions. If there is no alternative treatment to the one under study, blinding may be accomplished by using a placebo treatment.

When there is not another effective treatment, it would be ethical to offer a placebo treatment to the control group. A placebo is a substance that is indistinguishable from the agent being administered to the treatment group, but is inert. There is always a chance that some participants may find out they are taking the placebo, however.

The issues mentioned above should be carefully considered during the conduct of a clinical trial. It is usually not feasible to have a large sample size in clinical trials due to the physical and financial resources needed. The ignorance of the epidemiologic principles would decrease the **power** and **efficiency** of these studies.

Non-experimental studies are more common because experimental studies mentioned above are not always ethical and cost efficient. Another name for non-experimental studies is observational studies. Most of the evidence about the effectiveness of various orthodontic treatment techniques comes from observational studies. Studies without any controls and studies of expert opinion are considered to provide the least evidence for treatment effectiveness. The inclusion of controls and omission of clinical opinions still do not resolve all the weaknesses of observational study designs.

In these studies, the investigator usually does not have any control over treatment assignment. The clinician initiates or has initiated treatment that he deemed appropriate for the best patient care based upon his knowledge. Especially in the retrospective study designs, control of treatment protocol is not as strict as it is in the randomized clinical trials. These facts may introduce various biases that can influence study outcomes and conclusions. Different types of observational study designs and their strengths as well as weaknesses are discussed below.

5.2 COHORT STUDIES

In a cohort study, the risk of an outcome is measured in two or more study cohorts. The ratio of risk of disease in exposed subjects to the ratio of risk of disease in unexposed subjects is called the **relative risk**. One has to remember, however, that the number of individuals is used in the denominator to calculate the average risk. It may not always be possible to determine the average risk if a certain number of subjects are lost to follow-up during the study period. **Incidence rates** can still be estimated, because **person-time** is used in the denominator to calculate incidence rates. Then, an individual can contribute person-time to one or more of the cohorts and would not necessarily have to be included for the entire study period. In this type of study it is harder to determine the exposure status, because one person may be classified as a member of the different exposure groups at different times during the study period.

Study cohorts are two or more groups defined in terms of their exposure status. There is at least one group that is exposed, referred to as the exposed cohort, and one group that is not exposed, referred to as the unexposed or the reference cohort. At the beginning of the study, none of the subjects have developed the outcome being studied. The outcome is observed and/or measured in each of these groups as the study progresses and incidence rates or average risks are compared to each other; thus, one can conclude whether or not the exposure was present before the outcome as well as the presence or absence of an **association** between the **exposure** and outcome.

The time of the occurrence or measurement of the outcome needs to be precisely defined. A clear definition is even more important, if subjects will be contributing person-time to various exposure groups. In order to be able to have an appropriate definition, a certain level of knowledge about the study outcome is required.

There are two types of cohort studies. In prospective cohort studies, the sample and their exposure status is determined at the beginning of the study and this sample is followed for a specified period of time to observe the absence or presence of the outcome. Depending on the outcome being studied, a long follow-up period may be necessary. Indeed, retrospective cohort studies are preferred when a long follow-up period is needed. In this type of cohort study, historical data are used to identify the exposure status, then outcome is measured as the retrospective cohort study begins.

A sufficient sample size is required for valid results. It is very expensive to increase the sample size in cohort studies. Monitoring a large sample for a long period of time increases the cost of these studies greatly. These studies can get so expensive that it may not be feasible to conduct them anymore. It is not efficient to study the effect of exposures with long **induction periods** in a cohort study. The efficiency of the study is further reduced if the outcome being investigated is rare.

There are a number of ways to reduce the costs of a cohort study. The use of **registries** or historical cohorts would simplify the monitoring of the cohorts. In these retrospective cohort studies, however, past records may have poorly collected and/or missing information. Then, the study may suffer from recall bias as well as selection biases, if the reason that certain individuals' records are missing is associated with the study variables. Besides, one may use information from existing records of data on the general population instead of having a reference cohort. In this case, there would be no control over the quality of the already-collected data. The investigators would be limited with the available data for the reference group, even though they may be able to measure other variables in the exposure cohort. Furthermore, it is not feasible to use general population records for rare exposures. Finally, one may conduct a case-control study—nested case-control study—with a fraction of the cohort. These studies cost less than a cohort study and have valid findings.

A source population that represents a hypothetical study population is defined, in which a cohort study might have been conducted. If the population the study is being carried out in is a well-defined cohort, this type of a case-control study is called a nested case-control study. Using an already established cohort increases the efficiency of the study.

5.3 CASE-CONTROL STUDIES

At the beginning of a case-control study, cases are identified and their exposure status is determined. Then, a control group of study subjects is sampled from the entire source population that gave rise to the cases. Because the control group is used to estimate the distribution of exposure in the source population, the basic requirement of control selection is that the controls must be sampled independently of their exposure status. Indeed, if the distribution of the exposure in the control group is equal to the distribution of the exposure in the source population, incidence rate ratios can be calculated from a case-control study. If this criterion is not met, one can still calculate an **exposure odds ratio** from a case-control study. Unfortunately, the incidence rate ratio estimates are not as precise as the estimates from a cohort study. **Precision** could be increased by selecting more controls per case.

Although a case-control study has a simple definition, it is possible to come across a lot of studies in the medical and orthodontic literatures that are named case-control studies but do not meet the definition of a case-control study. Although one should not be too concerned about a title as long as the conclusions are valid, inappropriate selection of controls and/or cases leads to wrong findings and conclusions. For instance, patients treated by a single orthodontist in his/her clinical practice may be included as the cases in a case-control study. In many instances, historical controls are used for comparison. As mentioned above, the controls should be coming from the source population for the cases. Most of the time, it is very difficult to identify that population. When the controls do not come from the same population that the cases come from, bias occurs in the selection of controls.

There are various sources for controls. If cases are representative of all the cases that may occur in the population, this type of study is named a population-based case-control study. Ideally, controls should be randomly sampled from this population. Random selection of controls from the population is not always possible or feasible. Then, other sources may be used for selection of the controls.

When the whole population cannot be identified, controls may be selected from a variety of sources. Neighborhood controls are selected from the neighborhood of the case. Being a neighbor does not necessarily mean that this control is in the source population for cases. This fact should be taken into account before using neighbors as controls in a study. Another approach is random digit dialing. This random selection of phone numbers allows investigators to reach people with unlisted phones, but individuals without phones do not get a chance to be included in the sample as controls. Also, some researchers choose to use friend controls. There are certain problems with the use of friend controls as well. Cases may be friends with controls because of an activity that they participate in and that activity may be related to the exposure. Furthermore, choice of controls is decided by the cases, because the cases need to give a list of friends' names to the investigator. Although the investigator may identify the controls from this list by random selection, the involvement of the cases in this process adds bias to the selection of controls. Another problem with using friends as controls is that friendship groups are not mutually exclusive, meaning that popular individuals would be overrepresented in the control group.

If a case-control study is being conducted in a clinic, controls should be selected among the patients in that clinic or hospital that are not cases. These controls are **hospital controls.** Some investigators use disease registries and define their controls as patients with other diseases. Obviously, these other diseases should not be related to the exposure under study. In addition, in studies that cases are dead, dead controls may be used. Using dead controls in other instances may lead to various types of biases, because they are not representative of the source population for living cases. If information other than what is available on the death certificate is needed, the comparability of the groups could be jeopardized.

It is claimed the data collected from cases and controls should be of comparable accuracy, so that any misclassification that occurs would be nondifferential and would bias the estimates toward the null value. Nondifferential misclassification of the exposure does not always mean that the bias will be toward the null, however. One may say that the comparability of the information is useful when measurement error is very little.

It is true that case-control studies are more susceptible to bias than the cohort studies. There are times, however, case-control studies are more feasible. It is more practical to carry out case-control studies for rare diseases, for example. As long as valid epidemiologic principles are adhered to, valuable conclusions can be reached from case-control studies. As a result of many poorly conducted case-control studies, this type of study design developed an unfavorable reputation.

5.4 CROSS-SECTIONAL STUDIES

In cross-sectional studies, also called "**prevalence** studies", exposure and outcome status is determined at the same time in a representative sample of the **target population** to describe the population at that point in time. Ideally, these studies should be carried out for descriptive information. Still, there are many cross sectional studies with etiologic objectives. Before any conclusions are drawn about etiology of an outcome from cross sectional studies their limitations should be considered.

Because the sample is defined at one point in time, subjects who have the outcome for the longest time are overrepresented. The exposure measurement is only available for that point in time when the subjects' outcome status is identified. There may not be a causal connection between the current exposure and the outcome. This problem could be reduced if the exposures studied do not change in time.

5.5 ECOLOGIC STUDIES

In ecologic studies, aggregate measurements are made. In other words, variables are measured for a group of people; thus, individual measurements are not available. Instead, there are averages for a group of individuals. Consequently, the degree of exposure-outcome association does not reflect individual level associations. Use of **proxy measures** distort these associations further. Besides, data are unavailable to control for **confounding** in the analysis. As a result, findings may not be valid. Any results of an ecologic study that suggests an association between an exposure and outcome should be further investigated.

In all the study designs mentioned above, the goal is to estimate the parameter that is the object of measurement with as little error as possible. Principles of study design emerge from consideration of approaches to reducing error. Sources of error in estimation may be classified as random or systematic. Rothman and Greenland (1998) discuss precision and validity as they relate to random and **systematic error**, respectively.

6. PRECISION AND VALIDITY

6.1 PRECISION

Lack of **random error** is **precision**. Random error is introduced into a study during **sampling** and variable measurement; thus, increasing the sample size and efficiency of the study would reduce random error.

Indeed, estimates become more precise as the number of the study subjects increases. There are formulas for **sample size determination** that take into consideration the study design, study population, and the power desired to calculate the ideal sample size for a particular study. The value of the information acquired from the study with a certain sample size is not factored into these calculations, however. As more subjects are included in a study, the cost increases. Reduction in random error should be sufficient to justify the greater cost.

In addition to the sampling considerations, there are other aspects of a study design that affect precision. A study may be more efficient if one considers the distribution of the study variables among the subjects, such as sufficient number of cases for valid conclusions. Otherwise, increasing the sample size could be merely inflating the number of controls, whereas there may be very few cases. Modification of the composition of such a sample may increase efficiency and decrease random error.

6.2 VALIDITY

After reducing random error, the investigator has to make sure systematic error is minimized as well for the study to be valid and reliable. **Validity** is lack of systematic error. There are two kinds of validity. "**Internal validity**" refers to the validity of the study conclusions for the population that study subjects are sampled from. "**External validity**" refers to the validity of the study conclusions when they are extrapolated beyond the population that study subjects are sampled from.

Any bias that affects the true estimation of an epidemiologic measure reduces validity. Rothman and Greenland (1998) discuss **selection bias, information bias**, and **confounding** as the three biases that should be minimized for valid estimates. The distinction between these three biases is not always very straightforward. For example, confounding factors may be associated with selection bias.

6.2.1. **Selection Bias**

Selection bias means that the **association** observed in the study participants is systematically different than the association that would be observed in all the individuals eligible for the study. Reasons why people may or may not want to participate in a study, as well as the selection procedures, lead to selection bias.

A hypothetical example would be that children with **cleft palate** go to the dentist at an earlier age and more often than children without cleft palate; therefore, cleft palate children may be diagnosed as having caries more frequently. This fact may lead to an **apparent association** between cleft palate and caries. Also, including only people who have a job in an investigation would lead to a selection bias called the "**healthy worker effect**". In general, working individuals tend to be healthier than those who do not.

During the design stage of the study, any confounder that may be associated with selection bias should be identified. Complete follow-up and high **response rates** help reduce selection bias, but may not be sufficient by themselves. It is possible to have complete follow-up and high response rates and not be able to eliminate the selection bias that is inherent in the study.

6.2.2. Confounding

The effect of the exposure on the outcome becomes distorted because the effect of an extraneous **factor** is intertwined with the effect of exposure being studied. Confounding may bias results toward the null or it may overestimate the effect of exposure. Controlling for confounding reduces bias.

In order to be able to control for confounding, one has to identify possible confounders of the relationship under study. A factor should meet the following criteria to be a confounder:

1. There must be a causal relationship between the confounder and the outcome under study.
2. The exposure of interest should be associated with the confounder.
3. Exposure and/or the outcome must not affect the confounder. For instance, the confounder should not be in the causal pathway between the exposure and outcome (Figure 10-1).

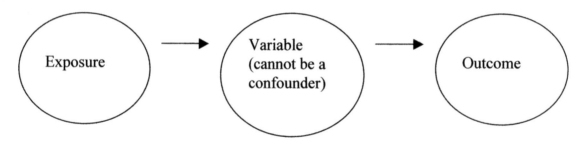

Figure 10-1

Once a **risk factor** meets the above criteria, it can be controlled for in the analysis. For instance, in a hypothetical prospective cohort study of the effect of twin block therapy on Class II correction, the crude (without controlling for any confounders) relative risk is 4 (Table 10-2), meaning that the treatment group who had the twin block therapy was 4 times more likely to achieve a Class II correction than the control group that received no therapy.

Table 10-2. Effect of Twin Block treatment on Class II correction

Outcome	Type of treatment	
	Twin Block	No Twin Block
Class II correction	400	100
No Class II correction	400	700

$$\text{Relative risk} = \frac{(400/800)}{(100/800)} = 4$$

The investigators may want to control for gender and observe if the same association still exists. The adjusted relative risks for males and females are both 2 (Tables 10-3 and 10-4). Although the magnitude of the relationship is the same for males and females, it is different than the crude relative risk. If there was no confounding, the adjusted relative risks should have been the same as the crude relative risk. One may conclude that gender is a confounder in this case.

Table 10-3: Effect of Twin Block treatment on Class II correction in females

Outcome	Type of treatment	
	Twin Block	No Twin Block
Class II correction	400	200
No Class II correction	400	600

$$\text{Relative risk} = \frac{(400/800)}{(200/800)} = 2$$

Table 10-4: Effect of Twin Block treatment on Class II correction in males

Outcome	Type of treatment	
	Twin Block	No Twin Block
Class II correction	300	150
No Class II correction	500	650

$$\text{Relative risk} = \frac{(300/800)}{(150/800)} = 2$$

On the other hand, if the adjusted relative risks for males and females were 3 and 2 respectively (Tables 10-5 and 10-6), it indicates confounding as well as **effect modification**. The effect of twin block therapy differs for the two categories of gender. If a factor is a confounder, it is controlled for in the analysis. Effect modification, however, is a biological phenomenon and must be reported as it is.

Table 10-5: Effect of Twin Block treatment on Class II correction in males

Outcome	Type of treatment	
	Twin Block	No Twin Block
Class II correction	300	100
No Class II correction	500	700

$$\text{Relative risk} = \frac{(300/800)}{(100/800)} = 3$$

Table 10-6: Effect of Twin Block treatment on Class II correction in females

Outcome	Type of treatment	
	Twin Block	No Twin Block
Class II correction	200	100
No Class II correction	600	700

$$\text{Relative risk} = \frac{(200/800)}{(100/800)} = 2$$

6.2.3. Information Bias

Information bias is misclassification that occurs as a result of incorrect measurement of exposure and/or outcome. Misclassification could be differential or nondifferential. In differential misclassification, subjects are misclassified on either the exposure or outcome. Misclassification of exposure changes across the different categories of outcome, or the misclassification of the outcome changes across the different categories of exposure. Differential misclassification can bias the results toward the null or away from the null. The second kind of information bias is nondifferential misclassification. Here, misclassification of a variable does not depend on the values of other variables. Nondifferential information bias usually biases the results toward the null. If the misclassification error is too high, however, bias may exceed the null value and go in the other direction.

Possible sources of information bias are faulty diagnostic procedures, incorrect data sources, and indices that do not measure what they intend to measure. An example of an incorrect data source as a result of recall bias would be that mothers of cleft palate babies are more likely to recall any exposure during their pregnancies than mothers of healthy babies. As a result of this differential recall, an apparent association may be observed between a specific exposure and cleft palate occurrence.

The relevance of the epidemiological principles and study designs to research is evident in an example the late Stephen Jay Gould (1996) gave in his book "Mismeasure of Man". He discusses the research Samuel George Morton conducted to establish ranking of races by measuring the cranial cavity of the human skull. Unfortunately, Morton's personal biases distort the results of the study and lead to false conclusions. Gould refers to Morton's work as "…a patchwork of fudging and finagling in the clear interest of a priori convictions." Also, Gould mentions that Morton published his data and that he made mistakes inadvertently as a victim of his prejudices. For instance, he was so sure that the cranial size reflected mental ability that he never considered alternate hypotheses. Thus, an objective attitude is necessary along with the adherence to the epidemiological principles and study designs.

All the methods of clinical epidemiology were developed to find answers to clinically relevant questions. The application of research results into clinical practice relies on the judgment of the experienced clinicians so that a treatment is not applied to all patients regardless of the appropriateness of this treatment for the individual patient.

Collaboration between researchers and clinicians is necessary so that the clinicians can easily find and incorporate the best evidence into their treatment decisions. Otherwise, clinicians are left with clinical judgment that is comprised of uncontrolled clinical experience. For instance, new orthodontic treatment techniques and appliances are mostly developed empirically. Empirical evidence may mean that a certain treatment technique worked well in the hands of a few orthodontists. Neither its efficacy nor effectiveness is rigorously tested prior to its clinical usage. In turn, researchers could also benefit from the clinicians' input and concerns about what kind of outcome measures need to be developed from the point of the clinician as well as the patient. No one should forget that orthodontics is both an "art" and a "science". To ignore either is a disservice to patients.

7. SUGGESTED READINGS

Introduction

Feinstein AR. Clinical Judgment. Huntington, NewYork: Robert E. Krieger Publishing Company, 1967.

Fletcher HR, Fletcher SW, Wagner EH. Clinical Epidemiology: The Essentials. Baltimore, Maryland: Williams & Wilkins, 1996.

Last JM. A Dictionary of Epidemiology. New York: Oxford University Press, 2001.

Causal Inference and Multifactorial Etiology

Holland JH. Hidden Order: How Adaptation Builds Complexity. Persus Books Group, 1995.

Rothman KJ, Greenland S. Causation and Causal Inference. In: Rothman KJ, Greenland S, editors. Modern Epidemiology. Lippincott-Raven Publishers, 1998; pp 7-28.

Sackett DL, Haynes RB, Guyatt GH, Tugwell P. Clinical Epidemiology: A Basic Science for Clinical Medicine. Little, Brown and Company, 1991.

Weiss NS. Clinical Epidemiology: The Study of the Outcome of Illness. Oxford: Oxford University Press, 1996.

Diagnosis

Bader J, Ismail A. A Primer on Outcomes in Dentistry. J Public Health Dent 1999; 59(3):131-135.

Bennett E, Michaels C, Very D, O'Brien K, Weyant RJ, Vig KWL. Psychometric considerations in the assessment of orthodontic treatment expectations. In: Orthodontic treatment: outcome and effectiveness. Eds., Trotman CA, McNamara JA. Center of Human Growth and Development, University of Michigan, Ann Arbor, 1995.

Birkeland K, Boe OE, Wiath PJ. Orthodontic concern among 11-year-old children and their parents compared with orthodontic treatment need assessed by Index of Orthodontic Treatment Need. Am J Orthod Dentofac Orthop 1996;110:197-205.

Brook PH, Shaw WC. The development of an index of orthodontic treatment priority. Eur J Orthod 1989;11:309-20.

Burt BA. Evidence-Based Dentistry, Its Development and Use in Clinical Practice. NYSDJ 1999;:34-40.

Comer RJ, Piliavin JA. The Effects of Physical Deviance Upon Face to Face Interaction: the Other Side. J Pers Soc Psychol 1972;23:33-39.

Cons NC, Jenny J, Kohout FJ. DAI: The dental aesthetic index. Iowa City: College of Dentistry, University of Iowa, 1986.

Draker HL. Handicapping labio-lingual deviations: a proposed index for public health purposes. Am J Orthod Dentofac Orthop 1960;46:295-305

Farina A, Allen JG, Saul BB. The Role of the Stigmatized Person in Affecting Social Relationships. J Pers 1968;36:169-182.

Feinstein AR. The Clinician as Scientist. In: Vig PS, Ribbens KA, editors. Science and Clinical Judgment in Orthodontics, Monograph 19, Craniofacial Growth Series. Center for Human Growth and Development, The University of Michigan, 1986:1-14.

Goffman E. Stigma: Notes on the Management of Spoiled Identity. Prentice Hall, Englewood Cliffs, NJ, 1963:1-147.

Gordis L. Assessing the Validity and Reliability of Diagnostic and Screening Tests. In: Gordis L, editor. Epidemiology. W.B. Saunders Company, 1996:58-76.

Grainger RM. Orthodontic treatment priority index. PHS Publication no.1000, Series 2, No 25, Washington: US Government Printing Office, 1967.

Hunt RJ, Slade GD, Strauss RP. Differences between racial groups in the impact of oral disorders among older adults in North Carolina. J Public Health Dent 1995;55(4):205-9.

Miotti FA. Orthodontics within the public health system. In: Orthodontic treatment: outcome and defectiveness. Eds., Trotman CA, McNamara JA. Center for Human Growth and Development, University of Michigan, Ann Arbor, 1995.

Sackett DL, Haynes RB, Guyatt GH, Tugwell P. Clinical Epidemiology: A Basic Science for Clinical Medicine. Little, Brown and Company, 1991.

Salzmann JA. Handicapping malocclusion assessment to establish treatment priority. Am J Orthod 1968;54:749-65.

Summers CJ. The occlusal index: A system for identifying and scoring occlusal disorders. Am J Orthod 1971;59:552-67.

Vig PS, Vig KD. Decision Analysis to Optimize the Outcomes for Class II Division 1 Orthodontic Treatment. Sem Orthod 1995; 3 (1):139-148.

Vig KWL, Weyant R, O'Brien K, Bennett E. Developing Outcome Measures in Orthodontics that Reflect Patient and Provider Values. Semin Orthod 1999;5:85-95.

Treatment Decision

Bader J, Ismail A, Clarkson J. Evidence-based dentistry and the dental research community. J Dent Res 1999;78(9):1480-1483.

Harrison JE, Deborah A, Lennon MA. An analysis of papers published in the British and European Journal of Orthodontics. Br J Orthod 1996;23:203-209.

Hume D. A Treatise of Human Nature. Oxford University Press, 1888; 2nd ed, 1978.

Sackett DL, Haynes RB, Guyatt GH, Tugwell P. Clinical Epidemiology: A Basic Science for Clinical Medicine. Little, Brown and Company, 1991.

Study Designs

Gordis L. Assessing the Efficacy of Preventive and Therapeutic Measures: Randomized Trials. In: Gordis L, editor. Epidemiology. W.B. Saunders Company, 1996:pp 89-97.

Gordis L. Randomized Trials: Some Further Issues. In: Gordis L, editor. Epidemiology. W.B. Saunders Company, 1996:pp 98-113.

Rothman KJ, Greenland S. Types of Epidemiologic Studies. In: Rothman KJ, Greenland S, editors. Modern Epidemiology. Lippincott-Raven Publishers, 1998; pp 67-78.

Rothman KJ, Greenland S. Case-Control Studies. In: Rothman KJ, Greenland S, editors. Modern Epidemiology. Lippincott-Raven Publishers, 1998; pp 93-114.

Precision and Validity

Gould SJ. In: The Mismeasure of Man. American Polygeny and Craniometry Before Darwin. New York: W. W. Norton and Company, 1981:pp 30-72.

Kleinbaum DG, Kupper LL, Morgestern H. Key Issues in Epidemiologic Research: An Overview. In: Kleinbaum DG, Kupper LL, Morgestern H, editors. Epidemiologic Research: Principles and Quantitative Methods. New York: Van Nostrand Reinhold, 1982: pp 1-13.

Riolo ML, Moyers RE and TenHave TR. Imprecision and bias in orthodontic treatment. Am J Orthod 1988;93:138-142.

Rothman KJ, Greenland S. Precision and Validity. In: Rothman KJ, Greenland S, editors. Modern Epidemiology. Lippincott-Raven Publishers, 1998; pp 115-134.

Rothman KJ, Greenland S. Accuracy Considerations in Study Designs. In: Rothman KJ, Greenland S, editors. Modern Epidemiology. Lippincott-Raven Publishers, 1998; pp 115-145.

Section III
Examination and Diagnosis

This section includes analyses of the musculature and skeleton of the face, the dentition, and the dental occlusion. Other topics include the orthodontic examination, diagnosis, and treatment planning.

Chapters:

CHAPTER 11

Orthodontic Examination and Diagnosis

G. Frans Currier

1. INTRODUCTION

The basis of planning and delineating orthodontic treatment is found in a sound database of information. It needs to be consistent, predictable, and transferable. However, the first step in the process is to determine if there is a problem in the particular case. When one initially screens, or evaluates, a patient, there are three steps one needs to consider: Is there a problem orthodontically? Do I treat the patient now or wait? Do I need to remove teeth to correct the problem? Most students have cases already selected for them. That is not true in practice. With more experience, this initial evaluation becomes more clear and exacting. Initially, this is a large problem because the expertise of the doctor might not be as broadbased as one would see with more experience and with a greater understanding of various treatment

outcomes, including less-than-acceptable or excellent results in certain types of cases. What is normal at one stage is not normal at another. There are definitive extraction cases and definitive nonextraction cases. There is a broad band in between. The later one treats in the development of the skeleton, dentition, occlusion and in **adolescence**, the more often the need for extractions. In the adult, extraction considerations are different than with the adolescent. Non-extractions, or **asymmetrical** patterns, predominate in the adult, while arch symmetry is the mainstay with younger patients.

Orthodontic databases include:

1.) A thorough history.
2.) A detailed clinical examination with various evaluations or measurements.
3.) A set of excellent study models with full facial depth extensions, with or without mounting on an articulator.
4.) Panoramic/cephalometric radiographs with appropriate, selected bitewing and/or periapical radiographs.
5.) Photographs, both extraoral to supplement the cephalometric evaluation and intraoral to compare and contrast to the study models. The photographs more clearly present the expression of the soft tissues.

All radiographs are prescriptive. There are no routine radiographs. Lateral cephalometric films without tracing analysis offer deficient documentation or plans. Study models need excellent apical, or root, extensions to determine torque or axial inclination needs of the patient. Occlusal surface study models offer limited diagnostic value.

The evaluation of the patient includes the face in addition to the dentition and occlusion. One treats to the face. Evaluation is needed both in the frontal and lateral views. Understanding what is normal at different stages of development, besides the variability seen in different racial groups and between males and females, makes this much more difficult than when one just considers the analysis of a generic case. Different ages with different genders and with different ethnic or racial groups give different plans of action, or observation. To treat to one view of dentofacial excellence is limiting. There are usually multiple treatment plans from the same database.

With each evaluation there needs to be an orientation to the three tissue groups (teeth, bones, and muscles) and the three planes of space (transverse, sagittal, and vertical). These tissues and planes need evaluation in the fourth dimension, which is time. Each person needs to be evaluated such that each component of the skeletal-dental-muscular system is analyzed. For example, all openbite malocclusions will have a neuromuscular component. Malocclusions should have neuromuscular components with A-P, or anteroposterior, slides in centric or movements over one millimeter in the front to back direction from maximum **intercuspation**, or **centric occlusion**. Certain Class II or Class III malocclusions have a skeletal basis to the problem; some have problems in the maxilla (Asian Class III deficient), some the mandible (Black Class III excess), and some both. However, a variety are orthognathic, i.e., balanced facial pattern in the sagittal, or A-P, plane.

The soft tissue drape of the facial profile usually does not mirror the underlying bone, or hard tissue, profile. In fact, there can be a favorable or unfavorable soft tissue compensation for the underlying facial skeleton. One might assume that Class I malocclusions might have the same facial patterns. That is not true. One variable of the face, frontally or in profile, can express itself vastly differently than the pattern of malocclusion. Angle's system is a dental classification of malocclusion, not a skeletal or neuromuscular one. A factor analysis of the three tissues needs to be considered for each patient.

The other important orientation is relative to the three planes of space. As mentioned previously, they are the transverse, sagittal, and vertical planes, and in that order. The sequence is the pattern of maturation of the skeleton in the dentofacial complex. One needs to evaluate the face in the three dimensions as well as the dentition and occlusion. They do not mirror each other.

The **transverse plane** matures the earliest. It is, therefore, the first plane of space to be treated as the child ages through **adolescence** into adulthood. Preschoolers are usually five years of age or younger, while early (6-8), middle (8-10), and late childhood (10-12) includes the grade school years. Early adolescence (12-14) includes junior high, while middle (14-16) and later (16-18) adolescence includes high school. The young adult period is from 18-22 years of age. In fact, most orthodontic treatment regimens now specifically address the transverse plane first and, if necessary, again prior to addressing the needs in the sagittal or vertical planes. The more expansion realized in the anterior portion of the buccal segments, the more favorable the effect (increase) on the **arch perimeter**.

The **sagittal plane** is the basis of Angle's classification of occlusion. The system is keyed to the position of the maxillary permanent first molar. A different orientation is usually developed over time for the clinician toward the buccal or lateral segments, away from the permanent first molars. This is especially true in the adolescent dentition (28 permanent teeth erupted) or in the correction of malocclusions with all permanent teeth. Prior to the eruption of the permanent first molars at six years of age, the distal surface, or terminal plane of the primary second molars, is used to classify the occlusion in the preschooler (five years of age or below). The absence of permanent first molars in adolescents or adults forces one to use the buccal segment orientation in classification. That is, to orient one along the side of the bite, or lateral aspect, of the occlusion from back to front. It is also more common than one might expect to have differences on one side as compared to the other. These left/right differences are heavily influenced genetically and express themselves as unilateral or **subdivision** malocclusions. These patterns present unique biomechanical interventions due to the **asymmetrical** nature of the problem.

The vertical pattern is the most complex plane to treat. It is the least understood in orthodontics. The face is particularly important here as we all start out as preschoolers with short face syndrome. This is a powerful non-extraction orientation. The face is separated into an anterior and posterior face. The anterior pattern can easily be evaluated from a profile view with three parts: superior above **Nasion**, or near the eyebrow (the neural face), the middle from the eyebrow to underneath the nose (in **cephalometrics**, the upper face), and the lower face (below the nose to the bottom of the chin). In preschoolers, the neural face is large, and the rest of the face is short. Children at five years of age that have vertical proportions of the face that one would see at 10 years of age have an adverse facial pattern. The same is true for a 10 year old who has the profile or proportion of a 15 year old. This, too, is unfavorable. An adult long face pattern is easier to identify early than one that is with a future short vertical face.

Short face syndrome adolescents do not have the same pattern as seen with the preschoolers. The anterior eyebrow to the base of the chin distance is shorter than normal, while the dimension below the nose is much smaller. However, even with this, the nose is actually larger vertically than normal. Short-face individuals are predominately non-extraction orthodontic cases. The longer face patients usually manifest themselves later. However, if seen early, it is an unfavorable sign that the pattern will only develop more in that specific direction. **Long-face** individuals have a long eyebrow-to-chin distance, a normal vertical nose height, but a long vertical distance inferior to the nose to the bottom-of-chin distance. The thickness of the soft tissue profile is larger for the long face and thinner in the short face. This seems like a method of natural compensation for the discrepancy.

The posterior portion of the vertical face lies inferior to the ears, not at the back of the head. It is determined from the junction of the mandible at the **cranial base** down to the gonial, or posterior, angle of the mandible. This is short in preschoolers but usually becomes longer or larger vertically with age for the anterior short face patterns and remains relatively shorter in anterior long faces with time. There is almost always an inverse correlation in the adolescent or the adult as compared to the child. This increase in the posterior vertical face height is related to the S curve of change (**Scammon's general or somatic curve**) that is seen with the airway or the neuromuscular system.

The understanding of various rates of dentofacial growth now become more apparent, especially when one attempts to diagnose cases during growth (increase in size) and development (increase in complexity).

The four **Scammon curves** are 1.) lymphoidal (peaks in middle childhood at eight to 10 years of age and then decreases as seen with tonsils and adenoids, 2.) neural (highest growth velocity early as cranium, eyes, and tongue), 3.) gonadal or genital (highest growth later as testes/penis, breasts, nose and chin), and 4.) general or somatic (sigmoidal or S curve, as skeletal, neuromuscular component, airway, and dentitions).

In evaluating a patient relative to the need for orthodontic care, there needs to be awareness of a patient's five ages: chronologic, dental, skeletal (bone or physiologic), mental, and emotional. The **chronologic age** is taken from birth, rather than conception, and it is used in years and months, i.e., CA=4-3, or 9-7, or 14-0. This age does not correlate well to the other ages. Dental age is a radiographic evaluation of the teeth that evaluates crown and root development for each tooth. Understanding the timing and usual sequence for the dentitions is essential in diagnosis. Dental age does not correlate well to chronologic age, especially under 10 years of age. The sequence of tooth growth and development needs to be recalled: initiation/proliferation, morphodifferentiation/histodifferentiation (shape before cellular changes), apposition, mineralization (calcification is the pathologic model of mineralization as seen with pulp stones, condensing osteitis, diminished pulp/chambers, salivary duct sialoliths, kidney stones, etc.) eruption (**ectopic eruption**, **ankylosis**, impactions, etc.), attrition, and in cases of primary teeth, resorption and exfoliation. The anomalies of the teeth predominate in Class I or end-to-end malocclusions.

Dental age should not be confused with the stage of the dentition: primary, transitional, young permanent (only permanent teeth present clinically but not all **succedaneous** teeth), adolescent (all 28 permanent teeth clinically present), and adult dentitions (permanent dentition after **adolescence** with or without third molars erupted). The primary dentition is usually from six months to six years ($\pm$ 1 year) while the **transitional dentition** is from six years to 12 years ($\pm$ 2 years). The adolescent dentition involves all 28 permanent teeth clinically. Teeth erupt most at night, and it usually takes four to six months after tissue emergence to erupt into occlusion.

Another age that is determined radiographically is the bone or skeletal age. It is sometimes also referred to as physiologic age. The left hand is used unless the child is under six years of age when both hands are used. The feet can be used, but it is easier for the hands because of accessibility. The left hand is considered the non-working hand, even with approximately 10-15% of the population left-handed. There are numerous heads and shafts of the long bones of the hand that help in the analysis, as well as the eight bones of the hand (carpals). There is a sequential change of the head from disc shape to cap shape to fusion with the shafts of metacarpals. The medial ulnar sesamoid bone in the inside portion of the thumb usually ossifies six to 12 months prior to maximum facial growth. There are boy and girl standards and a rather consistent order in the mineralization pattern. The analysis is done with the knowledge that the variability is $\pm$ one year. Height accounts for approximately 50% of bone growth as a predictive factor and should be measured in all orthodontic patients. It is the centile reading that is important. Children above the 95th and below the 5th centile need **bone age** determination. Is the patient a late or early maturer? Earlier maturers grow shorter in the long run, after growth completion. Late maturing girls happen to coincide more closely with male peak velocity. However, late maturing boys present unique self-image problems that do not resolve themselves well unless properly addressed.

Weight correlates poorly to skeletal age, except obese children usually have advanced skeletal age. The concern with weight is specifically related to Caucasian girls and **anorexia** or **bulimia**. If the skeletal age is advanced, limitations are placed in maxillary orthopedics. If delayed, the concern is related to mandibular prognathia.

Mental age can usually be easily determined by asking the grade in school. Most school systems in the United States follow the **Dewey system**, which has a strong social component as well as academic achievement orientation. Independent of **chronologic age**, predictable cooperative behavior is usually seen more clearly while the child is in the middle of the second grade. There is a shift cognitively that occurs from a more egocentric pattern to one where the child can reverse actions, can understand series of actions, and can apply the concepts of whole versus the part. This period is approximately in the second to seventh grades. A removable **orthodontic appliance** under the age of seven years is fraught with problems. The problems in adolescent behavior are more about the change in cognitive thinking centered about abstract thought, deductive thinking, and all possible ways for solution. The best period of overall cooperative behavior that is predictable is from seven to eight years to 11 to 12 years of age for both boys and girls.

Emotional age is more difficult to accurately ascertain. However, it is part of the regular grade school system. This may be related to males and the Y chromosome. There is **dyslexia**, hyperactivity, and short attention span associated with it. Increased use of psychological altering drugs rather than drugs used to control bacterial infection seems to be a new, complicating factor in orthodontic compliance. For boys, early entry into school may not be recommended and that a delay in school admission might be better than holding back after he has started in school.

There are a few initial helpful hints that can be observed that will help determine a need for an orthodontic database in growing individuals:

1.) Mis-matched dento-skeletal parameters.
2.) Retrusive lips, especially with a large chin, in the presence of malocclusion.
3.) Concave profile (chin ahead of forehead-maxillary line) or anterior divergence (anterior chin position on a facial plane that is near 90 degrees relative to Frankfort horizontal).
4.) Anomalies of the teeth, especially number problems such as supernumeraries or congenital absence, and problems in eruption such as ectopic position, **ankylosis**, impaction, and **transposition**.
5.) Anterior and/or posterior crossbites.
6.) Anterior protrusion or openbites after eight to nine years of age.
7.) Anterior midline problems without crossbites after seven to eight years of age.
8.) Moderate to severe arch perimeter crowding, either clinical or predicted, after eight to nine years of age, usually seen in the mandibular arch.

With this background orientation to diagnosis, a more detailed analysis of the orthodontic database should be completed prior to a follow-up discussion in the identification of problems or the variation from the normal range and a greater understanding of the specifics in diagnosis.

2. THE HISTORY

It is important for the clinician to identify the main concern, or chief complaint, that is presented. This aspect of the history is usually best described through a fill-in-the-blank orientation. What the doctor sees and what the patient wants many times do not initially match. There can also be two views, one from the patient and one from the parent. They are not always the same. With adults, the main concerns need to be identified and discussed with patient and spouse or significant other. It is necessary for the chief complaint to be addressed in the treatment plan. It might be the primary or secondary or tertiary factor, but it must be incorporated in the plan. If one fails to address this issue, successful treatment is qualitatively limited.

The personal family background is important, because orthodontic problems have a strong genetic basis. Anterior parts of the dentition and the occlusion have greater effects from such environmental variables as habits, crowding, trauma, etc., while the posterior regions are more resistant. Information relative to whether other members of the family have had orthodontic treatment, and if teeth were removed, are important in planning orthodontic therapy for the patient. The best method to determine the familial pattern is to see the older siblings. It is important to make sure, however, that the children have the same biological parents. Usually the variation in the dentofacial complex is less severe than what one sees with the parents.

Parents can predict their child's behavior rather well. Therefore, it is important to ask questions about their compliance, or cooperation. "I don't know" or fair-to-poor prediction needs closer examination. If the patient does not wish orthodontic care, even if the parents want it for the child, orthodontic intervention should be delayed until the child or adolescent is ready. If the adult patient wants orthodontic care, but the spouse does not concur, resolution of this difference is essential before initiating treatment.

The triad of walking, talking, and toilet training seen at two to three years of age is the classic landmark between inpatient dental services under general anesthesia and outpatient services in the dental office. Menarche in the U.S. averages about 12 to 12 and a half years of age with maximum facial growth approximately six to 12 months before it. The growth period for girls is usually two years earlier than for boys. Growth for girls usually stops more quickly after maximum growth rate than that seen with boys. Premature birth, or systemic problems that raise the body temperature, can create **hypoplasia** or hypocalcification problems of the teeth that are developing at the time of the insult. The pattern of attack will affect multiple teeth as compared to the physical trauma one sees to the anterior teeth. The common pattern of primary incisor trauma is intrusive, with displacement toward the lingually placed succedaneous incisor that will be marked or injured on the facial surface. Severe trauma can cause dilacerations of the crown or root of the permanent incisor.

Oral habits can be identified not only clinically, but also through the history. Two-finger or single-finger habits as well as thumb habits should be noted. The general pattern of non-nutritive sucking is very common with over 50% frequency at birth, and it decreases naturally over time to less than 10% for seven to eight year old children. The habit is usually extinguished by competitive, favorable reinforcements and shaping the behavior from diurnal (daytime) to nocturnal (nighttime). Relapse in the habit can occur in middle childhood if the child moves or is otherwise traumatized psychologically and regresses to an earlier, more secure stage. Oral habits are most related to anterior openbite or posterior quadrant crossbite malocclusions. The triad of the habit, which is a variation of an applied biomechanical force system, is frequency, duration, and intensity. Two of these factors are time related. Therefore, oral habits present different patterns of malocclusions, but they usually manifest themselves on the side of the persistent digit habit if there is one. There are three major speech problems: speech articulation distortion, dyslexia, and stuttering. Mature articulation of speech is seen around the age of eight years. If an openbite malocclusion exists, speech articulation can be affected adversely with distorted "s", "th", and "z" sounds. Not all openbite malocclusions have associated speech articulation problems. Correction of openbite malocclusions does not necessarily correct the speech articulation distortion. Speech therapy needs to be added to a plan of action. The openbite malocclusion that is not related to an obvious extraoral habit is more complex. There are the neuromuscular deficiencies, as seen with cerebral palsy or muscular dystrophy. With these children, the tongue with its active, frequent, and powerful thrusting overwhelms the buccal musculature that has a more passive, continuous, and lighter force system. The cheeks are not strong enough, and the tongue moves the dentition outward.

Tongue thrusting is usually considered compensatory to oral habits and openbite malocclusions in childhood. Openbite malocclusions that are related to habits and are seen up to eight years of age are usually Class I problems. In the adolescent population, the problem is different and demonstrates more a skeletal Class II or Class III problem.

Tonsils and/or adenoids are not commonly removed in the present day. They do contribute to variations in dentofacial growth and development if persistently large and debilitating enough to create open-mouth breathing patterns. If the airway is severely restricted and/or altered with adverse downward and backward positions of the mandible that are consistent over time, then evaluation for their removal should be considered. This becomes a greater concern for posterior divergent faces with high mandibular plane angles.

A detailed model of a history form with proper recall schedules is presented in Figure 11-1.

Specific areas of content should include the following:

PERSONAL

Patient's name, nickname, gender, date of birth, patient/parent occupation and employment.

MEDICAL

Patient's physician, address, and phone number, date of last medical exam, and condition being treated. List of medications, any allergies or any hospitalizations. All immunizations, any diseases/conditions including tonsillectomy/adenoidectomy. Family medical history, and milestones of development, i.e., sit up alone, walking, talking, toilet training, stopping bottle feeding, and voice change (boys)/first menstrual period (girls).

DENTAL

Patient's dentist, address, and phone number. Past injuries, use of mouth protectors for contact sports, any oral habits, i.e., lip biting/sucking, nail biting, finger/thumb/blanket sucking, tongue thrusting, cheek biting, teeth grinding/clenching, constant mouth breathing, and jaw click/pain/restricted opening, fluoridated water supply/toothpaste, frequency of brushing/flossing, and type of between-meal snacks.

SOCIAL/BEHAVIORAL

Reaction to past medical/dental care (very good, moderately good, moderately poor, very poor). How parent/patient will react to orthodontic care, description of patient as advanced in the learning process, progressing normally in the learning process, or slow learner, best description of patient (calm, moody, shy, active, spoiled, sickly, defiant, fearful, suspicious, talkative, friendly, healthy, temper tamptrums, high-strung, cooperative, and compulsive). Hobbies, special interests, pets at home and their names. List of other children in family with their gender and age.

ORTHODONTIC

Reason for seeking orthodontic care (needs to be fill-in-the-blank), anyone else in the family with a similar orthodontic condition, and/or who has received orthodontic care, type of care wished (minor correction, comprehensive treatment, consultation or recommendation only), and patient's anticipated reaction to orthodontic treatment (excellent, good, fair, poor, I don't know).

Figure 11-1: Patient Information Form.

3. CLINICAL EXAMINATION

The ideal clinical examination form is one that is a blank slate that the clinician completes from a patterned, rational protocol. However, that takes years to develop for the clinician. Therefore, a structured approach is the better initial plan. A detailed model of a clinical exam form is presented in Figures 11-2A and 11-2B.

Orthodontic Clinical Examination:

THE FACE

1.) What is the soft tissue angle of convexity (8° to 11° larger than hard tissue angle of convexity)?
2.) What is the facial divergence (2° to 3° larger than hard tissue facial divergence): posterior divergent, orthognathic (non-divergent), anterior divergent.
3.) What is the mandibular plane to Frankfort Horizontal, or FMA: low angle, average angle, high angle.
4.) Symmetrical/asymmetrical face.
5.) Pleasing smile: no teeth showing (low smile line), average, excessive gingiva (high smile line).
6.) Sizes of nose and chin: small, average, and large.
7.) Lip position: apart at rest, hyperactive mentalis, mouth breather, and short upper lip.
8.) Classification of occlusion expected from patient's profile: Class I or end-to-end, Class II division 1, Class II division 2, and Class III.

MAXILLARY AND MANDIBULAR ARCHES

1.) Arch form/symmetry: ovoid, square, tapered.
2.) Clinical anterior/posterior crowding/spacing. Consider curve of Spee (deep, average, or reverse) for mandibular arch.
3.) Extra or missing teeth: supernumerary, congenital absence, or extracted.
4.) Size/shape/texture of teeth: macrodont, microdont, hypocalcification, and/or hypoplasia that is localized or generalized (genetic vs. environmental cause).
5.) Disturbances in eruption: abnormal or unfavorable sequence, ectopically positioned, ankylosis, severe rotation, over-retained, impacted.
6.) Decalcification/caries/fistulous tract/abscess.
7.) Traumatized/fractured teeth.
8.) Adverse periodontal conditions, including marked frena or midline diastema (maxilla).
9.) Expected tooth size/arch perimeter deficiency/excess.

TRANSVERSE PLANE

1.) Maxillary/mandibular tooth midline.
2.) Posterior crossbite in retruded contact position: Yes/No. Bilateral with shift or without shift.
3.) Buccal or lingual version: Yes/No. Which teeth?

SAGITTAL PLANE

1.) Overjet in millimeters.
2.) Anterior crossbite in retruded contact position: Yes/No. Which teeth?
3.) Slide over 1mm from retruded contact position to maximum intercuspation: Yes/No. Which teeth?
4.) Primary/permanent, right/left, canine relationship: Class I, end-to-end, Class II, Class III.
5.) Primary second molar right/left relationship (no permanent first molars): mesial step, flush terminal plane, distal step, super mesial step.
6.) Permanent first molar right/left relationship: Class I, end-to-end, Class II, Class III.
7.) Subdivision malocclusion (unilateral): Yes/No. Left/Right, Class II/Class III.
8.) Pseudo Class II or Pseudo Class III malocclusion (shift of permanent first molar due to primary molar loss): Yes/No, Left/Right. Class II/Class III.

VERTICAL PLANE

1.) Overbite in percentage.
2.) Anterior/posterior bite depth: open (no contact of opposing teeth), normal, deep (50% or more overlap clinically), impinging (lower teeth touch palate).

HABITS

1.) Patient/parent mention of habits: Yes/No.
2.) Tonsils/adenoids present/removed.
3.) Clinically observed habits: Finger/thumb/blanket sucking. Lip sucking/biting, nail biting, teeth grinding/bruxism/clenching, tongue thrusting, constant mouth breathing, speech articulation distortion, TM joint clicking/crepitation/pain/limited movement.

Figure 11-2A: Name of patient, age in years and months, grade in school (if appropriate), date of examination.

Orthodontic Clinical Examination - Recall Patients:

1.) Changes in facial convexity, divergence, and smile.
2.) Maxillary/mandibular arches crowded/spaced current and prediction for future.
3.) Anterior/posterior crossbites in retruded contact position and/or maximum intercuspation: Yes/No coincident midlines. Which teeth?
4.) Openbite/oral habits/abnormal eruption.
5.) Functional disturbances: excessive wear, slide in centric, TM joint clicking/crepitation/pain/limited movement.
6.) Overbite/overjet.
7.) Canine/molar classification for right and left side that becomes buccal segment orientated with premolar eruption.
8.) Classification of occlusion/malocclusion and predicted future problems.

Figure 11-2B: Recall Patient's age in years/months, grade in school (if appropriate), date of examination.

If possible, it is best to see the patient walk into the examination room or clinical setting. Observation allows one to identify restrictions in gross and fine motor movements. In time, a more precise evaluation of height at different ages allows one to estimate height centiles, i.e., tall for age, short for age or about average for age. Height is a reasonable indicator for **skeletal age**, or facial bone development.

When the patient is seated, it is best that the patient sit upright in the chair, not lying back. The patient's hands need to be observed prior to the dentofacial examination. The hands develop at the same time that the face develops. Anomalies of the hands and fingers can show appropriate signs related to the head and face. The hands are placed in front of the patient with the doctor's hands as models. The hands are observed from both the dorsal and ventral sides. The pattern allows one to evaluate the patient's vision, hearing, and attention to a non-threatening behavior pattern. Oral habits can be observed with the appropriate finger/thumb being cleaner, more wrinkled, bent, and/or having shorter fingernails. Unusual scarring or trauma patterns of the arms or hands need further explanation to eliminate abuse concerns. The length of digits is important, as foreshortened or elongated digits are signs of genetic disturbances or medical problems.

The curved, smallest finger is a classic sign of a craniofacial problem. If the finger/thumb nail beds are bulging out, i.e., clubbing, there can be a problem with a chronic respiratory or cardiac condition, i.e., cystic fibrosis or congenital heart disease. When looking at the palms of the hands, a simian crease (a single crease rather than the common double crease) is found in only one percent of normal but over 50% of craniofacial anomaly patients. This examination of the hands should be completed in all patients, independent of chronologic age.

3.1 THE FACE

It is necessary for proper evaluation of the face that the head be positioned so that the Frankfort horizontal is parallel to the floor or ground. The ear needs to be exposed with the hair placed over the back part of the pinna. Some clinicians prefer natural head position, which is a head positioned so that the patients can see themselves frontally in a mirror. There are usually a few degrees of difference between the Frankfort horizontal position and the natural head position. However, any cranial base reference to the facial analysis leads to distorted and incorrect analysis of face position on the head.

A lateral view from the patient's right side allows evaluation of the profile in the sagittal and vertical planes. One needs to evaluate both the anterior and posterior vertical face heights. One cannot detect from the profile what the posterior height is without palpation. There are three positions that are possible from palpation with a tongue blade or patient mirror handle at the base of the lower jaw from anterior (**Menton**, anteriorly below the symphysis along the inferior border of the mandible toward the **gonial angle** in the posterior) into the occiput of the skull. One needs to use the left thumb on the posterior, or the outer inferior position of the skull, to help demonstrate the line from the blade or handle. If the blade or mirror handle intersects into the skull, which is higher than the thumbnail position, it is a high mandibular plane angle, or high angle (FMA). If the blade or mirror handle falls outside the skull, or below the thumbnail position, it is a low mandibular plane angle. If the blade or mirror is **tangent** to the skull border, or intersects into the thumbnail, it is normal or average. The adult usually has a low angle while the preschoolers will consistently have a high angle. If a child has a low angle, it will only get lower. This is a classic sign of a non-extraction protocol and is independent of Angle's classification of malocclusion. It is common for the mandibular plane angle to drop (more posterior than anterior) due to the S curve of change through growth and development of the airway (Scammon's general or visceral curve).

The observation of the anterior portion of the face is more complex. There are 3 areas of particular interest: 1.) the nose-lips-chin pattern, 2.) the position of the chin relative to nasal bridge-maxillary line, and 3.) the position of the chin referenced from facial plane to Frankfort horizontal. In other words, what are the esthetic lines, the convexity-straightness-concavity of the profile (**angle of convexity** over (+) five degrees, between 0 degrees and five degrees, and less than 0 degrees) and evaluation of the face as posterior divergent (**facial angle** below 85 degrees), anterior divergent (facial angle over 90 degrees), or balanced as orthognathic (facial angle between 85 degrees and 90 degrees). The vertical height of the anterior face has a profound effect on these parameters. There is another factor that makes the clinical evaluation of the face very difficult. One assumes that what one sees in the profile is the same exact pattern as the underlying hard tissue profile. Many times this is not true. The soft tissues over the nasal bridge (Nasion) are usually fairly consistent for males and females, independent of age. However, above the nasal bridge at the forehead, the male adolescent phenomenon of frontal bossing of the sinuses usually begins to occur so that the protuberance of the forehead at **glabella** becomes more common as seen with adult males. That is why it is usually observed that the eyes are recessed in adult males compared to adult females and adolescent boys and girls.

The thickness of the soft tissue glabella is the same for the males and females, independent of age. The nose and chin are not prominent in children. If they are, then they usually will be even longer or larger as they progress through **adolescence**. This can be manifested as lips that are behind the nose to chin line, which is called the esthetic line (E-line) or plane. If the lips are behind the line, the E-lines have a negative millimeter valence. If the lips are in the front of the nose-chin line, the E-lines have a positive valence. Children under eight years of age should have positive E-lines. If a child has lips behind the line, i.e., relatively retrusive lips, it is a good sign for a non-extraction protocol. Some practitioners use the line from the chin up to the outer part of the lips to intersect into the base or inferior border of the nose, with a middle position at the nose base, the most harmonious for the lips, chin, and nose as a unit. The growth of the nose and chin have not reached maximum velocity, and they are already prominent in the face. The lips follow tooth position with a complex response that is not a direct one-to-one ratio of lips to teeth. The upper lip is affected by both maxillary and mandibular tooth movements at a 3:2 ratio, with the lip change less than the tooth change. In fact, if the lips are thick, or redundant, lip position change is very small. If the lips are thinner, the changes are more pronounced. The lower lip position can affect closer to a one-to-one change with certain types of malocclusion. Thick lips, or marked protrusion, can distort the response. The thickness of the upper lip is greatest with adolescent males but decreases with age. It is normal for adolescent males to have a thicker upper lip. The thickness of the soft tissues over the chin can be very misleading. Often, the soft tissues compensate for bony deficiencies. Therefore, soft tissue prominence does not necessarily mean a bony prominence. One can have small bony and large soft tissue protuberances, others large bony and small soft tissue patterns, and still others that are combined large or small. It mostly depends upon familial tendency. It is species specific with Caucasian males but not with Black males. The average is (+) 2 mm to (+) 4 mm bony chin in adolescent Caucasian males from NB line (Nasion to B point) to **Pogonion** and 0 mm to (+) 2 mm in adolescent Caucasian females. In Blacks, the chin button is behind, or posterior, to this Nasion-B point line. Usually with children eight years of age, there is no bony chin in front of the hard tissue facial plane (Nasion-Pogonion line or plane). If there is any Pogonion in front of this plane, it is positive in valence and is a classic sign of a non-extraction protocol. If a child who is less than 10 years of age has a bony chin protuberance, it will become large during adolescence. This is most commonly seen in Caucasian males. The soft tissue convexity is greater than its hard tissue counterpart by eight degrees to 11 degrees, independent of age or malocclusion. The degree of difference slightly decreases as age increases and in going from Class III to Class I to Class II division 2 and to Class II division 1.

The patient's profile should be evaluated in a manner that will give an estimate of what the underlying malocclusion may hold. The majority of occlusions, normal or otherwise, should be Class I, independent of gender or race. Class II patterns vary markedly and are considered syndrome patterns. Class II division I malocclusions should most likely have convex, posterior divergent facial patterns if there is mandibular **retrognathia**, or convex non-divergent patterns with either a protrusive maxilla and orthognathic mandible, or a balanced maxillary/mandibular relationship. The Class II division 1 malocclusion is more common in Caucasians than in Blacks or Asians. The Class II division 2 malocclusions usually manifest themselves as convex, orthognathic profiles with stronger chin buttons and low mandibular plane angles. These are more similar to Class I skeletal deepbite malocclusions rather than posterior divergent, convex patterns usually seen in Class II division 1 patients. Class II division 2 malocclusions are seen in Caucasians, but are rare in Blacks and Asians. However, Class II malocclusions present a spectrum of patterns, and each case needs detailed analysis. Soft tissue facial angles are greater than hard tissue facial angles by an average three degrees.

The Class III profile has been so oriented toward mandibular prognathia that the failure has been to understand the more common maxillary deficiency problem. The Asian population commonly has maxillary retrognathia and a mandibular balanced pattern. Many Caucasians have maxillary retrognathia and a mandibular balanced pattern. Many Caucasians have maxillary hypoplasia with or without mandibular prognathia, while most Blacks have mandibular hyperplasia. Class III malocclusions are more common in Asians and Blacks than complete, or full step, Class II malocclusions that have five mm to six mm deviation sagittally. This is not true with Caucasians, who have more Class II patterns than Class III ones.

From the frontal view, it is important to evaluate the **smile line**. This is difficult for many adolescents, especially males. Many adolescent males have been conditioned over time not to smile. It is supposedly a sign of toughness not to smile, or they have been asked to wipe that smile off their face. This is an unfortunate, non-verbal cue. The frontal view of the face and smile does not give one the same perception as the lateral view of the face or smile. One should not view the smile from the lateral position. The upper lip lengthens with age, especially in males, and therefore the lower incisor smile is the predominant pattern in middle age adult males. The most frequent pattern shows the facial surfaces of the incisors in the smile while the uncommon pattern is to show less than half the incisor in the smile. The least common pattern is the high smile line. However, dentists are very oriented to this pattern due to the gingival response in esthetic dentistry. If the smile line presents excessive gingiva, evaluation of a short upper lip is needed. Currently, there is no method that is widely accepted to surgically lengthen the upper lip. This smile evaluation is essential in orthodontic treatment. Low smile lines with anterior deepbite malocclusions present problems, as maxillary incisor intrusive mechanics is limited; the problem needs to be addressed more in the lower arch. High smile lines with anterior openbite malocclusions are probably surgical cases. The smile dictates the pattern of anterior intrusive mechanics.

The breadth of the smile is important in the evaluation. Is the upper arch narrow? Can it be expanded? The dark spaces at the corners of the mouth are usually not esthetic. It is a sign of narrow arches.

Early in one's professional development, one is impressed by the symmetry of the smile or the arches. However, in time, the more experienced clinician becomes impressed by a more common pattern of asymmetry. Asymmetry is normal. The question is its degree. There is at least 0.5 mm to 1.0 mm difference in the condyles that allows slides in centric that are one mm or less to be considered as normal. If one takes frontal facial images and splices them to be left/left or right/right rather than left/right or right/left, the images will not match. A general pattern in the facial analysis should orient the clinician from normal, early short face syndrome to more balanced faces with asymmetries. We all start out like the character Charlie Brown. We have round heads and round faces. The mandible follows the general, or S curve of growth, while the maxilla more equally blends the neural and general curves. This vertical skeletal increase is very important to develop adult facial patterns. The soft tissue growth of the face is most noticeable sagittally with the growth of the nose and chin. Short face syndromes are classic non-extraction patterns. That is why almost all preschoolers have a non-extraction orientation. This pattern is important to understand. The sequence of early detection is that girls are easier to identify variations in than boys, because girls mature earlier. Long face patterns are easier to detect early than the short face patterns, as that pattern is normal at the earlier ages. Therefore, the sequence of identification from easiest to most difficult is long face girls, long face boys, short face girls, and lastly, short face boys.

3.2 THE ARCHES

The intraoral examination requires not only observation but also palpation, especially for unerupted teeth, specifically the permanent canines, by seven to nine years of age. The sequence of the exam includes both arches and then the three planes of space with the dentition in occlusion. The **arches** need to be identified relative to symmetry/asymmetry as well as shape or form, crowding/spacing, and evaluation for anomalies of the dentition. Most arches are usually symmetric. Rare, marked asymmetry cases present unique challenges with etiologic factors important in the treatment.

Arch forms are commonly labeled as ovoid/elliptical, tapered/V-shaped, or square/block. Most occlusions or malocclusions, independent of Angle's classification, have ovoid mandibular arches. The second most common mandibular pattern is the square arch. It is rare to see a V-shaped lower arch. In classic orthodontics, one treats to the lower arch, as it is the more difficult one to treat, i.e., the mandibular midline suture fuses at one year, therefore limited orthopedic treatment is available. The lower arch is the contained arch with a general pattern of facial root placement or torque for all the permanent teeth but to varying degrees, and **anchorage** is more difficult to use or maintain due to the absence of the palatal shelves of bone and the need for lateral molar root anchorage.

The most common maxillary arch form is also ovoid. The maxillary arch presents different patterns, depending upon the type of malocclusion. Class II division 1 and Class III patterns will many times present as V-shaped arches while the Class II division 2 pattern more commonly is square. The lower jaw that is allowed to slide forward from Class II division 1 to a Class I position can present itself with bilateral **posterior crossbite** with maxillary posterior constriction.

If there is a midline discrepancy of the arches, the problem is usually in the lower arch. Therefore, one must identify that the maxillary arch is coincident with the facial midline. Using the frenum attachment has limited value. If the midline discrepancy is in the maxilla, the orthodontic correction is more complex.

The arches should be divided not only left versus right, but also anterior versus posterior. In the adolescent dentition, the posterior section can be further divided into middle versus posterior. A common area for **anomalies of teeth** is the maxillary anterior segment, i.e., **mesiodens**. However, it is the maxillary permanent lateral incisor that is most variable in the spectrum of anomalies. The 20 primary teeth have their usual 20 succeeding permanent teeth, which are called succedaneous teeth. The permanent molars erupt between six and 21 years and are called **accessional teeth**.

The 12 permanent molars have a natural tendency to drift toward the midline; or, it is said that they have a mesial component of force. The permanent canines naturally erupt mesially in most cases. The primary teeth and the premolars do not have this marked natural tendency to drift mesially. The mandibular permanent incisors usually collapse lingually while the maxillary permanent incisors drift toward the midline. A high FMA (Frankfort Mandibular Plane Angle) has a greater anterior vector of force during occlusion that allows more rapid space closure, while a low FMA has a more vertical vector of movement that inhibits space closure.

Total leeway space is the mesiodistal crown width differences between the 10 primary teeth versus the 10 succedaneous teeth per arch. It is usually a negative 1.5 mm to 0 mm exchange in the lower arch and a negative five mm to 6.5 mm exchange in the upper arch. The difference in mesiodistal crown widths between the four primary incisors and four permanent incisors is called **incisor liability**. It usually has a negative exchange of 5 mm to 5.5 mm in the lower arch and a negative exchange of 6.5 mm to 7.5 mm in the upper arch. The difference in the mesiodistal crown widths of the permanent canine-premolars is labeled **posterior leeway space**, which gives a surplus in the lower arch during the exchange of plus 4 mm to 5 mm, and in the upper arch a surplus of plus 1 mm to 1.5 mm. It is more common to have clinical crowding in the anterior segment of the arches than in the posterior segments. Posterior crowding is usually related to early or unfavorable loss of primary molars.

The ectopic eruption of the permanent first molar into the primary second molar at about age six years is seen in two percent to three percent of the population. Some self correct with the root near or at the CEJ of the primary second molar with a loss of a dentin wedge, while others need separation orthodontically to be corrected. The older use of the brass wire separator has been followed by various new separating springs, i.e., the T P metal separator, or elastomeric radiopaque separator. This is usually a sign of an arch perimeter deficiency in the dentition. Maxillary permanent first molars that erupt distally prior to the mandibular ones can indicate developing Class II malocclusions.

Congenital absence or loss of maxillary teeth can present crossbite problems, especially for maxillary permanent incisors. It is more common to maintain or regain the space in congenital absence of maxillary permanent lateral incisors (75%) than it is to close the space orthodontically (25%).

Congenital absence of mandibular second premolars and retention of mandibular primary second molars presents unique problems. The usual difference in width of these two teeth is about (+) 2 mm to 3 mm in the exchange per side. The removal of the primary second molars in these cases is more dependent on other facial or occlusal factors than on pure congenital absence of the second premolar (50% extraction with closure versus 50% without closure). The factors that might lead to their removal are related to anterior clinical protrusion, high mandibular plane angles, and more Class II malocclusion patterns. Congenital absence of permanent teeth does not mean extraction orthodontics. Other important factors are the determining variables such as clinical crowding, protrusive anterior teeth, and/or **apical base** discrepancies.

Ankylosis of primary molars is a common phenomenon that is presented as a progressive disorder in the transitional dentition during the normal cycle of a primary tooth. If an anterior primary tooth is ankylosed, the chances of the successor erupting properly are poor without intervention. These **ankylosed** teeth are commonly removed. If a primary molar becomes ankylosed, there is a need for conservation of arch perimeter due to the mesial eruption of the permanent first molar over the crown of the ankylosed primary second molar. It is more common to have ankylosed primary molars in the lower arch than the upper, and it is more common to have the primary first molars affected than the primary second molars. Ankylosed permanent teeth are rare and present unique orthodontic problems. Ankylosed teeth cannot be moved orthodontically. They are anchorage units with the adjacent teeth moved toward them. Most ankylosed teeth are removed prior to orthodontic therapy. Some have attempted to remove the **alveolar bone** that is causing the ankylosis. This bony union is near the alveolar crest.

It is necessary to highlight some unfavorable patterns of tooth eruption. It is common for the mandibular permanent incisors to erupt around the same time as the permanent first molars. That is not true for the maxillary arch, where the permanent first molars erupt first. If a permanent lateral incisor erupts prior to a permanent central incisor, it is unfavorable. Depending on the arch, this could be either mandibular congenital absence of a permanent central incisor or a maxillary succedaneous supernumerary tooth (mesiodens, usually) preventing normal eruption. The permanent canine-first premolar eruption sequence is variable. However, it is essential to palpate the unerupted permanent canines facially at about eight to ten years of age. If they cannot be palpated facially, then they should be presumed to be palatal or lingual, which is not normal. Further radiographic evaluation is essential. The removal of the primary canine in the affected area is usually the plan of choice to redirect the eruption of these lingually positioned permanent canines. Lingually positioned permanent canines are usually non-permanent tooth extraction cases involving Class I malocclusions.

The eruption of permanent second molars prior to primary tooth loss marks another important, unfavorable pattern. These permanent molars are superior anchorage units and have mesial components of force. They do not move distally well even with adequate orthodontic force systems, and this is especially true in the mandibular arch. It is common in males to have the permanent second molars erupt prior to the mandibular second premolars. It is an older genetic pattern and should not be considered favorable.

If one observes one tooth anomaly, i.e., small shaped permanent lateral incisors, it is best to review the case for other anomalies such as impactions of adjacent permanent canines, ankylosis of primary molars, or congenital absence of second premolars.

There are midline and lateral frena that should be observed. In the mandible they are usually found in the lingual midline area and on the facial in the canine-premolar region. If a pull creates ischemia to the free gingival margin, surgical intervention is usually recommended. In the maxilla, the frena are usually facial both at the midline and in the canine-premolar area. A maxillary midline **diastema** usually is not corrected until after the eruption of the permanent canines as they usually help to naturally close the space because of their mesial pattern of eruption. A midline space over 1.5 mm will probably not self correct if the permanent lateral incisors have erupted. Congenital absence of permanent lateral incisors can give large anterior diastemata. Midline spaces need periodic radiographic evaluation to identify fibrous or muscular bands of tissue between the left and right maxillae, which present as an inverted, dark V shape on a radiograph. In general, one closes these spaces orthodontically first, and then surgical intervention is completed to remove the band of tissue. The cause of the midline space is rarely the frenum itself. It is a tooth-size/arch perimeter problem.

3.3 THE TRANSVERSE PLANE

The transverse plane of the face does not always mirror the transverse plane of the occlusion. A broad face does not necessarily give a broad arch, but usually a narrower face gives a narrower arch. Three important aspects of transverse discrepancies are related to 1.) **facial midline**-dental midline problems, 2.) posterior crossbites with their variations of buccoversions or linguoversions, and 3.) axial inclinations of the buccal segments, i.e., the uprightness or the tipping of the maxillary crowns facially and/or the mandibular posterior crowns lingually.

Usually, the maxillary dental midline is coincident to the facial midline, and it is the mandibular midline that is off compared to the maxillary due to lower anterior clinical crowding. Most maxillary midline problems are related to congenital absence or early loss of teeth in that arch. Congenital absence of one maxillary permanent central incisor, i.e., the cyclopian incisor, is extremely rare. Extraction of contralateral primary teeth does not allow self-correction of the problem in the maxilla. Mandibular midline discrepancies are usually related to **incisor liability** problems favoring one side of the arch with premature loss of one of the primary canines. The extraction of the contralateral mandibular primary canine can assist in self-correction of this lower midline problem, usually followed by a lingual arch for space maintenance.

Posterior crossbites are usually found in less than 10% of the population. They are much more common in the primary dentition as compared to **anterior crossbite**s in this dentition. The cause of most posterior quadrant crossbites in the primary or transitional dentition is the maxillary primary canines which are constricted in their **intercanine width**, which cause the mandibular teeth to shift to one side or the other. Almost all early posterior crossbites have lateral slides in centric. The lower midline is off to the side of the problem. If one places the lower midline so it is coincident with the maxillary midline, there usually is a bilateral posterior expression of the crossbite in **centric relation**, or retruded contact position. Therefore, most of these crossbites are treated bilaterally rather than on just one side. If, in the Class II division 1 malocclusion the lower teeth are allowed to shift forward, a bilateral posterior crossbite can be identified in many of these cases due to the constricted, V-shaped maxillary arch. Posterior quadrant crossbites that are not treated until growth is near completion can present unique asymmetric mandibular problems. These crossbites can be treated in the primary through the **transitional dentitions**. Most posterior quadrant crossbites are treated in the maxilla rather than the mandible.

There are a few unique crossbites that are more related to problems in permanent tooth eruption. The **succedaneous teeth** normally develop lingually as compared to their primary teeth. That is why it is common for the permanent incisors and premolars to erupt lingually in a malposed position. The permanent canines can be facial or lingual, depending upon the width of the arch and the extent of crowding. If there is posterior arch loss in either arch, the second premolars usually are blocked out lingually. They are considered in linguoversion, which is where the problem is, i.e., the facial cusp is lingual to the opposing teeth. The permanent second molars express their crowding problems differently. Usually the maxillary permanent second molar erupts into a **buccoversion**, i.e., the lingual cusp is facial to the lower second molar, as the maxillary permanent molars, the **accessional teeth**, erupt in a distal direction due to the posterior development of the maxilla and its displacement anteriorly. In the mandibular arch, the ascending ramus prevents this from occurring on the facial with permanent second molar eruption in a linguoversion. These bucco- or linguo- versions are expressions of middle or posterior arch shortages.

The primary teeth erupt into upright positions in the arches. This is not true for the permanent teeth. The four maxillary permanent incisors erupt with the crowns outward, or facial, and their roots lingual. This is called facial crown torque, or lingual root torque. These are the only permanent teeth that naturally do this. The other permanent teeth are more upright with the crown lingual and the roots facial. The lower permanent incisors are usually upright. However, the permanent canine to permanent second molar segments have their crowns lingual and their roots facial as a normal pattern. It is usually less so in the maxilla and mildly more so in the mandible. If the buccal segments are inclined in the direction of the crown out and root in for the maxilla, expansion of the arch should be considered. The cause of much of the crowding in the arches is not related to large teeth but to narrow arches, which have a strong genetic basis.

The mandibular midline suture fuses at one year after birth, but the maxillary midline suture is patent, or open, until at least the teenage years. Maxillary orthopedics, or the movement of the left and right maxillae, is possible; it is not possible in the lower arch without surgery. The transverse plane matures the earliest of the three planes and therefore needs to be treated first, or earliest. It is common in correction of an entire malocclusion that this plane is treated first, and separately, prior to intervention in the sagittal and/or vertical planes. Expansion of the maxillary arch increases arch perimeter with the premolar expansion affecting arch perimeter more so than the molar region.

If the posterior problems are related to **anterior crossbites** or anterior openbite malocclusions, the posterior is treated first. Most posterior crossbites, if left untreated, become arch perimeter problems and are resistant to change in adults.

3.4 THE SAGITTAL PLANE

Angle's classification is a dental classification of permanent first molars. It cannot be applied in the primary dentition, so a terminal plane relationship of the primary second molars is used. Unilateral problems of the occlusion are expressed as subdivision problems to the side of the problem. If the left side is Class I and the right side is Class II, the malocclusion is a Class II subdivision right with a label to the side of the disharmony. One cannot use the permanent second molars to classify the occlusion. The permanent canine relationship can be used as an adjunct to express the anterior portion of the occlusion. Evaluation of the buccal segment as a whole is best, especially in the adolescent or adult. Other components that need to be assessed in this plane are overjet and **anterior crossbite**.

There are three aspects of the position of the maxillary permanent first molars that need to be evaluated: 1.) the mesiobuccal cusp of the maxillary permanent first molar relative to the buccal groove of the mandibular permanent first molar (Class I), 2.) the mesiolingual cusp of the maxillary permanent first molar relative to the central fossa of the mandibular permanent first molar (Class I), and 3.) the distal surface of the distobuccal cusp of the maxillary permanent first molars relative to the mesial surface of the mesiobuccal cusp of the mandibular permanent second molar (Class I).

Class I canines demonstrate that the maxillary canines are distal to the mandibular canines with good intercuspation. If the maxillary canines fall on top of the mandibular canines without intercuspation, they are considered end-on-end, i.e., two mm to three mm off from Class I. If the maxillary canines are mesial to the mandibular canines with good intercuspation, this is a Class II canine relationship, i.e., five mm to six mm from Class I. If the maxillary canine is distal more extensively without good intercuspation, it is a Class III canine relationship. At this stage, there is usually an anterior crossbite of the incisors, but this is not always the case.

There is a distance between Class I and Class II that is midway facially, but not so lingually. That is the end-to-end permanent first molar relationship that expresses itself with cusp-on-cusp position facially, but the mesiolingual cusp of the maxillary permanent first molar occludes in the central fossa of the mandibular first molar as seen with Class I problems. If the permanent first molars are Class II, the mesiolingual cusp would be in the embrasure between the permanent first molar and the primary second molar, or second premolar if it were present. Some consider these half step **Class II malocclusions**, because the mechanics to correct the problem are in a Class II direction. However, they really are variations of a Class I molar relationship. The buccal segment anterior to the molar up to the canine can be end to end, Class I, or Class II. Each case is different. To concentrate only on the permanent first molars can be misleading, without including anterior evaluation.

The distobuccal cusp of the maxillary permanent first molar should touch the mandibular permanent second molar in the adolescent dentition, i.e., 28 permanent teeth erupted. This is part of Andrew's six keys to the occlusion.

If one removes excessive mandibular growth and adverse variations in tooth eruption or crowding or spacing of the arches, the most commonly found pattern of flush terminal plane occlusion in the preschool, independent of race or gender, gives rise to an end-to-end permanent first molar relationship. If there is **mandibular primate space** (2 mm to 3 mm space distal to mandibular primary canine), an early shift of the permanent first molar might give a Class I molar relationship. If crowding is present, no shift occurs. Differential mandibular growth relative to the maxilla can assist in developing a Class I molar relationship over time. The **maxillary primate spaces** (mesial to the primary canines) are used for correction of problems in maxillary incisor liability. Therefore, end-to-end permanent first molars might stay that way, might shift to Class I, or might shift to Class II if there is an unfavorable eruption of permanent teeth. A Class III molar relationship would result in future mandibular prognathia.

With the end-to-end permanent molars, there can be another pattern. With early loss of the maxillary primary second molar and a shift of the maxillary permanent first molar, it will be Class II. But because of this shift, it is labeled as a **pseudo Class II**. A premature loss of a mandibular primary second molar with a Class I molar can result in a lower molar shift and a **pseudo Class III** molar relationship.

The change in molar relationship after the preschool years is most common with end-to-end permanent first molars from the flush terminal plane of the primary second molars. It can stay end-to-end, or shift to Class I (favorable), or Class II (unfavorable), but rarely Class III during childhood. The less common mesial step of the primary second molars initially gives Class I permanent first molars at six years of age and usually holds there throughout childhood. The distal step from the terminal plane of the primary second molars consistently gives a Class II permanent first molar that does not self correct. The rarer super mesial step of the primary second molars at age six years gives a Class III permanent first molar relationship. Adverse or unfavorable eruption sequences in addition to adverse mandibular growth can alter the molar relationship during childhood.

Overjet is measured in millimeters from the facial of the incisors or from their incisal edges. Usually the normal adult dentition has two mm to three mm overjet throughout the whole dentition, not just the anterior segment. Those that use this reference use the facial surface reference in the lower arch. Protrusion of the dentition is usually labeled in the six to 12 mm range and is most common in the Class II division 1 pattern. Class II division 2 patterns have the maxillary permanent central incisors with a lingual crown position that is upright or retroclined with minimal overjet.

Anterior crossbites related to Class III malocclusions and Class II division 2 malocclusions can present unusual developmental patterns for the permanent central incisors. If one views from the side the development of these teeth, there is a normal crown to root angle that is five to seven degrees. This is the **collum angle** of the tooth. However, if this incisor is held behind the lower or is adversely retroclined, the angle of the root to the crown becomes much larger than normal, i.e., 12 degrees to 18 degrees. The problem with this development is that if one places the crown in correct esthetic position to the face with tooth movement, the root is placed too far to the lingual. In fact, one cannot correct the inclination enough as the root touches the palatal plate of cortical bone. The teeth look too upright. **Class III** anterior crossbite malocclusions and Class II division 2 malocclusions need growth-mediated earlier treatment protocols.

Anterior crossbites need to be treated early. They are rare in the primary dentition, but if present, can be treated. The more common problem with the anterior crossbite pattern is with the eruption of the permanent incisors. The most common incisor to be in crossbite is the maxillary permanent lateral incisor. However, if the permanent central incisors are in crossbite, a bilateral expression is as common as the unilateral problem.

Most anterior crossbites are treated in the maxillary arch rather than mandibular. If done in the transitional dentition, a 2 to 3 mm overlap of the incisors (overbite) is helpful. As one moves the maxillary incisors out facially (therefore, increasing **arch length**), the mandibular incisors move back, or to the lingual (therefore, decreasing arch length). The overbite usually becomes less with treatment until the incisors can erupt more. Therefore, shallow, initial overbite cases become problems in retention after the correction of the anterior crossbite. Correction of the anterior crossbite usually necessitates that a second step of maxillary incisor alignment will be needed.

There is another unique problem with crossbites and time. If left untreated, not only are there periodontal and traumatic tooth wear problems, but arch perimeter problems develop. If the adjacent teeth collapse and leave deficient room to move the incisor facially, then the arch perimeter must be increased prior to crossbite correction. A general rule during growth is that if you make room for the tooth it will erupt by itself. Proximal enamel removal of permanent teeth in the transitional dentition is not indicated, but proximal enamel removal of primary teeth can be indicated.

If anterior crossbites have anteroposterior shifts, the prognosis for the case improves. There is a neuromuscular component to the malocclusion with this shift, and that is favorable. One needs to consider posterior arch expansion with anterior crossbite problems. Usually there is a constriction around the whole arch rather than just the anterior region. Posterior biteplane therapy to assist in correction of these crossbites to prevent anterior traumatic occlusion is usually recommended.

3.5 THE VERTICAL PLANE

The vertical plane of the occlusion in the anterior segment is more susceptible to environmental effects than the posterior segment. The use of percentage **overlap** of the maxillary incisors over the mandibular incisors allows evaluation of the primary incisors as well as the permanent incisors. Unless one is using a cephalometric study, the criteria for overlap is **clinical crown** overlap rather than **anatomic crown** overlap. Therefore, overbite can change with the amount of enamel that is exposed. There is rarely anatomic incisor expression clinically in the child or adolescent.

There are numerous descriptions of **overbite**. Usually it is used almost exclusively in the anterior region. If it is seen in the posterior segments, it is usually labeled as an openbite related to **ankylosis** of primary molars or to a normal stage of eruption, or labeled as supraeruption with their antagonists. Normal bite is more than 10% and less than 50% overlap. Fractions or values less than 10% intervals are overly detailed for this measurement. If the incisors do not overlap, it is labeled an openbite with the amount of open space divided by the amount of lower incisor that is exposed clinically. It is a negative percentage. If the incisors do not contact but there is overlap, there is also an open bite. This type of openbite has many different names: sagittal openbite, non-contact openbite, or hidden openbite. These can be difficult malocclusions to treat, because the sagittal malocclusion has a neuromuscular component to it. Openbite malocclusions seen in the transitional dentition are usually Class I while those in **adolescence** are more complex with both Class II and Class III patterns involved. Openbite dental malocclusions need be related to the skeletal pattern. All high FMA cases have skeletal openbite tendencies or patterns, and are more difficult to treat. Openbite malocclusions also have strong relapse tendencies.

If the lower incisors touch the palate, the malocclusion is impinging. It is common to have deepbite malocclusions (50% or more overlap) where the lower incisors touch the palate. Those cases are deep and impinging. However, impinging malocclusions do not have to have deepbite; these cases usually have marked protrusion. All deepbites are 50% overlap or more.

Deepbite malocclusion is a common orthodontic problem. It is not commonly observed by patients or parents as a chief complaint. The most common orthodontic problem that is presented by patients or parents is clinical crowding. Deepbite malocclusions present challenging problems, because one needs to evaluate the facial photographs and the status of the mandibular second molars. If a bite needs to be opened, the extent of the smile needs to be evaluated. Low smile lines do not need upper incisor intrusion, but high smile lines do. Incisor intrusion is more predictable in the upper arch than the lower arch. Incisor intrusion uses very light forces (20 to 25 grams per tooth) and is slow (0.3 mm per month). It is correctly assumed that the amount of force to extrude is the same as to intrude, which is very light. Lower incisor intrusion is usually expressed more with incisor flaring than intrusion. The mandibular permanent second molars are used to help open the anterior bite through **extrusion** of the first molars and second premolars and intrusion of the second molars and incisors.

Deepbite, impinging malocclusions might have lateral tongue biting or thrusting problems that are difficult to treat and maintain. All low FMA cases should be considered skeletal deepbite patterns.

The vertical plane is the most complex plane in orthodontics and has been only recently extensively studied. It is the last plane to treat in the posterior region of the arch with the transverse first, but it can be treated first in the anterior region depending on its relationship to the sagittal problem and the particular problems in the case.

3.6 HABITS AND OTHER ANOMALIES OF THE TEETH

Most oral habits related to orthodontics are related to airway considerations, adverse vertical growth, anterior gingivitis with mouth breathing, and openbite malocclusions. The hands help with identification of **oral habits** involving the fingers or thumbs, as the hands develop at the same time as the face. One should ask non-threatening questions and use a non-judgmental orientation. However, it is necessary to get accurate information. "Which thumb do you like best?" is a reasonable approach. It could be left or right finger or thumb, or both. The digits related to the oral habits usually are cleaner than the other digits, usually along with smaller fingernails. The digit can also be bent. Most oral habits follow a decreased frequency from home life to grade school with an effect from peer pressure, and from daytime (**diurnal**) to night (**nocturnal**). Stress can express itself with recurrent oral habits. Not all digit habits present openbites. If there is no openbite, there is no need for intervention of the habit from an orthodontic point of view. An openbite can remain after cessation of the digit habit. Orthodontic appliances used in the presence of continued digit habits will not succeed.

There has been confusion about oral habits as they relate to tongue thrusting. Usually oral habits will create circumscribed anterior openbites to the side of the habit. The **tongue thrust** is compensatory to fill in the space, with the lips closing to prevent saliva from coming out of the month. In fact, the lower lip can become very involved, with increased hyperactivity around the chin. Mentalis muscle insertion into the soft tissues below the skin creates a dimpled effect. This is hyperactive mentalis muscle activity related to anterior openbites.

The common time for openbites to appear is around seven to eight years of age with the exchange of incisors. The treatment of openbites at this time is usually delayed until the permanent incisors can erupt. If the habit persists after eight years of age with the eruption of the maxillary permanent central incisors, then either removable or fixed orthodontic appliances can be introduced. Usually openbites related to thumb habits in preschoolers are not treated with orthodontic appliances unless there is a posterior quadrant crossbite also involved. Then a modified quadhelix appliance can be used if the child assists and wishes to stop the habit.

The timing for most openbite intervention is after the second grade with the child's approval. Openbites in middle childhood are related more to Class I malocclusions, while openbites seen in adolescence are more related to skeletal Class II and Class III patterns. They are not the same kind of openbite.

Most adolescent and adult patients can open their lower jaw to 40 mm or more and move it laterally eight mm to 10 mm. Children can usually open to at least 30 mm. Restriction of 20 mm vertical opening or less is a problem and is a sign of the temporomandibular (TM) joint dysfunction, which seems to be heavily based on adverse neuromuscular patterns, as seen in stressful circumstances. **Myofascial** pain can also be stress related and is a sign of TM joint dysfunction. The problem is that the longitudinal evaluation of TM joint dysfunction does not stay consistent, with some children or adolescents getting it new while others who had TM joint dysfunction lose it. It is a variable pattern over time.

Most children and adolescents growing up today now have their tonsils and adenoids present. If the tonsils touch each other ("kissing tonsils"), they are considered plus five tonsils. The range is from 0 to five. There is currently a general consensus to not remove tonsils and/or adenoids. It has been shown that these large adenoid tissues can redirect facial growth downward and/or backward. Specific adverse facial patterns would benefit from improved airways with tonsillectomy and/or adenoidectomy (T & A). Unusual wear facets on the canines or incisors can be related to functioning occlusion. Marked lateral disclusion, that is, canine rise, can wear the canines. This is usually not seen in lateral group functioning patterns. There should be no steep canine-rise lateral function, but a gradual rise. It is usually easier to gain an orthodontic occlusion, that is, canine rise, than group function. Unusual incisor wear patterns can be seen in either anterior crossbites or lateral disclusions, as with Class II division 1 patterns.

The pattern of dental hypoplasia (deficient matrix) and dental hypomineralization (deficient calcification) is important to determine systemic or local etiology. Patterns on individual incisors are classic for primary incisor intrusion during the time one learns how to walk at two years of age, while generalized patterns can be associated with fluorosis or various types of **amelogenesis imperfecta** (hypoplasia as thin enamel or as pitted enamel, while hypomineralization is loss of minerals). Decalcification of teeth demonstrates normal enamel which became carious, while hypomineralization never was normal in the first place. Fluorosis is a form of hypomineralization, not hypermineralization.

4. RADIOGRAPHIC EXAMINATION

A child's height has a good correlation to **bone age**, but if one needs specific documentation, a radiograph of the hand is indicated to determine skeletal, or bone age. Figure 11-3A-D presents orthodontic evaluation forms, which can be used after a database has been established, and Figure 11-4A-D is the height-weight charts for boys and girls.

GENERALIZED INFORMATION
Name, record number, and age in years and months, gender, and race.

RADIOGRAPHIC EXAMINATION FROM PANORAMIC AND/OR INTRAORAL SURVEY.
1.) Missing teeth: Yes/No, which teeth? Congenital absence/extracted/unknown.
2.) Supernumerary: Yes/No, which teeth?
3.) Unusual sequence of eruption: Yes/No, which teeth?
4.) Unusual path of eruption: Yes/No, which teeth?
5.) Other tooth anomalies: Yes/No, which teeth?
6.) Horizontal or vertical bone loss: Yes/No, which teeth?
7.) Cysts or other pathologic conditions: Yes/No, which areas?

CAST ANALYSIS
With radiographic supplement for maxillary and mandibular arch form/symmetry.
1.) Symmetry/right asymmetry/left asymmetry.
2.) Arch form: average (elliptical or ovoid), square, tapered (V-shaped).
3.) Alignment: anterior/posterior clinical crowding/spacing.
4.) Tooth anomalies: congenital absence, tooth removal, supernumeraries, small/large sized teeth, small/large shaped teeth, abnormal eruption sequence, ectopic eruption, rotations (15-45°, 45-90°, and over 90°), submerged teeth, over-retained teeth, impacted teeth.

Figure 11-3A

ARCH ANALYSIS
1.) Measure the mesiodistal widths of all teeth clinically present.
2.) Permanent Dentition Analysis. For the maxilla and mandible with comparison of arch perimeter/ circumference required (mesiodistal widths of succedaneous teeth) versus arch perimeter/ circumference available (adjacent tooth comparisons, not brass wire around arch; do not alter arch form). Excess/deficiency in millimeters: less than 3 mm mild, 3 to 7 mm moderate, and over 7 mm severe per arch.
3.) Transitional Dentition Analysis. Measure mesiodistal widths of mandibular four permanent incisors, and total these four teeth. Use this summed total to find the predicted space available for the permnent canine and both premolars. This is done for both quadrants in the mandibular arch and both quadrants in the maxillary arch. Space required for each of the four quadrants is determined after the incisor midlines are coincident to the face and the incisors have either been aligned or consolidated. Space required is measured from the mesial of the permanent first molars to the distal of the aligned lateral incisors. Excess is a positive value while a deficiency is a negative value. The two quadrants per arch are summed for a determination of arch perimeter excess or deficiency.

Figure 11-3B: Orthodontic evaluation forms needed to analyze the orthodontic database (continued on next page).

Sum of 4 lower permanent incisors	Maxillary Space Required canine/premolars (75%)	Mandibular Space Required canine/premolars (75%)
19.5 mm	20.6 mm	20.1 mm
20.0 mm	20.9 mm	20.4 mm
20.5 mm	21.2 mm	20.7 mm
21.0 mm	21.5 mm	21.0 mm
21.5 mm	21.8 mm	21.3 mm
22.0 mm	22.0 mm	21.6 mm
22.5 mm	22.3 mm	21.9 mm
23.0 mm	22.6 mm	22.2 mm
23.5 mm	22.9 mm	22.5 mm
24.0 mm	23.1 mm	22.8 mm
24.5 mm	23.4 mm	23.1 mm
25.0 mm	23.4 mm	23.1 mm
25.5 mm	23.7 mm	23.4 mm
26.0 mm	24.2 mm	24.0 mm
26.5 mm	24.5 mm	24.3 mm
27.0 mm	24.8 mm	24.6 mm
27.5 mm	25.0 mm	24.8 mm
28.0 mm	25.3 mm	25.1 mm
28.5 mm	25.6 mm	25.4 mm

4.) Curve of Spee correction: measure the deepest point to the cusp tip along the incisor-molar plane on the right side of the lower cast. Do the same for the left. Add both and divide by 2 to get the average. Add 0.5 mm and total to determine normal, flat, deep, or reverse curve. To level the curve usually reduces arch length and arch perimeter, as the incisors are advanced. Therefore, it is labeled as a negative value because one needs room to level.

5). Calculation of the total mandibular arch discrepancy:
       a.) Arch perimeter/tooth mass discrepancy: excess/deficient.
       b.) Curve of Spee (if leveled): deficient.
       c.) Molar relation correction excess/deficient (end-to-end usually deficient 2-3 mm if lower molar forward and 5-6 mm if Class II to I).
       d.) Relocation of lower incisor: excess/deficient (cephalometric correction factor with incisor backward taking room, therefore, deficient and incisor forward, excess).
       e.) Total net discrepancy sum of four variables above.

Figure 11-3B: Orthodontic evaluation forms needed to analyze the orthodontic database.

ORTHODONTIC CEPHALOMETRIC ANALYSES

6.) Skeletal (Steiner/Downs Analyses): facial angle (N-Pog/FH), hard tissue angle of convexity (N-A-Pog), SNA, SNB, ANB, GoGn/SN, FMA Y-Axis (S-Gn/FH).

7.) Dental (Steiner/Downs/Williams analyses): 1/to SN, 1/to NA and /1 to NB (mm and degrees), Pog to NB (mm), /1 to mandibular plane, 1/1, /1 to Pog (mm).

8.) Soft tissue analyses: Upper lip and lower lip to esthetic line (nose-chin line) in (mm), and Z-angle (most protrusive lip from mandible to Frankfort horizontal).

Steiner Chevrons:

ANB	-2°	0°	+2°
1/ to NA	8 mm/26°	6mm/24°	4 mm/22°
/1 to NB	3 mm/21°	3.5 mm/23°	4 mm/25°

ANB	+4°	+6°	+8°
1/ to NA	2 mm/20°	0 mm/18°	-2 mm/16°
/1 to NB	4.5 mm/27°	5 mm/29°	5.5 mm/31°

9.) Identify findings outside the normal range.
10.) Attempt to determine the growth pattern.

Figure 11-3C: Evaluation forms needed to analyze the orthodontic database.

V. ORTHODONTIC CEPHALOMETRIC ANALYSES

Form Completed by: _____ Date: _____ Month _____ Day _____ Yr.

Patient Name: _____ Record No. _____

Age: _____ Years ___ Months   Birthdate: _____ Month ____ Day ____ Year   Sex: _____ Male ____ Female   Race: _____

	DATE					
SKELETAL (Steiner/Downs Analyses)	AGE					
Facial Angle (N-Pog/FH)	(degrees)					
Angle of Convexity (N-A-Pog)	(degrees)					
SNA	(degrees)					
SNB	(degrees)					
ANB	(degrees)					
GoGn/SN	(degrees)					
FMA	(degrees)					
Y-Axis (SGn/FH)	(degrees)					
DENTAL (Steiner/Downs/Williams Analyses)						
1/ to SN	(degrees)					
1/ to NA	(mm)					
1/ to NA	(degrees)					
/1 to NB	(mm)					
/1 to NB	(degrees					
Pog to NB	(mm)					
/1 to Mandibular Plane	(degrees)					
1/1	(degrees)					
/1 to A-Pog	(mm)					
SOFT TISSUE ANALYSIS						
Upper Lip to E Line	(mm)					
Lower Lip to E Line	(mm)					
Z-Angle (protrusive lip-chin/FH)	(degrees)					
TWEED ANALYSIS						
FMA	(degrees)					
IMPA	(degrees)					
FMIA	(degrees)					

STEINER CHEVRONS

ANB	(−)2°	0°	(+)2°	(+)4°	(+)6°	(+)8°
1/ to NA	26° 8mm	24° 6mm	22° 4mm	20° 2mm	18° 0mm	16° −2mm
/1 to NB	21° 3mm	23° 3.5mm	25° 4mm	27° 4.5mm	29° 5mm	31° 5.5mm

Which findings are obviously at variation? _____

_____

What do you expect the growth pattern to be? _____

_____

Figure 11-3D: Orthodontic evaluation forms needed to analyze the orthodontic database.

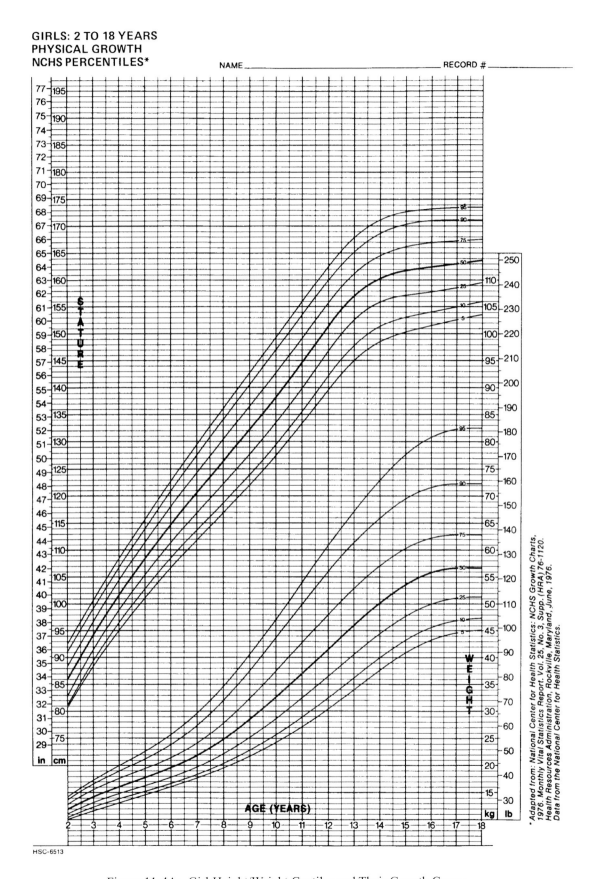

Figure 11-4A: Girl Height/Weight Centiles and Their Growth Curves

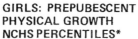

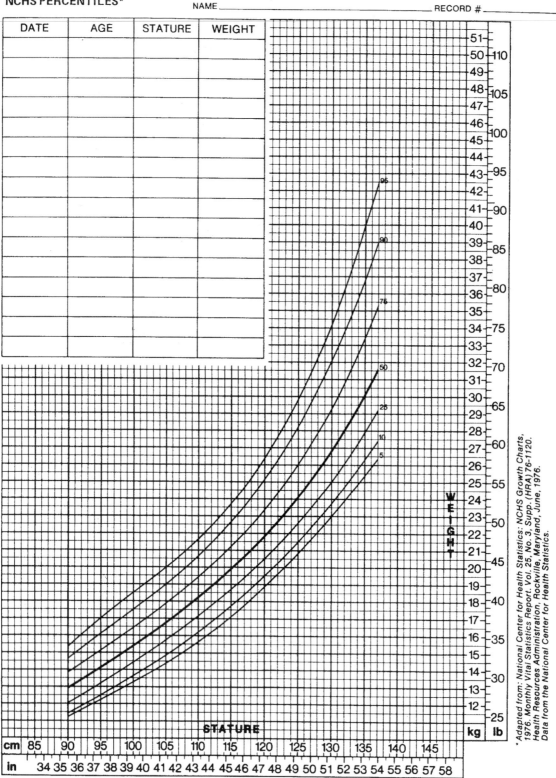

Figure 11-4B: Girl Height/Weight Centiles and Their Growth Curves

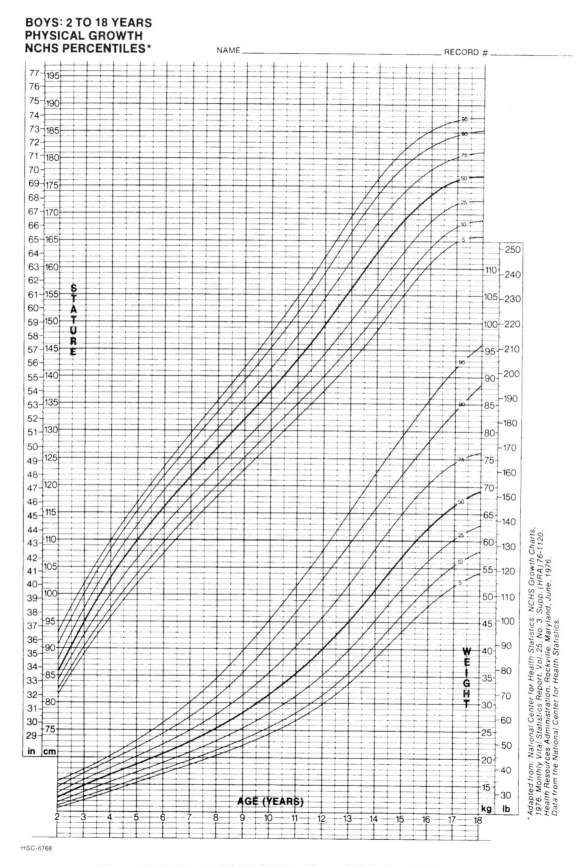

BOYS: 2 TO 18 YEARS PHYSICAL GROWTH NCHS PERCENTILES*

Figure 11-4C: Boy Height/Weight Centiles and Their Growth Curves

HSC-6768

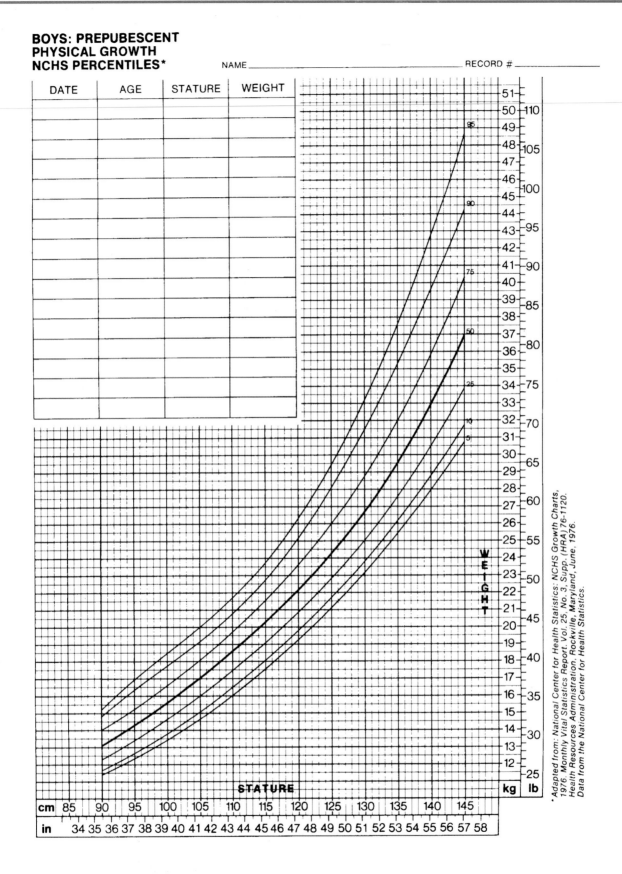

Figure 11-4D: Boy Height/Weight Centiles and Their Growth Curves

4.1 THE PANORAMIC FILM

The panoramic film is indicated in all growing individuals, independent of any specific problem or malocclusion status, at least twice: once as late as eruption of permanent incisors to check for anomalies of number or position of teeth, and another after eruption of permanent second molars to check for third molar anomalies, including cysts. The panoramic film is a laminograph that does not accurately assess sizes of the teeth or those teeth outside the plane of the cut. Severely malposed teeth facial or lingual might not be seen accurately. Supplemental intraoral periapical films might be needed. One cannot accurately measure widths of teeth from this laminograph. One should not mark over the hard or soft tissues of radiographs with a pen or pencil.

Supernumeraries that are primary teeth usually erupt into the arch, and are most commonly seen in the anterior segments. Neonatal teeth are usually early erupting primary incisors, not supernumeraries. The more common succedaneous **supernumerary teeth** are found in the maxillary anterior segment between three and eight years of age. Most of these teeth do not erupt. They can, in fact, be inverted. The timing for their removal is related to the actual disturbance in the eruption of the normally affected incisor, usually around seven to eight years of age. These succedaneous supernumeraries are most often lingual or palatal. Some practitioners remove succedaneous supernumerary teeth in the primary dentition stage.

The studies that have been done have placed the frequency of either supernumerary or congenital absence of teeth in this order from most frequent to least: congenital absence of permanent teeth (3.8% to 6.1%), supernumerary permanent teeth (2% to 3%), supernumerary primary teeth (0.3% to 1.8%), and congenital absence of primary teeth (0.1% to 0.4%).

The most common congenitally missing permanent teeth are related to the last tooth in its group: third molar more common than second molar more common than first molar. The first molar is more commonly absent than has been previously reported due inadequate radiographic documentation, improved fluoridation, and the lack of understanding in identifying tooth crown/root morphology. The second premolar is more commonly missing than the first premolar, which is rarely missing. The maxillary lateral incisor is the most anomalous succedaneous tooth. It can be absent, peg-shaped, small-sized, and have dens-evaginatus (talon cusp) or dens-invaginatus (dens in dente). The cyclopian maxillary central incisor is a very rare finding with congenital absence of a single maxillary central. The most common missing lower permanent incisor is the central incisor, not the larger lateral incisor. It seems that is related to the mandibular midline suture.

Hypodontia (Latin) and **oligodontia** (Greek) mean missing teeth, usually congenitally missing, and they have the same meaning. **Anodontia** means that no teeth developed, and that is extremely rare. There is no such thing as partial anodontia: part of nothing is still nothing.

The rank order from most to least common congenital absence of permanent teeth is: third molars, second premolars (both arches), maxillary lateral incisors, second molars, mandibular central incisors, and first molars. The least commonly absent are the maxillary central incisor, then first premolar, canine, and mandibular lateral incisor.

Congenital absence of permanent teeth does not mean that they are extraction orthodontic cases. The most commonly extracted tooth in dentistry is the third molar. The most commonly extracted tooth in orthodontics is the first premolar, which is related to crowding and/or protrusion. The more severely rotated premolar should be the preferred tooth to remove if extractions are indicated.

4.2 THE LATERAL CEPHALOMETRIC RADIOGRAPH

The lateral cephalometric film enables one to evaluate the dentofacial complex by observing the soft tissue drape over the teeth and bones. Orientation of the film should be either close to Frankfort horizontal or natural head position being parallel to the bottom of the radiograph. A film that is taken without the soft tissue profile screen, which is easily identified as the accessory on the cassette itself, has little diagnostic value.

The use of a cranial base reference to use with sequential cephalometric tracings is beneficial, but it is not beneficial for the analysis of the face with one film. Facial plane is the Nasion-Pogonion line and is a major vertical reference, with Nasion-**A point** and Nasion-B point minor variations of this plane.

Sella-Nasion is a major horizontal cranial reference, Basion-Nasion or Ethmoid Triad with the greater wings of the sphenoid bone to supplement Sella can also be used. The reference **Frankfort horizontal plane** is a reasonable reference to the face. It is valid to use in facial analysis, but it does have its limits due to reliability (**reproducibility**). It is necessary to use anatomic Porion rather than machine Porion, as machine Porion is dependent upon the individual who places the patient in the cephalostat. Anatomic or true Porion is at the same level as the head of the **condyle**. If machine is off from true Porion, it is usually in the inferior and/or anterior position.

If the **facial angle** is greater than 90 degrees, one has an anterior divergent skeletal facial profile. A large bony chin button can create anterior divergence of the mandible rather than a mandible that is hypertrophic or prognathic. Soft tissue facial angle is usually three degrees larger than hard tissue facial angle, and if Glabella is used superiorly, the angle is only one degree higher.

If the facial angle is less than 85 degrees, the skeletal profile is considered to be posterior divergent. If it is the 85 degrees to 90 degrees range, it is considered non-divergent or orthognathic.

Other major horizontal reference planes are mandibular planes, either measured to GoGn (posterior and anterior outer inferior borders of the mandible) as measured to SN or FMA (**Menton** tangent to the angle of the mandible to Frankfort horizontal).

Angle ANB is a measurement that is calculated from SNA minus SNB. If it is negative, one has a concave skeletal profile. If it is positive, one has a straight or convex profile. **Angle of convexity** uses NA line and positions Pogonion to that line. The vertex of the angle is at A point, not Nasion. If Pogonion is ahead of the NA line, the profile is concave. A protrusive Pogonion can give one a concave profile due to a large bony chin button, rather than an apical base discrepancy (negative ANB). If Pogonion is behind the NA line, and Pogonion to Nasion line is 0 degrees to five degrees from NA line, it is a straight profile (usually ANB+1 degrees to +3 degrees). If Pogonion-A point line intersects N-A point line at greater than five degrees, it is a convex profile. It is common to have a skeletal convex profile in children and most adolescents. Late adolescent Caucasians and adult Caucasian males can have concave skeletal profiles. The soft tissue **angle of convexity** is usually eight degrees to 11 degrees higher than the hard tissue angle of convexity.

The Y-Axis assists in determining the growth pattern of the patient. If measured to Frankfort horizontal, the anterior inferior angle should be in the range of 57 degrees to 59 degrees. Low 50 degrees readings translate to horizontal growth patterns, while middle to higher 60 degrees readings represent more vertical growth patterns.

A balanced upper permanent incisor to the face is demonstrated by an upper incisor long axis that intersects into the ascending portion of the orbit. If the facial plane were a straight vertical line, then many acceptable faces would have the long axis of the upper incisor about 25 degrees off the vertical and the lower incisor about 25 degrees off the vertical. The **interincisal angle** would be approximately 130 degrees. For primary teeth, the interincisal angle is 150 degrees with 15 degrees for the lower primary incisor and 15 degrees for the upper primary incisor off the vertical reference.

The use of the lower incisor edge to A point-Pogonion line (/1 to APog) describes the positioning of the lower incisor for various positive ANB problems. The incisal edge is usually on that line for Class I and Class II patterns. This reference presents high values for Class III malocclusions and for Blacks, due to the position of Pogonion.

The use of **Steiner chevrons** assists in assessment of dentoalveolar compensations of apical base discrepancies. The greater the sagittal difference between the maxillary and mandibular bases, the more the upper incisor is upright and moved backward while the more the lower incisor is proclined (degrees) and made more procumbent (millimeters). The reverse is true if the mandible is ahead of the maxilla in a sagittal skeletal position.   The upper incisor becomes more proclined (degrees) and procumbent (mm) while the lower incisor becomes more retroclined and retrocumbent. The chevrons show calculated compromised positions of the incisors for a sagittally malaligned maxilla and mandible.

5. ORTHODONTIC STUDY MODELS AND PHOTOGRAPHS

The orthodontic study models are important in the analysis of a specific case after it has been determined that an individual needs to be worked up orthodontically and obtain a database. There are two basic methods for preparing orthodontic models, with one using the classic or standard method of orthodontic models while the other is a strong proponent of mounted study models. The classic model will be presented here. Figure 11-5A and B outlines two methods of model trimming.

A. Considerations Prior to Model Trimming.

1.) Remove interfering bubbles on the occlusal surfaces or the posterior extensions that prevent the casts from occluding.
2.) Check the wax bite wafer for articulating the lower cast with the upper to remove any extensions beyond the anatomy of the arches.
3.) Do not grind off the teeth at any stage of trimming. If the upper anterior teeth present with marked proclination and a tapered arch, alter the anterior cut from 25º to 35º or 45º.
4.) Use the canine eminence most in line with the occlusion. If the teeth on both sides are not symmetrical, cut the side on which the teeth appear most normal or in better position.
5.) Do not leave any lip of stone on the sides. The depth of fold is carved flat from the base of the fold to the edge of the cast.
6.) Flatten and smooth the tongue space from the depth of the lingual vestibule to the edge of the heel of the cast.
7.) The lateral and back corner slices should be symmetrical and equal per cast. The casts need to have only a flush surface from a superior or top view at the heels or backs of the set of casts.

Figure 11-5A

B. The Model Trimming Sequence.

1.) Start with maxillary cast. Trim occlusal plane parallel to the base or top of upper cast, about 2 inches thick.
2.) One can next either trim the maxillary cast to the heel or back, perpendicular to the mid-palatal raphe (not anterior dental midline or maxillary midline frenum), or trim a 25° front slice at the midpoint of the palatal raphe to the depth of the fold. Do not trim any teeth. At this point, one can continue with the maxillary cast (3) or start on the mandibular (3a).
3.) Maxillary cast. Trim 65° lateral slice. Stop at canine eminence and depth of fold.
4.) Maxillary cast. Be sure 25° slices are equal in length and end at midline, canine eminence, and at depth of fold.
3a.) Mandibular cast. Use bite wafer here. Trim lower cast so that lower heel or back and the upper heel are in the same plane. Be sure one keeps the upper cast at right angles to its base or top of cast.
4a.) Mandibular cast. Separate the casts and trim the lower cast so that its base, or bottom, is perpendicular to the lower cast back or heel.

If one used 3A and 4A mandibular, do 3 and 4 maxillary now.

5.) The anterior of the lower cast should now be rounded with a front curvature at the depth of the fold that should stop at the lower canine eminence.
6.) Trim the lower cast at a 55° lateral slice that stops at the canine eminence and depth of fold.
7.) Trim the lower and upper casts at a 115° back corner slice. The left and rights of each cast should be equal in length and about 1/2 inch wide (±1/8 inch)
8.) Upper and lower casts together should be 2 3/4 inches in height (2 inches if primary dention). If needed, reduce the casts so that at the canine eminence, it is 2/3 anatomy and 1/3 art for each cast.
9.) Final occlusion of the casts is checked on their heels or backs, without the wax bite wafer, to determine proper intercuspation. The casts should not rock. If minor adjustment is needed, trim the cast at the heels without the wafer.
10.) After smoothing, sanding, filling voids, and (if done) inscribing patient information , the casts should be dried prior to soaping.
11.) Typed labels should be placed on the heels of the casts. If there is inadequate room on the heel of one cast, place the labels on both bases.
12.) The label should include:
 a.) Last name, first name of patient.
 b.) Chronologic age of patient at time of the impressions in years and months, i.e., C.A. = 10-1.
 c.) Date impressions were taken in month and year, i.e., June 2003.
 d.) Orthodontic chart number.

Figure 11-5B

To assist in determining the problem, it is essential that the art portion of the casts be standardized so that the anatomic portion is presented as the variable. Because primary dentitions are smaller than the transitional or permanent dentitions, the heights of their casts are smaller at two inches or 50 mm, while the other casts are 2 3/4 inches or 70 mm.

The angular patterns are the same for all dentitions and all malocclusions, unless there is an extremely narrow maxillary arch with protrusion, as seen with some Class II division 1 malocclusions. Then the anterior angles for the maxilla are narrowed. It is important that no anterior teeth, or fully erupted posterior teeth, are cut during the model trimming.

The maxillary cast is the basic reference for the set of casts. The maxillary occlusion is the reference in trimming to the top of the cast. Then the posterior heel is cut perpendicular to it and also to the mid-palatal raphe. The sides are cut equal at 115 degrees, 65 degrees, and 25 degrees with the anterior point at the midline of the casts, which is supposed to be coincident to the midline of the face. That is an important feature that needs to be done at chairside with the patient present. Usually midline discrepancies are off from the mandibular arch, not the maxillary. The use of the maxillary midline frenum is not a good reference to determine the maxillary midline. The lateral cuts are to the depth of the vestibule.

The mandibular cast is trimmed to the maxillary cast. The reference used is the posterior border of the maxillary cast, so that both back or heel portions are in the same plane. The wax bite registration should assist in this process. If there is a slide in centric that is over 1.5 mm, two wax bite registrations should be used. Maximum intercuspal position (centric occlusion or intercuspal position means CO or IC) should be used to trim the models. If one trims the models in retruded contact position (centric relation or retruded contact means CR or RC), the casts can easily be broken when they are held together.

The mandibular cast has two lateral cuts and a rounded anterior segment from canine eminence to canine eminence. The lateral cuts are 115 degrees and 55 degrees. The only parts of the cast that should be flush from a superior position is the heel or back, while it could be preferred at the lateral, but it is not essential.

If one trims the models to the lower arch, there is difficulty in relating the arches to the face as well as differences in overbite. The **curve of Spee** is much more pronounced in the lower arch than the upper arch.

The two casts should also be analyzed separately. One should evaluate symmetry versus asymmetry (most are symmetrical), **arch form** (ovoid, square, or tapered), and alignment (clinical crowding versus spacing). Most lower arches are ovoid while some are square. Lower arches are seldom tapered. The maxillary arch is usually ovoid but can be tapered (Class II division 1 and Class III) or square (Class II division 2).

There is a difference between clinical crowding and predicted crowding. The same is true for spacing. This is an important consideration in the transitional dentition. The method to determine crowding and/or spacing is fraught with error. The analysis of the specific arch should be as the arch presents. The determination should be done without changing arch form or attempting to predict where the teeth should be if a tooth had not moved. In the primary and permanent dentition, each specific area between teeth should be analyzed and calculated so that one can sum the parts for the whole arch. The former use of the brass wire or a string to determine this process had too much variability and presented a clinically unacceptable error of measurement.

The transitional dentition presents problems in prediction as compared to what the actual current clinical circumstance presents. The segment of the arch occupied by the canine and two premolars is the problem. The use of the four mandibular permanent incisors are used to predict the space required for the canine-premolars. The same lower four teeth are used to predict the space required for the maxillary canine-premolars. The maxillary permanent incisors are not used to predict this due to the wide variability in the sizes of the permanent lateral incisors. There is no use of prediction from primary tooth sizes for permanent tooth sizes as they have different genetic codes. It is analogous to tooth eruption and tooth exfoliation. These are governed by different genetic codes.

The great error in determining predicted crowding/spacing in the transitional dentition is related to incisor liability that is not properly addressed. It is essential to align the incisors prior to determining space available. Many determine the canine-premolars dimension (posterior leeway space) without addressing the alignment needs of the incisors first (incisor liability).

The use of quadrants is recommended versus the arch as a whole, as one cannot regain and hold more than approximately two to three mm in one mandibular quadrant, independent of the type of orthodontic intervention. That is not true in the maxilla. One can regain five to six millimeters in one maxillary quadrant.

The Rule of 21 can be applied to the lower arch. The average combined permanent mandibular incisor mesiodistal widths is 21 mm (5.0mm for the central and 5.5 mm for the lateral), while the average permanent canine-premolars width is 21 mm per side (7.0 mm each for all three teeth). The maxillary permanent canine-premolars segment is 21.5 mm (1/2 mm larger due to size of permanent canine).

Tooth anomalies have a profound effect on arch perimeter (circumference). Congenital absence of permanent teeth affects space required. The primary second molars can be retained rather than removed if the mandibular second premolar is absent. This second premolar has a greater variation in its timing to initiate mineralization. Normally it should start to mineralize at about two to three years after birth. However, there have been cases where it develops much later. One should plan that if it is not mineralizing by age nine years, it will not develop.

Congenital absence of second premolars presents unique problems as there is a 50:50 chance to remove them and close spaces versus hold the space. The space for the absent maxillary permanent lateral incisor is usually maintained rather than closed with the maxillary canine as the lateral incisor (75% open vs. 25% closed). It is dependent upon the type of malocclusion and gender (girls more often open, and boys more often closed).

Other variables in the cast analysis with radiographic supplement include supernumeraries, large sized/small sized teeth (macrodontia/microdontia), ectopic eruption (2% to 3% maxillary permanent first molars into the primary second molars with conservative treatment recommended), eruption sequence (eruption of permanent second molar prior to the loss of primary teeth should be considered unfavorable), rotations, ankylosis or submerged teeth (mostly primary molars as a progressive disorder of eruption that effects the mandible more and the primary first molars more), and impactions (last succedaneous teeth to erupt with mandibular second premolar lingual and the maxillary permanent canine facial). It is essential that the permanent canines be palpated facially by eight to 10 years of age. If they are not, they should be evaluated further for their lingual or palatal position. If the permanent canine is malpositioned over half the mesiodistal width of the root of the permanent lateral incisor, the primary canine should be removed.

The **curve of Spee** can affect arch perimeter needs. If one levels the curve in the lower arch, the mandibular incisors can be advanced to alter the mandibular arch discrepancy. The average of the left and right curves (molar-incisor line usually to depth of premolar) plus 1/2 mm measures the negative effect on arch perimeter. The reverse curve of Spee should not be considered an excess in leveling. This mandibular reverse curve is rare and is usually seen in openbite malocclusions. One usually does not level the arches in openbites.

Molar relation correction is the effect calculated if one corrected the permanent first molar relationship only in the lower arch. This is seldom the case. If the permanent first molars are bilaterally Class I, there is no correction for molar relation. If the permanent first molars are end-to-end on one side, a measurement is made from the mesiobuccal cusp tip of the maxillary permanent first molar to the buccal groove of the mandibular permanent first molar with the casts together. That distance is usually two to four mm. The total of the left and right sides are combined and placed as the molar correction factor.

If the permanent first molars are Class II, the distance from maxillary permanent first molar cusp tip to mandibular permanent first molar buccal groove is measured in occlusion. It is usually five to six mm per one side, or 10 to 12 mm for both sides. The Class III molar relationship is usually only half the correction of a Class II at two to three mm per side, or four to six mm per arch. Class III molar correction should not be labeled as excess. Class II molar correction, or an end to end molar relationship, should be labeled as a deficient mandibular arch problem if the problem is treated in the lower arch.

Relation of the lower incisor, or cephalometric correction factor, is an important consideration for the position of the lower incisor and its effect on lower **arch perimeter** and **arch length**. If one retracts the lower incisors orthodontically, the arch length is decreased. If one advances the lower incisors orthodontically, the arch length is increased. One may use the facial plane (N-Pog line) or **mandibular plane** (FMA) to determine this value. The classic ratio was for first premolar extractions and standard edgewise-orthodontic therapy, with one degree retraction in lower incisor position decreasing 0.8 mm of arch length. However, there is little change in non-extraction cases (1 degree of change effects only 0.2 mm arch length), and there are different results depending on second premolar removal (0 degrees to 5.0 mm) and first premolar removal (1 degree to 4.0 mm). Relocation of the lower incisor has high variability and allows greater differences among different orthodontists than from almost any other factor in diagnosis and treatment.

6. THE ORTHODONTIC DIAGNOSIS

Age, gender, and ethnicity enable one to more accurately place a patient's findings in the correct reference position. The history and chief complaint, along with the pertinent clinical and radiographic documentation, supplemented with the study models and photographs allows one to identify a problem oriented list in the diagnosis. Figure 11-6 presents a form for orthodontic diagnosis, treatment plan, prognosis, and records. The classification of the malocclusion need not only be intraoral with cast/arch analysis, but also extraoral (sagittal/vertical with transverse). Classification helps in clarification of treatment. Class II division 2 cases are classic non-extraction, growth-timed treatments. Most Class III cases are non-extraction cases. Crowding is associated with Class I cases. One treats to the face, and its analysis is essential in proper treatment planning.

STUDENT NAME _____   PATIENT NAME _____
INSTRUCTOR S SIGNATURE _____   DATE OF SIGNED TREATMENT PLAN _____
PATIENT AGE: ____YRS ____MOS   SEX: ____MALE ____FEMALE   RACE: _____   HEIGHT_____ HT. CENTILE _____

ORTHODONTIC DIAGNOSIS

CHIEF COMPLAINT:

HISTORY:

CLINICAL FINDINGS:

RADIOGRAPHIC FINDINGS:

CEPHALOMETRIC ANALYSIS: FACIAL ANGLE:____ ANB:_____ FMA:_____ IMPA:_____ /1A to POG:_____
                         OTHER:

CAST ANALYSIS:

ARCH ANALYSIS:

CLASSIFICATION OF THE FACE AND OCCLUSION:

ORTHODONTIC TREATMENT PLAN AND PROGNOSIS

TREATMENT OBJECTIVES   TREATMENT PLAN INCLUDING ALTERNATIVES

SEQUENCE OF FIRST SIX APPOINTMENTS   ESTIMATED TREATMENT TIME WITH ANY RE-EVALUATION AND
                                         THE PROGNOSIS WITH ANY APPLIANCES

ORTHODONTIC RECORDS

	Date	Date	Date	Date	Date	Date
A. STUDY MODELS						
B. PANORAMIC RADIOGRAPHS						
C. INTRAORAL PA RADIOGRAPHS						
D. LATERAL CEPHALOGRAM						
E. P-A CEPHALOGRAM						
F. PHOTOGRAPHS						
G. HEIGHT						
H. OTHER						

Figure 11-6: Orthodontic Diagnosis, Treatment Plan, Prognosis, and Records

The objective of treatment needs to be stated, as well as alternate treatment plans. There is seldom one treatment plan from the same database. Alternate plans need to be presented to the child or adolescent along with the parents. Rationale for one plan as compared to another needs presentation.

The sequence of the first six appointments includes case presentation, tooth separation for posterior banding (one week prior to banding), and prescription for tooth removal (use names of teeth primarily with supplemental tooth numbers). Most fixed active orthodontic appliances are seen monthly, but removable ones may be monitored at two week to six week intervals, depending upon the plan. Passive orthodontic holding appliances can sometimes become active, so a schedule at four month intervals might be reasonable. Fixed mandibular lingual arches that are not heat-treated may create bilateral **posterior crossbites** that have an **iatrogenic etiology**.

Estimated treatment time is important with a determation of prognosis. **Interceptive orthodontic treatment** for children, i.e., crossbites or openbites, should be no more than one year. Sometimes, with crossbites, four to six months. Retention periods need to be built into the time considerations. Adjunctive orthodontic procedures for adult patients, i.e., molar uprighting, should be about one year or less, but no more than 18 months. Preventive orthodontics that uses lower fixed lingual arches or upper Nance holding arches are long range treatments. Because of this, primary second molar lingual arches should be considered as the initial holding appliance, followed by the permanent first molar design at a time closer to mandibular primary second molar exfoliation. First phase corrective orthodontics should be limited to 12 to 18 months. Adolescent corrective orthodontics should be closer to 24 months, while adult corrective orthodontic cases should take six to 12 months longer. Adult orthognathic surgery cases are supposed to have a shorter period of time than regular adult corrective orthodontic cases.

It is important to develop the habit of re-evaluating an orthodontic case every time the patient is seen in follow-up. This is particularly true for active tooth movement. One should re-diagnose the case each time the patient returns. If one does not meet specific goals at specific times, one should address where the problem is. Is it the treatment mechanics? Is it cooperation? Is it the diagnosis? The concept of chaos is important here. It has come from observations of the weather. It means that slight changes along the way can give different results over time. Therefore, one must re-evaluate at each step. The concept of chaos is used at regular intervals by persons who do orthodontics.

After treatment is completed, follow-up records and evaluation are needed to reflect on changes from the original diagnosis and the treatment so one can improve one's diagnostic acumen. It is a life-long process.

7. SUGGESTED READING

INTRODUCTION

Ackerman JL, Proffit WR: The Characteristics of Malocclusion: A Modern Approach to Classification and Diagnosis. Am J Orthod 1969; 56:443-454.

Andrews LF: The Six Keys to Normal Occlusion. Am J Orthod 1972; 62:296-309.

Angle EH: Classification of Malocclusion. Dental Cosmos 1899; 41:248-264, 350-357.

Angle EH: Treatment of Malocclusion of The Teeth, Angle's System, 7th Edition, Philadelphia, SS White Co., 1907.

Heikinheimo K, Salmi K, Myllarniemi S: Long Term Evaluation of Orthodontic Diagnosis Made at the Ages of 7 and 10 Years. Eur J Orthop 1987; 9:151-159.

Otuyemi OD, Jones SP: Methods of Assessing and Grading Malocclusion: A Review. Aust Orthod J 1995; 14:21-27.

Proffit WR, Ackerman JL: Rating the Characteristics of Malocclusion: A Systematic Approach For Planning Treatment. Am J Orthod 1973; 64(3):258-269.

Sheats RD, McGorray SP, Keeling SD Wheeler TT, King GJ; Occlusal Traits and Perception of Orthodontic Need in Eighth Grade Students. Angle Orthod 1998; 68(2):107-114.

Tipton RT, Rinchase DJ: The Relationship Between Static Occlusion and Functional Occlusion in a Dental School Population: Angle Orthod 1990; 61:57-66.

Yang EY, Kiyak HA: Orthodontic Treatment Timing: A Survey of Orthodontists. Am J Orthod Dentofac Orthop 1998; 113:96-103.

Wagenberg BD: Periodontal Preparation of the Adult Patient Prior to Orthodontics. Dent Clin North Am 1988; 32:457-480.

Wolsky SL, McNamara JA: Orthodontic Services Provided By General Dentists. Am J Orthod Dentofac Orthop 1996; 110:211-217.

CLINICAL EXAM

Hintze H., Wenzel A., Williams S: Diagnostic Value of Clinical Examination for the Identification of Children in Need of Orthodontic Treatment Compared with Clinical Examination and Screening Pantomography. Eur J Orthod 1990; 12:385-388.

Wallen T, Bloomquist D: The Clinical Examination: Is It More Important than Cephalometric Analysis in Surgical Orthodontics? Int J Adult Orthod Orthognath Surg 1986; 3:179-181.

THE FACE

Ackerman JL, Proffit: Soft Tissue Limitations in Orthodontics: Treatment Planning Guidelines. Angle Orthod 1997: 67(5):327-336.

Arnett GW, Bergman RT: Facial Keys to Orthodontic Diagnosis and Treatment Planning. Part I. Am J Orthod Dentofac Orthop 1993: 103:299-312.

Bishara SE, Burkey PS, Kharouf JG: Dental and Facial Asymmetries: A Review. Angle Orthod 1994; 64(2):89-98.

Blanchette ME, Nanda RS, Currier GF, Ghosh J: Longitudinal Growth Study of Soft Tissue Facial Profile of Short and Long Face Subjects. Am J Ortho Dentofac Orthop 1996; 109(2): 116-131.

Czarnecki ST, Nanda RS, Currier GF: Perceptions of a Balanced Facial Profile. Am J Orthod Dentofac Orthop 1993; 104:108-187.

Formby WA, Nanda RS, Currier GF: Longitudinal Changes in the Adult Facial Profile. Am J Orthod Dentofac Orthop 1994; 105:464-476.

Lyndstrom A, Lyndstrom F, Lebret LM, Moorrees LF: Natural Head Position and Natural Head Orientation: Basic Considerations in Cephalometric Analysis. Eur J Orthod 1995; 17:111-120.

Michiels G, Sather AH: Validity and Reliability of Facial Profile Evaluation in Vertical and Horizontal Dimensions from Lateral Photographs. Int J Adult Orthod Orthognath Surg 1994; 9:43-54.

Strauss RA, Weis BD,. Lindauer SJ, Rebellatro J, Isaacson RJ: Variability of Facial Photographs for Use in Treatment Planning for Orthodontics and Orthognathic Surgery. Int J Adult Orthod Orthognath Surg 1997; 12:197-203.

THE ARCHES

Bimstein E, Machtei E, Becker A: The Attached Gingiva in Children: Diagnostic, Developmental and Orthodontic Considerations for Its Treatment. J Dent Child 1988; 55:351-356.

Bishara SE, Staley RN: Mixed-Dentition Mandibular Arch Length Analysis: a Step-by-Step Approach Using the Revised Hixon and Oldfather Prediction Method. Am J Ortho 1884; 86:130-135.

Bolton WA: The Clinical Application of a Tooth-Size Analysis. Am J Orthod 1962; 48:504-529.

Edwards JC: The Diastema, the Frenum, the Frenectomy: a Clinical Study. Am J Orthod 1977; 71:489-508.

Fanning EA: Effect of Extraction of Deciduous Molars on the Formation and Eruption of Their Successors. Angle Orthod 1962; 32:44-53.

Gianelly AA: Leeway Space and the Resolution of Crowding in the Mixed Dentition. Sem Orthod 1995; 1:188-194.

Godney E: Studies of the Eruption of the Permanent Teeth. III. Connections Between the Shedding of the Deciduous and the Eruption of the Succedaneous Teeth. Acta Genet 1952; 3:249-261.

Gron AM: Prediction of Tooth Emergence. J Dent Res 1962; 41:573-585.

Harris EF, Hassankiadeh S, Harris JT: Maxillary Incisor Crown-Root Relationships in Different Angle Malocclusions. Am J Orthod Dentofac Orthop 1993; 103:48-53.

Hixon EH, Oldfather RE: Estimation of the Sizes of Unerupted Cuspid and Bicuspid Teeth. Angle Orthod 1958; 28(4):236-240.

Hotz RP: Guidance of Eruption Versus Serial Extraction. Am J Orthod 1970; 58:1-20.

Hurd AG, Currier GF: Space Analysis and Prediction in the Transitional Dentition. J Dent Res 1998; 77: 267.

Lo RT, Moyers RE: Studies in the Etiology and Prevention of Malocclusion. I. The Sequence of the Permanent Dentition. Am J Orthod 1953; 39:460-467.

Mass E, Sarnat H: Single Maxillary Central Incisors in the Midline. J Dent Child 1991; 58:413-416.

Moorrees, CFA, Gron A-M, Lebret LM, Yen PKJ, Frohlich FJ: Growth Study of the Dentition: A Review. Am J Orthod 1969; 55:600-616.

Nowlin R, Currier GF: Criteria for Premolar Extraction in Orthodontics. J Dent Res 1999; 78:197.

Staley RN, Kerber RE: A Revision of the Hixon and Oldfather Mixed-Dentition Prediction Method. Am J Orthod 1980; 78:296-302.

Tanaka MM, Johnston LE: The Prediction of the Size of Unerupted Canines and Premolars in a Contemporary Orthodontic Population. J Am Dent Assoc 1974; 88(4):798-801.

ANOMALIES

Beiderman W: Etiology and Treatment of Tooth Ankylosis. Am J Orthod 1962; 48: 670-684.

Dahlberg AA: Concepts of Occlusion in Physical Anthropology and Comparative Anatomy. J Am Dent Assoc 1953; 46:530-535.

Primosch R: Anterior Supernumerary Teeth-Assessment and Surgical Intervention in Children. Pediatr Dent 1981; 3:204-215.

Teel TT, Henderson HZ. Ectopic Eruption of First Permanent Molars. J Dent Child 1989; 56:467-470.

Thuer U, Kuster R, Ingeruall B: A Comparison Between Anamnestic, Rhio Manometric and Radiographic Methods of Diagnosing Mouth-Breathing. Eup J Orthop 1989; 11:161-168.

Wyatt WN, Currier GF: Incidence and Treatment for Congenitally Absent Permanent Teeth. J Den Res 2000; 79:241.

TRANVERSE

Adkins M, Nanda RS, Currier GF: Arch Perimeter Changes upon Rapid Palatal Expansion. Am J Orthop Dentofac Orthop 1990; 97(3):194-199.

Jerrold L, Lowenstein LJ: The Midline: Diagnosis and Treatment. Am J Orthod Dentofac Orthod 1990l 97:453-462.

Osborn WS, Nanda RS, Currier GF: Mandibular Arch Perimeter Changes with Lip Bumper. Am J Orthod Dentofac Orthoped 1991; 99(6): 527-532.

OPENBITES

Brackett RL, Currier GF: Incidence and Treatment of Openbite Malocclusion in Two Orthodontic Populations. J Den Res 2000; 79:501.

Currier GF: The Smile, The Vertical, and Time. J SE Soc Ped Dent 1999; 5(3):36-39.

Nielsen IL: Vertical Malocclusions: Etiology, Development, Diagnosis and Some Aspects of Treatment. Angle Orthod 1991; 61(4):247-260.

Richardson A: A Classification of Openbites. Eur J Orthod 1981; 3(4):289-296.

Subtelny JD, Sakuda M: Openbite: Diagnosis and Treatment. Am J Orthod 1964; 50:337-358.

PANORAMIC RADIOGRAPHS

Ferguson JW, Evans PIW, Cheng LHH: Diagnostic Accuracy and Observer Performance in the Diagnosis of Abnormalities in the Anterior Maxilla: A Comparison of Panoramic with Intraoral Radiography. Brit Dent J 1992; 173-265-271.

Lindauer SJ, Rubinstein LK, Hang WM, Anderson WL, Isaacson RJ: Canine Impaction Identified Early with Panoramic Radiographs. J Am Dent Assoc 1992; 123:91-97.

Neal JJD, Bowden PEJ: The Diagnostic Value of Panoramic Radiographs in Children Aged Nine to Ten Years. Brit J Orthod 1988; 15: 193-197.

Revels MJ, Currier GF: Anterior Linear and Archial Analysis of Bitemark Identification. J Dent Res 2000; 79:500.

CEPHALOMETRICS

Altemus LW: A Comparison of Cephalometric Relationships. Ange Orthod 1960; 30:223-240.

Broadbent BH Sr, Broadbent BH Jr, and Golden WH: Bolton Standards of Dentofacial Developmental Growth. St Louis, Mosby, 1975.

Downs WB: Variation in Facial Relationships: Their Significance in Treatment and Prognosis. Am J Ortho 1948; 34:812-840.

Higley LB: Cephalometric Standards for Children 4 to 8 years of Age. Am J Orthod 1955; 40:51-59.

Hurmeriintra K, Rahkamo A, Haavikko K: Comparison between Cephalometric Classification Methods For Sagittal Jaw Relationships. Eur J Oral Sc 1997; 105:221-227.

Jacobson A: The "Wits" Appraisal of Jaw Disharmony. Am J Orthod 1975; 67:125-138.

Lyndstrom F, Lyndstrom A: Natural Head Position as a Basis for Cephalometric Analysis. Am J Orthod Dentofac Orthop 1992; 101:244-247.

Nanda RS: The Rates of Growth of Several Facial Components Measured from Serial Cephalometric Roentgenograms. Am J Orthod 1955; 41:658-673.

Riedel RA: An Analysis of Dentofacial Relationship. Am J Orthod 1957; 43:103-119.

Riolo ML et al.: An Atlas of Craniofacial Growth: Cephalometric Standards From The University School Growth Study. Ann Arbor, Michigan. University of Michigan Center for Human Growth and Development, 1974.

Riolo ML, Brandt DJ, TenHave TR. Associations between features of occlusion and signs and symptoms of TMJ dysfunction in children and young adults. Am J of Orthod 1987;92:467-477.

Snodell SF, Nanda RS, Currier GF: A Longitudinal Cephalometric Study of Transverse and Vertical Craniofacial Growth. Am J Orthod Dentofac Orthop 1993; 104:471-483.

Steiner CC: The Use of Cephalometrics as an Aid to Planning and Assessing Orthodontic Treatment. Am J Orthod 1960; 46:721-735.

Tweed CH: The Frankfort-Mandibular Incisor Angle (FMIA) in Orthodontic. Diagnosis, Treatment Planning and Prognosis. Angle Orthod 1954; 24:121-169.

CASTS

Du SQ, Rinchuse DJ, Zullo TG, Rinchuse DJ. Reliability of Three Methods of Occlusion Classification. Am J Orthod Dentofac Orthop 1998; 113:463-470.

Katz MI: Angle Classification Revised 2: A Modified Angle Classification. Am J Orthod Dentofac Orthop 1992; 102:277-284.

Shaw WC, Richmond S, O'Brien: The Use of Occlusal Indices: A European Perspective. Am J Orthod Dentofac Orthop 1995; 107:1-10.

Turner SAM: Occlusal Indices Revised. Brit J Orthod 1990; 17: 197-203.

Younis JW, Vig KWL, Rinchuse DJ, Weyant RJ: A Validation Study of Three Indexes of Orthodontic Treatment Need in the United States. Community Dent Oral Epidemiol 1997; 25:358-362.

DIAGNOSIS

Alexander SA: Diagnosis and Treatment Planning in Orthodontics. Current Opin Dent 1992; 2:9-13.

Bajada SB: Differential Diagnosis in Orthodontics. Aust Ortho J 1994; 13(3): 193-194.

Cisneros GJ: Diagnosis and Treatment Planning in Orthodontics. Current Opin Dent 1991; 1:595-597.

Hammond RS, Freer TJ: Application of a Case-Based Expert System to Orthodontic Diagnosis and Treatment Planning. Aust Dent J 1997; 14(4):229-234.

Gottlieb EL, Nelson H, Vogels DS: 1986 JCO Study of Orthodontic Diagnosis and Treatment Procedures. Part 2 Selected Breakdowns. J Clin Orthod 1986; 20(10):694-709.

Gottlieb EL, Nelson AH, Vogels DS: 1990 JCO Study of Orthodontic Diagnosis and Treatment Procedures. Part 1 Results and Trends. J Clin Orthod 1991; 25(3):145-156.

Merrified LL, Klontz HA, Vaden JL: Differential Diagnostic Analysis System. Am J Orthod Dentofac Orthop 1994; 106:641-648.

Ngan P, Fields H: Orthodontic Diagnosis and Treatment Planning in the Primary Dentition. J Dent Child 1995; 62(1):25-33.

Riolo ML, Brandt DJ, Tenhave TR. Etiologic role of occlusion in children: Associations between features of occlusion and signs and symptoms of TMJ dysfunction in children and young adults. TMJ 1998;6(1):6.

Riolo ML, TenHave TR, Clinical Validity of the Relationship between TMJ Signs and Symptoms in Children and Youth. Journal of Dent Child 1988;55(2):110-113.

Sarver DM, Weissman SM, Johnston MW: Diagnosis and Treatment Planning of Hypodivergent Skeletal Pattern with Clockwise Occlusal Plane Rotation. Int J Adult Orthod Orthognath Surg 1993; 8(2):113-121.

Vaden JL, Kiser HE: Straight Talk About Extraction and Non-Extraction: A Differential Diagnostic Decision. Am J Ortho Dentofac Orthop 1996: 109:445-452.

Vig KD, Ellis E: Diagnosis and Treatment Planning for the Surgical-Orthodontic Patient. Dent Clin North Am 1990; 34(2):361-384.

CHAPTER 12

Section I	Section II	Section III	Section IV
1. Developmental, Psychosocial, Behavioral, and Compliance Aspects of Care 2. Prenatal Craniofacial Growth 3. Postnatal Caniofacial Growth 4. Growth of the Craniofacial Skeleton 5. Development of the Dentition and Occlusion	6. Classification and Terminology 7. Etiology of Malocclusion 8. Force Systems and Tissue Response 9. Tissue Engineering in Orthodontics 10. Clinical Epidemiology and Malocclusion	11. Orthodontic Exam and Diagnosis 12. Analysis of Orofacial and Jaw Musculature 13. Analysis of Dentition and Occlusion 14. Dental Dysmorphogenesis 15. Analysis of Orofacial Skeleton 16. Planning Orthodontic Treatment	17. Preadolescent Treatment 18. Adolescent Treatment 19. Adult Treatment 20. Treatment of Patients with Craniofacial Anomalies 21. Retention, Relapse and the Recurrence of Malocclusion 22. The Adverse Effects of Orthodontic Treatment

TMD and Related Pain Conditions: The Orthodontic Perspective

Christian S. Stohler

1. INTRODUCTION

Painful conditions affecting the temporomandibular joint (TMJ) and the muscles of mastication are encountered in combination with planned, ongoing or recently completed orthodontic treatment. Because these conditions can be observed in the context of orthodontic consultation and therapy, appropriate diagnostic and management competencies are required. The clinical scenarios can be challenging and advanced understanding of these pain conditions is useful.

In the case of planned orthodontic treatment, the question arises whether an existing jaw condition constitutes a contraindication for orthodontic treatment. The patient may also want to undergo orthodontic therapy in the hope that alignment of teeth and/or jaws may resolve craniofacial pain and jaw dysfunction. If jaw pain develops during orthodontic treatment, the orthodontist must determine what actions are to be taken with respect to pain and jaw dysfunction and whether the condition has any bearing on the delivery of orthodontic therapy. The experience of pain often raises questions in the patient's mind regarding the rendered care. In case craniofacial pain and jaw dysfunction occur after completion of orthodontic treatment, the provider is often faced with the question whether there is a connection between those symptoms and the recently completed orthodontic therapy. This chapter is intended to provide the conceptual framework in support of clinical decision-making and actions for scenarios encountered in orthodontic practice.

What Are the Clinical Conditions Referred to as TMD?

The clinical presentations referred to as temporomandibular disorders (TMD) embrace a family of musculoskeletal conditions with common craniofacial signs and symptoms. In this respect, TMD should be understood as a collective term for a number of clinical manifestations associated with the TMJ and adjacent musculoskeletal tissues, rather than a specific diagnostic label. These conditions are considered as a major source of non-dental pain in the craniofacial complex. They are identified by clinically observable attributes. At this time, there are no established biomarkers of exposure or effect that would permit valid and reliable case ascertainment. Given this situation, it should not be surprising that prevalence figures depend on the employed TMD case definition.

Jaw ache or pain constitutes the chief complaint of all forms of TMD with the corresponding pain sensation being frequently characterized by words, such as "aching", "tight", "throbbing" and "tender" (Turp, Kowalski, et al., 1997). Pain, the most prominent symptom linked to these musculoskeletal conditions, is not always accompanied by visible trauma and/or disease. In fact, TMD pain ranges from an early response to simple injury to complaints of persistent, localized to regional and even widespread involvement without obvious cause. Most people with TMD have relatively mild forms, but not insignificant numbers must endure more persistent and even debilitating TMD pain. As for many pain conditions other than TMD, the personally most devastating and clinically most challenging forms occur in females in much greater number than males (Unruh, 1996).

Besides TMD pain, (1) inability to freely move the jaw due to pain and soft or hard tissue interference, (2) sounds originating from the jaw joint, and (3) the disturbing perception of teeth not meeting properly represent the other shared concerns of TMD patients. Among the clinically observable TMD signs, the presence of pressure allodynia constitutes the hallmark feature of all forms of TMD. Pressure allodynia, the experience of pain in response to pressure that is not painful for healthy subjects when subjected to palpation pressures applied to matched tissues, is observed in regions within which TMD patients experience pain. Inability to move the jaw freely is quantified by measurements of the mandibular range of motion and expressed by maximum left and right excursive mandibular movements, and maximum protrusion and mouth opening capacity. Joint sounds are often linked to mechanical events between moving articular structures, such as the temporal component of the TMJ, the **articular disc** and the **condyle**.

It is important to note that all present TMD taxonomies place emphasis on these types of clinically recorded signs and symptoms rather than on etiologic and/or pathogenetic factors, including the use of suitable biomarkers. From a taxonomy point of view, different diagnostic TMD subsets are delineated with case distinctions being based on the anatomical substrate believed to generate clinically observable signs and symptoms. To standardize diagnosis, the National Institute of Dental and Craniofacial Research (NIDCR), headed by the Pain Research Group at the University of Washington, has sponsored the development of a comprehensive taxonomy for TMD (Dworkin and LeResche, 1992). Using the Research Diagnostic Criteria for TMD (RDC/TMD), members of the TMD family can be distinguished with respect to three major subsets: Group I. Masticatory **myofascial** pain, Group II. TMJ internal derangements, and Group III. TMJ arthritides (Figure 12-1).

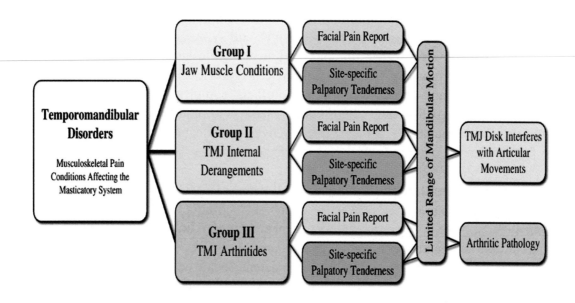

Figure 12-1: TMD family members as defined by the Research Diagnostic Criteria for TMD (RDC/TMD). Pain, palpatory tenderness and impaired range of mandibular motion constitute the case-defining attributes. Impaired range of motion is attributed to limitation caused by muscle and/or articular obstruction. The reader is encouraged to study the original reference for essential detail regarding the examination and diagnosis of TMD (Dworkin and LeResche, 1992).

Evidence-based and, in case of insufficient data complemented by experts' consensus, the RDC/TMD diagnostic system permits the classification of major TMD subtypes, allows assignment of several diagnoses to a single case, exhibits features that are useful for epidemiological description and research, and demonstrates properties in support of the inexperienced practitioner having to define the care requirements of a particular TMD patient. Given the importance of this work for the TMD field, the reader should review this key reference for understanding of the RDC/TMD construct, including its history and examination forms and related specifications (Dworkin and LeResche, 1992).

Although other taxonomies are in use, the RDC/TMD are considered superior over other classification systems in terms of many methodological and clinical considerations (Ohrbach and Stohler, 1992). An important feature of this classification system is its unique dual axes construct. While Axis I distinguishes the three major TMD categories as defined above, Axis II criteria serve to assess pain intensity, pain-related disability, and emotional symptoms linked to pain. Application of this dual-axes diagnostic system has solidified the understanding that more than one Axis I diagnosis is often applicable in a given case, that Axis I conditions are not necessarily stable over time, and that significant variation exists with respect to Axis II findings, even within a given Axis I diagnostic subset (LeResche, Dworkin, et al., 1991; Truelove, Sommers, et al., 1992;Huggins, Dworkin, et al., 1996; List and Dworkin, 1996; Ohrbach and Dworkin, 1998).

2. TMD SEVERITY, CHRONICITY AND COMPLEXITY

With case severity, chronicity and complexity being critical factors in decision-making when faced with TMD, their assessment constitutes a clinical necessity. Severe pain intensity has implications on the extent to which treatment is pursued. Chronicity, including the lack of favorable response to previous interventions, is suggestive of a required treatment focus broader than the alignment of teeth and/or jaws. Finally, the presence of co-morbid conditions determines in major ways the care setting within which treatment is offered to a given TMD patient. Comorbid health issues of advanced TMD cases consist of sleep disturbances, cardiovascular, gastrointestinal and reproductive system complaints, weight loss or weight gain, swelling, numbness, sweating and flushing, and concerns regarding loss of libido, drive, attention and memory.

In most cases encountered in orthodontic practice, TMD symptoms represent a transient nuisance. On occasion, however, acute complaints can be so severe that they require immediate action. There also exists a smaller case subset in which pain persistence and the impact of comorbid conditions significantly influence the life of the affected patient. This type of patient, in the search for cures, may seek advice and/or help from the orthodontist because of desperation that nothing short of the alignment of teeth and/or jaws may be able to provide relief.

Although shared case features within a single anatomical complex, such as the craniofacial complex, support diagnostic taxonomies and ease communication among concerned clinicians, it needs to be recognized that critical pieces of information regarding comorbid pains that are observed outside the region of interest are often missed. Indeed, TMD pain is not always limited to the face, and individual TMD pain distributions fall into one of three case clusters based on involvement of (a) trigeminal dermatomes (V_{1-3}), (b) trigeminal and upper cervical (C_{2-6}) dermatomes, and (c) pain sites in addition to the ones listed above (Figure 12-2).

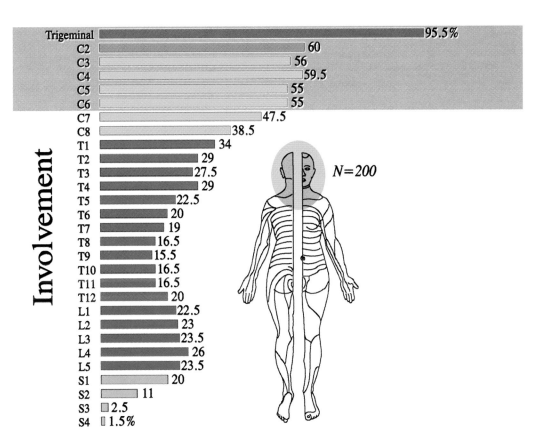

Figure 12-2: Likelihood of pain involvement outside the trigeminal dermatomes as reported by 200 patients encountered in an academic referral center. (Adapted after Turp, Kowalski, et al., 1998a).

Pain conditions that are observed in combination with TMD include systemic arthritides, headache, regional myofascial pain involving neck and shoulders, and widespread pain as seen in the fibromyalgia syndrome. TMJ arthritides can occur in isolation or be part of a systemic joint disease, such as juvenile rheumatoid arthritis (Figure 12-3). RDC/TMD Group I conditions, referred to as masticatory myofascial pain, are not always limited to the face (Krause, Tait, et al., 1989; Blasberg and Chalmers, 1989; Hagberg, 1991; Allerbring and Haegerstam, 1993; Hagberg, Hagberg, et al., 1994). Fibromyalgia, a clinical disorder that is characterized by pain on left and right sides of the body and pain above and below the waist for at least 3 months, and tenderness to 4 kilograms of pressure at 11 of 18 anatomically pre-defined body sites (Wolfe, Smythe, et al., 1990) can also affect the muscles of mastication in ways that such cases meet the diagnostic criteria of TMD. As far as the relationship of TMD and fibromyalgia is concerned, recent studies performed in academic referral centers have shown significant overlap between these pain conditions (Hedenberg-Magnusson, Ernberg, et al., 1997; Korszun, Papadopoulos, et al., 1998).

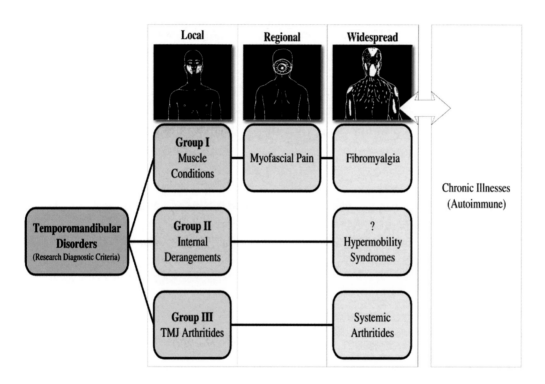

Figure 12-3: Overlap of TMD with diseases of regional and widespread pain involvement. Complex TMD cases can exhibit similar comorbid symptoms as reported by patients with autoimmune diseases.

Epidemiological studies also report a high **association** between TMD and tension-type headache and migraine headache (Agerberg and Carlsson, 1973). Because of this association, some authors went as far as considering headache part of the TMD symptom complex (Magnusson and Carlsson, 1980). Since these headaches exhibit peri-cranial tenderness, with greater frequency in tension-type headache than migraine headache cases (Forssell and Kangasniemi, 1984a; Forssell and Kangasniemi, 1984b), it becomes clear that the diagnostic boundaries between these headache types and TMD are not very distinct.

Pain severity, spread and impact, and the presence of co-morbid conditions vary considerably from case to case. Differences in treatment response of TMD cases encountered in different care settings also need to be emphasized. Between 65 to 95 per cent of patients with TMD, experiencing the condition for the first time, appear to improve with an array of therapies (Wessberg, Carroll, et al., 1981;

Magnusson and Carlsson, 1983; Okeson and Hayes, 1986; Wedel and Carlsson, 1986; Randolph, Greene, et al., 1990). On the other hand, patient pools encountered in academic referral centers comprise an overwhelming number of case histories, which exhibit a persistent condition that was not satisfactorily controlled by often more than one attempt (Turp, Kowalski, et al., 1998b).

Although physical features appear to be comparable between cases in primary and tertiary care settings with respect to case-defining physical attributes, differences concerning severity, persistence and impact exist between these patient pools. Also important is the fact that the proportion of women among TMD cases increases from community-based observations to primary and tertiary care settings with patient populations containing up to 90+% women in academic referral centers (Figure 12-4). Among women, prevalence rates are higher for subjects of reproductive age than subjects in post-menopausal years (Von Korff, Dworkin, et al., 1988;Von Korff, Wagner, et al., 1991). In children and pre-puberty adults, however, gender differences are not clear (Riolo, Brandt, et al., 1987; Pilley, Mohlin, et al., 1992).

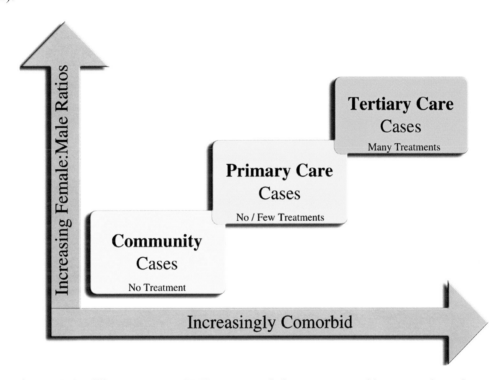

Figure 12-4: Differences among TMD case populations encountered in community, primary care and tertiary care settings with respect to gender distribution, the presence of comorbid complaints and the number of treatments received (Adapted after Stohler and Zarb, 1999).

3. TMD CAUSATION AND PATHOGENESIS

Although the literature is full of theories and speculations regarding causes of TMD, including many heated arguments about the role of the dental occlusion, it is reasonable to conclude that their exact causation has not been established yet. The confusion on this subject matter is compounded by reports and studies that employ very different diagnostic criteria and, not surprisingly, often reach opposite conclusions regarding the significance of presumed factors. Although the presumed relationship between occlusal disharmonies and TMD has been the cornerstone of traditional orthodontic thinking about these disorders, it has increasingly become clear that TMD problems constitute medical orthopedic conditions that have little to do with occlusal morphology or maxillo-mandibular relationships (Greene, 1988). Instead, it is now understood that alterations in the occlusion represent the effect of the disease and not its cause.

What appears to be increasingly clear is that the frequency of TMD cases is highest in the reproductive years, that women seem to be more susceptible, and that trauma appears to be a predisposing factor, at least in a subset of TMD cases. With respect to age, prevalence rates are lower among older subjects. Initial care-seeking in both men and women is more likely to occur before age 50 than later in life. Although less likely in later life, TMD can still occur in the elderly (Hiltunen, Schmidt-Kaunisaho, et al., 1995). This means that onset for the overwhelming case majority coincides with the time in life within which orthodontic treatment is administered. Prevalence rates are higher for women of reproductive age than in postmenopausal years (Von Korff, Dworkin, Le Resche, and Kruger, 1988; Von Korff, Wagner, Dworkin, and Saunders, 1991). The likelihood of seeking treatment for TMD increases by 77% with the use of supplemental estrogen in the postmenopausal years, or by 19% in subjects on oral contraceptives that were common in the late 80s and early 90s (LeResche, Saunders, et al., 1997). According to the 1989 National Health Interview Survey, prevalence rates for facial and jaw pain is 7% for Whites and 5% for Blacks that are not of Hispanic origin (Lipton, Ship, et al., 1993).

Although the sequence of events that leads to the development and persistence of TMD symptoms remains largely unknown, common attributes such as (1) tenderness to palpation, (2) limitation in mandibular range of motion, and (3) perceived and/or clinically manifest alteration in the dental occlusion can be explained by pain and/or structural changes linked to disease, such as loss of articular support (Figures 12-5, 12-6). Many TMD symptoms and signs have now been linked to basic processes, such as the sensitization of peripheral tissue, central neuroplasticity and sensitization in pro-nociceptive and anti-nociceptive systems, neuroendocrine and autonomic stress effects, and the consequences of pain on motor function, emotionality and cognition (Stohler, 1999).

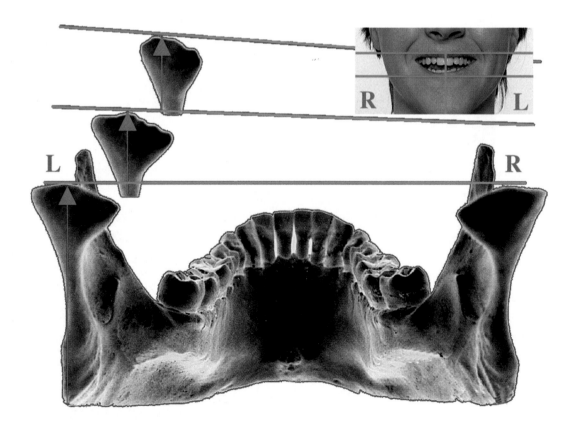

Figure 12-5: Loss of articular support results in changes of the plane of occlusion and frontal open bite.

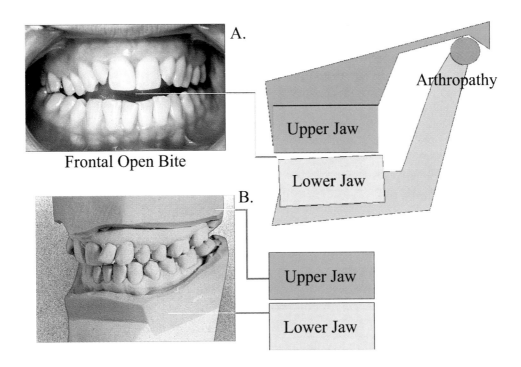

Figure 12-6: A.) Frontal open bite caused by loss of articular support. B.) Upper and lower casts, placed in maximum inter-cuspation, reflect the original intra-oral situation.

4. SPATIAL PAIN INVOLVEMENT AND GRADED CHRONIC PAIN STATUS

An integral part of good clinical practice involves the assessment of pain, including its spatial distribution. This includes the careful documentation of areas reported as painful within the regions covered by trigeminal and upper cervical dermatomes. The use of a template, similar to the one provided in Figure 12-7 is suggested.

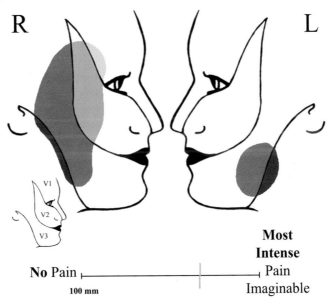

Figure 12-7: Template used to capture the spatial pain involvement in the craniofacial complex. Besides shading painful areas, patients are also asked to rate the present pain intensity on the visual-analog scale with endpoints marked as "no pain" and "most intense pain imaginable". Abbreviations V1, V2 and V3 denote the trigeminal dermatomes. R= Right, L= Left.

Patients with persisting and/or severely impacting TMD pain may want to undergo orthodontic therapy in the hope that alignment of teeth and/or jaws may resolve TMD pain and jaw dysfunction. In some, significant malocclusion is present that unmistakably would improve with orthodontic therapy. However, experience teaches that treatment of such cases has to focus on pain and that any consideration of orthodontic treatment has to be postponed until the status of the patient has improved.

The RDC/TMD history form provides the necessary questions to assess the Graded Chronic Pain Status, permitting the assignment of a severity grade to pain conditions lasting for 6 months or more (Von Korff, Ormel, et al., 1992). This type of assessment can help the practitioner to get important information in support of strategic decision-making, such as precluding Grade 3 and 4 cases from orthodontic treatment. Instead, such patients should receive appropriate pain management and respective referrals be initiated.

5. ASSESSMENT OF MECHANICAL ALLODYNIA

RDC/TMD specifications provide the basis for clinicians' training and calibration. With pain to palpation being a key component in TMD assessment, reliable and reproducible measurement is crucial. The examiner should keep in mind that diagnostic assignment is based on counts of pressure-pain reports at specified measurement sites that are clearly defined in the RDC/TMD. Because agreement of examiners is less likely to occur with the assessment of palpatory tenderness than range of mandibular motion, strict adherence to specifications is required. Assessment of intra-oral testing sites also tends to be even less reliable than extra-oral measurements (Dworkin and LeResche, 1992).

Examiners are instructed to press on specified muscle sites using the fingertips of the index and third fingers (or the spade-like pad of the distal phalanx of the index finger only) with 2 lbs. of pressure and with the muscle in a relaxed state. Similarly, 1 lb of pressure is applied to the lateral aspect of the TMJ. The patient is requested to indicate if the palpation pressure hurts or if he/she just feels pressure. If it hurts, he/she is asked to report whether the pressure-pain is mild, moderate or severe. During digital palpation, the opposite hand should brace the head to provide stability. To achieve greater accuracy in application of mechanical stimuli, pressure algometers are often employed in a research context (Figure 12-8).

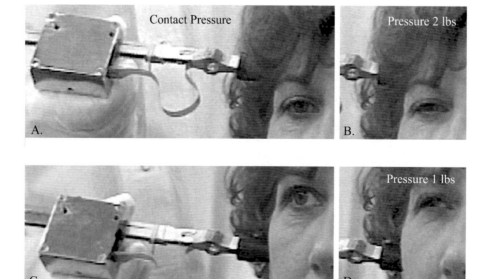

Figure 12-8: A.) and C.) Pressure algometer is applied to the skin overlying the anterior temporal muscle and the TMJ. B.) and D.) capture the subject's response at measurement pressures specified by the RDC/TMD.

6. FRAMEWORK FOR DECISION-MAKING

Because TMD conditions are observed in the context of orthodontic consultation and therapy, a framework for detection, diagnosis and action of this potential complicating condition should be adopted. This includes scenarios involving planned, ongoing or recently completed orthodontic therapy (Figure 12-9) (Collett and Stohler, 1994). The dismissal of past theories regarding the presumed relationship between occlusal disharmonies and TMD, once considered the cornerstone of traditional orthodontic thinking about these disorders, has fundamentally changed the interface between TMD and orthodontic practice. Therefore, orthodontists must discard past beliefs and practices, replacing them with modern understanding of musculoskeletal pain and pain-related dysfunction, in order to best serve their patients with TMD (Greene, 1988).

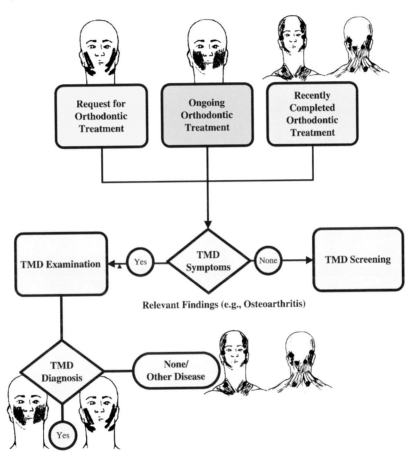

Figure 12-9: TMD screening and examination. When faced with symptoms that are suggestive of TMD, the patient should receive a comprehensive TMD examination as outlined in the RDC/TMD. Patients without complaints suggestive of TMD should be screened for TMD and those with signs of potential TMD should be subjected to a more elaborate examination as illustrated in the flowchart.

When active TMD is present, there is little justification for orthodontic treatment. On the other hand, previous TMD may have left the patient with significant malocclusion in need of correction for functional and/or esthetic reasons. Although orthodontic treatment does not cause TMD, it is possible that orthodontic therapy may act as an aggravating factor, or that TMD manifests by chance during orthodontic therapy. If TMD pain arises during orthodontic treatment, it is considered prudent to reduce and/or remove any extra-orally applied forces, such as those administered by **headgear** or chin-cap devices. Similarly, inter-arch wires may be reduced or removed (Collett and Stohler, 1994). If TMD symptomatology is encountered after recent completion of orthodontic therapy, TMD management should be administered (Figure 12-10).

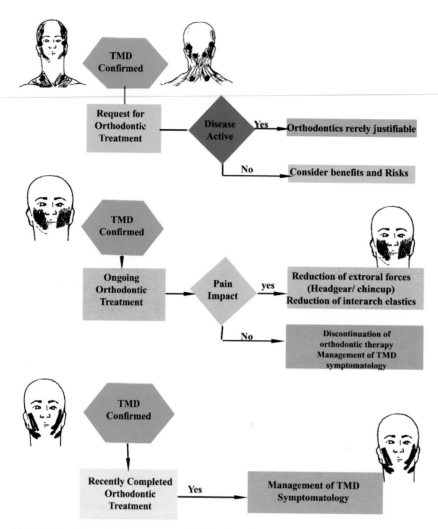

Figure 12-10: Decision tree in support of clinical actions.

7. SUMMARY

Painful conditions affecting the temporomandibular joint and the muscles of mastication are encountered in combination with planned, ongoing or recently completed orthodontic treatment. The clinical scenarios can be challenging and advanced understanding of these pain conditions is useful. These pain conditions are considered as a major source of non-dental pain in the craniofacial complex. Pain ranges from an early response to simple injury to complaints of persistent, localized to regional and even widespread involvement without obvious cause. Among all clinically observable signs, the presence of pressure allodynia constitutes the hallmark feature of all forms of temporomandibular disorders. Case severity, chronicity and complexity represent critical factors in decision-making and their assessment constitutes a clinical necessity. This chapter is intended to provide the conceptual framework in support of clinical decision-making and actions for scenarios encountered in orthodontic practice.

8. CONCLUSIONS

Because temporomandibular disorders can be encountered in the context of orthodontic consultation and therapy, appropriate diagnostic and management competencies are required. These diseases and disorders are characterized by pain, inability to freely move the jaw, joint sounds and the disturbing perception of teeth not meeting properly. Members of the TMD family are identified and distinguished with respect to particular TMD subsets and named according to the type of craniofacial structure explaining the clinical presentation. Because case severity, chronicity and complexity shape clinical decisions and actions, their assessment constitutes a clinical necessity.   Diagnostic assignment depends on the examiner's familiarity and adherence to the protocol accompanying the TMD diagnostic system. As for any medical/dental care, appropriate assessment and diagnosis constitutes the foundation for good clinical judgment and actions.

9. SUGGESTED READINGS

Agerberg G, and Carlsson GE. Functional disorders of the masticatory system. II. Symptoms in relation to impaired mobility of the mandible as judged from investigation by questionnaire. Acta Odontol.Scand 1973;31:337-347.

Allerbring M and Haegerstam G. Characteristics of patients with chronic idiopathic orofacial pain. A retrospective study. Acta Odontol.Scand 1993;51:53-58.

Blasberg B, and Chalmers A. Temporomandibular pain and dysfunction syndrome associated with generalized musculoskeletal pain: a retrospective study. J Rheumatol.Suppl 1989;19:87-90.

Collett T and Stohler CS. The orthodontic/TMD patient: review of the literature and an introduction to structured clinical decision making. Australian Orthodontic Journal 1994;13:188-193.

Dworkin SF and LeResche L. Research diagnostic criteria for temporomandibular disorders: review, criteria, examinations and specifications, critique, J Craniomandib.Disord, 6 (1992) 301-355.

Forssell,H. and Kangasniemi,P., Mandibular dysfunction in patients with migraine. Proc Finn Dent Soc 1984a;80217-222.

Forssell H and Kangasniemi P, Mandibular dysfunction in patients with muscle contraction headache. Proc Finn Dent Soc 1984b;80:211-216.

Greene CS. Orthodontics and temporomandibular disorders. Dental Clinics of North America 1988;32:529-538.

Hagberg C. General musculoskeletal complaints in a group of patients with craniomandibular disorders (CMD). A case control study. Swedish Dental Journal 1991;15:179-185.

Hagberg C, Hagberg M, and Kopp S. Musculoskeletal symptoms and psychosocial factors among patients with craniomandibular disorders. Acta Odontologica Scandinavica 1994;52:170-177.

Hedenberg-Magnusson B, Ernberg M, and Kopp S. Symptoms and signs of temporomandibular disorders in patients with fibromyalgia and local myalgia of the temporomandibular system. A comparative study Acta Odontologica Scandinavica 1997;55: 344-349.

Hiltunen K, Schmidt-Kaunisaho K, Nevalainen J, Narhi T, and Ainamo A. Prevalence of signs of temporomandibular disorders among elderly inhabitants of Helsinki, Finland. Acta Odontol.Scand 1995;53:20-23.

Huggins KH, Dworkin SF. Saunders K, Von Korff M, and Barlow W. Five-year course for temporomandibular disorders using RDC/TMD.   J Dent Res 75(Special Issue) 352. 1996. Ref Type: Abstract.

Korszun A, Papadopoulos E, Demitrack M, Engleberg C, and Crofford L. The relationship between temporomandibular disorders and stress-associated syndromes. Oral Surgery, Oral Medicine, Oral Pathology, Oral Radiology, & Endodontics, 1998:86:416-420.

Krause SJ, Tait RC, and Margolis RB. Pain distribution, intensity, and duration in patients with chronic pain. J Pain Symptom.Manage 1989;4:67-71.

LeResche L, Dworkin SF, Sommers EE, and Truelove EL. An epidemiologic evaluation of two diagnostic classification schemes for temporomandibular disorders. J.Prosthet.Dent 1991:65131-137.

LeResche L, Saunders K, Von KM, Barlow W, Dworkin, and SF, Use of exogenous hormones and risk of temporomandibular disorder pain. Pain 1997;69:153-160.

Lipton JA, Ship JA, and Larach-Robinson D. Estimated prevalence and distribution of reported orofacial pain in the United States. Journal of the American Dental Association 1993;124: 115-121.

List T, and Dworkin S F. Comparing TMD diagnoses and clinical findings at Swedish and US TMD centers using research diagnostic criteria for temporomandibular disorders. Journal of Orofacial Pain 1996;10:240-253.

Magnusson T, and Carlsson GE. Changes in recurrent headaches and mandibular dysfunction after various types of dental treatment. Acta Odontologica Scandinavica 1980;38:311-320.

Magnusson T and Carlsson GE. A 21/2-year follow-up of changes in headache and mandibular dysfunction after stomatognathic treatment. Journal of Prosthetic Dentistry 1983;49:398-402.

Ohrbach R, and Dworkin SF. Five-year outcomes in TMD: relationship of changes in pain to changes in physical and psychological variables. Pain 1998;74:315-326.

Ohrbach R, Stohler CS. Current diagnostic systems. In: S.F.Dworkin and L.LeResche (Eds.), Research Diagnostic Criteria for Temporomandibular Disorders: Review, Criteria, Examinations and Specifications Critique. J Craniomandibular Disorders: Facial Oral Pain 1992;6:307-317.

Okeson JP, and Hayes DK. Long-term results of treatment for temporomandibular disorders: an evaluation by patients. J Am.Dent Assoc 1986;112:473-478.

Pilley JR, Mohlin B, Shaw WC, and Kingdon A. A survey of craniomandibular disorders in 800 15-year-olds. A follow- up study of children with malocclusion. Eur J Orthod 1992:14:152-161.

Bandolph CS, Greene CS, Moretti R, Forbes D, and Perry HT. Conservative management of temporomandibular disorders: a posttreatment comparison between patients from a university clinic and from private practice. American Journal of Orthodontics & Dentofacial Orthopedics 1990;98:77-82.

Riolo ML, Brandt D, and TenHave R. Associations between occlusal characteristics and signs and symptoms of TMJ dysfunction in children and young adults. Am J Orthod Dentofacial Orthop 1987;92:467-477.

Stohler CS. Muscle-related temporomandibular disorders. Journal of Orofacial Pain 1999;13:273-284.

Stohler CS and Zarb GA. On the management of temporomandibular disorders: a plea for a low-tech, high-prudence therapeutic approach. Journal of Orofacial Pain 1999;13:255-261.

Truelove EL, Sommers EE, LeResche L, Dworkin SF, and Von Korff M. Clinical diagnostic criteria for TMD. New classification permits multiple diagnoses. J.Am.Dent.Assoc 1992;123:47-54.

Turp JC, Kowalski CJ, O'Leary TJ, and Stohler CS. Pain maps from facial pain patients indicate a broad pain geography. J Dent Res, 1998a;77:1465-1472.

Turp JC, Kowalski CJ, and Stohler CS. Pain descriptors characteristic of persistent facial pain. J Orofacial.Pain 1997;11: 285-290.

Turp JC, Kowalski CJ, and Stohler CS. Treatment-seeking patterns of facial pain patients: Many possibilities, limited satisfaction. J Orofacial.Pain 1998b;12:61-66.

Unruh AM. Gender variations in clinical pain experience. Pain 1996;65:123-167.

Von Korff M, Dworkin SF, Le Resche L, and KrugerA. An epidemiologic comparison of pain complaints. pain 1988;32:173-183.

Von Korff M, Ormel J, Keefe FJ, and Dworkin SF, Grading the severity of chronic pain 1992;50:133-149.

Von Korff M, Wagner EH, Dworkin SF, and Saunders K. Chronic pain and use of ambulatory health care, Psychosom.Med 1991;53:61-79.

Wedel A, and Carlsson GE. A four-year follow-up, by means of a questionnaire, of patients with functional disturbances of the masticatory system. Journal of Oral Rehabilitation 1986;13:105-113.

Wessberg GA, Carroll WL, Dinham R, and Wolford LM, Transcutaneous electrical stimulation as an adjunct in the management of myofascial pain-dysfunction syndrome. J Prosthet.Dent 1981;45:307-314.

Wolfe F, Smythe HA, Yunus MB, Bennett RM, Bombardier C, Goldenberg DL, Tugwell P, Campbell SM, Abeles M, Clark P, and et al. The American College of Rheumatology 1990 Criteria for the Classification of Fibromyalgia. Report of the Multicenter Criteria Committee Arthritis Rheum 1990;33:160-172.

CHAPTER 13

Analysis of the Dentition and Occlusion

Deborah Priestap
Michelle J. Thornberg
Michael L. Riolo

1. INTRODUCTION

"In every case of malocclusion presented for treatment, the importance of a thorough study and a correct diagnosis cannot be overestimated. Otherwise any plan of treatment will be very uncertain as to results; with all of its embarrassments."

Edward H Angle

Nothing is as fundamental to the specialty of orthodontics as the analysis of the dentition and the analysis of the occlusion. The very term "orthodontics" is defined in the Websters Dictionary as, "the branch of dentistry concerned with diagnosing, correcting, and preventing irregularities of the teeth and poor occlusion." The tooth sizes, shapes, and positions themselves and within their respective dental arches, the dental **arch form** and symmetry, and the inter-relationships of the dental arches and jaws all combine to create and define the occlusion. In order to facilitate any discussion of irregularities in the dentition or the occlusion, it is necessary to have a uniformly recognized standard for comparison. Hence, not only does the ideal dentition and occlusion need to be defined, but so too do the various anomalies involving the dentition and skeletal relationships, which ultimately result in a deviation from this ideal goal, thus necessitating orthodontic intervention.

As important to recognizing the various characteristics of the dentition and the skeletal components of occlusion is to the orthodontist, so too is our understanding of the various factors or reasons for problems pertaining to the occlusion. If the etiology of the malocclusion can be identified, orthodontic treatment strategies can be implemented to address and correct the particular problems, leading to optimal treatment results.

When assessing the dentition and the occlusion, the orthodontist must rely upon certain diagnostic tools that facilitate evaluation and aid in the treatment planning phase of patient care. Using the obtained diagnostic data, the clinician can then determine not only the problems contributing to the malocclusion, but also possibly gain some insight into the etiology of the malocclusion, thus leading to a treatment plan tailored by objective findings.

2. DIAGNOSTIC DATA

Perhaps the single most important component to a successful orthodontic result is the accurate compilation and subsequent assessment of the diagnostic records. From this data, the clinician hopes to gain the knowledge necessary to interpret a particular patient's malocclusion, define specific orthodontic objectives, and design an appropriate corrective treatment plan. When these records are systematically collected and thoroughly evaluated, the probability of a successful treatment result is enhanced.

Orthodontic diagnostic records and their interpretation target three basic areas of evaluation. They are:

1.) those designed to evaluate the individual teeth or intraoral tissues
2.) those designed to evaluate the occlusion
3.) those designed to evaluate the facial and skeletal balance

Typically, the orthodontic records that provide the basic data necessary for sound clinical judgments include photographs or digital images, study cast data, and the appropriate radiographic images. It should be said, however, that some clinicians prefer, and some situations dictate, further data to address a particular concern.

2.1 THE CLINICAL EXAM

In addition to the standard orthodontic record battery, a clinical exam and interview are equally essential to an accurate evaluation. From the clinical exam and interview, the orthodontist is able to assess the patient's speech, swallowing patterns, and TMJ status. Further information can be gained by exploring the chief complaint, attitude toward orthodontic treatment, and treatment goals and expectations. Many times standard records do not adequately reveal morphological and functional subtleties that can be detected very easily by the clinical exam.

Initially, the orthodontist will observe the patient's facial esthetics, profile, balance or proportionality, symmetry, soft tissue drape, lip posture, incisor prominence, skeletal/dental midline positions, and **smile line**. Speech, oral, and temporomandibular joint functions will also be evaluated to detect any irregularities that may complicate the treatment plan or affect the orthodontic outcome. This allows the orthodontist and the patient an opportunity to discuss alternative options and set realistic expectations prior to treatment initiation.

Following this, an intraoral exam will be conducted. This is done to evaluate such conditions as the status of the dentition (i.e., the presence of caries, enamel abnormalities, restorative history, wear patterns, etc.), developmental stage of the patient, and the number of teeth present. Additionally, the soft tissues and mucosa will be examined for any pathologies or evidence of ancillary habits, while the periodontium will be evaluated for evidence of disease or anomalies. Tongue size, shape, function, and posture will also be assessed, as will the general oral hygiene status of the individual.

2.2 DENTAL CASTS

Dental casts (Figure 13-1) are an important source of information for the orthodontist, so the time one devotes to them to obtain an accurate representation of the dental morphology and occlusal relationships is time well invested. A good three-dimensional representation of hard and soft tissues can show the alignment of the teeth, the alveolar processes, and the soft tissue morphology with exceptional detail. From the occlusal perspective, the **arch form** can be assessed, which is clinically very important to the orthodontist. One can also measure accurately the arch dimensions, arch asymmetries, dental alignment, palatal vault shape, tooth sizes, shapes, and rotations. When relating the casts in the usual occlusal position (as determined by a wax bite registration taken in **centric relation** occlusion), one can observe the occlusal relationships of all the teeth, the coincidence of the dental midlines, attachments of the frenula, the nature of the occlusal curve, eruptive anomalies, spacing requirements, and the rotations and inclinations of the teeth.

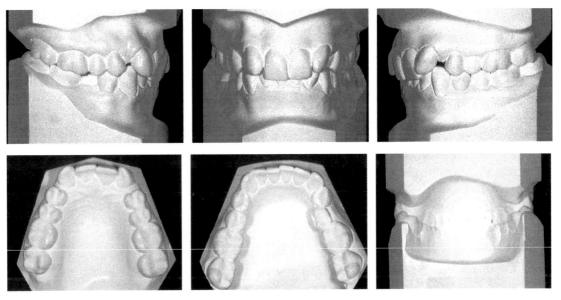

Figure 13-1

2.3 RADIOGRAPHIC IMAGES

Panoramic Radiographic Image

The panoramic radiographic image (Figure 13-2) is an essential orthodontic diagnostic tool that gives the clinician an overall view of not only the status of the dentition, but also any developmental anomalies associated with the dentition, pathological lesions, and gross periodontal and dentoalveolar conditions. Collectively, the patient's teeth can be related to pertinent growth standards, allowing the orthodontist to assess their developmental progress while visualizing the relationships of both dentitions, both jaws, and both temporomandibular joints simultaneously. Individual teeth can be compared to each other to identify any personal disharmonies. Additionally, the congenital absence of teeth, impactions, **supernumerary teeth**, and the stage of development can all be advantageously studied. One can also view the maxillary sinus region as well as the mandibular **condyle** for any evidence of abnormalities that would warrant further evaluation.

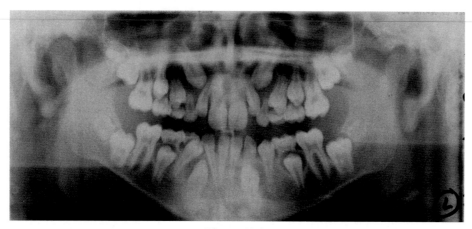

Figure 13-2

An added advantage of the panoramic radiographic image is that it requires less radiation than a full series of intraoral radiographs, whose specific detail is infrequently needed. When, however, situations necessitate closer examination, such as where there is evidence or suspicion of interproximal decay, **root resorption**, or periodontal disease, bitewing or periapical radiographs are an appropriate adjunct in addition to the panoramic radiograph for such detection.

Lateral Cephalometric Radiographic Image

As with the panoramic radiographic image, the lateral cephalometric radiographic image (Figure 13-3) is also a crucial diagnostic tool used by the orthodontic clinician. From this radiograph, the patient's craniofacial and dental relationships and proportions can be evaluated. Hence the anatomical basis for the malocclusion can frequently be determined from the information gained. Lateral cephalometric radiographic images allow the orthodontist to evaluate what role the major functional components of the face (the **cranial base**, the maxilla and the mandible, and the dentition) play in the presenting malocclusion. This is important because the positions of the jaws to the cranial base, the relationship of the jaws to each other, and the positions of the teeth all combine to create one's occlusion. When any of these components is not within an acceptable range, a malocclusion will result. The interplay of these relationships can best be determined with the

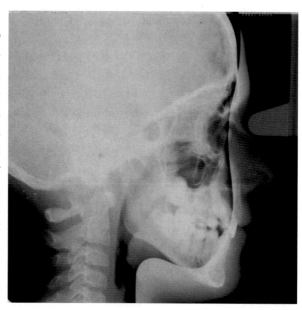

Figure 13-3

lateral cephalometric radiograph. No other diagnostic record allows one to effectively visualize all the parts of the whole as does the cephalometric radiographic image. It is not uncommon for the orthodontist to see two apparently similar malocclusions, as defined by the dental casts, which turn out to be two very different situations when evaluated with the lateral cephalogram.

In addition to establishing the initial craniofacial and dental components of a malocclusion, the lateral cephalometric radiographic image can be a dynamic tool that allows the clinician to monitor the skeletodental changes that can occur during or as a result of growth and development or orthodontic treatment. Thus, an individual patient's response to a particular treatment regime can be objectively assessed, verified, or altered as the situation dictates. Furthermore, long-term changes that occur following orthodontic treatment can be documented leading to improvements in the predictability of future orthodontic treatment results.

To quantify craniofacial and dental discrepancies, the orthodontist will measure well-defined radiographic landmarks and intersections between the bony components of the jaws to create reference points. Lines and angles are then drawn on an acetate page overlay of the cephalogram and measured to compare a particular patient to a previously developed standard that represents an ideal. This is called a **cephalometric analysis** (Figure 13-4). It should be remembered that there is not just one recognized or widely used cephalometric analysis. Doctors Tweed, Steiner, Downs, Bjork, Enlow, Sassouni, Harvold, Ricketts, and McNamara, to name a few, have all developed their own versions of cephalometric analyses which are used today. When making clinical decisions, many orthodontists will use more than one analysis in their evaluation, thus enhancing their understanding of a particular malocclusion.

Cephalometric analyses can be roughly categorized into two groups. The first group is comprised of those analyses that compare a patient to a specific set of ideal values. In doing so, the cephalometric analysis defines the patient's particular malocclusion, the ultimate treatment goal, and hence the direction of the orthodontic treatment plan. Examples of these include the Steiner and the Tweed cephalometric analyses. The second group of cephalometric analyses includes those designed to understand the etiology of a particular malocclusion, whether it is dentoalveolar, skeletal, or a combination of both, and the influences that the antero-posterior and vertical dimensions have upon it. These include the Bjork and the Downs cephalometric analyses.

In addition to allowing the quantitative measurements of a malocclusion via the **cephalometric analysis**, the lateral cephalometric radiographic image is also used for a predictive analysis of the skeletal and dental relationships, as well as profile changes following orthodontic or orthognathic surgical treatment. This predictive analysis is called a **Visual Treatment Objective** or **"VTO"** (Figure 13-5), and is used by the orthodontist to predict both antero-posterior and vertical changes that will occur as a result of changes in the denture bases and positions of the teeth. This is frequently useful when considering various treatment options and their subsequent outcomes.

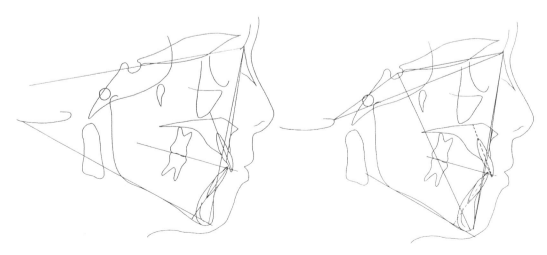

Figure 13-4

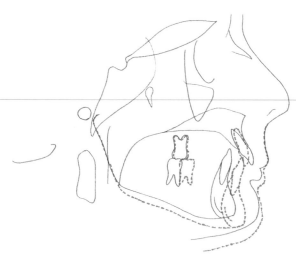

Figure 13-5

Postero-Anterior Cephalometric Radiographic Image

In cases where a patient presents with a suspected skeletal or **facial asymmetry**, a frontal or postero-anterior cephalometric radiograph image (Figure 13-6) is indicated. This is also useful in those patients with transverse skeletal disharmonies where the relative **apical base** widths can be visualized simultaneously. Because this image reflects minor malpositions of the head more sensitively than does that of the lateral cephalometric radiographic image, care must be taken when positioning the patient for this film. Since not every orthodontic patient clinically presents with a skeletal transverse discrepancy or an asymmetry, this radiographic image is typically not indicated for every patient. As with other ancillary diagnostic records, this image is typically reserved for specific circumstances.

Hand-Wrist Radiographic Image

Some clinicians use the hand-wrist radiographic image (Figure 13-7) to measure the skeletal age of a patient by using the ossification of the skeletal bones as markers for maturational assessment. Proponents believe that the sequence of ossification of the small bones within the hand and wrist is predictable, thus leading to an accurate assessment of the patient's developmental status and physical maturity. This knowledge is important to the orthodontist in situations where either growth modification or **orthognathic surgery** is contemplated and the physical growth status is in question.

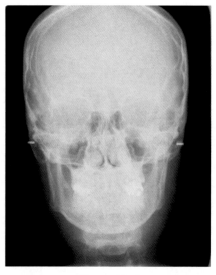

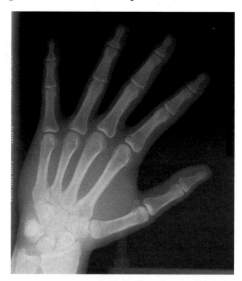

Figure 13-6   Figure 13-7

Occlusal Plane Radiographic Image

The occlusal plane radiographic image (Figure 13-8) is a useful adjunct for the orthodontist in locating supernumerary teeth at the midline, positions of unerupted and sometimes impacted maxillary canines, and anterior pathologies that could impact upon orthodontic treatment.

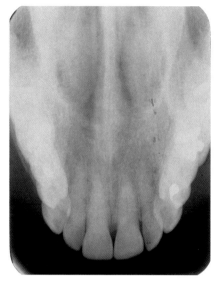
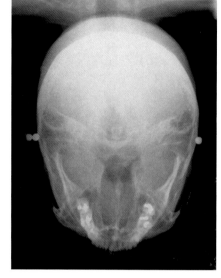

Figure 13-8   Figure 13-9

Submento-Vertex Cephalometric Radiographic Image

When the clinician feels that it is appropriate to evaluate the morphology and the horizontal symmetry of the mandible or the horizontal angulation of the condyles for any irregularities, a submento-vertex radiographic image (Figure 13-9) can be useful. Practically speaking, this is infrequently used by most orthodontists, and is usually reserved for those patients who have cranio-facial anomalies, or have had trauma to the mandible.

Trans-Cranial Radiographic Image

Some clinicians find a trans-cranial radiographic image to be beneficial in their evaluation of suspected temporomandibular joint dysfunction symptomologies such as pain, reduction in mobility, or possible disk displacements. This image is used to detect any abnormalities in the condylar position within the fossa, or morphological osseous changes on the condyles, such as those found in rheumatoid arthritis patients. The diagnostic **validity** of this image sparks significant controversy within the orthodontic community with regards to its accuracy in determining condylar positioning, with the balance of literature tending to discount its usefulness.

2.4 PHOTOGRAPHY/DIGITAL IMAGING

Photographic or digital imaging records are taken of the patient to allow a visual analysis of both extra-oral and intraoral features. Extraorally, a standard series of three views (Figure 13-10) are routinely taken:

1.) A non-smiling frontal facial view with the teeth in maximum **intercuspation** and the lips sealed. This image aids in detecting facial asymmetries of the various structures such as the eyes, nose, ears, and mandible. The clinician is also able to evaluate the soft tissue drape of the face and the perioral tissues for evidence of flaccidity.

2.) A smiling frontal facial view. This will allow the clinician to not only assess the **lip line** and gingival display of the patient, but also the comparative positions of the dental midline to that of the **facial midline**.

3.) A lateral facial view with the teeth in maximum intercuspation and the lips sealed. In using this image, the soft tissue profile of the patient in such areas as the contribution of the nose and chin to the face, as well as the competency or strain of the lips, can be critically evaluated.

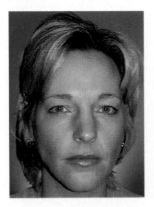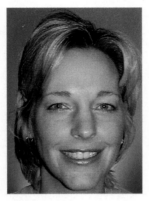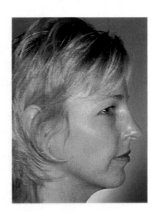

Figure 13-10

Additionally, some orthodontists elect to take other photographic or imaging views for greater insight into the facial esthetics and soft tissue balance. These views include a frontal facial image with the mandible in a **rest position** and the lips in repose, a lateral facial image with the mandible in a rest position and the lips in repose, and a three-quarters view image with the patient smiling (Figure 13-11).

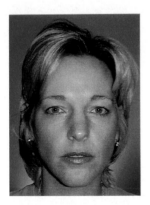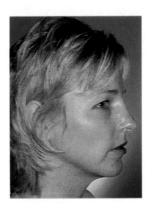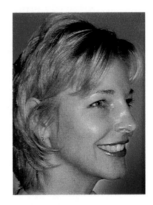

Figure 13-11

Intraorally, five views are typically used to visually evaluate the dentition and the surrounding oral mucosa. These images can be difficult to adequately capture due to the taut perioral tissues. Maximum lip retraction is necessary if quality and detail are to be attained. In addition, the clinician will frequently take these images with the aid of dental mirrors to enhance the detail and visual field. These views include:

1.) A right and left lateral intraoral view. These images are taken in the centric occlusion position and show the buccal occlusal relationships of the teeth and the dynamics of the hard and soft tissues.

2.) A frontal intraoral view with the teeth in centric occlusion. This image allows the orthodontist to assess for overbite relationships, dental midline discrepancies, and abnormal conditions of the enamel and surrounding gingival tissues prior to orthodontic treatment.

3.) Occlusal view of the maxillary and mandibular dentitions. The arch form and symmetry, restorative status of the dentition, and the palate and sublingual soft tissue conditions can all be examined using these images.

2.5 COMPUTERIZED DIAGNOSTIC ANALYSES AND TOOLS

.

Traditionally, the orthodontist evaluated the dental casts and radiographic diagnostic records through visual as well as mathematical examination. For example, the study casts were not only examined for arch form and symmetry, but also manually measured for spacing requirements and tooth size discrepancies. The lateral cephalometric radiograph afforded the clinician not only the visual relationships of the craniofacial, dental, and soft tissue components of the head, but also the objective ability to measure and compare a patient to a standardized set of ideals, termed a **cephalometric analysis** (Figure 13-4). This analysis was carried out using an acetate page placed on the radiograph to create a tracing, which was then measured with a ruler and protractor. Today, however, our diagnostic options have expanded. The new technological age has afforded today's orthodontist analytical tools unforeseen by our predecessors. Examples of these include:

Computerized Radiographic Analyses

Recently, the advent of electronic digitizing equipment has allowed an increase in diagnostic abilities for the clinician. Using either a **cephalometric tracing** or a digitized radiographic image, the orthodontist can either manually digitize a particular set of cephalometric landmarks, or allow for its computer-aided determination. From these landmarks, the computer can then mathematically calculate distances and angles based upon Cartesian coordinates, thus creating the particular cephalometric analysis desired by the clinician.

Proponents of computer assisted cephalometric analyses will cite the benefits of time savings, increasing accuracy, and concomitant improvements in diagnostic abilities as reasons to embrace this technology. They will also point out that this will allow more complex analyses of hard and soft tissue relationships, such as those found in the mesh diagram, to be readily available and clinically applicable in the private sector. Opponents argue that the manual digitization of landmarks is as error-prone and as subjective as traditional methods, since they both still rely upon human identification. Additionally, they say it is still time-consuming due to the fact that the number of landmarks necessary for a digitized computer analysis is high, tending to negate any time saving advantages.

Fully automated cephalometric landmark identification systems have the potential to save time, increase accuracy, and improve diagnostic abilities. In addition, they will allow a different set of mathematical descriptions of landmarks than have traditionally been used. This will provide the orthodontist with new cephalometric ways to evaluate the patient. At this time, however, there doesn't seem to be a diagnostic advantage to automated landmark identification, as preliminary results of accuracy show no significant differences between this and the traditional manual approach in selected landmarks only. In other landmark identifications, the manual approach was found to be statistically superior to that of the automated approach. Nonetheless, investigators remain confident that this technology can and will be significantly improved upon, thus leading to a faster and more highly accurate diagnostic tool with the promising ability to expand clinical knowledge.

Computerized Dental Cast Analyses

Attempts have been made to measure dental casts with computer aided programs to determine such factors as tooth sizes, arch forms, intercanine and intermolar distances, and dental spacing requirements. These have been done using photocopies of dental casts, and then digitizing and measuring specific landmarks found on the dental casts and reproduced on the photocopies. (Photocopies of the dental casts were used for ease of measurement and to reduce the high potential for operator error sometimes experienced with the direct measurement of three-dimensional objects.) At this time, this technology has not been shown to be as accurate as the traditional method of manually measuring the dental cast, as photocopies of the dental casts have not been shown to be accurate representations of the casts. Thus, computerized analyses using this approach have been disappointing. Nonetheless, investigative efforts continue to search for simple computer-assisted dental cast analyses to enhance our diagnostic armamentarium.

Computerized Visual Treatment Objective

The recent combination of computer technology and cephalometric interpretation has facilitated a better understanding of complex statistical analyses regarding craniofacial growth and dentoskeletal relationships. This has allowed the creation of a computerized visual treatment objective (VTO), which, as with the manually derived VTO, is used by the orthodontist to simulate and predict orthodontic and orthognathic surgical movements as well as the resultant concomitant esthetic and soft tissue changes. In addition, the clinician is afforded the ability to "view" different computer generated treatment results, and from these decide upon a particular plan that would best satisfy the initial treatment goals. These "morphed" or modified facial images can then be presented to the patient as a realistic goal of treatment, thus enhancing patient understanding, acceptance, and ultimately satisfaction with orthodontic treatment results.

3. ANALYSIS OF TOOTH SIZE

The sizes of the patient's teeth are important only when related to (a) the space available for them in the arch perimeter, (b) the clinician's ability to increase the space and, (c) when they are disharmonious with each other.

3.1 INDIVIDUAL TEETH

Individual tooth sizes can vary as a result of many factors. Environmental factors (nutrition, climate, and disease) have been identified as affecting the dentition during the prenatal period, but they seemingly have little impact on normal dental variation. General factors such as sex and race, as well as secular changes and bilateral asymmetry have all been shown to affect tooth sizes. When considering the sizes of the teeth, several measurements and concepts seem confusing. Some definitions may help clarify the important concepts involved. The **basal arch** is the arch formed by the maxillary or mandibular corpus. Its dimensions are probably unrelated by the loss of all permanent teeth and resorption of the alveolar process. It is the measurement of the **apical base arch** (Figure13-12), which is defined as the area of **alveolar bone** on a level with the root **apices** of the teeth. When the tooth sizes and the apical base morphologies complement each other, the possibilities for normal tooth positions, normal tooth axial inclinations, and dental spacing are most ideal.

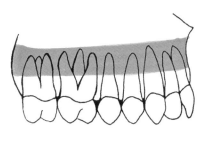 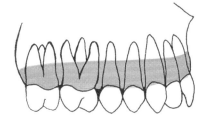

Figure 13-12   Figure 13-13

The **alveolar arch** (Figure 13-13) is the measurement of arc of the the alveolar process. The dimensions of the alveolar arch may not coincide with those of the **basal arch** if, for example, the teeth are tipped labially off the basal arch.

The **dental arch** (Figure 13-14) usually is measured through the contact points of the teeth. When the crowns are tipped markedly off the **basal bone**, the dental arch and alveolar arch are not coincident. Ideally, the sizes of the dental arches are coincident with the sizes of the alveolar and basal arches. Unfortunately, variations often occur resulting in dental and occlusal compromises. The combined mesiodistal widths of the teeth constitute still another measurement.

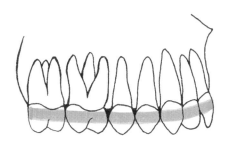

One aims, by orthodontic treatment, for all of the teeth to be so aligned that the combined widths of the teeth will be identical with the dental arch measurements and the dental arch will be positioned over the basal bone. Then gross differences in the dental arch, alveolar arch, and basal perimeters will not obscure cosmetics, or complicate occlusal function and stability.

Figure 13-14

For orthodontic diagnostic purposes, the sizes of the teeth are entirely a relative matter. Large teeth do not always result in a malocclusion, since the available space may be sufficiently large to include them nicely. Simple tooth size tells little. Comparisons of tooth size and available space, the effects of the size of the teeth on the overbite and overjet, and the identification of disharmonies of tooth size within the arch are, however, of great clinical importance.

3.1.1. Shape Discrepancies

Variations in individual crown sizes or shapes (Figure 13-15) can likewise contribute to occlusal disharmonies. The teeth most commonly affected by variations in crown sizes or shapes include the: 1.) third molars, 2.) maxillary lateral incisors, and 3.) the mandibular second bicuspid teeth.

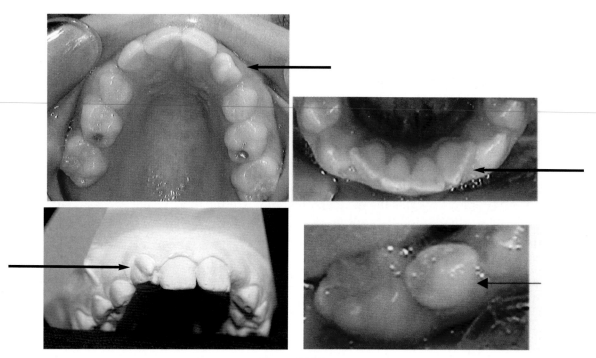

Figure 13-15

Although the third molar teeth are the most frequently affected, variations regarding the sizes and shapes of these teeth are really without any clinical importance. The maxillary lateral incisor teeth occasionally exhibit a more slender conical shape than expected. This morphology is referred to as a **"peg lateral" incisor** (Figure 13-16). Clinically this variation presents both occlusal and esthetic complications.

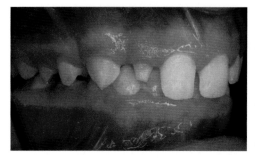

Figure 13-16

The mesio-distal dimension of the mandibular second bicuspid teeth also frequently vary. Increases in the widths of these teeth reduce the available **leeway space**, potentially resulting in crowding or unsatisfactory intercuspation.

Two specific morphological characteristics that have been studied among populations are shovel-shaped incisor teeth and the Cusp of Carabelli (Figure 13-17). The Asian and Indian populations have shown the greatest incidence of shovel-shaped incisors among populations, while the Cusp of Cararbelli most frequently found among Caucasoids.

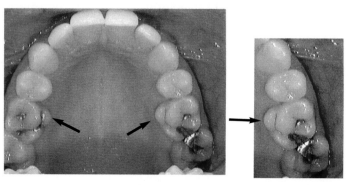

Figure 13-17

3.2 SIZE RELATIONSHIPS OF GROUPS OF TEETH

The precise alignment of teeth and attainment of perfect posterior intercuspation can be frustrating when crown size discrepancies are present. For example, it is not unusual to achieve a perfect Class I molar relationship during orthodontic treatment and yet not be able to achieve a similar cuspid intercuspation because of tooth-size discrepancies in the lateral segments. While left-right symmetry of size is usually assured, the anteroposterior tooth sizes are often not so harmonious. Not only can a single tooth's size discrepancy be troublesome, but also the accumulation of minor differences along the arch can produce overall difficulties in achieving a precise occlusion.

The examination of the dentition during treatment planning must include the identification of the effects of tooth size (both local and general), upon the ultimate overbite, overjet, and posterior occlusal relationships. To this end, orthodontists have used several methods to recognize inter-arch tooth size discrepancies. Some of the lesser methods include Howe's ratio of canine fossa width to total maxillary tooth width, Kesling's diagnostic set-up, and Neff's anterior coefficient. The most popular and highly recognized method, however, remains the **Bolton Tooth Ratio Analysis (or the Bolton Analysis)** (Figure 13-18).

3.2.1. **Bolton Tooth Ratio Analysis**

The Bolton Analysis is based on the ratio between the mesiodistal tooth diameter sums of the maxillary and mandibular teeth. The ratios for both anterior and overall dentitions were derived from 55 patients with perfect Class I occlusions.

Dr. W. A. Bolton studied the interarch effects of discrepancies in tooth size to devise a procedure for determining the ratio of total mandibular versus total maxillary tooth size, and anterior mandibular versus anterior maxillary tooth size. Studying these ratios will help in estimating the overbite and overjet relationships that will likely be obtained after treatment is finished, the effects of contemplated extractions on posterior occlusion and incisor relationships, and the identification of occlusal discrepancies produced by interarch tooth size incompatibilities.

The procedure is as follows: the sum of the widths of the mandibular 12 teeth is divided by the sum of the maxillary 12 teeth and multiplied by 100. A mean ratio of 91.3, according to Bolton, will result in ideal overbite-overjet relationships, as well as an ideal posterior occlusion. If the overall ratio exceeds 91.3 the discrepancy is due to excessive mandibular tooth material. In the chart, one locates the figure corresponding to the patient's maxillary tooth size. Opposite is the ideal mandibular measurement. The difference between the actual and the desired mandibular measurement is the amount of excessive mandibular tooth material when the ratio is greater than 91.3. If the ratio is less than 91.3, the difference between the actual maxillary size and the desired maxillary size is the amount of excess maxillary tooth material. A similar ratio (anterior ratio) is computed for the six anterior teeth (incisors and cuspids). An anterior ratio, 77.2, will provide ideal overbite and overjet relationships if the angulation of the incisors is correct and if the labiolingual thickness of the incisal edges is not excessive. If the anterior ratio exceeds 77.2, there is excessive mandibular tooth material; if it is less than 77.2, there is excess maxillary tooth material.

Over-all Ratio

Sum mandibular 12 ___mm. / Sum maxillary 12 ___mm. = ___ x 100 = ___ % (Over-all ratio)   Mean 91.3 = 0.26 S. D. (σ) 1.91 Range 87.5 - 94.8

Maxillary 12	Mandibular 12	Maxillary 12	Mandibular 12	Maxillary 12	Mandibular 12
86	77.6	94	85.8	103	94.0
86	78.5	95	86.7	104	95.0
87	79.4	96	87.6	105	95.9
88	80.3	97	88.6	106	96.8
89	81.3	98	89.5	107	97.8
90	82.1	99	90.4	108	98.6
91	83.1	100	91.3	109	99.5
92	84.0	101	92.2	110	100.4
93	84.9	102	93.1		

Patient Analysis

If the over-all ratio exceeds 91.3 the discrepancy is in excessive mandibular arch length. In above chart locate the patient's maxillary 12 measurement and opposite it is the correct mandibular measurement. The difference between the actual and correct mandibular measurement is the amount of excessive mandibular arch length.

_____ - _____ = _____
Actual mandibular 12   Correct mandibular 12   Excess mandibular 12

If over-all ratio is less than 91.3:

_____ - _____ = _____
Actual maxillary 12   Correct maxillary 12   Excess maxillary 12

Anterior Ratio

Sum mandibular 6 ___mm. / Sum maxillary 6 ___mm. = ___ x 100 = ___ % (Anterior ratio)   Mean 77.2 = 0.22 S. D. (σ) 1.65 Range 74.5 - 80.4

Maxillary 6	Mandibular 6	Maxillary 6	Mandibular 6	Maxillary 6	Mandibular 6
40.0	30.9	45.5	35.1	50.5	39.0
40.5	31.3	46.0	35.5	51.0	39.4
41.0	31.7	46.5	35.9	51.5	39.8
41.5	32.0	47.0	36.3	52.0	40.1
42.0	32.4	47.5	36.7	52.5	40.5
42.5	32.8	48.0	37.1	53.0	40.9
43.0	33.2	48.5	37.4	53.5	41.3
43.5	33.6	49.0	37.8	54.0	41.7
44.0	34.0	49.5	38.2	54.5	42.1
44.5	34.4	50.0	38.6	55.0	42.5
45.0	34.7				

Patient Analysis

If anterior ratio exceeds 77.2:

_____ - _____ = _____
Actual mandibular 6   Correct mandibular 6   Excess mandibular 6

If anterior ratio is less than 77.2:

_____ - _____ = _____
Actual maxillary 6   Correct maxillary 6   Excess maxillary 6

Figure 13-18

Although the Bolton Analysis is the most widely used method for detecting interarch tooth size discrepancies, it is not without criticism. For instance, because Bolton's sample consisted of 55 individuals with perfect Class I occlusion, estimates of variation were underestimated. More importantly, both the gender and the population composition of his sample group were unreported, implying a potential selection **bias**.

3.2.2. Sanin-Savara Tooth Size Analysis

The Sanin-Savara Analysis is based on the need to know the clinical implications of discordantly sized individual teeth.

Dr. C. Sanin and Dr. B. S. Savara and colleagues at the University of Oregon devised a simple and yet ingenious procedure to identify individual and group tooth size disharmonies. This procedure makes use of precise mesiodistal measurements of the crown size of each tooth, appropriate tables of tooth size distributions in the population, and a chart for plotting the patient's measurements. The teeth should be measured with a tooth-measuring gauge, architectural dividers, or a finely pointed Boley gauge.

3.2.3. Populations and Tooth Size Discrepancies

Individual tooth sizes and interarch tooth size relationships are population specific. Significant differences have been shown in the Bolton overall anterior, posterior and interarch ratios between Caucasoids, Mongoloids, and Negroids. This is primarily due to significant variations in the interarch tooth sizes of the mandibular central incisors, the maxillary lateral incisors, the second bicuspids, and the first molar teeth. Therefore, when an interarch **tooth size discrepancy** is suspected, these teeth should be examined first. Additionally, recognition should be given to the limitations of the population specific standards we utilize in clinical analysis.

The harmonious alignment of the teeth within the **dental arch** is fundamentally dependent upon the relationship between the dental arch size and the tooth size. Malocclusions exist when either of these factors is incongruent.

Many investigators have shown that population differences exist between tooth size and dental arch size. Negroids have been shown to have larger tooth size and greater arch widths and depths than Caucasoids. They have also demonstrated a closer degree of conformity between the maxillary and mandibular tooth dimensions and dental arch sizes than have Caucasoids, with Mongoloids being the intermediary. This is verified by the fact that malocclusions are more prevalent in the societies of North America and Europe than in the developing societies.

There is, however, little relationship between body size and tooth size among populations. A shorter statured person does not necessarily have shorter or smaller teeth. A classic comparison, which highlights this, is that of the Australian Aborigines and the Norwegian Lapps. While the Australian Aboriginal peoples are shorter in stature, they have much larger teeth than those of the taller Norwegian Lapps.

3.2.4. Gender and Tooth Size Discrepancies

Gender comparisons indicate the presence of sexual dimorphism. Males have larger tooth sizes than females with the largest difference being found in the cuspid teeth. These teeth have been shown to average up to six percent larger dimensionally in males, both buccolingually and mesiodistally, than in females.

Tooth sizes and their interarch tooth relationships have also demonstrated gender differences. This has been shown in both the posterior and overall Bolton ratios. Males have routinely exhibited larger Bolton ratios than females, regardless of the specific population, with Caucasoid females in particular having shown the closest ideal overall Bolton ratio of any group. Some researchers have referred to this finding to suggest that Bolton's original sample was most likely comprised of Caucasoid females.

3.2.5. Malocclusion Groups and Tooth Size Discrepancies

Several studies have examined the relationship between tooth size discrepancies and various malocclusion groups. These studies have shown that, although large numbers of tooth size discrepancies exist within the malocclusion groups, there were no significant differences in the incidence of tooth size discrepancies among the malocclusion groups. In other words, no specific malocclusion group was shown to contain a larger percentage of tooth size discrepancies.

3.3 RELATIONSHIP OF TOOTH SIZE TO THE SUPPORTING STRUCTURES

3.3.1. **Apical Base** Influences

Generally speaking, the space conditions in the dental arches are closely related to the adequacy of the bony support for the teeth (in the maxilla and mandible) in relation to the sizes of the teeth. As previously described, the **apical bases** are those areas of the alveolar bone that are in the same plane as the root apices of the teeth. When a balance exists between the apical base morphology and the tooth sizes, the potential for normal tooth axial inclination, dental spacing, and tooth positions is greatest.

Differing apical base sizes (Figure 13-19) can have a profound impact on the dentition and occlusion. A smaller **apical base** (in relation to tooth size) usually results in the abnormal positions of the root apices of the teeth, buccal/labial inclinations of the teeth, and dental crowding. This is most often apparent in the incisor region. A less frequent situation occurs when a large apical base (in relation to tooth size) is present, resulting in the teeth being characteristically more vertical in inclination, with generalized dental spacing.

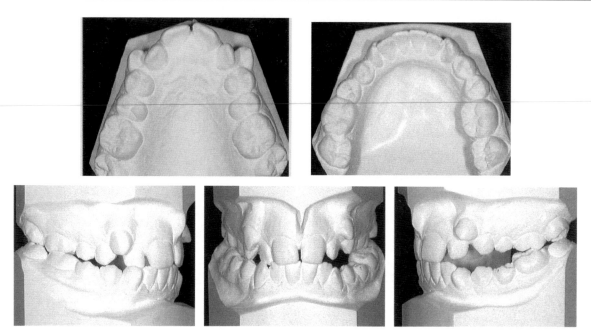

Figure 13-19

3.3.1.1. Howes Analysis

Dr. A. E. Howes drew attention to the fact that crowding could result not only from excessive tooth size, but also from inadequate apical bases as well. He devised a formula for determining whether the apical bases could accommodate the patient's teeth. Since this method was introduced, rapid palatal expansion has come into more common use, and clinicians have much more opportunity to alter the maxillary apical base than once was thought. Nevertheless, the Howes analysis is useful in treatment planning problems with suspected apical base deficiencies. Mandibular apical base restrictions are more difficult, and thus more critical than maxillary arch deficiencies, as they are much less amenable to change.

3.3.1.2. **Diagnostic Set-up**

It is useful in difficult space management problems to ascertain, before orthodontic treatment is begun, precisely the amount and direction each tooth must be moved. A popular and practical technique available to the clinician for visualizing such three dimensional space problems in the permanent dentition is that of cutting the teeth off of a set of working casts and resetting them in more desirable positions. This procedure is called a **diagnostic or prognostic set-up**. The record casts are not used for this technique, since they must be saved for comparison with the diagnostic set-up and with progressive record casts.

To achieve a diagnostic set-up, the clinician must do the following: Individually cut out the teeth destined to be positionally changed at the alveolar base level on the dental cast. (It is best not to cut off all the teeth so that the bite registration can be kept.) These teeth can then be re-aligned on the dental cast and waxed into the desired positions for a visual evaluation of the potential treatment outcome. In addition, the clinician can combine this with the knowledge gained by the cephalometric analysis and the prediction of incisal positioning and angulation to aid in assessing alignment stability, or potential profile changes resulting from treatment.

When extractions are contemplated as part of the orthodontic treatment, the diagnostic set-up will demonstrate vividly the amount of space created by the extractions and the tooth movements necessary to close the space. It will also aid in choosing which teeth to extract.

An even more accurate method of using the diagnostic set-up involves taking a wax bite in the retruded contact position, mounting the casts on an adjustable articulator, and finishing the diagnostic set-up within the limits of the jaw relationships thus imposed.

3.4 RELATIONSHIPS OF TOOTH SIZE TO THE AVAILABLE SPACE

Proper alignment of the teeth requires harmony between the tooth sizes and the space available within the dental arch. Sometimes the space available is not similar to the space required for the alignment of the teeth. It is thus important for the clinician to determine prior to the onset of orthodontic treatment the space requirements necessary for favorable results. To accomplish this, a space analysis must be done.

Several types of space analyses exist, dependent upon the development of the dentition. For younger children in the mixed dentition stage of development, several methods have been proposed to analyze spacing requirements. These analyses all rely not only upon the direct measurements of the erupted teeth, but also upon indirect measurements of the teeth yet to erupt. Individuals with permanent dentitions do not need to rely upon indirect measurements. Their teeth can be directly measured, thus reducing estimation error.

3.4.1. Permanent Dentition Space Analyses

Two practical ways exist to analyze the spacing requirements of the permanent dentition. The first way involves directly measuring the dental casts themselves. The second method involves computer digitizing and measuring the teeth and the dental arches from a two dimensional occlusal image. Regardless of which method is used, the space required and the space available values must be calculated.

The space available figure can be ascertained by measuring the **arch perimeter** from first molar to first molar. This can be achieved in one of two ways. The preferred approach is to divide the dental arch into four segments of straight-line approximations through the contact points of the posterior teeth and the incisal edges of the anterior teeth (Figure 13-20). Four linear measurements are thus taken: two involving the posterior arch segments and two involving the anterior arch segments. The total of these four sums represent the space available for alignment.

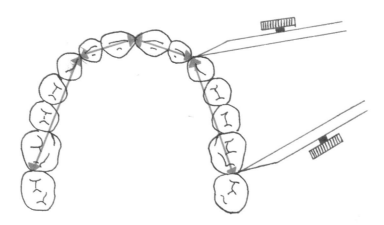

Figure13-20

A second way to measure the space available is to bend a piece of brass wire through the contact points of the posterior teeth and the incisal edges of the anterior teeth, on the occlusal plane of the dental casts (Figure 13-21). This wire can then be straightened out and measured.

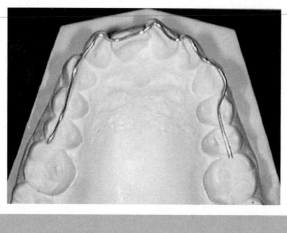

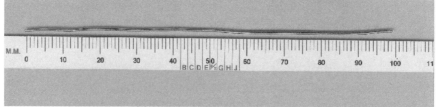

Figure 13-21

The sum totals of the individual teeth (as calculated by the mesiodistal tooth widths from first molar to first molar), represents the space necessary for alignment. This number can be derived by measuring each tooth (from contact point to contact point) with a dial caliper, architectural dividers, or a finely sharpened Boley gauge (Figure 13-22).

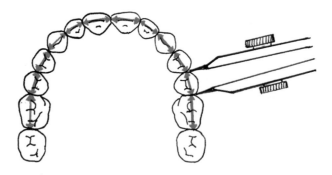

Figure 13-22

If the sum total of the widths of the teeth is greater than the arch perimeter, the individual is said to have a **space deficiency** (Figure 13-23). Likewise, if the sum total of the widths of the teeth is less than the arch perimeter, the individual is said to have **space excess** (Figure 13-24). Clinically the practitioner could expect to observe dental crowding and rotations in patients who have a space deficiency, and gaps between teeth in individuals with space excess.

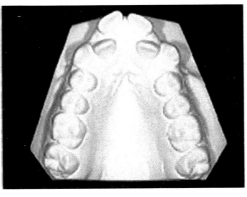 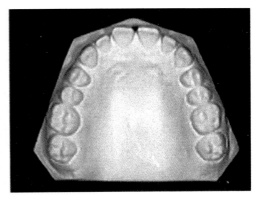

Figure 13-23   Figure 13-24

3.4.2. Limitations of Permanent Dentition Space Analyses

Situations can occur which could compromise the accuracy of the previously described permanent dentition space analyses. Dentally, if the angulation of the incisors is excessively proclined or retroclined, it will impart the appearance of alignment disharmonies. Proclined incisors will seem to diminish the dental crowding while retroclined incisors enhance the crowding. The irony is that both situations are really just an expression of the same situation; insufficient space for proper dental alignment. The prudent clinician will note any deviations in incisor position, either cephalometrically or by clinical exam, and weigh these factors in when using the space analysis.

Skeletally, in non-growing individuals, the arch perimeter or space available measurement would be expected to change very little. Likewise, in a child with a balanced skeletal growth pattern, there is only a remote chance that skeletal growth will displace the dentition. Unfortunately, in children with disproportionate skeletal jaw growth patterns (either in the anteroposterior or vertical dimensions), teeth can shift either anteriorly or posteriorly in response. For these individuals, space analyses will be of greater need, but of lesser accuracy.

3.4.3. Mixed Dentition Space Analyses

An important consideration for any clinician devising an orthodontic treatment plan for a child in the mixed dentition is, "how much space will the unerupted permanent teeth require for alignment?" The answer to this question can be critical to a sound treatment plan. Space maintenance, space reclamation, eruption guidance, and the need for extractions can all be addressed by knowing this value. To complete an analysis of the mixed dentition, three factors must be noted:

1.) The sizes of all the permanent teeth anterior to the first permanent molar
2.) The arch perimeter
3.) Expected changes in the arch perimeter that may occur with growth and development.

A **Mixed Dentition Space Analysis (or Mixed Dentition Analysis)** helps one estimate the amount of spacing or crowding which would exist for the patient if all the primary teeth were replaced by their successors the very day the analysis is done, not two or three years later. It does not predict the amount of natural decrease in arch perimeter, which may occur during the transitional period without the loss of teeth.

Many mixed dentition space analysis methods have been suggested; however, all fall into three strategic categories:

1.) Those in which the sizes of the unerupted cuspids and bicuspids are estimated from measurements of their radiographic images
2.) Those in which the sizes of the cuspids and bicuspids are derived from knowledge of the sizes of permanent teeth already erupted in the mouth
3.) A combination of the above approaches.

In all of the commonly used mixed dentition analyses, the mandibular permanent incisors have been chosen for measuring, since they are erupted into the mouth early in the mixed dentition, they are easily measured accurately, and they are directly in the midst of most space management problems. The maxillary incisors are not used in any of the predictive procedures since they show too much variability in size, and their correlations with other groups of teeth are of low predictive value. Therefore, the lower incisors are measured to predict the sizes of the upper as well as the lower cuspid and bicuspid teeth.

Commonly Used Mixed Dentition Space Analyses

3.4.3.1. Nance Mixed Dentition Space Analysis

In 1947 Dr. Hays N. Nance proposed a mixed dentition space analysis that involved measuring the mesiodistal widths of the unerupted mandibular cuspid and bicuspid teeth using a radiographic technique. This method involved taking radiographic images between the contact points of the yet unerupted permanent cuspid and bicuspid teeth while still in their crypts, and directly measuring them with architectural dividers. This number could then added to the sum total widths of the erupted mandibular central and lateral incisor teeth to represent the space necessary for alignment. Dr. Nance then measured with brass wire the arch perimeter from the mesiobuccal surface of one permanent mandibular first molar around to the mesiobuccal surface of the other permanent mandibular first molar to determine the amount of space available for alignment. Discrepancies in tooth size and **arch length** could thus be determined.

One of the recognized difficulties of this technique is that radiographic distortions will directly affect the accuracy of the measurements. If the contact points between the unerupted teeth have not been opened up, the mesiodistal widths of these teeth cannot be accurately assessed. To adjust for this, Dr. Nance suggested either using the measurement from the same tooth on the contralateral side, or if this was unavailable, referring to tooth size averages compiled by Dr. G. V. Black.

3.4.3.2. Hixson-Oldfather Mixed Dentition Space Analysis

Dr. E. H. Hixon and Dr. R. E. Oldfather developed a method in 1958 to predict the space required for the unerupted permanent cuspid and bicuspid teeth. This was based upon the directly measured sums of the mesiodistal widths of the permanent mandibular central and lateral incisor teeth. Radiographic measurements were then taken of the unerupted bicuspid teeth. These were compared to values derived by participants in the 1949 Iowa Facial Growth Study to predict the mesiodistal widths of the unerupted cuspid teeth.

While many investigators believe that this is the most accurate prediction method, criticism of this technique has also occurred. Some believe that the Hixon-Oldfather method under-predicts the widths of the bicuspid and cuspid teeth resulting in a consistently optimistic space analysis. A revised Hixon-Oldfather prediction method has subsequently been proposed which averages the variables from both sides of the lower arch, (as compared to just the left side as was originally done). Proponents of this new approach believe this revision results in a lower standard error, and thus a more accurate estimation. They also point out that while this may be an under-predictive space analysis, it would still result in a more conservative treatment approach, whereas over-predictive methods tend to exaggerate space requirements potentially resulting in unnecessary extractions.

3.4.3.3. Tanaka-Johnston Mixed Dentition Space Analysis

Dr. Marvin Tanaka and Dr. Lysle Johnston published in 1974 a mixed dentition space analysis that also uses the mesiodistal widths of the lower incisor teeth to predict the sizes of the unerupted cuspid and bicuspid teeth. Their method is recognized as the most convenient in that it relies neither on radiographic measurements, nor predictive tables, once the method is memorized. Additionally, it can be used in both the maxillary and mandibular arches.

The Tanaka-Johnston method works as follows: The combined mesiodistal widths of the four lower incisor teeth are added up. This number is then divided by two and added to either 11.0 for the maxillary cuspid-bicuspid segments, or 10.5 for the mandibular cuspid-bicuspid segments. The new number thus equals the predicted widths of the unerupted cuspid and bicuspid teeth within a segment, valid to the 75th percentile confidence interval.

The advantages to the Tanaka-Johnston method include simplicity, time savings, and ease of application with a predictability level virtually identical to the widely used Moyers Mixed Dentition Space Analysis. (In fact, it could be argued that many of the reasons offered for the popularity of the Moyers Mixed Dentition Space Analysis could also describe the Tanaka-Johnston method minus the inconvenience of the necessary predictive tables.) Critics of this analysis (and the Moyers method) believe that it over-predicts the space necessary for the unerupted cuspid and bicuspid teeth at the 65% to 95% levels of confidence. This over-prediction, they believe, could result in exaggerated space requirements, and subsequently unnecessary extractions.

3.4.3.4. Moyers Mixed Dentition Space Analysis

Probably the most widely recognized mixed dentition analysis is the one developed by Dr. Robert Moyers. This method was the first to use predictive tables for the combined widths of the unerupted cuspid and bicuspid teeth based upon the measured widths of the lower incisor teeth. Advocates of this method present the following reasons for its popularity: 1.) it has minimal systematic error and the range of such errors is known, 2.) it can be done with equal reliability by the beginner as well as the expert for it does not presume sophisticated clinical judgment, 3.) it is not time consuming, 4.) it requires no special equipment or radiographic projections, 5.) although it is best done on dental casts, it can be done with reasonable accuracy in the mouth, and 6.) it can be used for both dental arches.

The procedure to use this method in the mandibular arch is as follows:

1.) Measure with a pointed Boley gauge or architectural dividers the greatest mesiodistal width of each of the four mandibular incisors. Record these values on the Mixed Dentition Analysis form (Figure 13-25).

2.) Determine the amount of space needed for the alignment of the mandibular incisors. Set the

Boley gauge or dividers to a value equal to the sum of the widths of the left central incisor and the left lateral incisor. Place one point of the gauge at the midline of the alveolar crest between the central incisors and let the other point lie along the line of the dental arch on the left side. Mark on the tooth or the cast the precise point where the distal surface of the lateral incisor will be when it has been aligned. Repeat this process for the right side of the arch. If the cephalometric evaluation shows the mandibular incisor to be positioned too far labially, the Boley gauge tip is placed at the midline, but moved lingually a sufficient amount to simulate the expected uprighting of the incisors as dictated by the cephalometric evaluation.

3.) Compute the amount of space available after incisor alignment. To do this, measure the distance from the point marked in the line of the arch to the mesial surface of the first permanent molar. This distance is the space available for the cuspid and two bicuspids and for any necessary molar adjustment after the incisors have been aligned. Record the data for both sides on the Mixed Dentition Analysis form.

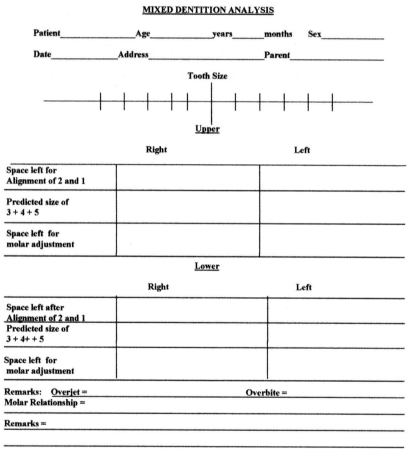

Figure 13-25

4.) Predict the size of the combined widths of the mandibular cuspid and bicuspid teeth. (Experienced clinicians may choose to use the 50% prediction since it is a more precise estimate. Those who are inexperienced or without the use of **cephalometrics** and a precision appliance method would do well to proceed more conservatively; i.e., use the 75% level of prediction.)

Prediction of the combined widths of the cuspid, first bicuspid, and second bicuspid teeth is done by use of probability charts (Figure 13-26). Locate in the left column of the mandibular chart the value that most nearly corresponds to the sum of the widths of the four mandibular incisors. To the right is a row of figures indicating the range of values for all the cuspid and bicuspid sizes that will be found for incisors of the indicated size. For example, note that for small incisors of 22.0 mm combined width, the summed mandibular cuspid and bicuspid widths range from 22.6 mm at the 95% level of confidence to 18.7 mm at the 5% level. This means that of all the people in the universe whose lower incisors measure 22.0 mm, 95 % will have cuspid and bicuspid widths totaling 22.6 mm or less. No one figure can represent the precise cuspid-bicuspid sum for all people, since there is a range of posterior tooth widths seen even when the incisors are identical. The value at the 75% level is chosen as the estimate, since it has been found to be the most practical from a clinical standpoint. In this instance, it is 21.4 mm, which means that three times out of four the cuspid and bicuspid teeth will total 21.4 mm or less. Note also that only five times in a hundred will these teeth be more than 1 mm greater than the estimate chosen (21.4 mm). Theoretically, one should use the 50% level of probability, since any errors would then distribute equally both ways. Clinically, however, we need more protection on the down side (crowding) than we do on the upside (spacing).

PROBABILITY CHART FOR PREDICTING THE SUM OF THE WIDTHS OF 345 FROM $\overline{21|12}$

$\overline{21|12}$ =	19.5	20.0	20.5	21.0	21.5	22.0	22.5	23.0	23.5	24.0	24.5	25.0
95%	21.6	21.8	22.1	22.4	22.7	22.9	23.2	23.5	23.8	24.0	24.3	24.6
85%	21.0	21.3	21.5	21.8	22.1	22.4	22.6	22.9	23.2	23.5	23.7	24.0
75%	20.6	20.9	21.2	21.5	21.8	22.0	22.3	22.6	22.9	23.1	23.4	23.7
65%	20.4	20.6	20.9	21.2	21.5	21.8	22.0	22.3	22.6	22.8	23.1	23.4
50%	20.0	20.3	20.6	20.8	21.1	21.4	21.7	21.9	22.2	22.5	22.8	23.0
35%	19.6	19.9	20.2	20.5	20.8	21.0	21.3	21.6	21.9	22.1	22.4	22.7
25%	19.4	19.7	19.9	20.2	20.5	20.8	21.0	21.3	21.6	21.9	22.1	22.4
15%	19.0	19.3	19.6	19.9	20.2	20.4	20.7	21.0	21.3	21.5	21.8	22.1
5%	18.5	18.8	19.0	19.3	19.6	19.9	20.1	20.4	20.7	21.0	21.2	21.5

PROBABILITY CHART FOR PREDICTING THE SUM OF THE WIDTHS OF $\overline{345}$ FROM $\overline{21|12}$

$\overline{21|12}$ =	19.5	20.0	20.5	21.0	21.5	22.0	22.5	23.0	23.5	24.0	24.5	25.0
95 %	21.1	21.4	21.7	22.0	22.3	22.6	22.9	23.2	23.5	23.8	24.1	24.4
85%	20.5	20.8	21.1	21.4	21.7	22.0	22.3	22.6	22.9	23.2	23.5	23.8
75%	20.1	20.4	20.7	21.0	21.3	21.6	21.9	22.2	22.5	22.8	23.1	23.4
65%	19.8	20.1	20.4	20.7	21.0	21.3	21.6	21.9	22.2	22.5	22.8	23.1
50%	19.4	19.7	20.0	20.3	20.6	20.9	21.2	21.5	21.8	22.1	22.4	22.7
35%	19.0	19.3	19.6	19.9	20.2	20.5	20.8	21.1	21.4	21.7	22.0	22.3
25%	18.7	19.0	19.3	19.6	19.9	20.2	20.5	20.8	21.1	21.4	21.7	22.0
15%	18.4	18.7	19.0	19.3	19.6	19.8	20.1	20.4	20.7	21.0	21.3	21.6
5%	17.7	18.0	18.3	18.6	18.9	19.2	19.5	19.8	20.1	20.4	20.7	21.0

Figure 13-26

The procedure to use this method in the maxillary arch is similar to that for the mandibular arch with two exceptions: 1.) a different probability chart is used for predicting the upper cuspid and bicuspid width sums, and 2.) allowance must be made for overjet correction when measuring the space to be occupied by the aligned incisors. Remember that the widths of the lower incisors are used to predict the widths of the upper cuspid and bicuspid teeth.

3.4.4. Limitations of the Mixed Dentition Space Analyses

A problem arises when considering the space left for molar adjustments. If this value in the chart is negative, that is, the predicted sizes of the cuspid and bicuspid teeth is greater than the space available after the alignment of the incisors, then crowding will occur in the arch even without any forward molar adjustment. When the first permanent molar teeth are in an end-to-end relationship (i.e., a flush terminal plane of the second primary molars), approximately 3.5 mm of space (one-half of a cusp width) is required to convert the occlusion to a Class I molar relationship. This needed 3.5 mm might be acquired without orthodontic intervention in any of three ways:

1.) 3.5 mm more **late mesial shift** of the mandibular first permanent molar than that of the maxillary first permanent molar;

2.) At least 3.5 mm more forward growth of the mandible than of the maxilla;

3.) Some combination of dental adjustment and differential skeletal growth.

Since we cannot yet predict accurately the amount of differential skeletal growth that will occur, treatment planning must be based upon dental adjustment factors. If differential skeletal growth occurs during this period, alterations in the molar relationship will result and the Mixed Dentition Analysis predictions must be altered accordingly. When there is a Class I molar relationship in the mixed dentition, (mesial step of the second primary molars), no part of the arch perimeter need be pre-empted for molar adjustment, and all the space can be made available for incisors, cuspids, and bicuspids.

It has become accepted in many mixed dentition analysis procedures to assume that every child will require precisely 1.7 mm of late mesial molar shift. Such fallacious reasoning is unfortunate, since it leads to errors in treatment planning. One cannot assume an average mesial shift or leeway space value any more than one can assume average tooth sizes. As was stated earlier, though some children will require no mesial shift of the first permanent molars (Class I molar relationship), the greatest number of children will require approximately 3.5 mm late mesial shift or differential skeletal growth (end-to-end molar relationship). It is best to quantify the amount of mesial shift necessary to bring the molars into a Class I relationship. The treatment plan is then devised to accomplish the precise amount of correction needed in each arch.

Mixed dentition space analyses do not reflect the position of the incisors with respect to the skeletal profile. There are a number of crude rules of thumb for determining how much arch perimeter reduction occurs for each degree or millimeter the incisor edge is changed in the cephalometric visualization of treatment. For example, one degree of tipping or 1 mm of lingual displacement of the mandibular incisal edge is said to be equal to 1 mm of arch shortening on each side. Useful as such estimates are, the simple truth remains: We must use some clinical judgment when applying the Mixed Dentition Space Analysis onto the facial skeleton with regards to both at the profile and the apical bases.

A problem is imposed when the occlusal curve is assumed to be a flat plane. Mixed dentition space analyses assume, by projection to a flat plane, no vertical occlusal curve. Often in the mixed dentition there is indeed a flat occlusal plane, but many times the **Curve of Spee** (Figure 13-27) is exaggerated or complicated.

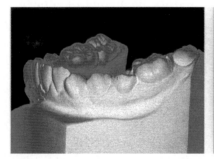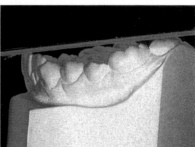

Figure 13-27

Enhanced and elaborated occlusal curves are, unfortunately, seen frequently with some of the most severe malocclusions. The arch perimeter is usually longer than it is measured, particularly when the Curve of Spee is exaggerated or shows complicated vertical curves. As a result, the clinician may assume that there is sufficient space for all the teeth, until the arch is made level during treatment. Then it becomes obvious that the Mixed Dentition Space Analysis is a two dimensional visualization of a complex three-dimensional problem.

The predictive mixed dentition space analyses that derive the sizes of the unerupted cuspid and bicuspid teeth from knowledge of the permanent teeth already erupted in the mouth (Hixon-Oldfather, Moyers, and Tanaka-Johnston), have all relied upon measurements compiled from predominantly Caucasian populations. The Hixon-Oldfather data was taken from forty-one children of "predominantly northwest European ancestry" who participated in the Iowa Facial Growth Study as their sample. The Moyers predictive tables were tabulated from "white American children", and Tanaka and Johnston based their findings on 506 orthodontic patients of "probable European ancestry". As a result, these analyses are probably accurate for Caucasoids, however they are of lesser value for other population groups. Tooth size differences between population groups (as was previously described) will have a direct impact on the accuracy of predictive space analyses that do not take these discrepancies into consideration. Likewise, sexual dimorphism of tooth size may also contribute to lesser predictive accuracies. Therefore, important variables such as population differences and sexual dimorphism in tooth size must be considered when using predictive mixed dentition space analyses.

Finally, the clinician should recognize that any mixed dentition analysis is simply a guide to a treatment decision. It would be erroneous to allow one number to ultimately dictate the totality of treatment. As one of many factors that we consider when making treatment decisions, a mixed dentition space analysis can be a useful adjunct in our diagnostic armamentarium.

4. ARCH FORM AND SYMMETRY

Over the last 100 years orthodontists have attempted to find the ideal arch form which was symmetric in nature and yet would aid in achieving one of the primary goals of orthodontic treatment: functional stability with optimum esthetics. Since that time, many investigators have attempted to come to an agreement regarding this universal **arch form**, believing that one ideal size and shape could effectively be used for all cases. Unfortunately, this goal has thus far been elusive due to the inherent variability and asymmetry found in nature.

4.1 DESCRIPTION OF ARCH FORM

Maxillary and mandibular arch forms have been described according to their shapes. Qualitative terms such as ovoid, trapezoid, squared, U-shaped, and tapered have all been used. Attempts have also been made to describe the shapes in mathematical or geometrical formulas, such as the ellipse, catenary curve, parabola, hyperbola, conic function, cubic spline, or polynomial function. Each of these descriptions or shapes has received both acclaim and criticism. Some are felt to be too simplistic in the "one size fits all" mode. Others are felt to be of higher accuracy, but of little clinical use. A few of these descriptions have been accepted as the basis for commercially produced arch forms.

Among the earliest arch forms to be used by orthodontists was the Bonwill-Hawley arch form (Figure 13-28). This was derived by the measurement of the anterior segment of the dental arch from cuspid to cuspid. The posterior segments of the **arch form** were then fabricated by extending a straight line back from either cuspid (Figure 13-29). Thus the created arch form was directly related to the sizes of the anterior teeth, and not the individual's original arch form. This unmodified method is rarely used today.

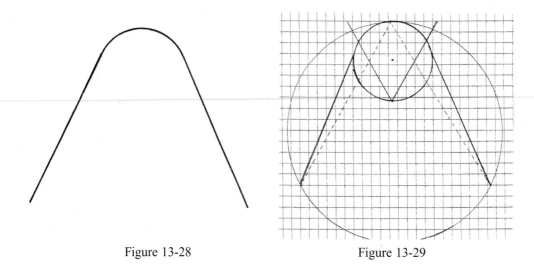

Figure 13-28   Figure 13-29

The Catenary Curve is one of the first mathematical formulas used to describe a natural arch form. One can visualize this curve by suspending a length of chain from two hooks and noticing the shape that it assumes (Figure 13-30). While this form has been shown to be fairly accurate for the anterior to premolars regions of many arches, it doesn't allow for the commonly seen lingual curvature that occurs in the molar regions of many individuals. Likewise in broader arch forms, this formula or shape is of lesser accuracy. The catenary curve remains, however, very popular with commercial orthodontic archwire manufacturers. Therefore, those practitioners who choose to use this preformed archwire shape perhaps would be wise to remember that compensatory wire bending in the molar regions may be appropriate to more accurately reflect the positions of the molar teeth in the **dental arch** of a specific patient.

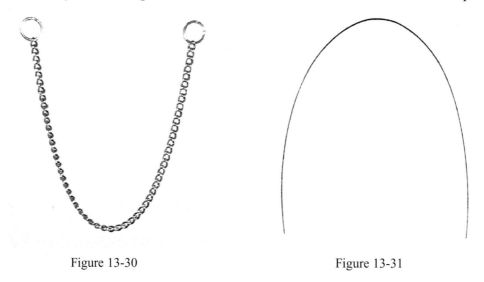

Figure 13-30   Figure 13-31

The Brader arch form is another mathematical formula used to describe the natural dental arch. This is based upon a trifocal ellipse that differs from the catenary curve shape by appearing slightly wider in the bicuspid region followed by a gradual constriction in the molar areas. This gives the appearance of a more "rounded" arch form (Figure 13-31). As with the catenary curve, this too has been popularized as a commercially available orthodontic archwire, and is promoted as a more compatible arch form in individuals who have undergone orthodontic expansion treatment. Thus far, however, no data has been supplied to support this assertion. Once again the practitioner should be reminded that any preformed archwire is based upon an average shape. When a preformed archwire is used, it should be appropriately contoured to match the individual arch variations of a particular patient.

It has also been suggested that certain shapes are more frequently represented in the maxillary arch form (the ellipse or parabola) than in the mandibular arch form, (which is more frequently represented by the catenary curve). Should this finding be borne out, it would further serve to complicate efforts to come to any agreement on the concept of an ideal arch form.

4.1.1. Individualized Arch Form

While it is important to understand that considerable research efforts have gone into identifying the ideal arch form, this is of little clinical use to the orthodontist who is faced with everyday decisions regarding the appropriate arch form for an individual patient. A patient specific or "natural" arch form can be determined by fabricating an **occlusal map** of an individual dental arch. To accomplish this, the occlusal surface of the dental cast is directly photographed at a 1:1 setting. By placing a piece of acetate paper over this photograph, the occlusal shapes of the individual teeth can be traced.   A second piece of acetate paper is then placed over the photograph with a dotted line being drawn through the mesiodistal widths of each tooth, and connected through the proximal contacts. This arc represents the natural arch perimeter. Even badly rotated or imperfect teeth won't impede the identification of this central arc. Finally, the original shapes of the individual teeth can be traced to an ideal position over the central arc perimeter to give the clinician an individualized ideal arch form.

This occlusal map can aid orthodontic treatment decisions in two important ways. The most obvious benefit is that it will allow the orthodontist to maintain, within reason, the individual's original arch form. The benefit of this can be found in the long-term retention studies that support the notion of the pretreatment arch form tending to return in the post-retention period, and maximum stability being greatest in those individuals whose arch form has been maintained.

Secondly, arch length discrepancies can be more readily identified and measured by using an occlusal map than by simply trying to eyeball the spacing requirements of the individual dental arch. As we know, the success of orthodontic treatment begins with an accurate diagnosis. An under-estimation of arch length could lead to unnecessary extractions. An over-estimation of arch length could lead to increased treatment time or unstable orthodontic results.

4.1.2. Malocclusions and Arch Form

Different malocclusions have also been suggested to influence the shape of the dental arches. Recently investigators measured the arch widths and depths of Class I, Class II, and Class III occlusal groups. Their data seemed to indicate that the maxillary arch forms of Class II malocclusions were narrower than those of maxillary Class I arches in the posterior segments. Class III arch widths, on the other hand, were found to be wider in the posterior segments that those of Class I arches. The maxillary arch depths remained relatively similar for all occlusal groups.

In addition to this, variability was found in the mandibular arch forms of Class I, Class II, and Class III occlusal groups. The mandibular Class III arch forms generally exhibited a smaller **arch depth** and a greater posterior arch width than those found in Class I occlusions. The mandibular Class II arch forms also differed from those of the Class I occlusal group by being reduced in both depth and posterior arch width.

We should remember that the notion of arch form variability among the occlusal groups has not been universally accepted. There have been other researchers who have been unable to verify these same conclusions. Further study in this area is obviously warranted.

4.1.3. Asymmetries in Arch Form

Perhaps one of the factors leading to our frustration in attempting to establish an ideal arch form is that we are expecting symmetry and balance in the dental arches. Any variation from this situation is considered an annoyance or an anomaly. We have to remind ourselves that symmetry in nature is predominantly a theoretical concept. Seldom are living things symmetrical. Thus we should expect that the shapes of the dental arches would likewise reflect this precept. Furthermore, if true arch symmetry is exceedingly rare or does not exist, shouldn't we ask ourselves if the pursuit of a symmetrical arch form is not an affront to nature and an unrealistic expectation, perhaps clinically increasing the chances of orthodontic relapse?

General Contributory Factors to Arch Form Asymmetries

Asymmetries affecting the general arch form (Figure 13-32) usually result from of one of three factors: genetics, the environment, or a combination of both. Examples of genetic factors that could influence the arch form would be craniofacial syndromes, (including clefting), **anodontia** (total congenital absence of teeth), **oligodontia** (partial congenital absence of teeth), and variations in tooth sizes and shapes. Environmental influences that likewise would affect the dental arch form include thumb or digital habits, trauma, and systemic diseases. A combination of genetics and the environment probably contribute to the arch form disparities seen among individuals with mouth breathing or tongue thrusting habits.

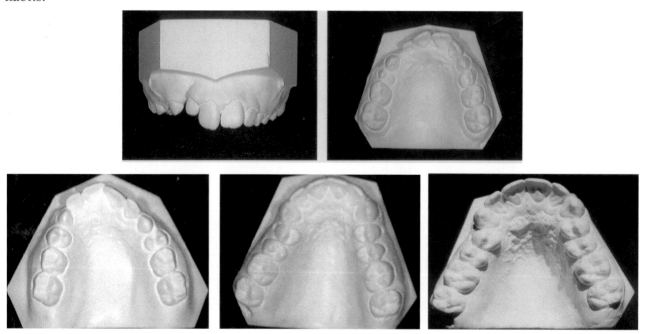

Figure 13-32

Local Contributory Factors to Arch Form Asymmetries

Dental relationships can likewise affect the developing arch form, thus potentially contributing to arch form asymmetries. For example, the **ankylosis** of primary teeth below the plane of occlusion permits the adjacent teeth to tip into the space where the **ankylosed** tooth is positioned. This results in a net loss of space or space deficiency, concomitant **asymmetrical** axial inclinations of the adjacent teeth (when compared to the contralateral side), and an asymmetrical molar relationship. Thus the ankylosis of an individual tooth (Figure 13-33) or a group of teeth could eventually result in a dental midline shift, adversely affecting the developing dental arch and leading to an asymmetry.

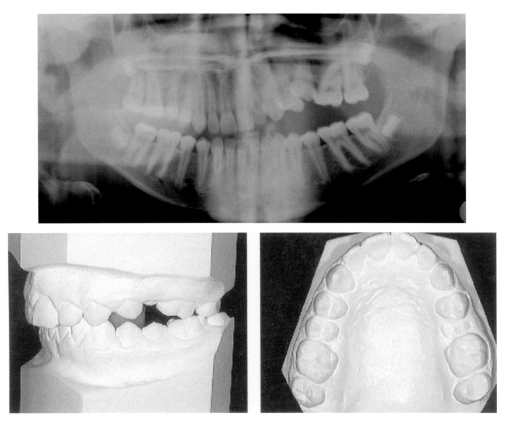

Figure 13-33

Ectopically erupting permanent teeth (Figure 13-34) can also impact the arch form symmetry. Specifically, the **ectopic eruption** of the maxillary first permanent molar has been shown to occur in between 4-5% of northern Europeans. If this is left untreated, the primary second molar is usually lost prematurely (unless space maintenance intervention is begun), resulting in the **mesial drift** of the permanent first molar and a subsequent space loss/arch form asymmetry.

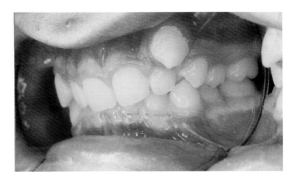
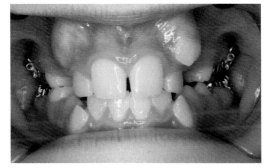

Figure 13-34

Interproximal caries can be an important cause of localized space loss in the **dental arch** (Figure 13-35), thus contributing to an arch form asymmetry. Particularly in the deciduous molar regions, interproximal caries can cause a reduction in the mesiodistal widths of the affected teeth, resulting in the mesial drift of the tooth distal to the affected tooth. This results in a shortened dental arch and ultimately an arch form asymmetry.

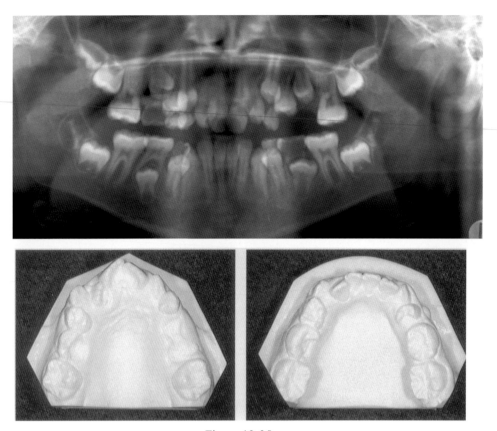

Figure 13-35

Early extractions of deciduous teeth (Figure 13-36) also contribute to the net loss of arch length due to the migrations of the adjacent teeth into the extraction spaces. The importance that early extractions of deciduous teeth have on the overall arch form depends upon the type of deciduous tooth that was extracted, the patient's age or dental development at the time of the extraction, and the relative arch length / spacing requirements within the dental arch itself. All of these variables should be taken into account prior to the removal of any deciduous teeth, as the sequela of any of these variables can adversely affect the developing arch form symmetry.

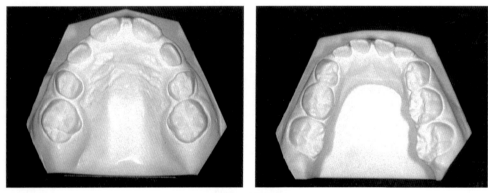

Figure 13-36

Tooth number disparities such as extra or supernumerary teeth or congenitally missing teeth both contribute to the development of asymmetric arch forms. Supernumerary teeth are found in about 1% of the population. They have been known to cause local eruption problems such as impactions or ectopic eruptions of the adjacent teeth. The resulting midline discrepancies are frequently cited as contributing to asymmetric arch forms. Likewise, congenitally missing teeth (Figure 13-37), which are found in approximately 5% of the population, also influence the arch symmetry by disrupting the occlusal relationships and contributing to midline discrepancies.

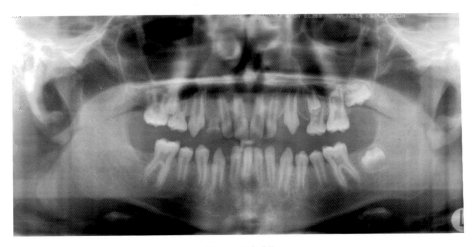

Figure 13-37

4.1.4. Maxillary Arch Asymmetry Analysis

A fairly simple method for determining tooth position asymmetries in the maxillary arch involves the use of a **symmetrograph** (Figure 13-38). This is a transparent plastic device with an inscribed grid, which may be either purchased or made. To determine maxillary arch asymmetry, place the dental cast on its base and carefully mark the median raphe with a series of tiny dots. The median raphe is a proper representation of the skeletal midline. Orient the symmetrograph so that its midline is directly superimposed over the median raphe and parallel to the occlusal surface. Total and partial arch asymmetries are quickly visualized and localized, as are drifting, tipping, and rotations of individual teeth. This simple step is most useful in planning individual tooth

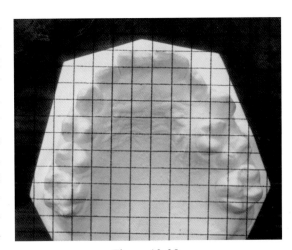

Figure 13-38

movements and determining appliance design. A similar analysis of the mandibular dentition is likely to be less precise, since mandibular landmarks are not as reliable as the median raphe.

4.1.5. Population differences in arch form

Differing factors are believed to impact upon an individual's arch form. The influence of the oral musculature on the positions of the teeth and the size and shape of the **basal bone** both contribute to the size and shape of the dental arches. In addition, tooth sizes exert an affect on the arch form, with the arch length being influenced to a greater extent than the arch width. Therefore, variations in the tooth sizes of a particular group would likely be responsible for the variations in the arch form or length within that group.

Recently several studies have been done to compare the arch form and length of African Americans to White Americans. What was found was that African Americans had significantly larger arch lengths and widths (approximately 10% greater) than White Americans, in addition to having larger tooth sizes. Spatial differences were also noted in the dental arches, particularly in the cuspid and first bicuspid regions. Specifically, African Americans exhibited more of a convex curvature in this region than

White Americans, who had a relatively straight line. This difference gave an overall rounded appearance to the arch form of White Americans as compared to African Americans, who exhibited a more squared shape. These differences are relevant to the success of individualized patient treatment plans, particularly if the arch form is standardized or modified and long-term stability is of concern.

4.1.6. Arch Form and Aging

An interesting concern to the clinician who treats children and adolescents is how growth, development, and maturity affect their treatment results. As most orthodontic patients are children, knowledge of these areas is imperative to understanding the probable long-term consequences of treatment. Not only are treatment results important to both the patient and clinician, but so too are the stability of the results. Therefore a greater understanding of foreseeable changes over time could aid both the patient and the orthodontist in determining realistic expectations for treatment, retention, and long-term stability.

Researchers have found that changes in the size and shape of the cranio-facial complex do not stop when biological maturity is reached. Even decades into adult life, changes have been shown to occur. The rate of growth and the direction of growth ("aging") is what differ when comparing changes between children and adolescents to adults.

Studies have been done on the arch size and shape of orthodontically untreated individuals from as young as 6 weeks to as old as to 68 years of age. From these studies, some consistent patterns of arch change have been noted:

-Before the complete eruption of the deciduous dentition, (between the ages of 6 weeks to 2 years), there were significant increases in the maxillary and mandibular anterior and posterior arch widths.

-By 8 years of age and after the eruption of the four incisor teeth, the mandibular intercuspid width was established.

-Between the ages of 3 to 13 years, the intercuspid and **intermolar width**s increased significantly in the maxillary arch. Once the permanent dentition had completely erupted, a slight decrease was noted in the dental arch widths, particularly in the intercuspid region, although a decrease was also evident in the intermolar region.

-From the age of 15 to 26 years, a decrease in arch depth was consistently noted, as was the inference of a decrease in arch length.

-Arch lengths and arch depths decreased significantly with time among individuals between the ages of 20 to 55 years of age. Arch width increases were noted in this group in the molar regions. These changes tended to occur most rapidly in young adulthood, however evidence of change was found even in later years.

Understanding how these natural aging or changing processes will affect the arch size and shape will aid the clinician in future dental/skeletal predictions for a particular patient. Overall what was found was that with age, both maxillary and mandibular arches tended toward a broader, shallower, and shorter morphology than was originally present. The speculative cause of these morphological changes is that bone growth or remodeling occurs in response to the affects of anterior and buccal occlusal forces. Once again, however, these longitudinal findings of arch form changes are not universally accepted, and thus demand continued research and analysis.

4.1.7. Alterations / Expansion of Arch Form

For many years the stability of the dental arch has been challenged. Studies have been conducted which seemed to show that any alteration in the arch widths at the cuspid and first molar regions, as a result of orthodontic treatment, would be unstable and should not be expected to be maintained in the post-retention phase of orthodontic treatment. The greater the treatment changes in arch form, the greater the tendency for a return to the pretreatment shape after retention. At best, these post-retention studies showed an occasional 2.0 mm expansion at the molar region, with the cuspid region never holding any increases. Therefore, expansion treatment approaches were considered to be risky and holding no scientific merit.

Recently, there has been a renewed interest in attempting to increase the widths of the dental arches (particularly the maxilla). In trying to avoid the failures of the past, closer attention has been paid to the accurate diagnosis of the location of the particular transverse problem and the skeletal maturity of the patient. Arch widths have been assessed at the dental, alveolar, and skeletal levels, using not only information provided by the clinical exam, or model analysis, but also a posteroanterior (PA) cephalometric radiograph. Some studies have suggested that expansion of the maxillary arch can occur, and can remain stable if the reason for the transverse discrepancy is identified and addressed appropriately. If the problem is deemed to be skeletal in nature, and is corrected at the midpalatal suture by applying a heavy force across the suture (thus stimulating increased bone formation) the long-term stability is believed to be enhanced. This is more optimally achieved in a younger child. Research has indicated that 50% of expansion gains in a younger child are skeletal in nature, with the other 50% being dental (tipping), when such forces are used. This ratio can unfavorably change as the child matures to an adolescent; then only 35% of expansion gains this way are believed to be skeletal in nature. Based upon these numbers, over-correction or over-expansion in children has been advocated to account for unwanted dental and alveolar changes, which can be expected to occur and likewise can be expected to ultimately relapse.

Sutural closing signals the end of any opportunity to non-surgically expand the maxillary arch. If non-surgical expansion is attempted after the palatal suture closes, unstable results and deleterious periodontal complications may develop, which could include complaints of pain, or adverse extrusions or tipping of the maxillary teeth. By surgically assisting the sutural opening in the mature maxilla, the clinician can expect to see a predominantly (84%) skeletal change occur. For this reason, over correction of these patients is not advised.

Attempts to change or widen the mandibular arch form have been, until relatively recently, discouraged for concerns about lack of stability. Some clinicians have reported success with a lip bumper; however, these changes are believed to be dentoalveolar as opposed to skeletal in nature. The lip bumper in combination with the tongue posture, proponents believe, can serve to broaden and reshape the mandibular arch, which some clinicians claim has excellent long-term stability. This contention is not without skeptics. Obviously additional research and long-term studies are needed in this very interesting area.

5. ANALYSIS OF TOOTH POSITIONS AND INTER-ARCH RELATIONSHIPS

Differences in the occlusal relationships between the dental arches and individual teeth can occur in three spatial planes: vertical, antero-posterior, and transverse. This is the result of complex genetic and environmental processes that influence tooth development, eruption, and jaw growth. Individual variations or failures in any of these areas can have a profound impact upon the developing occlusion, and can result in anomalies or compensatory changes in what would otherwise have been an acceptable occlusion.

5.1 TOOTH POSITIONS AND RELATIONSHIPS

In attempting to evaluate the occlusion of an individual, it is important to first note any abnormalities or irregularities in the arrangement of the teeth within the jaws. Dr. Edward H. Angle geometrically described the ideal arrangement of the teeth as the "line of occlusion", which he defined as, "the line with which, in form and position according to type, the teeth must be in harmony if in normal occlusion". Angle felt that there was only one true line of occlusion dictated by the length, width and characteristic curves of the dental arches, as well as the size and pattern of the individual teeth, cusps, and inclined planes composing the dental arches. This "line of occlusion" can be visualized as a symmetric curve that describes the position of the maxillary teeth (along the central fossa line) when "normally" occluded with the mandibular teeth (along their bucco-occlusal line). An individual tooth's spatial relationship within the arch can thus be explained.

Angle further described the orthodontic tooth movements that would be necessary to correct a malpositioned tooth to the line of occlusion. These were called **first, second,** and **third order positions**. A horizontal movement relative to the line of occlusion was termed a first order movement, a vertical movement relative to the line of occlusion was termed a second order movement, and a twisting or torsional movement relative to the line of occlusion was termed a third order movement. Since the introduction of pre-adjusted orthodontic brackets, these compensations have been built into the orthodontic appliances and have been casually termed as follows:

-"in-out" is used to define **first order positioning** (Figure 13-39) and describes the faciolingual or bucco-lingual relationship of the crown of the tooth to the line of occlusion.

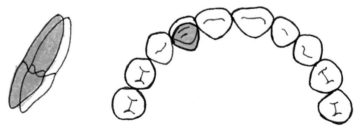

Figure 13-39

--"tip" or "angulation" is used to define **second order positioning** and (Figure 13-40) describes the mesial or distal inclination of the crown or root of the tooth to the line of occlusion

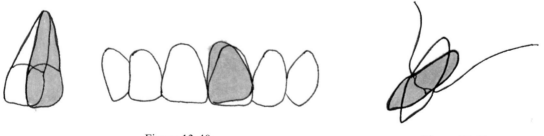

Figure 13-40

Figure 13-41

--"torque" is used to define the **third order positioning** (Figure 13-41) and describes the inclination of the crown or root of the tooth to the line of occlusion.

Additionally, today's clinician may consider two other factors when evaluating tooth positions within the **dental arch**. The first of these factors is the rotation of an individual tooth, as described by the proximal tooth contacts in relation to the line of occlusion. This is a sometimes referred to as an **offset**. The second factor is the cusp height or vertical position of an individual tooth, which is also evaluated in relation to the plane of occlusion. This has been termed cusp height positioning.

5.2 INTRA–ARCH AND INTER-ARCH RELATIONSHIPS AND CLASSIFICATION

Classification methods have been developed over the years by many orthodontists to describe the various interarch relationships and malocclusions they observed in their clinical practices. Such eminent orthodontists as Doctors Kingsley, Case, Dewey, Anderson, Hellman, Simon, Bennet, Elsasser, Ackerman and Profitt have all offered different approaches to describe the various interarch relationships they observed; however, thus far none of their methods have gained widespread acceptance. While many classification methods have been developed, the method developed by Dr. Angle over 100 years ago still remains as the orthodontic standard today.

One might ask, "Why is there a need for a classification system?" Classification systems are important to the individual clinician and to the specialty for three reasons. First, they help the individual clinician focus on the particular type and magnitude of the malocclusion. This will facilitate a successful diagnosis and treatment plan. For example, a malocclusion classified as a "Class III" requires entirely different types of treatment mechanics than that of a malocclusion classified as a "Class II". If the clinician fails to correctly identify and classify the malocclusion, he or she may begin inappropriate mechanics for that patient's particular problem, culminating in a less than ideal result.

Secondly, a classification system allows for a common descriptive language among all orthodontists. This is absolutely vital for communicating not only to other orthodontists, but also to fellow dentists, dental students, governmental agencies, and insurance providers the scope and magnitude of a particular patient's problem.

Thirdly, as one of the goals of orthodontic treatment is to treat the patient to an ideal result, there has to be an agreement among orthodontists as to what constitutes an ideal result. A common classification standard has to be accepted, to which all treatment results are aimed and evaluated. Without this, chaos would exist as no consistent goals for treatment outcome could be established.

5.2.1. Historical Descriptions of Normal Occlusion and New Methods

Today's clinician uses many parameters to evaluate their patient's occlusion. Proper dental alignment, relationship of the dental arches, skeletal pattern, and positions of the temporomandibular joint condyles within the **glenoid fossa** are all necessary for an acceptable occlusion. Additionally, the facial profile and soft tissue proportions of the patient must be taken into consideration when evaluating an occlusion or correcting a malocclusion, if today one is to say that a good orthodontic result has been attained.

Historically, however, these parameters have not always been used to differentiate an acceptable occlusion from a malocclusion. Early definitions of a proper occlusion involved only the dental alignment and the anteroposterior relationship of the dental arches. Two prominent orthodontists who have had a substantial impact on the orthodontic world in defining a proper or "normal" occlusion and, as a result, malocclusions, and who primarily focused their analysis of occlusion on the areas of dental alignment and the anteroposterior relationship of the dental arches were Dr. E. H. Angle and Dr. L. F. Andrews.

5.2.1.1. **The Angle Classification System**

Dr. Angle, in 1900, used the antero-posterior positions of the upper and lower first molars and the alignment of the teeth to the line of occlusion to describe for the first time not only malocclusions, but also normal occlusion. The descriptions he developed were as follows:

Normal occlusion was defined as a Class I relationship when the mesio-buccal cusp of the maxillary permanent first molar tooth occludes with the buccal groove on the mandibular permanent first molar tooth, and when the teeth are well-aligned and on the line of occlusion (Figure 13-42). When this occurs in permanent, intact dentitions (presumably without tooth size discrepancies), the posterior intercuspal relationships, overbite, and overjet would be expected to be ideal.

The Angle Class I malocclusion (sometimes referred to as **neutral occlusion**) was defined as when the maxillary permanent first molar tooth occludes in the buccal groove of the mandibular permanent first molar tooth, and teeth were not well aligned or on the line of occlusion (Figure 13-43).

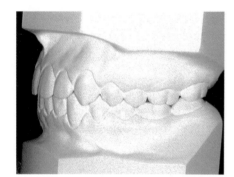

Figure 13-42

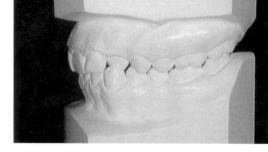

Figure 13-43

The Angle Class II malocclusion (sometimes referred to as **distoclusion** or **disto-occlusion**) was defined as a situation in which the mesio-buccal cusp of the maxillary permanent first molar occludes anteriorly to the buccal groove of the mandibular permanent first molar. Angle further described two types of Class II malocclusions. These include Class II division 1 malocclusions (Figure 13-44) and Class II division 2 malocclusions (Figure 13-45), dependent upon the angulations of the maxillary central incisor teeth. If the upper and lower dentitions are permanent, intact, and well aligned, (again presumably without tooth size discrepancies), the posterior intercuspal relationships, overbite, and overjet will all vary from the ideal (normal occlusion) in both Class II situations, with the degree of severity dictated by the amount of the discrepancy.

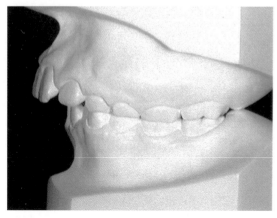

Figure 13-44

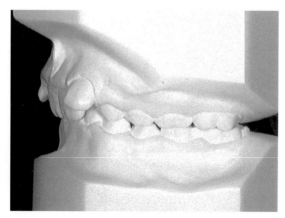

Figure 13-45

The Angle Class III malocclusion (sometimes referred to as **mesioclusion** or **mesio-occlusion**) was defined as a situation in which the mesio-buccal cusp of the maxillary permanent first molar occludes distally to the buccal groove of the mandibular permanent first molar (Figure 13-46). As with the Class I and Class II malocclusions, if the upper and lower dentitions are permanent, intact, and well aligned, (and again presumably without tooth size discrepancies), the posterior intercuspal relationships, overbite, and overjet will vary from the ideal, with the degree of severity dictated by the amount of the discrepancy.

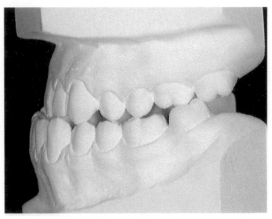

Figure 13-46

The **Angle classification** system has remained the most popular classification system in orthodontics. Even today the Angle classification system is the only universally accepted system to classify malocclusions. This is the system is used by such pre-eminent organizations as the American Board of Orthodontics (ABO) in their Phase III examination for Board Certification. It is not, however, a system without criticism. From its inception, critics have pointed out that it is a system that idealized the straight Caucasoid profile of an Apollo Belvedere while referring to the dentition in the skull of a prognathic Negroid male as the ideal, thus setting up an impossible situation where the two circumstances could never have coexisted in one individual.

Additional criticism has been aimed at the Angle classification system because of its failure to adequately address all possible malocclusion groups, for instance, those situations in which one side of the occlusion is one class, and the other side is another class of occlusion. Another example of this failure would be those situations in which analogous malocclusions having similar posterior relationships (yet requiring very different treatment approaches) are not recognized as such.

The greatest criticism of Angle's classification system is that it only addresses malocclusions in the antero-posterior or sagittal dimension. There is no consideration given for the vertical or transverse dimensions, let alone consideration for the positions of the condyles, or the soft tissue profile and face. It is widely recognized today that discrepancies can occur in any one or more of these areas, and while contributing to the malocclusion, must be recognized and addressed if a successful treatment outcome is to be expected.

5.2.1.2. The Six Keys To Normal Occlusion

Another important investigator who attempted to define "normal" or the desired occlusion was Dr. L. F. Andrews. In 1972, he wrote an article detailing six significant characteristics, involving both tooth alignment and the anteroposterior interarch relationship, that he felt were necessary for a "normal occlusion". Dr. Andrews determined these characteristics by examining what he termed 120 non-orthodontic normal models. The characteristics these models exhibited were considered to be the best in nature and were described in a paper entitled "The Six Keys To Normal Occlusion". They were as follows:

-Molar relationship
-Crown angulation or the mesiodistal "tip"
-Crown inclination
-Rotations (or the lack thereof)
-Spaces (or the absence of, resulting in tight dental contacts)

-The occlusal plane (varying from a flat Curve of Spee to a very slight curve)

The absence of any of these qualities he believed was, " a defect predictive of an incomplete end result". Likewise he felt that if the six keys were achieved, a final desired normal occlusion could be attained.

Although this was also cited as a landmark study, critics have pointed out that this too only described the static positions of the teeth within the dental arches, and the antero-posterior relationship of the dental arches as defined by the first molar teeth. As with Dr. Angle's classification system, no considerations were given in Dr. Andrews' paper for the vertical or transverse relationships of the dental arches, the facial profile, or the positions of the condyles, all of which today are considered necessary for an acceptable occlusion.

5.2.1.3. Diagnostics in OrthoCAD and emodels™

Recently introduced, the OrthoCAD software for 3D digital study casts contain several tools that facilitate pre-treatment diagnostics as well as post-treatment analysis and evaluation. A virtual caliper enables the user to make any type of point-to-point and point-to-plane measurements. In all instances, users mark the beginning and end of each measurement on screen, while data is collected for pre-determined analyses (Figure 13-47A).

Also recently introduced is the emodel™ software, which contains many diagnostic tools. The tools range from easy to use measurements to a complete setup tool called eplan™. The measurements consist of point to point, Bolton Analysis, and curve length measurements. Measurements are accomplished with ease using a point and click method. emodels™ are created through the non destructive laser scanning process that digitally transforms plaster study models into a high resolution image that ensures accuracy to ±.01mm. emodels™ offer extensive analysis tools enabling intuitive and precise measurements unavailable with plaster study models (Figure 13-47B).

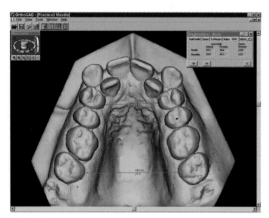 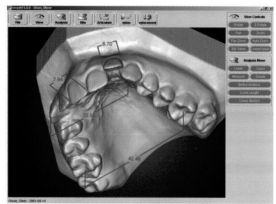

Figure 13-47A   Figure 13-47B

The Bolton analysis is a widely used tool, designed to evaluate the mesiodistal tooth size discrepancies between sets of corresponding maxillary and mandibular teeth. The software offers a built-in "Bolton calculator" to determine the difference between the actual case ratio and a user-defined "ideal ratio" (with the default value set on one standard deviation). The value obtained provides an estimate in millimeters of the severity of tooth size discrepancy between the arches. Additional formulas that are embedded in the software include width and length analyses, as well as Tonn's formula (Figures 13-48A and 13-48B).

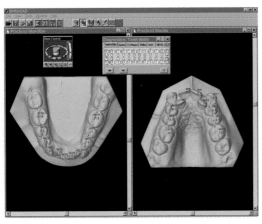 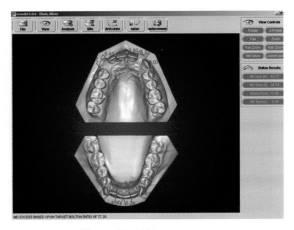

Figure 13-48A   Figure 13-48B

The virtual caliper can be used in a similar fashion to measure the overbite, or the degree of vertical overlap, of the mandibular incisors by their maxillary antagonists, and overjet, or the distance between the labial surface of the mandibular incisors and the labial aspect of the incisal edges of the maxillary incisors (Figure 13-49A). The ability to zoom in on points of interest can significantly increase measuring accuracy.

Using the emodel™ measurement tools is a simple way to take accurate overjet/overbite measurements (Figure 13-49B). With the ability to infinitely zoom in, measurement accuracy will increase and your measurements will be completed in a matter of seconds.

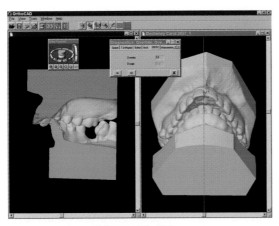 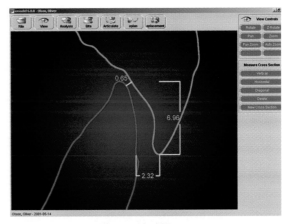

Figure 13-49A   Figure 13-49B

Digital casts can be sectioned in the midpalatal plane, defined by anatomical points on the palatine raphe, and the tuberosity plane, a parafrontal plane (Figure 13-50A). While the former mostly serves as a reference for assessment of transverse symmetry, the latter is traditionally associated with analysis of antero-posterior malpositions. From a diagnostic point of view, assessment of transverse symmetry is clinically relevant, particularly in cases of transverse malocclusions. Analyses of antero-posterior malocclusions are primarily utilized to diagnose mesial tooth shift. When there is no right-left asymmetry, the teeth are correctly positioned, or there has been symmetric migration.

emodels™ can be sectioned on any plane. Utilizing the vertical and horizontal cross-sectioning tools enables the clinician to check symmetry, overjet, overbite and complete measurements on any location or plane (Figure 13-50B).

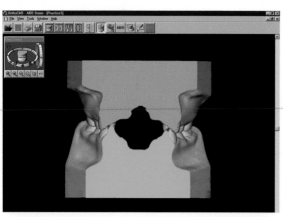 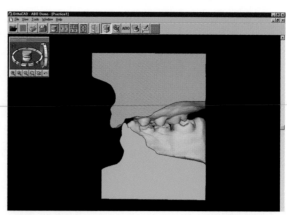

Figure 13-50A

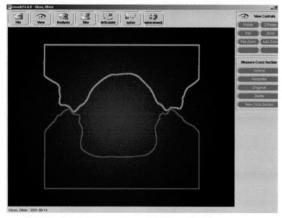 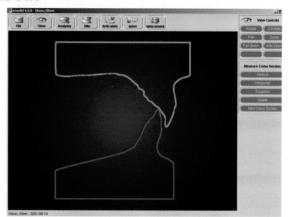

Figure 13-50B

One of the latest innovations in 3-D digital treatment planning is the eplan™ by GeoDigm Corporation. eplan™ is a segmented 3-D digital dental model that provides doctors with the ability to simulate multiple treatment options to determine the most effective treatment plan and to optimize patient outcomes. eplan™ treatment planning tools provide the ability to simulate accurate tooth rotation, movement, and extraction to assess various treatment options and outcomes with the simple click of a mouse. eplan™ enables patients to watch the movement of their own teeth from malocclusion view to post-treatment view, providing an unprecedented insight into the treatment process. In addition, eplans are effective communication tools that enable clear communication between doctors, patients, and referring practitioners (Figure 13-50C).

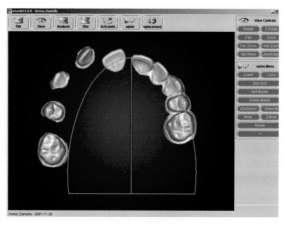

Figure 13-50C

The occlusogram in the OrthoCAD software is used to analyze occlusal relationships (Figure 13-51A). The image is color coded to allow for easier visual assessment of the occlusion.   This analysis is particularly useful in comparing and contrasting pre-treatment and post-treatment occlusal relationships and to aid in determining the efficacy of specific treatment regimens.   In addition, the bite registration may prove to be useful for some clinicians in their TMJ/TMD treatment.   The software also allows singling out full contacts only, in addition to a complete description of the occlusal relationship.

The Color Bite Mapping in emodel™ software allows the user to analyze occlusal relationships.   The color coded map shows where contact is happening and the severity of contact.   In combination with eplan™ this diagnostic tool will show the differences in bite registrations of various treatment plans. The color map can be viewed in any portion of the emodel™ software (Figure 13-51B).   This is useful when aligned with a digital cephalogram and then articulated.   The articulation will allow the visualization of the contact as it happens.   When color mapping is combined with eplan™ articulation and a ceph you will have all the tools needed to visualize the outcome of any treatment plan.

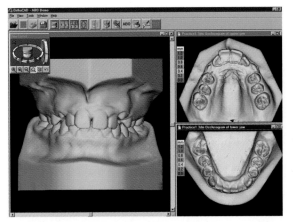 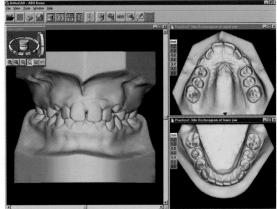

Figure 13-51A

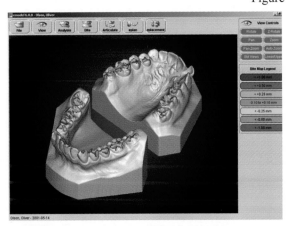 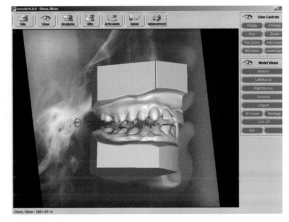

Figure 13-51B

Still utilizing the occlusogram feature, OrthoCAD provides for antero-posterior and transverse adjustments in the relationship between the maxillary and mandibular arches.   This feature enables the orthodontist to compensate for slight bite registration inaccuracies or to simply test the interdigitation potential of different antero-posterior or transverse positions.   Compare the original bite registration as seen in Figure 13-51A with Figure 13-52 where the mandible has been protruded by 0.6 mm.

The emodel™ software allows the user to adjust bite registration to alleviate any problems with the original bite registration without re-pouring a plaster model.   Used in combination with the Color Bite

Mapping the orthodontist can be sure that the emodel™ is accurate to the patient's true bite.

After the individual findings are compiled to form the comprehensive diagnostic assessment, this assessment can be represented digitally on the screen with the notes system. Three separate layers of information can be noted for:

1.) Case presentations
2.) Colleague-to-colleague and all other types of extra-office communications (case transfers, interdisciplinary cases, patients, insurances companies, etc).
3.) Intra-office guidelines.

All the information, including the diagnostic data and the notes, can be communicated electronically to colleagues and other dental specialists via e-mail or printed as a hard copy. In addition, users are able to relay the information as simple two-dimensional representations of the 3D model (Figure 13-53).

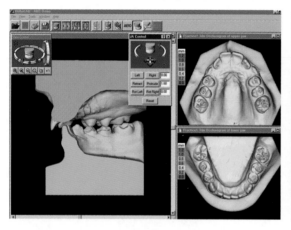
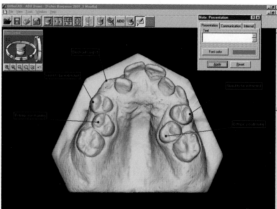

Figure 13-52   Figure 13-53

After the diagnostics are finished on an emodel™ the file can be saved for future reference. The file can also be emailed to a referring doctor for consultation. The referring doctor can view the emodel™ as if they were in the same location. The referring doctor can also make modifications to the treatment plan if desired and email the file back. This freedom allows diagnostics to be completed quickly and easily without leaving the office. It is also possible to save two-dimensional images for use in presentations, letters, and integrated into the office's imaging software. The combination of digital photos, digital x-rays, and emodel™ 3D digital models into one integrated system enables efficient diagnostic record management and retrieval.

5.2.2. Factors Influencing The Occlusion

5.2.2.1. Intra-Arch Relationships

An ideal occlusion relies on many factors, not the least of which are the teeth themselves. Variations in the size, shape, position, and number of teeth will all have an impact on the final occlusion, as will the crowding and spacing of these teeth within the dental arch. If we are to understand the impact any one of these situations could have on the occlusion we should examine each variable separately.

Individual Tooth Positions

The inappropriate angulation of an individual tooth may result in that tooth occupying a position other than its ideal position, with the apex of the tooth being in the correct place, but the crown being tilted away from ideal. This differs from the bodily displacement of a tooth, in that both the crown and the root have moved together to a compromised position. Vertical displacements of a tooth or some teeth, (extrusions and intrusions), can also occur, which negatively affect the occlusion. The failure of a tooth to erupt (an impaction), likewise will adversely affect the occlusion. Although this can occur with any of the teeth, it is most frequently seen with the maxillary cuspids (Figure 13-54) and the mandibular third molar teeth (Figure 13-55). Any of the preceding situations may involve only one tooth; however, the result would affect the entire dentition and the occlusion.

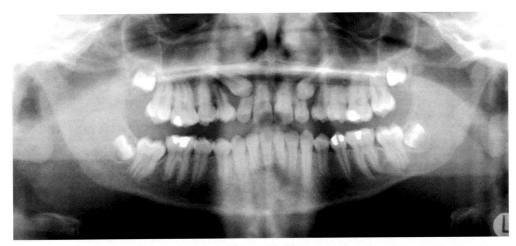

Figure 13-54

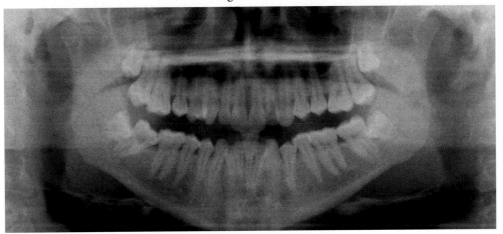

Figure 13-55

Tooth Size And Shape Variations

Tooth sizes frequently have an influence upon the perimeter size of the dental arches, and consequently on the occlusion. When, however, there is a variation in an individual tooth size (Figure 13-56), irregularities in dental positioning and occlusion can result. If a permanent tooth is too small, spacing will occur. If a permanent tooth is too large, crowding will occur.

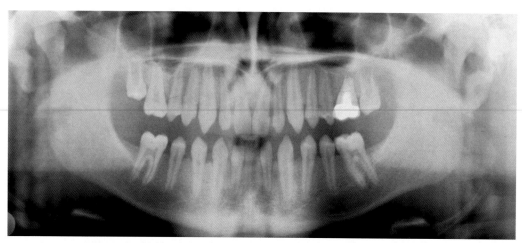

Figure 13-56

Anomalies in tooth shape can also negatively affect the overall occlusion. Probably the most frequently encountered example of this is the peg maxillary lateral incisor (Figure 13-57), which is an abnormally small tooth. When this occurs a dental spacing problem will result. Another commonly occurring tooth shape anomaly is seen in the mandibular second bicuspid teeth. The crowns of these teeth can occasionally present with two lingual cusps, thus resulting in an increased mesio-distal width, unsatisfactory intercuspation, and concomitant crowding. Additional dental morphological variations that can adversely affect the proper intercuspation and occlusion include claw form incisors, Hutchinson's incisors, fused teeth (Figure 13-58), taurodontia (Figure 13-59), gemination, and hypoplastic teeth.

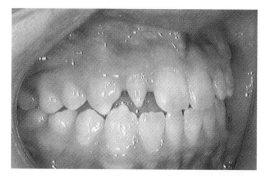

Figure 13-57

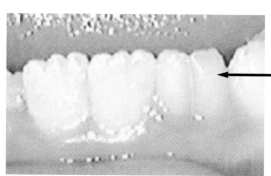

Figure 13-58

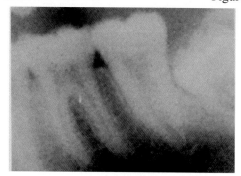

Figure 13-59

Tooth Number Variations

When a tooth fails to develop (tooth **agenesis**), a spacing problem is created. Interestingly enough, when one or more teeth are absent in an individual it is not uncommon to note a generalized reduction in the sizes of the remaining teeth (Figure 13-60), thus complicating an already difficult spacing and occlusion problem.

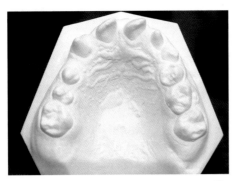
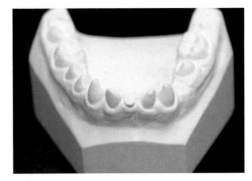

Figure 13-60

A supernumerary or extra tooth that has erupted into the dental arch will likewise compromise the occlusion. This occurs because the additional tooth mass will result in crowding and poor intercuspation. An unerupted supernumerary tooth can occasionally affect the occlusion by displacing the position of the adjacent tooth or teeth out of their appropriate alignment (Figure 13-61), thus resulting in a situation of crowding or poor intercuspation.

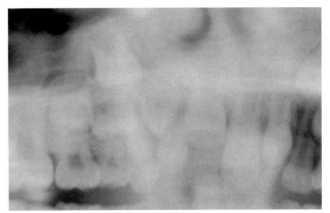

Figure 13-61

Exfoliation And Eruption Variations

The premature loss of a deciduous tooth or teeth can adversely affect the alignment of the permanent dentition, thus to the detriment of the occlusion. For example, the premature loss of a deciduous incisor tooth could result in the mesial tooth migration and subsequent space deficit for the erupting permanent incisor tooth. This would then appear as anterior tooth crowding. The premature loss of a deciduous molar can result in the mesial migration of the adjacent posterior tooth (Figure 13-62), once again manifesting as dental crowding. Occasionally, individual tooth **crossbites** or **scissorsbites** may be seen in these situations, reflecting the space loss.

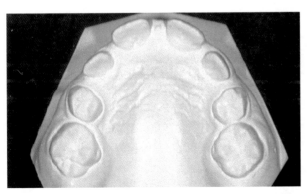
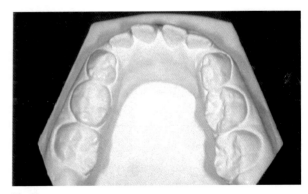

Figure 13-62

Situations can also occur where the deciduous teeth are not exfoliated in a timely manner. When this occurs, the eruption of the permanent teeth can be negatively affected. Ectopic eruptions and positional tooth displacements can result as a consequence of this adverse pattern. Hence, poor intercuspation and a compromised occlusion are usually found in these situations.

5.2.2.2. Inter-Arch Relationships

An individual's occlusion is directly affected by the inter-arch relationships that occur in the three spatial planes (antero-posterior, transverse, and vertical). Thus, for an occlusion to be deemed acceptable, balance must occur in all three dimensions. Likewise, disharmony in any one of these areas will lead to a less than desired occlusal situation. Frequently, the clinician will find that many patients present with two of the three spatial dimensions within acceptable parameters, however one is not, thus necessitating orthodontic intervention. Furthermore, discrepancies in these planes can have either a skeletal or a dental basis. For example, apertognathia or an **anterior open bite** could have a skeletal basis, as seen in those individuals with a divergent skeletal growth pattern (Figure 13-63). Conversely, a similarly appearing anterior open bite could have a dental origin, such as in those situations where the teeth have been intruded due to a thumb or digital habit (Figure 13-64). Obviously, careful assessment of not only the spatial problem, but also the underlying etiology, is necessary if a successful correctional treatment is to be rendered.

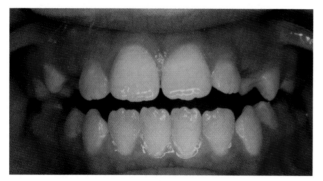

Figure 13-63

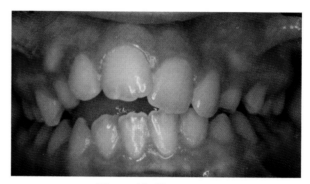

Figure 13-64

Antero-Posterior Malocclusions

The antero-posterior (A-P) occlusal relationships and classification system, as defined by Dr. Angle (and previously described), remain the most frequently used method to evaluate this inter-arch dimension. Because the A-P spatial dimension has been studied and documented for over 100 years, this aspect of a malocclusion is most frequently recognized and detailed by today's clinicians. When Dr. Angle was defining "normal occlusion" and malocclusions using this dimension, his basis was the dental relationship of the first molars, not the skeletal positions of the maxilla or the mandible. The terms he chose, however, to describe the malocclusions (**"neutral occlusion"**, **"disto-occlusion"**, and **"mesio-occlusion"**), referred to the position of the mandible in relationship to the maxilla, with the maxilla seen as the biological constant. He thus inadvertently recognized the potential for both dental and skeletal discrepancies in this dimension.

Today when the orthodontist evaluates a patient's antero-posterior spatial relationship, it is imperative that the etiology of the specific problem (whether dental, skeletal, or sometimes both) is identified, as treatment approaches are vastly different for a skeletal antero-posterior problem as opposed to a dental antero-posterior problem. Skeletal antero-posterior problems can be treatment time sensitive for the orthodontist, as differentiated by dental antero-posterior problems, which can usually be addressed with lesser concern for growth and development. When a skeletal A-P problem is identified in a growing patient, the preferred treatment approach is usually one of growth modification. Typically this is begun with consideration given to the circumpubertal growth spurt and remaining growth potential the particular individual may have. Because girls on average mature earlier that boys, their treatment timing is even more sensitive, as an under- or over-estimation of remaining growth could adversely affect one's expected orthodontic outcome.

When growth modification is not an option for correction of antero-posterior skeletal problems, either due to patient non-compliance or developmental maturity, treatment options can include dental camouflage (usually involving the incisor teeth), or surgical (orthognathic) interventions. Ideally, both of these options are usually reserved for the non-growing individual.

Dental antero-posterior problems are much easier for the orthodontist to correct than are skeletal antero-posterior problems, and unlike the skeletal antero-posterior problems, are much less treatment time sensitive. These situations usually involve arch length / tooth size discrepancies and are readily correctable with conventional orthodontic approaches.

In order for the orthodontist to appropriately analyze a patient in the antero-posterior spatial dimension, six fundamental relationships must be evaluated. These include the following:

  - The cranial base to the maxilla
  - The cranial base to the mandible
  - The maxilla to the mandible
  - The maxilla to the maxillary teeth
  - The mandible to the mandibular teeth
  - The maxillary teeth to the mandibular teeth

To adequately assess a patient's antero-posterior spatial relationship, the clinician will typically refer to specific orthodontic records, beginning with a lateral cephalogram, for analysis of the skeletal and dental/skeletal relationships that are otherwise not apparent upon clinical exam. (Many cephalometric analyses have been developed to aid the orthodontist in this area.) Additionally, examination of the dental models affords the clinician an opportunity to evaluate the dental relationships, the intercuspation of the teeth, and the occlusion. Finally, dental photographs or images are valuable to the practitioner for an overall perspective of the patient in this spatial dimension.

Transverse Malocclusions

An examination of the comparative widths of the dental arches, and any discrepancies therein, is the focus of what is considered a transverse analysis of the occlusion. In an ideal situation, the buccal cusps of the posterior mandibular teeth occlude within the fossa and the occlusal surfaces of the maxillary posterior teeth (Figure 13-65). When this occurs, a harmonious relationship between the widths of the corresponding maxillary and mandibular dental arches would be expected.

CROSSBITE   NORMAL   TELESCOPIC OR **SCISSORS BITE**

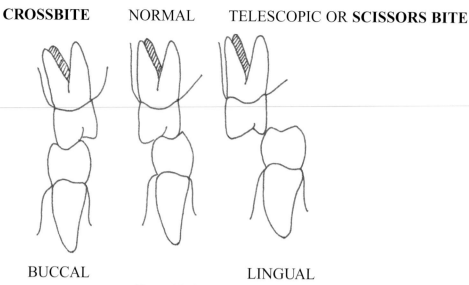

BUCCAL   LINGUAL

Figure 13-65

Occasionally, the buccal cusps of the maxillary posterior teeth occlude lingually to the buccal cusps of the mandibular posterior teeth, resulting in a situation termed a **posterior crossbite** (Figure 13-66). Conversely, an **anterior crossbite** (Figure 13-67) is defined as when the mandibular incisor teeth are situated anteriorly to the corresponding maxillary incisor teeth, when the patient is in centric relation occlusion. This malrelation is an antero-posterior dimensional problem. A **crossbite** can involve anywhere from a single tooth (sometimes also referred to as a single tooth crossbite) to many teeth. When a crossbite involves the posterior teeth, it can result in a compensatory functional shift of the mandible to the affected side.

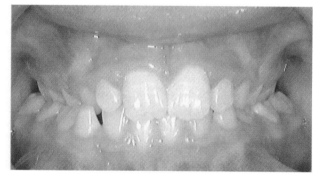

Figure 13-66

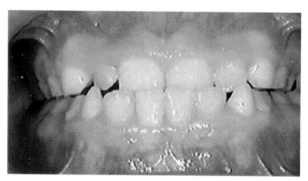

Figure 13-67

Similarly, a situation is occasionally seen where disharmony of the dental arches in the transverse dimension results in an occlusion termed a **buccal crossbite,** a **telescopic bite** or **scissors bite.** This occurs when one or more of the maxillary posterior teeth occlude completely buccally to the mandibular teeth (Figure 13-68), potentially resulting in the functional shifting of the mandible away from the affected area. This relationship is less frequently seen than that of the previously described crossbite, but it is potentially more difficult to correct, particularly when the entire mandible is affected.

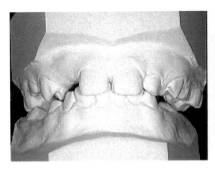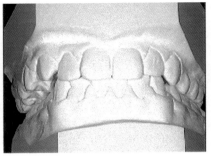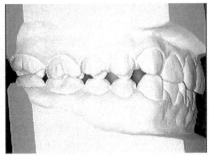

Figure 13-68

As in the antero-posterior dimension, a transverse spatial discrepancy can be either dental or skeletal in origin. For example, a skeletal basis for the disharmony of a posterior crossbite is seen when the maxillary apical base (as defined by the palatal vault evident on the dental casts) is constricted as compared to the corresponding mandibular apical base. In this situation, the dentition or the dentoalveolar processes of the maxilla may be either upright or lean outward in relation to the dentition or the dentoalveolar processes of the mandibular teeth, yet the maxillary teeth still remain in crossbite due to the narrowness of the maxilla itself (Figure 13-69). Occasionally, the asymmetric development of the maxillary or mandibular apical bases themselves results in a unilateral crossbite or scissors bite. This unusual situation is characterized by the absence of any mandibular functional shifting, and can likewise be difficult for the clinician to correct. What can be agreed upon is that the underlying constant for all skeletal transverse discrepancies is the comparative disharmonious widths of the maxillary and mandibular apical bases.

A transverse malocclusion of dental origin is seen when the comparative widths of the maxillary and mandibular apical bases are adequate, however a disparity in the dental arch relationships or the dentition is evident. Again using the example of a posterior crossbite, the dental origin for this could be that where the maxillary arch dentition has a lingual inclination to the corresponding mandibular dentition, the maxillary apical base (as viewed by the palatal vault) is adequate (Figure 13-70). Usually these situations appear unilaterally when the patient is in occlusion, however the clinician will notice that the individual's path of closure is often guided by interferences from the malpositioned teeth, resulting in a functional shift of the mandible into the corresponding posterior crossbite. Thus, the dentition at this time is compromised, but the skeletal component of the malocclusion is not. Treatment of these cases is deemed imperative, as this repetitious posturing of the mandible could lead to an asymmetric mandibular skeletal development and subsequent deleterious functional habits. Fortunately such dental transverse malocclusions are usually very amenable to orthodontic correction.

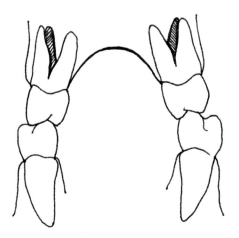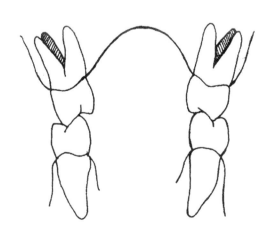

Figure 13-69   Figure 13-70

To adequately assess the transverse spatial dimension, the clinician will rely on several specific ortho-dontic records. These begin with the dental casts that are used to evaluate the **apical base** widths of the maxilla and the mandible, the inclinations of the dentition, and the static tooth positions within and between the dental arches. Additionally, intra-oral dental photographs or images allow the visual-ization of the dentition in occlusion, while extra-oral photos or images allow detection of gross skele-tal asymmetries. The lateral cephalogram is of limited use in the diagnosis of transverse occlusal dis-crepancies; however, some orthodontists rely upon the frontal or postero-anterior cephalogram to aid in the evaluation of transverse malocclusions. Arguably, the most important diagnostic tool the clini-cian will have to diagnose this spatial problem is the clinical exam. Only by watching the patient function during opening and closing movements can one detect the subtleties of the working occlu-sion, and detect any occlusal interferences and corresponding functional shifts. Again, the impor-tance of the correct diagnosis of the etiology of the problem is imperative to a successful orthodontic treatment plan and outcome.

Vertical Malocclusions

Historically, perhaps the least understood spatial dimension that an orthodontist considered when evaluating a malocclusion was that of the vertical dimension. This particular dimension has not been as intensely studied and classified for as long a period of time as has been the antero-posterior dimension. Likewise, the particular nuances of this dimension have not always been as readily appar-ent to the clinician as have those in the transverse and antero-posterior dimensions.   Nonetheless, the impact that this spatial relationship can have on the occlusion must not be overlooked or underesti-mated.

The vertical relationship is a measure dentally of the depth of the bite, and skeletally of the vertical position of the maxilla and the mandible to the cranial base. As with the other two dimensions, it is important that this be evaluated not only from a skeletal perspective, but also from the dental perspec-tive. A vertical malocclusion of skeletal origin is treated in a very different way from that of a simi-larly appearing malocclusion of dental origin.

In order for the orthodontist to clinically assess the vertical dimension, the same six relationships as for the antero-posterior dimension must again be considered. They are the following:

-The cranial base to the maxilla
-The cranial base to the mandible
-The maxilla to the mandible
-The maxilla to the maxillary teeth
-The mandible to the mandibular teeth
-The maxillary teeth to the mandibular teeth

From these relationships, cephalometric measurements and proportions, such as the occlusal plane, the **mandibular plane**, the **palatal plane**, the anterior facial height and the posterior facial height can be derived, which serve to guide the orthodontist in the decision making process involved in evaluat-ing the vertical dimension.

In addition, the relation of the anterior position of the maxilla or of the mandible (as measured in the antero-posterior spatial plane) to the vertical position of the maxilla or mandible (as measured in the vertical spatial dimension) has to be considered when evaluating the occlusion, as a deviation in the one dimension will directly affect the relationship in the other dimension. For instance, an increase in the vertical dimension of the mandible will result in a downward and backward rotation of the mandible to produce, in the antero-posterior dimension, a more Class II appearing occlusion and a clinically weaker appearing mandible in profile than had previously been evident, when the vertical dimension was not as great (Figure 13-71). Conversely, when the vertical dimension is lessened, one can expect to see the mandible auto-rotate forward, to produce a more Class III facial profile than before, and a more prominent appearing chin (Figure 13-72).

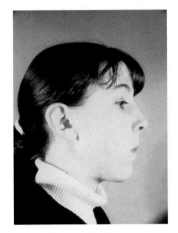

Figure 13-71

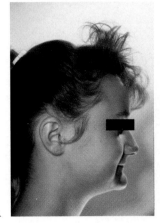

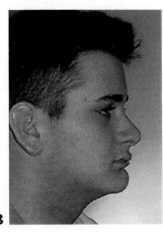

Figure 13-72

As was previously stated, a vertical malocclusion can have a skeletal etiology, a dental etiology, or a combination of both. Furthermore, when evaluating vertical malocclusions, one must remember that the clinical occlusal appearance can be, and frequently is, the same regardless of the etiology (whether skeletal or dental) of the problem.

The positions of the maxilla and the mandible relative to the cranial base will dictate the vertical skeletal dimension. If the maxilla is tipped up relative to the cranial base, one might expect to see a concomitant distal rotation to the mandible, and clinically an **anterior open bite**. If the maxilla is tipped down relative to the cranial base, the patient may display what is termed a **vertical maxillary excess**, or a "gummy smile" (Figure 13-73), with a concomitant deep bite. Likewise, the position of the mandible relative to the cranial base will also affect the vertical plane. When the mandible is tipped down relative to the cranial base, a more retrognathic facial profile should be expected clinically with a greater chance for the appearance of an anterior open bite. Conversely, when the mandible is tipped forward relative to the cranial base, a deeper overbite and a more prognathic facial profile should be expected. Combinations of any of the skeletal vertical positions discussed above can occur to further complicate the occlusion.

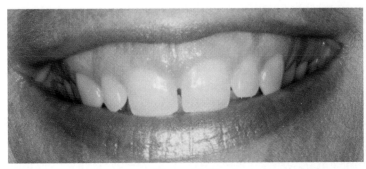

Figure 13-73

Dentally, the vertical relationships can appear as any one of four situations: an anterior deep bite (Figure 13-74), an **anterior open bite** (Figure 13-75), a posterior collapsed bite, or a **posterior open bite** (Figure 13-76). Eruptive disturbances of the teeth are frequently the cause of these problems. Supraeruption of the anterior teeth or the lack of eruption of the posterior teeth could be the cause for a dental deep bite. An anterior open bite could be the result of the supraeruption of the posterior teeth or a lack of eruption of the anterior teeth. The collapse of the posterior occlusion could be the result of a failure of the posterior teeth to erupt, however more likely it is caused by the loss of molar teeth. A posterior open bite (usually seen unilaterally) could be the result of a failure of the posterior teeth to erupt.

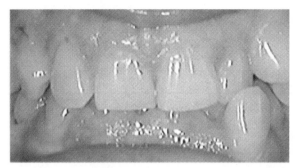
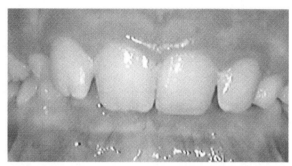

Figure 13-74

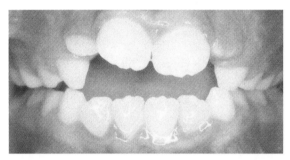
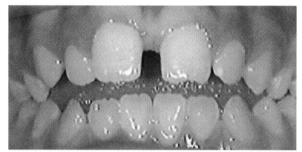

Figure 13-75

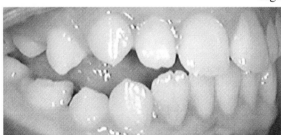
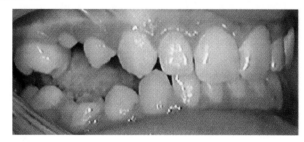

Figure 13-76

When assessing the vertical dimension, as with the antero-posterior and transverse dimensions, several specific orthodontic records are particularly helpful. The lateral cephalogram again proves to be an invaluable tool to quantify the skeletal relationships as well as the dental positions. Several classic cephalometric analyses have been devised to aid the clinician in this evaluation; however, there is not one popularly accepted standard for this dimension. (This may be a reflection of the difficulty we have in grasping all of the parameters of this spatial dimension.) In addition to the lateral cephalogram, the orthodontist typically will also rely upon the dental casts to aid in evaluating the tooth positions, as well as the intra-oral and extra-oral photographs or images. Again, however, the clinical exam is invaluable to the practitioner for detecting such important items as the smile or lip line, tissue drape, and mandibular posture, all of which are essential when addressing vertical spatial issues.

5.2.3. Congenital Anomalies and Condylar Pathologies of the Temporomandibular Joint

Pathological processes and **congenital anomalies** involving the mandibular condyle can contribute to occlusal relationship changes. These occur as a result of morphological changes in the size and shape of the condyles and their relationship within the glenoid fossa. While a fairly wide range of variability is normal and acceptable, significant alterations in condylar morphology (Figure 13-77) can have a tremendous impact upon the affected individual's occlusion.

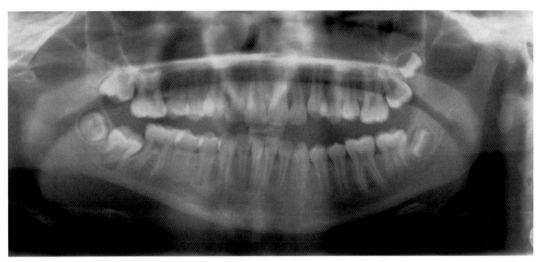

Figure 13-77

For example, congenital conditions can result in anomalies appearing as a bilateral diminution of the mandible, condyle, or temporomandibular joint. These congenital conditions include such syndromes as Pierre Robin syndrome or Robin sequence, Treacher-Collins syndrome, and Hallerman-Streiff syndrome. The individuals who have these syndromes are micrognathic in appearance, with hypoplastic mandibles resulting in an antero-posterior spatial plane discrepancy of the mandible.

Conversely, anomalies can occur that result in a hyperplasia of the mandible, usually affecting one side only (Figure 13-78). This unilateral mandibular hyperplasia is typically limited to one condyle only, and affects the occlusion in all three spatial planes resulting in a marked mandibular **facial asymmetry**.

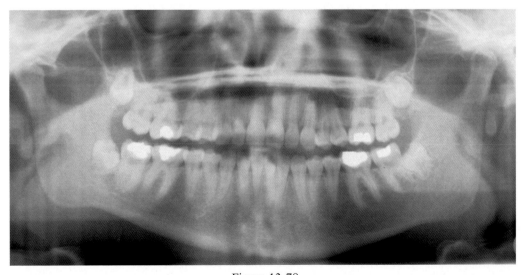

Figure 13-78

Dysplasias involving the temporomandibular joint are commonly grouped together under the term **hemifacial microsomia**, and usually involve the lateral two thirds of the face (with the exception of the median structures). The etiologies of these conditions are difficult to ascertain, but the adverse clinical effect to the occlusion can be seen in all three spatial planes. Interestingly enough, in some individuals with more severe asymmetries, the occlusion can be reasonably good as a result of dentoalveolar compensations. In others, vertical discrepancies will be seen on the contralateral side of the **dysplasia**.

Degenerative or traumatic changes to the condyle can also adversely affect the occlusion. The arthritic diseases, both osteoarthritis and rheumatoid arthritis, result in a deterioration and erosion of the condylar and soft tissue surfaces. As a result, occlusal changes can occur in the antero-posterior and vertical spatial planes. Commonly, patients enduring an acute bout of rheumatoid arthritis will present with a previously unseen anterior open bite.

Traumatic changes to the jaws or the temporomandibular joint will also obviously affect the occlusion. Dislocations, ankyloses, hypo- and hypermobility, as well as fractures of the jaws can all have an adverse effect upon an otherwise acceptable occlusion. Careful clinical evaluation is necessary to detect these changes prior to the onset of orthodontic treatment.

For additional information on the influences of the temporomandibular joints and their impact upon the dentition and occlusion, the reader is directed to Chapter 12.

6. SUGGESTED READINGS

Diagnostic Data

Ferrario V F., Sforza C., Schmitz J H., Miani, Jr. A., Serrao G. A three-dimensional computerized mesh diagram analysis and its application in soft tissue facial morphometry. Am J Ortho Dentofacial Orthop 1998: 114; 404-413.

Ferrario V F., Sforza C., Serrao G., Colombo A., Ciusa V. Soft tissue facial growth and development as assessed by the three-dimensional computerized mesh diagram analysis. Am J Ortho Dentofacial Orthop 1999: 116; 215-226.

Lui J K., Chen Y T., Cheng K S. Accuracy of automatic identification of cephalometric landmarks. Am J Ortho Dentofacial Orthop 2000: 118; 535-540.

Nickel J, et al: Validated numerical modeling of the effects of combined orthodontic and orthognathic surgical treatment on TMJ loads and muscle forces. Am J Orthod Dentofacial Orthop 2002; 121:73-82.

Rudolph D J., Sinclair P M., Coggins J M. Automated computerized radiographic identification of cephalometric landmarks. Am J Ortho Dentofacial Orthop 1998: 113; 173-179.

Sarver D M. Video cephalometric diagnosis (VCD): A new concept in treatment planning? Am J Ortho Dentofacial Orthop 1996: 110; 128-136.

Schirmer U R., Wiltshire W A. Manual and computer-aided space analysis: A comparative study. Am J Ortho Dentofacial Orthop 1997: 112; 676-680.

Thilander B., Ronning O. Introduction to Orthodontics – 2nd Edition. 1995, Forlagshuset Gothia AB.

Zarb G A., Carlsson G E., Sessle B J., Mohl N D. Temporomandibular Joint and Masticatory Muscle Disorders. 1994, Mosby – Year Book, Inc.

Analysis of Tooth Size

Bishara S E., Jakobsen J R., Abdallah E M., Garcia A F. Comparisons of mesiodistal and buccolingual crown dimensions of the permanent teeth in three populations from Egypt, Mexico, and the United States. Am J Ortho Dentofacial Orthop 1989: 96; 416-422.

Bishara S E., Staley R N. Mixed-dentition mandibular arch length analysis: A step-by-step approach using the revised Hixon-Oldfather prediction method. Am J Ortho 1984: 86; 130-135.

Bolton W A. The clinical application of a tooth-size analysis. Am J Ortho 1962: 48; 504-529.

Buschang P H., Demirjian A., Cadotte L. Permanent mesiodistal tooth size of French-Canadians. J Can Dent Assn 1988: 54; 441-444.

Crosby D R., Alexander C G. The occurrence of tooth size discrepancies among different malocclusion groups. Am J Ortho Dentofacial Orthop 1989: 95; 457-461.

Doris J M., Bernard B W., Kuftinec M M. A biometric study of tooth size and dental crowding. Am J Ortho 1981: 79; 326-336.

Freeman J E., Maskeroni A J., Lorton L. Frequency of Bolton tooth-size discrepancies among orthodontic patients. Am J Ortho Dentofacial Orthop 1996: 110; 24-27.

Frankel H H., Benz E M. Mixed dentition analysis for black Americans. Ped Dent 1986: 8; 226-230.

Gardner R B. A comparison of four methods of predicting arch length. Am J Ortho 1979: 75; 387-398.

Hassanali J., Pokhariyal G P. Anterior tooth relations in Kenyan Africans. Arch Oral Biol 1993: 38; 337-342.

Hixon E H., Oldfather R E. Estimation of the sizes of unerupted cuspid and bicuspid teeth. Angle Orthodontist 1958: 28; 236-240.

Howe R P., McNamara Jr. J A., O'Connor K A. An examination of dental crowding and its relationship to tooth size and arch dimension. Am J Ortho 1983: 83; 363-373.

Howes A E. Case analysis and treatment planning based upon the relationship of the tooth material to its supporting bone. Am J Ortho 1947: 33; 499-511.

Hunter W S. Application of analysis of crowding and spacing of the teeth. Dent Clinic of North Amer 1978: 22; 563-577.

Jaroontham J., Godfrey K. Mixed dentition space analysis in a Thai population. Eur J Ortho 2000: 22; 127-134.

Lavelle C L B. Maxillary and mandibular tooth size in different racial groups and in different occlusal categories. Am J Ortho 1972: 61; 29-37.

Nance H N. The limitations of orthodontic treatment. I. Mixed dentition diagnosis and treatment. Am J Ortho & Oral Surg. 1947: 33; 177-223.

Nance H N. The limitations of orthodontic treatment. II. Diagnosis and treatment in permanent dentition. Am J Ortho & Oral Surg. 1947: 33; 253-301.

Nie Q, Lin J: Comparison of intermaxillary tooth size discrepancies among different malocclusion groups. Am J Orthod Dentofacial Orthop 1999; 116: 539-544.

Pont A. Der Zahn Index, Orthodontic. Zeitshrift fur Zahnartzliche Orthopaedic

Santoro M., Ayoub M E., Pardi V A., Cangialosi T J. Mesiodistal crown dimensions and tooth size discrepancy of the permanent dentition of Dominican Americans. Angle Ortho 2000: 70; 303-307.

Smith S S., Buschang P H., Watanabe E. Interarch tooth size relationships of 3 populations: "Does Bolton's analysis apply?" Am J Ortho Dentofacial Orthop 2000: 117; 169-174.

Smith H P., King D L., Valencia R. A comparison of three methods of mixed-dentition analyses. J Ped 1979: 3; 291-302.

Staley R N., Hu P., Hoag J F., Shelly T H. Prediction of the combined right and left canine and premolar widths in both arches of the mixed dentition. Ped Dent 1983: 5; 57-60.

Tanaka M M., Johnston L E. The prediction of the size of unerupted canines and premolars in a contemporary orthodontic population. J Am Dent Assn 1974: 88; 798-801.

Yuen K K., Tang E L., So L L. Mixed dentition analysis for Hong Kong Chinese. Angle Ortho 1998: 68; 21-28.

Arch Form and Symmetry

Alavi D G., BeGole E A., Schneider B J. Facial and dental arch asymmetries in Class II subdivision malocclusion. Am J Ortho Dentofacial Orthop 1988; 93; 38-46.

Araujo T M., Wilhelm R S., Almeida M A. Skeletal and dental arch asymmetries in Class II division I subdividion malocclusions. J Clin Ped Dent 1994: 18; 181-185.

Araujo T M., Wilhelm R S., Almeida M A. Skeletal and dental arch asymmetries in individuals with normal dental occlusions. Int J Adult Orthod Orthognath Surg 1994: 9; 111-117.

BeGole E A. Application of the cubic spline function in the description of dental arch form. J Dent Res 1980: 59; 1549-1556.

BeGole E A., Lyew R C. A new method for analyzing change in dental arch form. Am J Ortho Dentofacial Orthop 1998: 113; 394-401.

Bishara S E., Jakobsen J R., Treder J., Nowak A. Arch width changes from 6 weeks to 45 years of age. Am J Ortho Dentofacial Orthop 1997: 111; 401-409.

Bishara S E., Treder J E., Jakobsen J R. Facial and dental changes in adulthood. Am J Ortho Dentofacial Orthop 1994: 106; 175-185.

Bishara S E., Burkey P S., Kharouf J G. Dental and facial asymmetries: a review. Angle Ortho 1994: 64; 89-98.

Braun S., Hnat W P., Fender D E., Legan H L. The form of the human arch. Angle Ortho 1998: 68; 29-36.

Buschang P H., Stroud J., Alexander R G. Differences in dental arch morphology among adult females with untreated Class I and Class II malocclusion. Eur J Ortho 1994: 16; 47-52.

Burris B G., Harris E F. Maxillary arch size and shape in American blacks and whites. Angle Ortho 2000: 70; 297-302.

De La Cruz A., Sampson P., Little R M., Artun J., Shapiro P A. Long-term changes in arch form after orthodontic treatment and retention. Am J Ortho Dentofacial Orthop 1995: 107; 518-530.

Felton J M., Sinclair P M., Jones D L., Alexander R G. A computerized analysis of the shape and stability of mandibular arch form. Am J Ortho Dentofacial Orthop 1987: 92; 478-483.

Ferrio V F., Sforza C., Miani Jr. A., Tartaglia G. Mathematical definition of the shape of dental arches in human permanent healthy dentitions. Eur J Ortho 1994: 16; 287-294.

Ferrario V F., Sforza C., Poggio C E., Serrao G., Colombo A. Three-dimensional dental arch curvature in human adolescents and adults. Am J Ortho Dentofacial Orthop 1999: 115; 401-405.

Harris E F. A longitudinal study of arch size and form in untreated adults. Am J Ortho Dentofacial Orthop 1997: 111; 419-427.

Hassanali J., Odhiambo J W. Analysis of dental casts of 6-8 and 12-year old Kenyan children. Eur J Ortho 2000: 22; 135-142.

Hnat W P., Braun S., Chinhara A., Legan H L. The relationship of arch length to alterations in dental arch width. Am J Ortho Dentofacial Orthop 2000: 118; 184-188.

Howe R P., McNamara Jr. J A., O'Connor R H. An examination of dental crowding and its relationship to tooth size and arch dimension. Am J Ortho 1983: 83; 363-373.

Kirschen RH, et al: The Royal London Space Planning: An integration of space analysis and treatment planning Part I: Assessing the space required to meet treatment objectives. Am J Orthod Dentofacial Orthop 2000; 118:448-455.

Kirschen RH, et al: The Royal London Space Planning: An integration of space analysis and treatment planning Part II: The effect of other treatment procedures on space. Am J Orthod Dentofacial Orthop 2000; 118:456-461.

Kronmiller J E. Development of asymmetries. Seminars in Ortho. 1998: 4; 134-137.

Kula K., Esmailnejad A. Dental arch asymmetry in children with large overjets. Angle Ortho 1996: 68; 45-52.

Lavell C L B., Plant C G. Comparison between the right and left sides of the dental arch. J Dent Res 1980

Maurice T J., Kula K. Dental arch asymmetry in the mixed dentition. Angle Ortho 1998: 68; 37-44.

Merz M L., Isaacson R J., Germane N., Rubenstein L K. Tooth diameters and arch perimeters in a black and a white population. Am J Ortho Dentofacial Orthop 1991: 100; 53-58.

Mutinelli S., Manfredi M., Cozzani M. A mathematical-geometric model to calculate variation in mandibular arch form. Eur J Ortho 2000: 22; 113-125.

Sillman J H. Dimensional changes of the dental arches: Longitudinal study from birth to 25 years. Am J Ortho 1964: 50; 824-842.

Rose J M., Sadowsky C., BeGole E A., Moles R. Mandibular skeletal and dental asymmetry in Class II subdivision malocclusions. Am J Ortho Dentofacial Orthop 1994: 105; 489-495.

Pirttiniemi P M. Associations of mandibular and facial asymmetries – a review. Am J Ortho Dentofacial Orthop 1994: 106; 191-197.

Varnarsdall Jr. R L. Transverse dimension and long-term stability. Seminars in Ortho 1999: 5; 171-180.

Woods MG. Mandibular arch dimensional and positional changes in late mixed-dentition Class I and II treatment. Am J Orthod Dentofacial Orthop 200;122:180-188.

Analysis Of Tooth Positions and Inter-Arch Relationship

Angle E H. Classification of malocclusion. Dent Cosmos 1899: 41; 248-264, 350-357.

Andrews L F. The six keys to normal occlusion. Am J Ortho 1972: 62;296-309.

Brin I., Weinberger T., Ben-Chorin E. Classification of occlusion reconsidered. Eur J Ortho 1999: 21; 169-174.

Du., S Q., Rinchuse D J., Zullo T G., Rinchuse D J. Reliability of three methods of occlusion classification. Am J Ortho Dentofacial Orthop 1998: 113; 463-470.

Katz M I. Angle classification revisited 1: Is current use reliable? Am J Ortho Dentofacial Orthop 1992: 102; 173-179.

Katz M I. Angle classification revisited 2: A modified Angle classification. Am J Ortho Dentofacial Orthop 1992: 102; 277-284.

Katz M I., Sinkford J C., Sanders Jr. C F. The 100-year dilemma: what is a normal occlusion, and how is malocclusion classified? Quintessence Int 1990: 21; 407-414.

Moyers RE, Vanderlinden FPGM, Riolo ML, McNamara JA Jr. Standards of human occlusal development, Monograph 5, Craniofacial growth series. Ann Arbor, Michigan, Center for Human Growth and Development, University of Michigan, 1976.

Nojima K, et al: A Comparative Study of Caucasian and Japanese Mandibular Clinical Arch Forms. Angle Orthodontist 2001; 71 (3): 195-200.

Thilander B., Ronning O. Introduction to Orthodontics – 2nd Ed. 1995, Forlagshuset Gothia AB.

CHAPTER 14

Dental Dysmorphogenesis

Robyn S. Silberstein

1. INTRODUCTION

Congenital variations in dental morphology occur as a result of **agenesis**, aplasia or **dysplasia** of the tooth germ. These include anomalies of number, size, shape and position. More anomalies occur in the permanent than the primary dentition, and in the maxilla than the mandible.

The most common agents associated with dental anomalies are genetic; however, viewing a genetic mutation as a specific etiologic mechanism resulting in a specific disease entity may be misleading. **Dysmorphogenesis** is the product of both its unique genetic background and the environment in which this background is forced to operate. There is constant interaction between the genome of a developing fetus, the **epigenetic** microenvironment, the intrauterine environment and the external milieu, or environmental insults (Melnick 1982). Poswillo (1976) states that single gene mutations are not mechanisms in themselves but agents that may initiate mechanisms of malformation or disease at the subcellular, cellular or tissue levels.

2. DENTAL DYSMORPHOLOGY

2.1 ANOMALIES

2.1.1. Number

Anodontia

Complete failure of the teeth to develop is rare. Gorlin reported isolated instances of complete anodontia due to an autosomal recessive gene that affects the permanent dentition. Missing teeth are correlated largely with familial hereditary patterns (Figure 14-1).

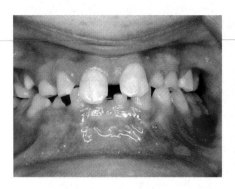
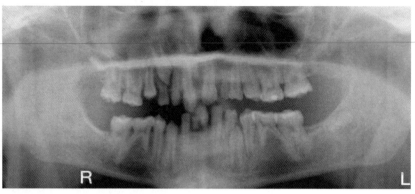

Figure 14-1: Oligodontia in an 11 year old male. There are 13 missing teeth including molars, premolars, cuspids and incisors. His 13 year old brother is missing six teeth.

Excluding third molars the incidence of congenitally missing teeth ranges from 1.5% to 10%. Including third molars incidences of 20% are reported. A study that evaluated 1702 children reported 5% of the children were missing teeth in the permanent dentition other than the third molars. The maxillary third molars then the mandibular third molars are the most commonly missing permanent teeth. The next most frequently occurring absent permanent tooth is the mandibular second premolar, closely followed by the maxillary lateral incisor; each one is approximately 1-3% (Figure 14-2).

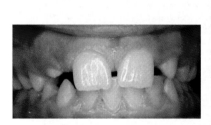
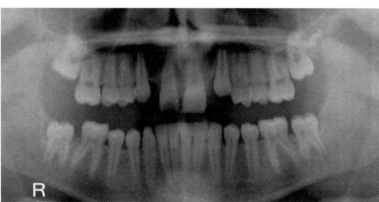

Figure 14-2: Hereditary missing bilateral maxillary lateral incisors. Excluding the third molars, second premolars and lateral incisors are the most common missing teeth with a prevalence of approximately 1-3%.

There is a high correlation between primary tooth absence and permanent tooth absence. There are several genes associated with non-syndromic familial missing teeth, including Msx, Dlx and Pax. Syndromes that demonstrate multiple congenitally missing teeth include ectodermal dysplasia, chondroectodermal dysplasia, achondroplasia, Rieger, incontinenti pigmenti and Seckel. In addition to hereditary patterns producing missing teeth, physical disruption of the **dental lamina** may affect tooth number. There is an increased incidence of missing teeth with alveolar clefting (Figure 14-3).

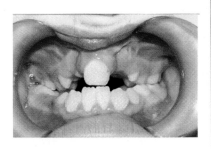
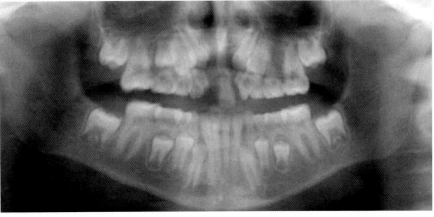

Figure 14-3: Cleft palate patient with 3 missing incisors. Incomplete fusion of the frontonasal and maxillary processes may disrupt a continuous dental lamina. Clinically there is an increased incidence of missing/misshapen maxillary incisors.

A recent study reported a **hypodontia** prevalence of 77%, excluding third molars, in a sample of 278 cleft patients (Shapira, et al., 2000). This incidence is significantly higher than has been reported previously. One can appreciate the significance of a continuous dental lamina in the formation of a complete dentition. There is a physical disruption or lack of dental lamina in the cleft area. An interesting study reported an increase in missing teeth outside of the cleft area (canine and post-canine area) of more than 24%, excluding third molars, in cleft palate repaired children, (Lekkas, et al., 2000). The authors felt there was likely a physical disruption to the dental sacs at the time of early palate surgery, roughly between 10 months and 2 1/2 years. This congenital absence of teeth was previously attributed to some general disturbance to the physiologic process of tooth development. In the study of 266 dental casts of fully unoperated adult cleft patients there was no absence of permanent teeth in the canine and molar area of the upper jaw.

Supernumerary

An increase in tooth number can occur in both primary and permanent dentitions. Incidence values are as high as 3%, males being affected twice as frequently as females. Up to 98% of supernumerary teeth occur in the maxilla. The most common is the **mesiodens**, which occurs in the palatal midline, generally palatal to the central incisors. Extra molars or fourth molars have been reported. Supernumerary teeth in the mandible are generally fourth molars or extra first premolars (Figure 14-4).

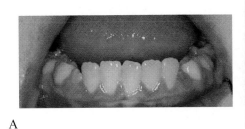
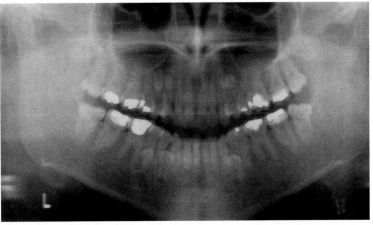

A
B

Figure 14-4: Supernumerary teeth. Easily identified when clinically erupted (A), supernumerary teeth can sometimes be discovered in a case work-up in a non-syndromal non-symptomatic orthodontic patient (B).

Syndromes involving **supernumerary teeth** include Apert, Cleidocranial dysplasia, Gardner, Downs, Crouzon, Sturge-Weber, Oral-facial-digital, and Hallermann-Streiff.

2.1.2. Shape

Odontoma

The abnormal proliferation of cells of the enamel organ can produce an odontogenic tumor, or odontoma. It appears to be a continued budding of the primary or permanent tooth germ, in which case the odontoma replaces the normal tooth, although it is not always the case (Figure 14-5).

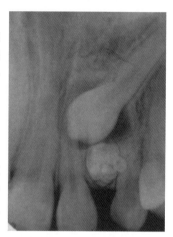

Third Molars

The maxillary third molars have the most variable crown shape ranging from a small peg shaped crown to a multicusped malformed tooth. The mandibular third molars display the next greatest variation in crown shape.

Figure 14-5: Odontoma.

Peg Laterals

The most common anomaly in the anterior region of the permanent dentition is the peg-shaped permanent maxillary lateral incisor, occurring in 1-2% of the population. The phenotype is generally small, conical and tapered to a point at the incisal (Figure 14-6).

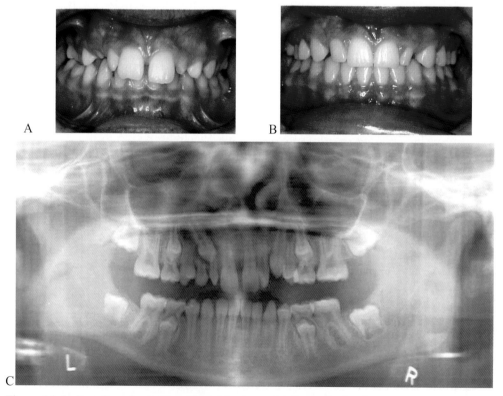

Figure 14-6: Peg shaped maxillary lateral incisors. A.) Pre-orthodontic treatment. B.) Post-orthodontic treatment and pre-prosthetic. C.) Initial Panorex.

Studies of identical twins demonstrate both missing and peg-shaped lateral incisor teeth, indicating they may be varied expressions of the same genetic influence.

Gemination

Gemination results from the splitting of a single tooth germ. Clinically, it appears as double or fused teeth, however, these teeth generally have a single root and pulp canal with a notch in the crown. This occurs in less than 1% of the population, frequently in the anterior region. The normal complement of teeth is generally seen, counting the geminated tooth as one (Figure 14-7).

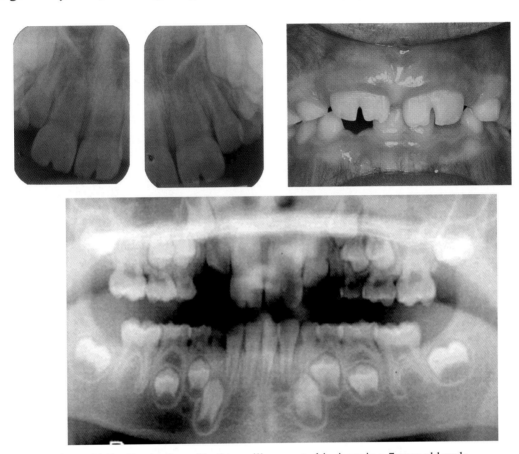

Figure 14-7: Gemination of both maxillary central incisors in a 7 year old male.

Fusion

Fusion is clinically similar to gemination except that fusion results from the union of two adjacent tooth germs involving the dentin. There are usually two separate roots and pulp chambers. There is generally one less individual tooth than the normal complement (Figure 14-8).

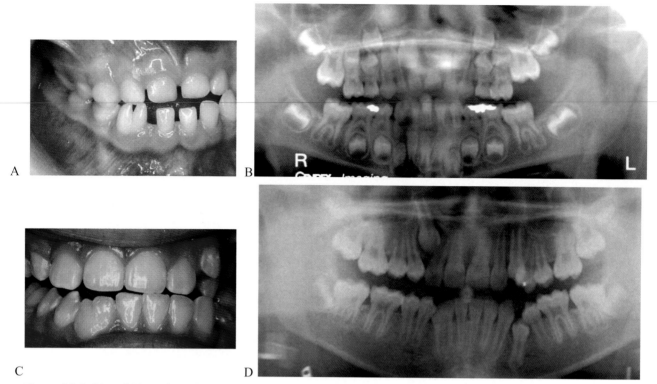

Figure 14-8: (A and B) Fusion of the primary mandibular right cuspid and lateral incisor. (C and D) Fusion of the permanent mandibular right cuspid and lateral incisor. There is one less tooth in both the primary and permanent dentition.

Accessory cusps/tubercles

Enamel pearls are small nodules of enamel with a core of dentin found frequently on the distal of third molars and the buccal root furcation of molars. The enamel will not allow normal connective tissue attachment, making it a potential periodontal problem area. Talon cusps are small enamel projections in the cingulum area of anterior permanent teeth that have a pulp horn. Removing this cusp from maxillary incisors for occlusion purposes may require endodontic treatment (Figure 14-9).

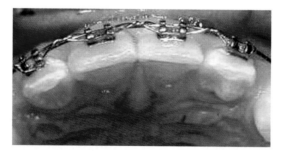

Figure 14-9: There is a talon cusp on the lingual of the maxillary left lateral incisor. Root canal treatment was required to remove the cusp and allow for an ideal overbite and overjet relationship.

Shovel

Pronounced lingual ridges and cingulums of permanent anterior teeth give the appearance of a shovel-shaped incisor. There is an increased frequency of shovel-shaped maxillary incisors in Asian, Eskimo and American Indian populations. Often it is extremely helpful to reduce the upper anterior lingual ridges for final finishing of ideal overbite and overjet.

Pre-eruptive coronal resorption

Pre-eruptive "caries" has been recognized as a radiolucent defect on an unerupted crown of a permanent tooth in the apparent absence of infection (Figure 14-10). It is treated when accessibility permits as caries, and is restored if possible or removed.

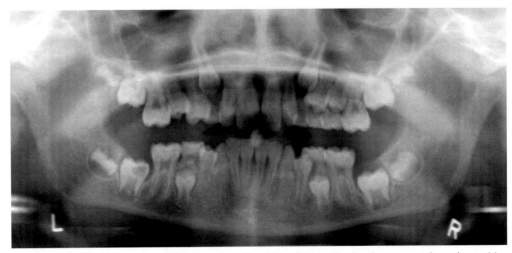

Figure 14-10: Pre-eruptive caries noted at the time of the orthodontic case work-up in an 11 year old patient. The mandibular left second molar was removed and the patient has had periodic radiographs to reevaluate the mandibular right second molar.

Taurondontia

Elongated crown shape and pulp chambers at the expense of the root, with little to no constriction at the **cementoenamel junction**, is seen in approximately 0.1% of the population and is referred to as taurondontia.

Dilaceration/Flexion

A severe bend of a tooth root is termed dilaceration (Figure 14-11). A sharp curvature or twist to a root is termed flexion (Figure 14-12).

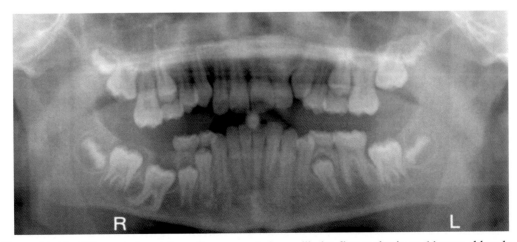

Figure 14-11: Dilacerated root tips of an unerupted mandibular first molar in an 11 year old male.

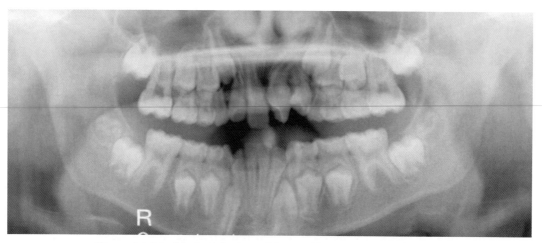

Figure 14-12: Marked flexion of the maxillary left central incisor.

Dens in Dente

The development of a "tooth within a tooth" results from the enamel organ invaginating within the crown, extending into the dentin and root of the tooth. It can occur in the primary or permanent dentitions, although it is more common in permanent teeth, specifically maxillary laterals. Dens in dente are suspected where there are deep lingual pits. There is a familial tendency and a possible autosomal dominant inheritance pattern with variable expressivity and minimal penetrance.

Concrescence

Concrescence is the joining of two adjacent teeth at the cementum only. The teeth develop separately but are joined by cementum deposition. This is distinguished from hypercementosis, which is the excessive production of cellular cementum, more commonly seen as a response to trauma from occlusal forces and chronic periapical inflammation.

Accessory Roots

Supernumerary or accessory roots are also reported in the literature, although they are rare. They are most often seen on third molars and can potentially develop a cyst, resulting in a **dentigerous** cyst.

2.1.3. Size

Normal tooth size has been studied using twin methodology. Every tooth (except the mandibular second molars) showed evidence for significantly greater discordance in dizygotic than in monozygotic cotwins. This provides strong evidence for significant genetic determinants of tooth size variability in humans.

Microdontia

Small but normally shaped teeth can occur as a single tooth, several teeth or an entire dentition. Dwarfism may affect maxillary lateral incisors and third molars. **Hemifacial microsomia** and Down syndrome also demonstrate an increased incidence of one or more abnormally small teeth.

Macrodontia

Large but normally shaped teeth can occur as a single tooth, several teeth or an entire dentition. Gigantism can demonstrate one or more teeth that are abnormally large or long rooted and most frequently involves incisors and canines. Facial hemihypertrophy can demonstrate larger teeth on the affected side. Otodental syndrome can also display macrodontia.

2.1.4. Position

Transposition

Occasionally teeth erupt in a transposed position. This occurs most frequently with teeth at the border of a series; for example, the maxillary canine and lateral incisor or first premolar (Figure 14-13).

Winged Incisors

Rotation of the maxillary central incisors in a mesiolingual direction ("wing teeth") or distolingual direction ("counter-wing teeth") is an autosomal dominant dental trait (Figure 14-14). There is no significant relationship between this phenotype and the width of the incisors, **available arch length** or **arch width**. There is an increased incidence of this trait in American Indian and Asian populations.

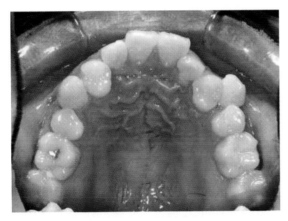

Figure 14-13: Bilateral transposition of the maxillary cuspids and first premolars. Transpositions occur in less than 1% of the population and are generally seen at the border of a series, e.g., incisors/cuspids or cuspids/premolars.

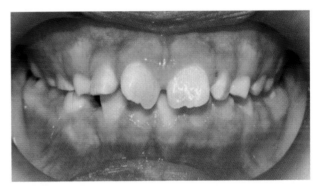

Figure 14-14: Wing teeth. This patient demonstrates mesiolingual rotation of the maxillary right central incisor. Note the absence of marked arch length discrepancy.

2.2 ENVIRONMENTAL AGENTS AFFECTING TOOTH DEVELOPMENT

The developing teeth have only a limited number of ways to respond to an environmental insult. While there are over 200 agents that can potentially affect the developing tooth adversely, the number of mechanisms and resultant defects are dramatically less. The defect is related to the nature of the substance (affecting developing tissues differently), degree of deficiency or excess, developmental time frame as well as the individual embryonic milieu. The majority of enamel defects are enamel opacities, pitting and discoloration. Incidence reports vary, the range approaching 60% or more of the population exhibiting a clinically apparent enamel defect.

2.2.1. Trauma

Individual permanent teeth may exhibit a hypoplastic or hypocalcified area on a crown resulting from infection or trauma. Infection of a primary tooth can extend toward the developing permanent tooth bud. A traumatic blow to an anterior primary tooth that is displaced apically can interfere with matrix formation or calcification of the underlying permanent tooth. The trauma or periapical infection can produce defects on the labial surface of the permanent incisor (Figure 14-15). Thus, retaining an infected primary tooth, even if asymptomatic, is not advisable. There is evidence of local trauma from laryngoscopy and endotracheal intubation of premature newborns, which results in localized enamel **hypoplasia** of the maxillary anterior teeth.

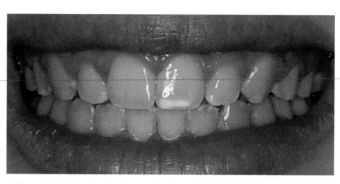

Figure 14-15: Enamel opacity on the incisal third of the maxillary left central incisor. The patient's mother reported trauma to the primary central incisor as a toddler. Enamel opacities are very common.

2.2.2. Nutrition

Nutritional Deficiencies

Deficiencies in vitamins A, C, and D, calcium, and phosphorus are related to an increased incidence of enamel hypoplasia. Vitamin A affects enamel and dentin formation, however, primary effects appear to be on enamel formation. Vitamin C deficiencies affect primarily dentin development, and also cementum. Vitamin D deficiencies affect mineralization, and hypoplastic and hypomineralized areas of enamel, dentin and cementum are seen. Parathyroid hormone irregularities can be seen as hypocalcified/hypercalcified zones. The appearance of enamel can be affected by excessive fluoride intake. There is a clear **association** between the level of ingested systemic fluoride and incidence of enamel hypoplasia, both in the primary and permanent dentitions. While there is evidence that fluoride can cross the placenta, it is thought that the fluoride is incorporated into the enamel during the maturative stage of amelogenesis, which is longer for the permanent dentition. Thus, if fluorosis is noted in the primary dentition, fluoride intake should be evaluated and perhaps changed so that mottling in the permanent teeth can be avoided. There is wide variability in the phenotypic expression of fluorosis. Usually, primary teeth show evenly whitened areas and permanent teeth have generalized, symmetrical, diffuse, lacelike opacities (Figure 14-16).

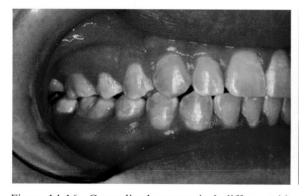 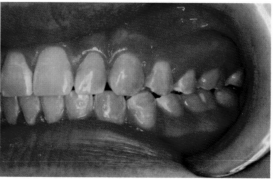

Figure 14-16: Generalized symmetrical, diffuse and lacelike enamel opacities. The mottled areas show irregularity of enamel rods. In some cases this can contribute to decreased bond strength, and a booster to increase the chemical bond is advised.

The mottled areas may or may not be mineralized and show irregularity of enamel rods. While diffuse, symmetrical white opacities are pathognomonic for fluorosis, not all diffuse opacities are fluoride induced. Fluorosis has a distinctive defect, although not unique. There is evidence that mild fluorosis can occur in as little as 1 part per million (ppm), which is the recommended level. The optimal level of fluoride is perhaps closer to 0.5 ppm, since anticariogenic effect is 0.5 ppm with no mottling reported. The **phenotypic variation** may be in part due to metabolic and genetic factors. Also, fluorides are found in infant foods, vitamins, formula, carbonated beverages and fish products, of which individual intake varies and individual bioavailability varies. At high levels, such as 6 ppm, there is a 90% chance of some degree of dental fluorosis.

2.2.3. Birth and Childhood Diseases

Neonatal and postnatal disturbances are expressed mainly at the cervical level of the crown in primary teeth and the incisal portion of the permanent teeth. There does not appear to be an increased incidence of dental anomalies with premature birth in itself; however, the association appears to be with the attending complications of premature births. Complications include metabolic disturbances, hypocalcemia, hypoxia, prolonged jaundice, nutritional deficiencies, fever and traumatic injuries due to laryngoscopy and intubation. The highest correlation of enamel hypoplasia and opacities in the primary dentition is with low-birth-weight infants. Further, complications due to hypoxia can contribute to hypoplasias and opacities associated with cerebral palsy. Systemic diseases such as cystic fibrosis also report increased incidence of enamel defects. Enamel, dentin and cementum development can be arrested in children who receive excessive x-radiation in treatment of malignancies, depending on the stage of dental development, in spite of the fact that ameloblasts are generally resistant to x-radiation.

Lead poisoning

There is an increased incidence of pitting hypoplasia in children exposed to lead poisoning, as well as delays in eruption of primary teeth in children of lead poisoned mothers (lead readily crosses the placenta).

2.2.4. Teratogens

Rubella Virus

Rubella virus infection in utero is associated with congenitally missing primary incisors, altered cuspal morphology, microdontia, enamel hypoplasias and delayed tooth eruption.

Tetracycline

In utero fetal exposure to tetracycline during the second and/or third trimester is frequently associated with a yellow to gray-brown pigmentation in horizontal bands in the primary dentition. Primary dentition susceptibility begins at the 4th month in utero and extends throughout the first year of life.

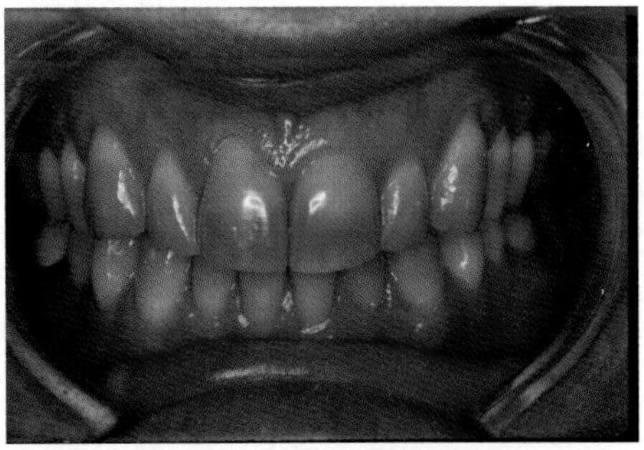

Figure 14-17: Tetracycline staining in an adult female.

Permanent dentition susceptibility also begins at approximately 5 months in utero and extends through 12 years of age. If tetracycline is present during mineralization, it is deposited in the mineralizing dentin, enamel, cementum and bone. Discoloration is most commonly seen (Figure 14-17), although hypoplasia can also result.

2.3 GENETIC DISEASES AFFECTING TOOTH STRUCTURE

Inherited defects of enamel and dentin may occur as part of a syndrome, or as a condition affecting specifically enamel or dentin. The most current reference of syndromes associated with an increased prevalence of enamel and dentin defects is found in the Web site On-line Mendelian Inheritance in Man, http://www.ncbi.nlm.nih.gov/omim.

There are features that distinguish heretibility as opposed to an isolated defect. First, there is an identifiable family history. Second, there is a generalized effect on the dentition, usually affecting both primary and permanent dentitions. Third, there is no relationship to time or environmental factors.

With enamel defects, however, this is complicated by the fact that enamel defects approach normality in the overall population and phenocopies clearly exist. Further, there is extreme phenotypic variability within the same family identified with amelogenesis imperfecta, and even within the same individual (the defect is not necessarily expressed in a generalized pattern as in Figure 14-18).

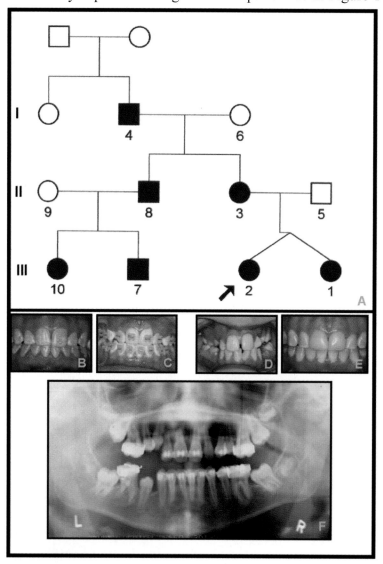

Figure 14-18: (A) Pedigree of family ascertained with autosomal dominant amelogenesis imperfecta, hypoplastic type I. The proband (III-2) is indicated with an arrow. (B-E) Intraoral photographs demonstrate varying severity of enamel defects and yellow-brown and white-yellow lesions. (E) Bonding of maxillary incisors where the enamel has chipped. (F) Panorex of proband demonstrating root resorption, impactions and eruption problems consistent with hypoplastic type I ADAI.

2.3.1. Amelogenesis Imperfecta

Amelogenesis imperfecta (AI) is an inherited disorder that affects enamel formation in the primary and permanent dentitions and is clinically and genetically diverse. The prevalence of all forms of AI has been reported at 1:14,000 in the U.S., 1:8,000 in Israel and 1:4,000 in Sweden. Based on clinical appearance, radiographic characteristics and microscopic features there are three major types of AI: 1.) hypoplasia; 2.) hypocalcification; and 3.) hypomaturation. In type 1, enamel hypoplasia, the enamel is hard and well calcified but defective in amount. This can be generalized (all the enamel) and localized (specific areas of pits and grooves). In type 2, hypocalcification, the enamel is soft and mushy and wears away easily. In type 3, hypomaturation, the enamel has relatively normal thickness and hardness with discoloration and reduced radiographic density. There are 14 different subtypes of AI recognized, based on mode of inheritance and clinical appearance and characteristics. There are autosomal dominant forms, autosomal recessive, X-linked dominant and X-linked recessive, all demonstrating various forms of hypocalcification, hypomaturation and hypoplasia. The X-linked hypoplastic form is associated with mutations in the amelogenin gene. There is a family with autosomal dominant hypoplastic type genetically linked to chromosome 4 reported in the literature and several families excluded from this region. The existing nosology reflects the genetic and phenotypic diversity of AI.

AI can also occur as part of a syndrome. For example, AI has been identified with tricho-dento-osseous syndrome (TDO), taurodontism and curly hair. It is autosomal dominant and displays a four-basepair deletion in the DLX3 gene on chromosome 17. The AI is fully penetrant in affected individuals although the hair features are variably expressed.

Treatment of enamel defects can be handled most effectively based on diagnosis and specific phenotype. For example, hypoplastic enamel is well mineralized and treated effectively with bonding procedures. Severely hypomineralized enamel is treated with full coverage crowns.

2.3.2. Dentinogenesis Imperfecta and Dentin Dysplasia

Dentinogenesis Imperfecta (DI) is a dentin defect inherited as an autosomal dominant trait and occurs about 1 in 8000 people. DI affects the primary and permanent dentition. There are three types of DI. Type I DI occurs in **association** with Osteogenesis Imperfecta. The dentin defect results from a **collagen** defect. Type II DI occurs as an isolated trait and is not related to a collagen defect but is likely related to a mineralization defect. One form has recently been linked to a Chinese family. Type III DI is seen in an inbred Brandywine, Maryland population in which collagen and mineralization is affected. DI type II and type III have been linked to chromosome 4.

There are two types of dentin dysplasia. Type I, **radicular** dentin dysplasia and type II, coronal dentin dysplasia. In type I both dentitions are affected and it is an autosomal dominant trait. Roots are short and pointed with an absence of the root canals and pulp chambers. The color and morphology of the crowns are normal, although they may be opalescent and radiolucencies may be present radiographically. Scanning electron microscopy of these teeth demonstrates normal enamel, a thin layer of normal dentin at the dentinoenamel junction, and dysplastic dentin throughout the rest of the crown and root. Type II is also an autosomal dominant trait. The primary dentition appears opalescent, but the permanent dentition has normal color and exhibits a thistle tube pulp with pulp stones radiographically. Scanning electron microscopy shows highly irregular and disorganized dentin. Given the similar phenotypes, the candidate gene for Dentinogenesis Imperfecta may also be a candidate gene for Dentin Dysplasia type II due to different alleles at the same locus. In addition to the two major groups of primary disorders of dentin published by Shield, et al., (1973), hereditary systemic conditions such as hypophosphatasia include abnormal dentin formation.

3. Suggested Readings

Dental Dysmorphology

Avery JK. Agents affecting tooth and bone development. In: Avery JK editor. Oral Development and Histology. New York: Thieme, 1994: pp 130-143.

Bixler D, Hartsfield JK. Clinical genetics for the dental practitioner. In: McDonald RE, Avery DR, editors. Dentistry for the Child and Adolescent. Mosby, 2000: pp 82-104.

Burzynski N, Escobar V. Classification genetics of numeric anomalies of the dentition, Birth Defects 1983, 13: 95-106.

Dummett CO. Anomalies of the developing dentition. In: Pinkham JR, editor. Pediatric Dentistry: infancy through adolescence. WB Saunders, 1999: pp 43-53.

Forsman K, Lind L, Backman B, Westermark E, Holmgren G. Localization of a gene for autosomal dominant amelogenesis imperfecta (ADAI) to chromosome 4q. Human Molec Genet 1994; 3:1621-1625.

Gorlin RJ, Herman NG, Moss S. Complete absence of the permanent dentition: an autosomal recessive disorder. Am J Med Genet 1980; 5:207-209.

Graber LW. Congenital absence of teeth: a review with emphasis on inheritance patterns. J Am Dent Assoc1978; 96: 266-275.

Karrman C et al. Genetic heterogeneity of autosomal dominant amelogenesis imperfecta demonstrated by its exclusion from the AIH2 region on human chromosome 4q. Arch Oral Biol 1996; 41: 893-900.

Lekkas C, Latief BS, Rahe SPN, Kuijpers-Jagtam AM. The adult unoperated cleft patient: absence of maxillary teeth outside the cleft area. Cleft Palate-Craniofacial Journal 2000;37(1):17-20.

MacDougall M, DuPont R, Simmons D, Reus B, Krebsbach P, Karrman C, Holmgren G, Leach R, Forsman K. Critical region for autosomal dominant Amelogenesis Imperfecta at chromosome 4q21. Genomics 1997; 41:115-118.

McDonald RE, Avery DR, Hartsfield JK. Acquired and developmental disturbances of the teeth and associated oral structures. In: McDonald RE, Avery DR, editors. Dentistry for the Child and Adolescent. Mosby, 2000: pp 105-150.

Melnick M. The Doctrine of Multifactorial Association: Gene-Environment Interaction. In: Melnick M, Shields ED, Burzynski NJ, editors. Clinical Dysmorphology of Oral-Facial Structures. Littleton: John Wright, PSG Inc., 1982: 28-35.

Melnick M, Burzynski NJ, Escobar VH. Oral Dysmorphology and Genetics. In: Melnick M, Shields ED, Burzynski NJ, editors. Clinical Dysmorphology of Oral-Facial Structures. Littleton: John Wright, PSG Inc., 1982: 447-473.

Shapira Y, Lubit E, Kuftinec MM. Hypodontia in children with various types of clefts. Angle Orthodontist 2000; 70(1):16-21.

Small B, Murray J. Enamel opacities: prevalence, classification and aetiological considerations. J Dent 1978; 6:33-42.

Woelfel JB, Scheid RC. Dental Anomalies. In: Dental Anatomy: its relevance to dentistry. Williams & Wilkins, 1997:345-374.

Warren JJ, Kanellis MJ, Levy SM. Fluorosis of the Primary Dentition: what does it mean for permanent teeth? JADA 1999; 130: 347-356.

Witkop C, Sauk JJ. Heritable Defects of Enamel. In: Oral Facial Genetics. Steward RE, Presscott GH, editors. St. Louis, Mosby Co.1976; pp 151-226.

Wright T. Normal formation and development defects of the human dentition. Ped Clin N Am 2000; 47:(5)975-1000.

CHAPTER 15

Analysis of the Orofacial Skeleton
W. Stuart Hunter

1. INTRODUCTION

The purpose of this chapter is to provide basic information about **cephalometrics**, which will enable a clinician to:

1.) undertake an "entry level" analysis of a lateral cephalogram in order to answer such questions as: Is there a skeletal component to the malocclusion? and if so, is it mild, moderate or severe?

2.) understand an orthodontist's explanation of those aspects of the patient's malocclusion explained by the **cephalometric analysis**, such as the relative contribution of the skeletal and dental components of the malocclusion.

3.) interpret to parents the implications of proposals by orthodontists and/or surgeons with respect to (proposed) surgical alterations to the face and jaws of the patient. For example, how much improvement is expected? Generally, when the skeletal improvement after surgery is expected to be less than 2 - 3 mm, surgery may not be the preferred option.

What constitutes an entry-level analysis and what is its purpose? An entry level analysis will include the identification of approximately 12 cephalometric landmarks and how they are used to quantify the severity of a skeletal malocclusion in terms of: 1.) the antero-posterior relationship of the mandible to the face and head, and 2.) the antero-posterior relationship of the maxilla to the mandible.

There are many qualifying measures used by orthodontists which are meant to refine the measures of those two relationships. Some are of more significance than others. For example, the anterior angle that the **mandibular plane** makes with a cranial plane such as Sella - **Nasion** suggests the future growth direction of the mandible, whether forward (small angle) or down (large angle). The probable direction of growth of the mandible is of great interest to the orthodontist since downward growth is believed to be less helpful to treatment than forward growth (See discussion of Direction of Growth, outline item 11, page 411).

When surgical repositioning of the mandible is being contemplated for the correction of a moderate to severe skeletal Class II malocclusion, from the surgeon's point of view, the purposes of the cephalometric analysis are threefold:

1.) to determine the amount of mandibular deficiency that exists and, from that, to decide how much advancement is needed,

2.) to relate the proposed position of the mandible to the existing position of the maxilla to determine whether the maxilla also needs to be moved, and

3.) to determine the amount of correction which can be accomplished using surgical procedures that correct the vertical proportions of the face.

In an unpublished Master's thesis "Skeletal Measures used in Mandibular Advancement Surgery (1991)", Low concluded that the initial planning for antero-posterior changes which can be accomplished by surgical lengthening of the mandible need consider only two cephalometric measures - one which relates the mandible to the face as a whole (such as Na Perpendicular) and one which relates the maxilla to the mandible (such one that relates as the **A point** to B Point or Wits).

He noted another factor of at least equal importance: the amount of advancement of the mandible that can be accomplished by surgery is limited by the amount of overjet reduction available at the time of surgery. Therefore, although the initial surgical planning need not involve complex cephalometric analysis, orthodontic treatment planning may require quite sophisticated cephalometric evaluation to determine how the amount of overjet required for the surgical correction can be accomplished. The overjet limitation also explains why orthodontic treatment in preparation for surgery has quite different objectives than when non-surgical treatment is the procedure of choice. Preparation for surgery may even involve increasing the overjet to permit the amount of mandibular advancement planned.

In that context, it is often assumed that the position of the mandible observed when the patient with a severe Class II Division 1 maloccclusion postures his mandible forward represents the relationship that will be seen after successful **activator** (monobloc) treatment. That, unfortunately, is not so. The major effect of activator treatment is retraction of the maxillary dentition. Mandibular advancement is usually only a millimeter or so more than normal growth.

2. EQUIPMENT & ENLARGEMENT

An x-ray film of the head is called a cephalogram when it has been obtained using a fixed frame having rounded plastic ear plugs which position the subject so that his/her head is in exactly the same posture for each exposure. The frame is constructed so that for a lateral cephalogram the **sagittal plane** of the head is precisely 60 inches from the actual source of the x-rays and the axis of the two ear plugs is aligned with the point source of the x-rays. As a result, a pre-treatment lateral cephalogram can be compared with the post-treatment lateral cephalogram and the changes resulting from treatment (and/or growth) evaluated.

As a consequence of the alignment of the **central ray** with the axis of the two ear plugs, the subject's head posture (chin up or chin tucked in) may differ as much as 5 degrees between successive films without significantly affecting the angles or distances measured on those films. On the other hand, when a posteroanterior cephalogram is obtained, the tilt of the head is very important because when the chin is raised, the vertical dimensions are decreased and when the chin is lowered, the vertical dimensions are inflated. For that reason, postero-anterior films are used only for the evaluation of asymmetries.

It is helpful to remember that almost everyone is asymmetric by 2% to 5% of whatever dimension is considered.

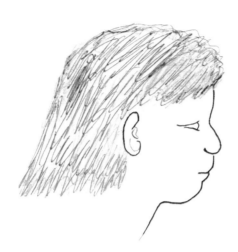

Figure 15-1: A severe Class II malocclusion.

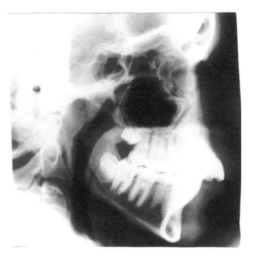

Figure 15-2: Lateral cephalogram for the subject in Figure 15-1.

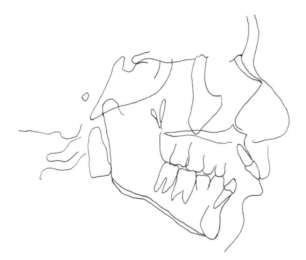

Figure 15-3: Tracing of the cephalogram in Figure 15-2.

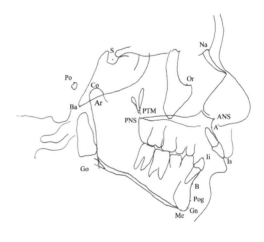

Figure 15-4: The cephalometric landmarks defined below.

In theory, because the 60-inch cephalometric source-to-subject distance is widely adhered to in North America, the differences between cephalograms should be the result of differences between subjects; or the result of growth if between different ages for one subject. Unfortunately, the necessity of maintaining a standard distance between subject and film has not been accepted worldwide, and **enlargement** may range from 5% to 15%. Since many clinical planning and evaluation procedures involve several size measures, a difference in enlargement of 5% between initial and end-of-treatment measures may result in misleading conclusions.

Although many orthodontists have their own equipment for obtaining cephalograms, others prefer to use the services of a nearby medical radiographic unit. In that case, much confusion and misdirection can be avoided by insisting that a constant distance between subject and film be maintained (and documented) by the x-ray technician involved. That is not a trivial matter, because for medical purposes, x-ray technicians are trained to obtain crisp and clear images that facilitate a qualitative evaluation of pathology by radiologists. To some extent, the closer to the head the film is, the better the image, with the result that the enlargement often varies from film to film when the cephalogram has been obtained by a medical x-ray unit.

3. TRACING vs VIDEO IMAGING FOR LANDMARK IDENTIFICATION

The invention of the **cephalometer** (an initial version of which was described by Broadbent in 1931) permitted the comparison of the relationship of the mandible to the maxilla, as seen in the pre-treatment **headfilm**, with that relationship as seen in the post-treatment headfilm. Because one cannot simply superimpose one film over another to evaluate growth or treatment changes, the procedure called tracing was devised. Since the surfaces of a bone such as the mandible maintain their basic shape as the bone increases in size, they can be traced on a sheet of frosted acetate which is temporarily attached to the headfilm on an illuminated surface or light box. The increase in size of the mandible from age 10 years to 14 years is then represented by the increase in the distance between the most posterior superior surface of the **condyle**, called **Condylion**, and a point on the outline of the **symphysis** of the mandible, called **Gnathion**, as measured on the tracings at 10 and 14 years.

A tracing of a cephalometric headfilm is an artistic abstract of a headfilm, wherein various landmarks are identified by their relationship to adjacent bony structures, most of which are on a bony surface. Thus Nasion is where the fronto-nasal suture ends at the surface of the frontal bone.

However, the use of film as a medium for recording and storing x-ray images is declining rapidly, as the techniques for digital imaging and storage become commonplace.

The acquisition of an x-ray image in digital format is accomplished indirectly by means of an intensifying screen (or directly by excitation of a photoelectric panel). The crystalline structure of the intensifying screen "glows" less or more in proportion to the amount of x-rays passing through it. The resulting light image is converted to a **digital image** by an associated scanning device. The digital image is loaded into a computer for display on its video screen. When the indirect method is used, regular film procedures can be used as well, whereas the direct method can produce only digital images. The monitor image is not suitable for tracing, but the landmarks can be located and marked on the **digital image** using the same definitions and appropriate software (which includes line drawing capabilities when needed for landmark location). A more detailed account of digital imaging for cephalometry may be found in the chapter by B. Holly Broadbent in "Essentials of Facial Growth" by Enlow and Hans (1998).

The future is therefore almost upon us, and tracing as an essential step between film and analysis would appear to be en route to extinction. However, tracings are at this time the best available way of learning how to recognize and correctly locate landmarks. As the digital version of x-ray imaging becomes more available, the methods for learning how to identify landmarks will probably involve the familiar self directed "Correct, proceed / wrong, go back" procedure in video format.

3.1 LANDMARK IDENTIFICATION PROCEDURES

The next section in this chapter contains the landmark definitions and illustrations that may be traced and compared with the adjacent tracings provided for that purpose by superimposing your tracing on the adjacent tracings. The landmarks have been grouped according to their location into five areas shown in Figure 15-5A. The definitions of the landmarks in each Section are followed by a print of the radiograph for that section and a tracing with the landmarks identified. The student will have no diffi-culty in tracing the outlines on a sheet of .003 frosted acetate. Back lighting is not required.

It should be emphasized that accuracy in the location of landmarks depends largely upon knowing what to look for and where to look. Your tracing should superimpose on the tracing provided as part B of Figures 15-6 through 15-16.

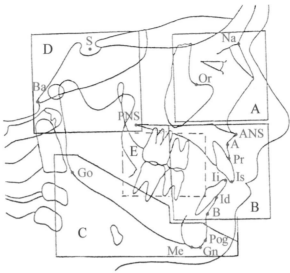

Figure 15-5A: The tracing divided into five sections for the defi-nitions which follow.

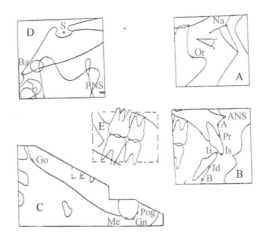

Figure 16-5b. Exploded view of Figure 16-5a.

Figure 15-5B: Exploded view of Figure 15-5A.

4. LANDMARKS

4.1 MIDLINE

Since our objective is to provide "entry level" information, we need define only the landmarks essen-tial for some very basic analytic procedures. The following landmarks are midline except for **Gonion**, **Articulare**, **Condylion** and **PTM**.

4.1.1. Section A   Upper Anterior

Nasion (Na): junction of the fronto-nasal suture at the most posterior point on the concave curve at the bridge of the nose, or simply (by default, if the suture is not visible) the most posterior point on the curve.

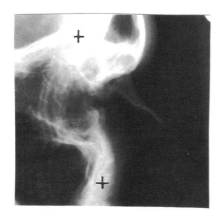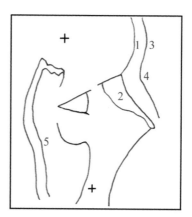

Figure 15-6A and B: Part A is the radiograph for Section A, Figure 15-5A. Part B is the tracing for Section A. The numbers are explained in the text below.

Figure 15-6B: The surface of supra orbital ridge is at 1, the nasal bone at 2, the soft tissue over supraorbital ridge at 3, but the soft tissue over nasion at 4 is seldom seen. Posterior surfaces of the **zygomatic arches** are at 5.

It is suggested that tracing begin with the bony outline of the supraorbital ridge down to its junction with the nasal bone (1). Next, draw in the nasal bone (2) including the jagged suture between nasal and frontal bones, if it can be seen. When the soft tissue can be seen, it is done next (3). Although the soft tissue over Nasion is not usually seen, the supraorbital part (4) is often connected to the part that becomes visible toward the tip of the nose. Some artistic license is allowed! The posterior surfaces of the zygomatic arches are usually visible at (5), but are not essential to any diagnostic procedure and need not be traced. Nasion is then identified.

4.1.2. Section B   Anterior Midface

Anterior Nasal Spine (ANS): the most anterior point on the maxilla at the level of the palate.

The next four landmarks are located using the "**tangent**" principle. Thus, for example, **Pogonion** is defined as the point on the anterior surface of the symphyseal outline that is tangent to a line from Nasion. The tangent is where the line just touches the symphyseal outline. When the outline is somewhat flat, the "just touches" rule means the center of the "touch", which may be 3 or 4 mm long. In anticipation of digital imaging and the location of landmarks using digital technology on a computer monitor, we assume that the software support for the location of landmarks will have the necessary line-forming capability so that a tangent can be constructed.

A point: the most posterior point on the concave curve between **ANS** and the teeth that is tangent to a line from Nasion.

A point is the only landmark on our list that is regularly confused by soft tissue, in this case, the cheeks. Other soft tissues such as the tonsils, tongue, soft palate, turbinates, nose, lips, etc., are not in conflict with bony landmarks. In Figure 15-8, both examples have two vertical lines extending above ANS. There is no problem with the anterior line. It is the more distal shadow that fades into the image of the bone over the middle third of the incisor that can be misleading.

B point: the most posterior point on the concave curve between the teeth and Pogonion which is tangent to a perpendicular from **Mandibular Plane (MP)** or tangent to a line from Nasion.

The incisor landmarks are illustrated in Figure 15-11B

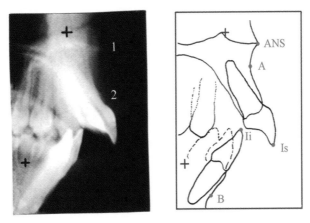

Figure 15-7A and B: Part A is the radiograph for Section B. Part B is the tracing for Section B.

Begin by identifying the converging arcs (1) that define ANS as shown in Figure 15-7B. Continue down to the **cementoenamel junction** of the maxillary incisors (2). This film has a "just discernible" layer of bone over the middle 1/3 of the incisor roots, but from the level of the root **apices** to ANS there is not a distinct line. The midline flange of bone is often so thin that a distinct edge is frequently not seen, but it is customary to "sweep" it in as though it can be seen. For such situations, **A point** may be located 2.0 mm mesial to the apical third of the incisor roots; that is the recommended default when there is no curve for the tangent to touch.

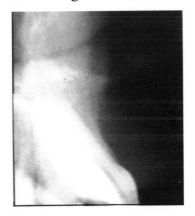
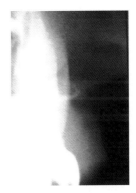

Figure 15-8: Cheek outlines superimposed on the bony septum from ANS to the maxillary incisors. Note that the cheek outlines extend above the palatal plane whereas the septal outline, if seen, does not.

4.1.3. Section C   The Mandible

Pogonion (Pog): the most anterior point on the symphyseal outline relative to the tangent of a line from Nasion.

Menton (Me): the most inferior point on the symphyseal outline tangent to the Mandibular Plane.

Gnathion (Gn): most distant from **Ar** or Co on the symphyseal outline (or the midpoint between Pog and Me).

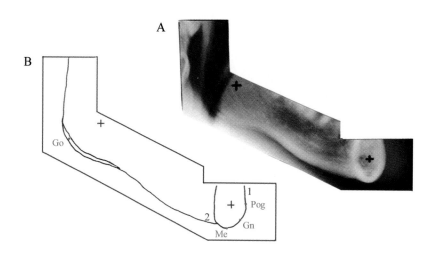

Figure 15-9A and B: Part A is the radiograph for Section C. Part B is the tracing for Section C. The numbers are explained in the text below.

4.2 BILATERAL LANDMARKS

Gonion (Go): usually a point at the most inferior, posterior point on the outline of the mandible. It is accurately determined as the intersection of the bisector of the angle Mandibular Plane makes with the Ramal Plane and the outline of the mandible. However, it may also be the intersection of Ramal and Mandibular Planes, in which case it is a "space mark".

Figures 15-9a and 15-9b show the x-ray and tracing for Section C. The outline of the symphysis (1) is a continuation of the line begun above at the cementoenamel junction of the lower incisors. Continue around its outline and up the **lingual** surface to the level of the **apices** of the canine and premolar roots. That outline represents the symphysis of the mandible. The outline of the inferior border of the mandible (2) is begun just posterior to Me on the symphyseal outline. It is swept in as smoothly as possible and continued up the **ramus** to the base of the skull.

Since there are right and left sides for the mandible, there are usually two lines diverging from the symphyseal outline to the Gonial area, where they may continue separately around the "Gonial corner" and be **offset** horizontally; or they may cross over one another and continue offset; or they may converge to a single superimposed line.

4.2.1. Section D The Base of the Skull

Articulare (Ar): the intersection of the Ramal Planes with the image of the base of the skull. Unless wide-open jaw films are available for accurate tracing of the heads of the condyles, this point is more reliable than Condylion. When there are two outlines as in Figure 15-10a, they are "averaged" visually.

Condylion (Co): the most posterior superior point on the outlines of the condylar heads, which are not usually seen when the teeth are in occlusion because the base of the skull obscures them.

In theory, a cephalogram taken with the jaw wide open can provide a clear image of the condyles (See Appendix A). In fact, a lateral view of the condyles does not reveal that they are cylindrical with their long axes oriented in a slightly posteriorly diverging direction. Further, it is seldom possible to establish which level of the cylinder (inner, central or outer) is portrayed. Thus, it is questionable whether the cost in time, material and exposure to radiation is justified by the somewhat dubious gain in information obtained from a "wide open" exposure.

Posterior Nasal Spine (PNS): the most posterior point at the **Sagittal plane** on the bony hard palate. Usually, it must be taken as the confluence of the posteriorly converging, inferior and superior surfaces of the bony hard palate (when they can be seen). It should not be used for antero-posterior measures. See ANS above and the maxillary length discussion below.

Sella turcica (S): the center of the pituitary fossa, determined by inspection; a subjective choice that has been found to be quite accurate. It is helpful to sketch in a curve from anterior to posterior clinoids giving an egg-shaped or round outline to the **hypophyseal fossa**, facilitating the choice of the center.

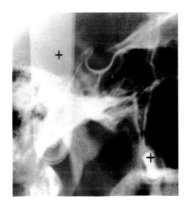 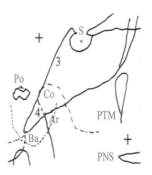

Figure 15-10A and B: Part A is the radiograph for Section D. Part B is the tracing for Section D. The numbers are explained in the text below.

Pterygomaxillary fissure (PTM): A bilateral, upside-down teardrop-shaped area of radiolucency, the anterior surfaces of which are taken as the posterior surfaces of the maxilla. PTM is taken at the inferior point of convergence.

Basion (Ba): There are at least 3 possible protocols for locating Ba as follows: 1.) the anterior margin of Foramen Magnum where the posterior surface of the **cranial base (clivus)** converges on the inferior surface of the cranial base, 2.) when the inferior surface of the skull <u>posterior</u> to Foramen Magnum can be seen, the continuation of its curve to the inferior surface of the cranial base <u>mesial</u> to Foramen Magnum should sweep past just below Basion, and 3.) the tip of the "**Odontoid process**" of C2 is usually about 5 mm from Basion and pointing to it.

The points listed above are on the mid-sagittal plane except for Gonion, Condylion, Articulare and PTM, which are bilateral. The procedure for bilateral points is to identify both and select the midpoint between them. When that is done, there is no need to identify left and right sides. Also, very often when a pre-treatment tracing is compared with the post-treatment tracing, the amount of **offset** is not the same and midlining is essential.

Figures 15-10A and 15-10B show the x-ray and tracing for Section D. The posterior surfaces of the rami shown in Figure 15-10A are slightly separated or offset. It is usually best to trace both since both are used to locate Gonion and the location of Ar halfway between the two is quite simple. The base of the skull is drawn in where it can be seen, especially from Sella posteriorly (3) and as it crosses the rami (4).

A Little Landmark Philosophy

Probably because cephalometric analyses feature angular and metric measures it is tempting to attribute a level of precision to the results not warranted by the accuracy (or inaccuracy) of location of the components. Thus, the identification of landmarks is a highly subjective procedure that is often undertaken with little (or very little) consideration given to the factors that contribute to that subjectivity. Thus, the location of A point as "the most posterior point on the concave curve between **Anterior Nasal Spine** and the maxillary incisors" assumes that:

1.) such a curve can be seen on the film or monitor image. Quite often, the image of the bone is only slightly lighter than the image of the soft tissue and the antero-posterior location of the curve has to be chosen as approximately 2 mm anterior to the incisor roots.

2.) the vertical location of A point is determined using the tangent from Na to the curve (and the principles of geometric tangents). Although the tangent principle provides some assurance of repeatability to the antero-posterior location of A point, there is less assurance with respect to its vertical location. Review the discussion on the "tangent" principle on page 390.

3.) the film is viewed under lighting conditions which are optimal for that investigator's visual physiology, and that the investigator is wearing glasses or contact lenses appropriate to his or her visual deficits.

4.) the investigators are using definitions for the landmarks which are generally agreed upon.

The last point raises the issue that there is considerable disagreement among those using landmarks as to the proper definitions for Gonion: (on the bone or at the junction of the Ramal Plane and the Mandibular Plane), Condylion: (most superior or most posterior or greatest distance from Gn or Me on the head of the mandibular condyle) and Basion, which is just simply hard to find. (Review the three protocols for locating Basion on page 393-394).

5. THE TEETH

5.1 INCISORS (see Section B)

Most cephalometric analyses include an evaluation of the relationship of the maxillary and mandibular central incisors to one another and to their supporting structures, and of maxillary and mandibular molars to one another and to their supporting skeletal structures.

For angular measures of incisor relationships a line connecting the incisal edge and the center of the apex of the root is ideal, but the apex is seldom as clear as in Figure 15-11A.

The crown of the most anterior maxillary central incisor is often (or usually) used to represent both incisors when they are not closely aligned. The maxillary incisors are unusually clear in Figure 15-11A because the left and right sides are perfectly superimposed. Since the incisor crowns are 'radio-opaque', tracing their radiographic images is not difficult, especially the labial surfaces. The **lingual** surfaces are often not clear, because the images of the lateral incisors are superimposed. However, one hopes that the recollection of their shape from one's exposure to dental anatomy will result in an acceptable outline.

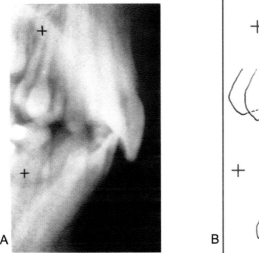
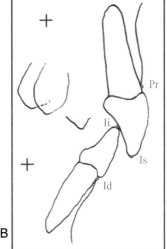

Figure 15-11A and B: Part A Radiograph for Incisors. Part B Tracing for Incisors.

Although occasionally of use, the landmark labels for the incisors are not entry-level information. **Incision superiorus (Is)** and **Incision inferiorus (Ii)** are the maxillary and mandibular incisal edges respectively. **Prosthion (Pr)** is supposed to be the tip of the alveolar bone between the maxillary incisors and is the same as the cementoenamel junction. **Infradentale (Id)** is the analagous point between the mandibular incisors.

5.2 Section E Molars

How the "offset" of molars affects the accuracy of molar location on a monitor has yet to be determined. It would seem that the availability of colors would simplify the procedure. In the following procedural suggestions, it is assumed that your landmark-locating software includes a line-drawing capability with color options. Therefore, for those using digital cephalometrics, "trace" should be translated as "draw".

In the suggested procedures that follow, it is assumed that the molar location is of concern because we want to know whether the molars have been moved distally or mesially (or not at all) and whether they have been intruded or extruded. When the outlines are as clear as in Figure 15-12A, the answers are easily provided. It is when the images such as those in Figure 15-16A are seen that the answers are provided with some difficulty.

Tracing (drawing) the molars is probably the most confusing component of the entire tracing procedure because the images of the left and right side molars seldom superimpose. The recommended procedure involves two principles:

    1.) if possible, trace one quadrant at a time.
    2.) begin with the most posterior erupted tooth in the quadrant being traced, because that tooth
        will provide at least one surface which is not ambiguous.

When there is no overlap or "**offset**", tracing the molars is quite straightforward. When there is either horizontal or vertical offset, tracing is not greatly more difficult, but when both horizontal and vertical offsets obtain, the task is daunting.

5.2.1 No Offset of the Molars

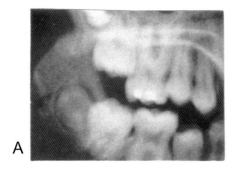
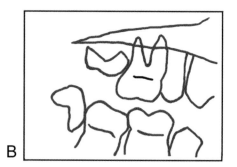

Figure 15-12A and B: Part A shows all molars superimposed. Part B is the tracing of Figure 15-12A

5.2.2 Slight Offset of the Molars

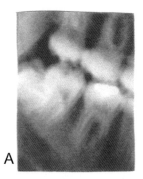
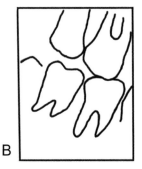

Figure 15-13A and B: Part A is a radiograph showing mandibular molars slightly offset. Part B is the tracing of the average between left and right sides.

Proceed as suggested above. Usually, the more anterior molar seems to be slightly wider than its

antimere because it is the right side molar and, therefore, enlarged more than the left side molar. However, it is not necessary to identify which side is right and which left. Indeed, when the overlap is slight, the averaging procedure can be accomplished without tracing both sides as seen in Figure 15-13B above.

5.2.3 Horizontal Offset of the Molars

When the horizontal offset is more than 1.0 mm, the "one quadrant at a time" procedure is advised. As shown in Figures 15-14B and 15-14C, the last molar, in this case the first molar, is traced and then the premolar. Repeat for the maxillary molars. The broken lines in Figure 15-15C are the other side. The average is then drawn in, using a colored pencil.

At this point, it is obvious that we have a plethora of lines. The "average" is meant to be a simplification. And it is, provided the initial outlines are removed, which is usually messy. It is tempting to average the outlines without tracing them. That may occasionally be possible, but for images offset both horizontally and vertically the usual result of such an attempt is confusion.

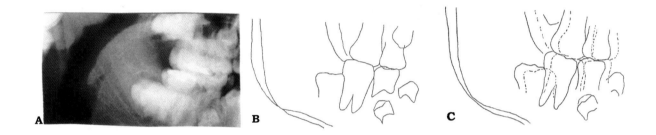

Figure 15-14A, B, and C: Part A: Note that the molar offsets match the ramus offset.
Part B: Tracing of the most posterior molars. Part C More mesial molars: broken lines.

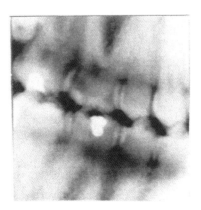

Figure 15-15: Remember that the proximal surfaces of the molars are not at right angles to the **Sagittal plane** of the head. These angled proximal surfaces double the density of the left side/right side offsets resulting in multiple radiopaque vertical ovals at the molar contact points.

5.2.4 Both Horizontal and Vertical Offsets

Quite often, as well as being 'offset' antero-posteriorly, one side is higher than the other. The last molars, if fully erupted, will be offset vertically and consistent with the other teeth on that side. The amount of vertical offset will decrease anteriorly until it vanishes at the central incisors.

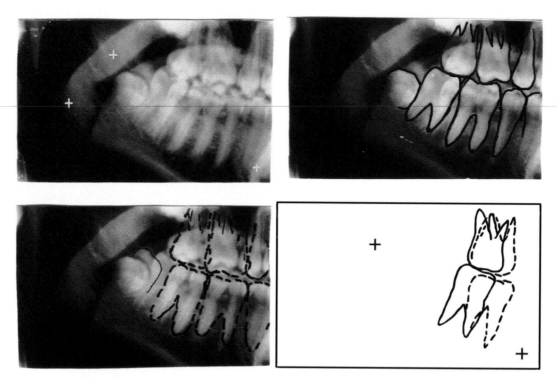

Figure 15-16A, B, C, and D: Part A Molars offset both horizontally and vertically. Part B The posterior and superior molars. Part C The anterior and inferi-
or molars and first premolars. Part D All first molars.

As with horizontal offsets, the most posterior, fully erupted molars provide the best clue as to the amount of vertical offset. Assuming that the teeth on each side are consistent with respect to the amount of vertical offset, begin as before, with the most posterior, fully erupted molar for either the maxilla or the mandible and proceed forward to include the second premolars. It is generally best to complete one side before attempting the other because, if correct, the first side maxillary occlusal surfaces will suggest where the mandibular occlusal surfaces should be.

When there is an unusual arrangement of the teeth, such as when a molar is missing, the plaster casts or the panoramic film should be studied to ensure a proper interpretation of the occlusal surfaces.

6. PLANES AND LINES

A **plane** may be thought of as a graphic summary of the skeletal or dental component in which the landmarks defining the plane are found. However, a plane has meaning only in relation to other planes. Thus, a large angle between **Sella-Nasion** (cranial base) and **Mandibular Plane** (the mandible) suggests that relative to the cranial base, the mandible is growing more downward than forward.

See this Chapter's Appendix B for illustrations of Mandibular Growth Direction.

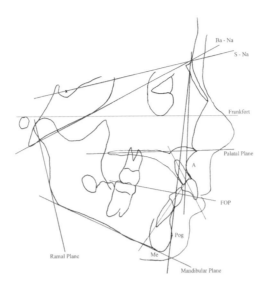

Figure 15-17: Major planes and lines.

Sella Nasion (S-N): representing the **anterior cranial base**. Although the surfaces adjacent to both landmarks have been shown to change by the addition or subtraction of surface bone, the amount of change is seldom in excess of 1 mm.

Basion - Nasion (Ba-Na): the cranial base from the anterior edge of Foramen Magnum to Nasion. Basion is not always easily located.

Frankfort Plane (FP): The use of Frankfort Plane as a reference plane derives from anthropometry of skulls at the turn of the last century, for which the superior surface of **Porion** and the inferior surface of the eye socket, called **Orbitale**, were easily accessible on a skull. The line or plane between them approximated the cant of the head when looking at the horizon (or was approximately parallel to the floor). The fact that neither landmark is reliably identified in lateral cephalograms has not deterred traditionalists from attempting to use it as a reference line.

Palatal Plane (Pal P): ANS to PNS. Maxillary length may be taken as the distance between the perpendiculars from Palatal Plane through PTM and A point.

A Little More Landmark Philosophy

Maxillary Length is occasionally defined as the distance between ANS and PNS. Because ANS is found at the convergence of inferior and superior arcs and PNS at the convergence of inferior and superior surfaces (when they are not obscured by the maxillary second molars), their anteroposterior location is somewhat subjective.

It is therefore recommended that the anterior terminus be defined as the point at which a perpendicular to Palatal Plane from A point intersects Palatal Plane. The posterior terminus is then the point at which a perpendicular to Palatal Plane from PTM intersects Palatal Plane.

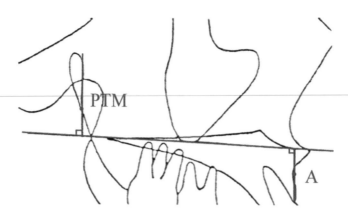

Figure 15-18: The anteroposterior length of the maxilla using perpendiculars from PTM and A point.

Occlusal Plane (OP): from the mid-occlusal point of the averaged maxillary and mandibular molars to the midpoint of the overbite of the incisors. Often this plane is called "Down's Occlusal Plane" simply because he appears to have been the first to define it.

Functional Occlusal Plane (FOP): from the mid-occlusal point of the averaged maxillary and mandibular molars to the mid-occlusal point of the averaged maxillary and mandibular first premolars. See also the discussion of FOP on page 403.

Mandibular Plane (MP): tangent to the posterior portion of the inferior border of the mandible and to the symphyseal outline.

Broadbent ('98) listed 4 definitions of MP:

- A tangent to the lower border of the mandible.
- A line joining Gonion and Gnathion.
- A line joining Gonion and Menton.
- A line from Menton tangent to the posteroinferior border of the mandible.

None of these is helpful in the face of a Rocker mandible, the lower border of which has no **antegonial notch** and resembles the functional part of a rocking chair — the part that rests on the floor. When there are not two end points (or surfaces) for the determination of MP, the location of Gonion becomes questionable. The "best guess" estimate for the location of MP is utilized in such circumstances.

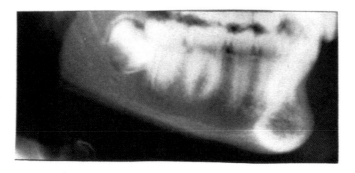

Figure 15-19: Rocker mandible.

Ramal Plane (RP): tangent to the posterior border of the **ramus** between Articulare and Gonion.

7. CRANIOFACIAL PLANES AND GROWTH DIRECTION
(OR, ON THE IMPORTANCE OF HAVING A STRONG CHIN)

Since the beginning of the cephalometric concept (around 1925 -30), there have been regular attempts to relate the increases in size of the various components of the craniofacial complex to the direction of growth of the face. Although seldom, if ever, stated, the underlying concern most likely has to do with the prominence of the chin as it relates to the rest of the face. For the Western component of Homo Sapiens, a prominent chin bestows upon its owner personality characteristics of strength, determination and independence. On the other hand, a deficient chin is usually associated with pusillanimity, weakness and frailty. Therefore, the treatment for a deficient chin (often associated with Class II malocclusion), is simply to move it forward. When the direction of growth of the mandible is forward, the correction, either orthodontic or surgical or both, is believed to be enhanced. On the other hand, when the direction of growth of the mandible is down, orthodontic correction of the deficiency is difficult and surgical correction is often a preferred choice. Hence the concern orthodontists have for the direction of growth is founded in clinical experience and enhanced by cultural standards.

For a time, from the mid thirties to the late sixties, there was considerable interest in the idea that there is one spot in the craniofacial complex which is neutral and from which all components move away during growth. More recently, the direction of facial growth, as it influences the appearance of the person involved, has focused on the direction of the change in the position of the chin from before treatment to after treatment (see Mair and Hunter '92). Figures 15-43, 15-44 and 15-45 (Appendix B) illustrate the differences between downward and forward direction of growth of the chin. In that context, the amount of change required for the change to be perceived has not been established. That is, the difference between a dental Class II and a dental Class I occlusion is readily observable, especially when a patient can move her mandible from Class II to Class I and can be seen without an examination of the dentition. On the other hand, because most of us are not able to identify a slide in centric of 2 mm at a distance of two meters, it is tempting to suggest that a horizontal advance of the chin of less than 4.0 mm is probably not discernible.

8. ANALYSES

The analysis of a headfilm image is actually an attempt to facilitate the conversion of subjective impressions of what is good (or bad) in the patient's face into numbers, which may be compared with averages for populations or into proportions that confirm or refute the original subjective appraisal.

Since surgical repositioning of the body of the mandible has become a practical procedure, confirmation of the severity of the mismatch between mandible and maxilla is of interest, if not essential. When, for example, the ANB angle is less than $3°$, simply aligning the teeth will most often serve the patient well. When the ANB angle is $4°$ or more, treatment options are: 1.) camouflage or 2.) surgical advancement of the mandible. And when the ANB is $8°$ or more, a non-surgical approach is seldom satisfactory.

Although the use of cephalometric x-rays of the head for diagnostic purposes was reported as early as 1922 in Spanish and European literature, Broadbent's 1931 report in the Angle Orthodontist was the first in an American journal to suggest their diagnostic potential. As both cross sectional and longitudinal data became available, many schemes were devised for the comparison of skeletal characteristics of malocclusion with those of good or ideal occlusion. In 1957, Krogman and Sassouni evaluated 45

cephalometric analyses that had been reported to that point in time. They identified ten different analytic procedures reported in English language journals between Broadbent's 1931 report and 1948 when
Downs published his analysis, which used 5 skeletal and 5 dental measures. Those ten measures proved
to be the right level of complexity and became the most popular cephalometric analysis for many years.
However, SNA and SNB were not included and his colleagues at Northwestern University added those
that same year and replaced **Frankfort Horizontal (FH)** with Sella - Nasion because the landmarks for
Frankfort are often obscure. Three of Downs' five skeletal measures are shown in Figure 15-20.

The ANB angle has become perhaps the most widely used measure of the severity of a skeletal malocclusion because its size is usually a reflection of what we see. An ANB angle of 2° means a straight or
orthognathic profile as shown in Figure 15-21A and an ANB angle of 11° means a severely retrognathic or convex profile as shown in Figure 15-21B. Jacobson (1985, pp. 63-67) has shown how an ANB
angle of 7° can occur with an ideal Class I dental relationship as well as with a Class II dental relationship, which substantiates the fact that although there is most often a close relationship between the
skeletal and dental classifications, it is not perfect.

Note that in addition to being part of the **ANB angle**, SNB usually provides an indication of the relationship of the mandible to the face as a whole. The average value is in the 78° - 80° range. Another
measure of the relationship of the mandible to the face (used by McNamara - see below) is the distance
from Pog to Nasion Perpendicular. Nasion Perpendicular is a line from Nasion perpendicular to FH.
Figure 15-22 illustrates that a **Facial angle** of 83° (Downs) would have a large measure of about 18 mm
between Nasion Perpendicular and Pogonion. The metric measure can then be used in the planning
process to estimate how much mandibular advancement is practical.

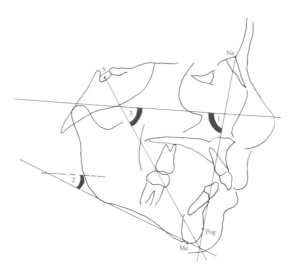

Figure 15-20. Downs' analysis. Three of the five skeletal measures from the
Downs Analysis: 1.) Nasion - Pogonion (Facial Plane) to Frankfort, 2.)
Gonion - Menton (Mandibular Plane) to Frankfort, 3.) Sella - Gnathion to
Frankfort (Y axis). The Downs analysis also includes five dental measures not
shown.

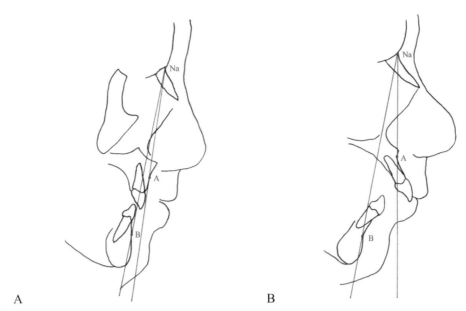

Figure 15-21. The Northwestern Analysis included six of Downs' measures and added SNA, SNB and ANB. Shown here at (A) is an ANB angle of 3° for a normal orthognathic profile, and at (B) an ANB angle of 11° for a severe skeletal Class II.

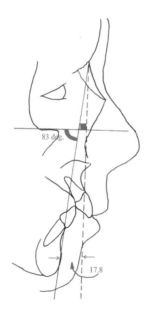

Figure 15-22. Facial Plane vs Nasion Perpendicular. The Facial Plane (Na - Pog) is measured in degrees. Nasion Perpendicular to Pogonion is measured in mm and is the distance from Pogonion to a line from Nasion perpendicular to Frankfort.

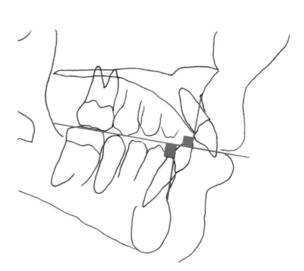

Figure 15-23. Wits analysis. Popularized by Jacobson (1985), who trained at Witswatersrand (hence the "Wits"). The concept appears to have been suggested originally by Jenkins in 1955.

In the **Wits analysis** the line from A point, which is perpendicular to FOP in an ideal face, is about 1 mm posterior to the perpendicular to FOP from B point for males and coincident with the line from B point for females.

The Wits analysis is based upon the **Functional Occlusal Plane**, which is supposed to represent something that is true and consistent about the dentition and its relationship to the face. When it is "functional" our intuition tells us that it has to be good and pivotal in the same way that Moss' Functional Matrix is intuitively central and significant. However, until how a curved surface (the Curve of Spee) can be converted to a straight line (the Functional Occlusal Plane) consistently has been clarified, the FOP may be seen as neither more nor less variable in its central position in the face than any other of the planes used to analyze the relationship of the mandible to the maxilla. That is, it may intuitively be more meaningful than Se - Na but it is not likely to be as reproducible or accurate.

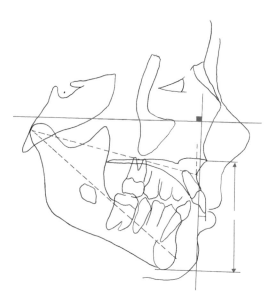

Figure 15-24: McNamara Analysis. It does not matter whether Co can be seen or not, so long as the same point in that location is used for end of treatment as for before treatment by superimposing the 2nd tracing over the first and marking the same point.

The values for Co-Pog, Co-A, Anterior Lower Face Height and A point to Na Perpendicular are listed in Table 15-1 below.

The McNamara analysis is based upon Harvold's appraisal of the difference between maxillary and mandibular lengths measured from Condylion. Harvold provided age-related values derived from the Burlington, Ontario, data which McNamara adapted as follows:

Table 15-1. Average values from McNamara and Brudon's Table 4 (which includes, in addition, SDs, ages 6, 16, 18, 20 and Maxillomandibular differentials). Data are from the Burlington Orthodontic Research Centre.

	MALES		FEMALES		LFH	
AGE	Mx	Md	Mx	Md	M	F
9	84.9	105.0	88.3	103.3	63.0	61.2
12	90.3	113.0	87.3	110.2	65.7	63.4
14	93.9	119.2	89.2	114.9	68.8	66.2

He suggests that **A point** to Na Perp should be about 1.1 mm for males and 0.4 mm for females and that Pog to Na Perp should be about -0.3 for males and -1.8 for females.

Thus, McNamara's analysis includes the three relationships, suggested by Low initially in this chapter, as basic to planning for orthognathic surgery: 1.) the relationship of the mandible to the maxilla, 2.) the relationship of the maxilla to the face (A point - Na Perp), and 3.) a measure of lower face height (LFH). In addition, the average for Na Perpendicular to Pog may serve as a check for the other values. McNamara also provides other values for use in orthodontic treatment planning. Note that all of the above measures are metric, thus emphasizing the need for consistency in **cephalometric enlargement**.

9. THE FUTURE OF IMAGING FOR ORTHODONTICS
Contributed by William Harrell, Jr., D.M.D.

The goal of medical and dental imaging has been to represent and display the anatomic truth of our patients. Historically, imaging has been confined to representations in only two dimensions. There are currently 3-dimensional imaging techniques, but they are still limited by the amount of information they can represent and by their static nature. The creation of a fully interactive three-dimensional model of patient anatomy would greatly improve the doctor's ability to predict and display different treatment results, monitor changes over time, i.e., the fourth dimension in areas such as: aging, treatment effects, degenerative changes, etc., and the ability to accurately measure treatment outcomes.

For decades and today in 2002, the only true 3-dimensional information orthodontists use for diagnosis and treatment planning are the plaster study models of the teeth that are created from impressions. Currently, there are techniques (OrthoCad & Emodels) that create accurate digital representations of the teeth on the computer monitor for orthodontic diagnosis and treatment planning, but these modalities are not merged with the other data such as: facial soft tissues or skeletal structures in three dimensions and impressions still have to be made for the 3D data input. There is an intra-oral scanner (Suresmile by OraMetrix) that uses a small intra-oral scanning device to create the three-dimensional information of the occlusal surfaces of the teeth without the need for impressions, but there is no information on the location and anatomy of the roots nor is this data merged with the soft tissues or skeletal structures of the face.

Acuscape International, Inc. (www.acuscape.com, Glendora, CA), has developed a method that combines the information from standard cephalometric radiographs, standard facial and intra-oral photographs and 3D information from either plaster study models or electronic study models of the teeth, to create a three-dimensional matrix, or a 3D digital representation of patient anatomy. Acuscape has been working with Science Applications International Corp, Advanced Technology Group (Huntsville, AL) to apply advanced image processing technology to fuse multiple image modalities on the basis of classified work performed for the Department of Defense for image recognition, manipulation, and archiving. These advanced technologies, when applied to orthodontics, orthognathic surgery, plastic and reconstructive surgery, forensics, facial recognition, and orthopedics, will allow for computer-assisted identification of anatomy and anatomic landmarks and the manipulation of the 3D data in a web-based environment.

Acuscape® is in the process of creating the Acuscape ® Universal Anatomic Database which will grow with the data mined from every new patient, creating a knowledge base that can be used for monitoring treatment over time, evaluating different treatment simulations, and enhancing and updating the general orthodontic database of anatomy for clinical and academic research. The database can be grouped into archetype 3D models and further divided by age, sex and race. These three-dimensional archetype models can then be compared with the patient-specific 3D digital model to arrive at a "mathematical measure of difference" between these two three-dimensional models for diagnosis, evaluation and orthodontic treatment planning.

The ability to view the 3D computer patient models stereoscopically, with binocular vision, allows the doctor to visualize true depth information, as we see with "real world" 3D objects, see Figure 15-41. The ability to "see depth" (stereopsis) is accomplished by humans having two eyes offset horizontally. Not only does stereopsis improve the qualitative aspects of visualization, but also improves the quantitative analysis of the information.

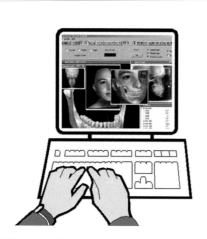

Figure 15-25: Acuscape® Clinician Software.

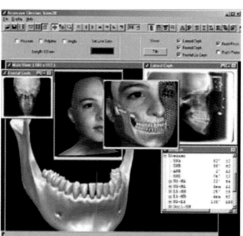

Figure 15-26: Acuscape® 3D Digital Patient Model & 3D Analysis.

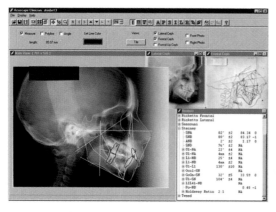

Figure 15-27: Traditional 2D Lateral Cephalometric Analysis.

The Clinician Software allows the clinician to interact with the 3D digital patient (Figures 15-25 and 15-26). The doctor can measure, move, try extraction vs non-extraction treatment plans along with interproximal reduction, expansion or surgical treatment plans, all in true three dimensional (3D) space. These can also be shared with other doctors involved with the treatment plan via the Internet for **interdisciplinary treatment** planning.

Traditional 2D Lateral Cephalometric Analysis. Bilateral structures are "averaged" to the "midline" losing the three-dimensional bilateral information. Differential magnification from right to left sides are created due to the geometric errors of projection.

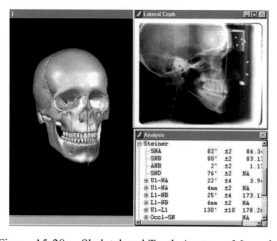

Figure 15-28: Skeletal and Tooth Anatomy Merged with Facial Soft Tissue of 3D Digital Patient.

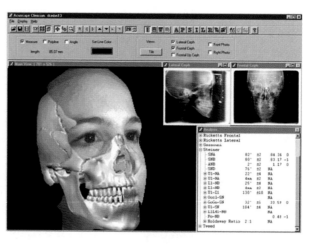

Figure 15-29: Skeletal and Tooth Anatomy of 3D Digital Patient.

Figure 15-28 is skeletal and tooth anatomy of the 3D digital patient derived from 3D data of traditional orthodontic records that are then merged using Acuscape ® Sculptor software.

Figure 15-29 is 3D skeletal and tooth anatomy merged with the facial soft tissue, for three-dimensional diagnosis and treatment planning.

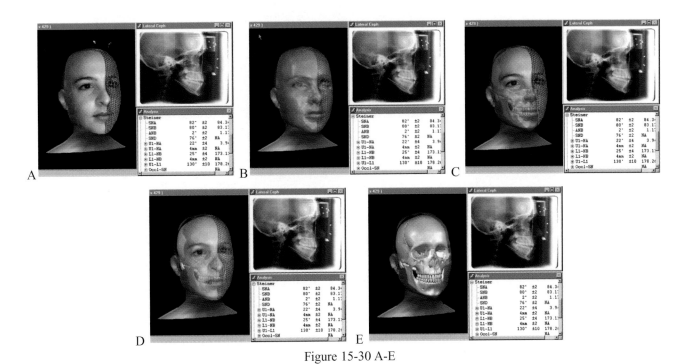

Figure 15-30 A-E

3D Virtual Patient, Figures 15-30A-E, in sequential stages of transparency from textured face in Figure 15-30A to underlying skeleton in Figure 15-30E.

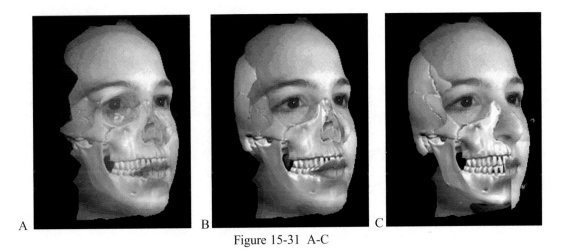

Figure 15-31 A-C

Figures 15-31A through 15-31C show the 3D Virtual Patient at various stages of transparency of the facial soft tissues. They show the relationship of the facial soft tissue to the underlying skeletal and tooth anatomy in anatomically true 3D relationships.

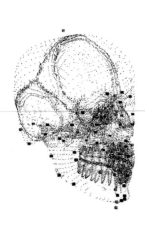

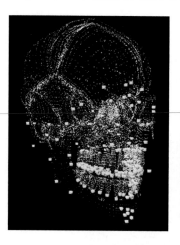

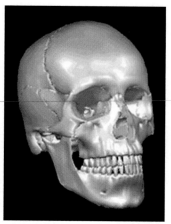

Figure 15-32: Acuscape® Sculptor dotPROfile.

Figure 15-33: Acuscape® Sculptor dotPROfile.

Figure 15-34: Textured dotPROfile

The swarm of three-dimensional landmarks that are created from the images that are taken of the patient are called a dotPROfile (pronounced dot PRO file). This dotPROfile is created by the Acuscape® Sculptor software from calibrated two-dimensional images.

The dotPROfile can be textured to look like a skull and teeth (Figure 15-16C).

Figures 15-35A and 15-35B show the face in a three dimensional perspective rotated to various degrees for analysis of the facial soft tissues.

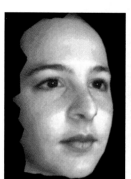

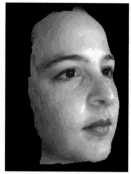

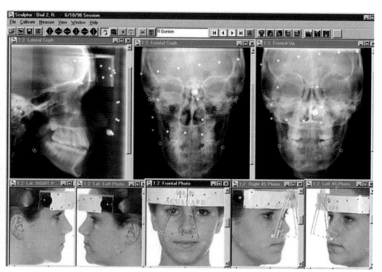

Figure 15-35A and B: A.) 3D Face, B.) 3D Face Rotated.

Figure 15-36: Acuscape® Calibrator and Sculptor software.

The lateral ceph, frontal ceph and frontal up ceph (head tilted 10-15 degrees "up") are calibrated with the facial photos by way of the Acuscape® Calibrator and Sculptor software.

The Calibrator is worn on the head and used by the Processing Center to calibrate and derive the 3D data from these images.

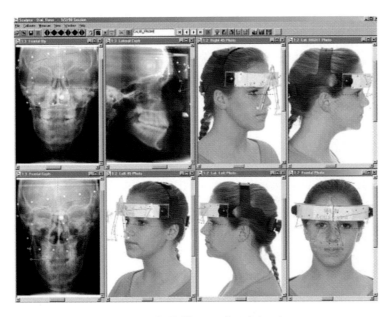

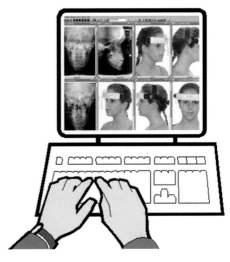

Figure 15-37: Acuscape® Calibrator (headpiece).

Figure 15-38: Calibration of Images in Acuscape® Sculptor Software.

The Acuscape® Calibrator (head piece) is being used to calibrate the X-rays and photographs, so that the true 3D information may be extracted. Software algorithms are used to remove size, rotational, and projection errors from the data so that true size 3D information is created.

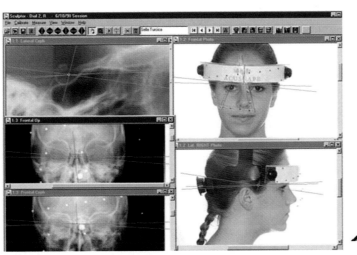

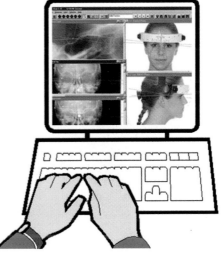

Figure 15-39: Cross-calibration of Landmarks in Acuscape® Sculptor.

Figure 15-40: Landmarks can be compared.

Landmarks can be cross-calibrated and the location of these landmarks can be viewed on other views as to their locations in true three-dimensional space. The limitations of traditional two-dimensional cephalometrics have been well documented and recently Dibbets 5 has studied the effects of magnification on lateral cephalometric studies.

Figure 15-41 shows an example of the possibilities on a Compaq Ipaq Pocket PC with a "stereoscopic" image, sticking out of the computer screen. By the use of stereoscopic glasses, newer retinal displays, or auto-stereoscopic displays, the doctor of the future will be able to bring up a patient's 3D model on their wireless pocket PC, and view the 3D virtual patient with true depth perception using binocular vision.

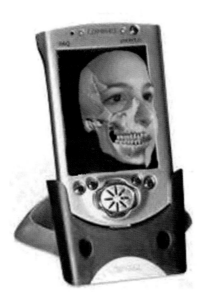

Figure 15-41: "Stereoscopic" image on Compaq Ipaq Pocket PC.

10. APPENDIX A. THE MANDIBULAR CONDYLE

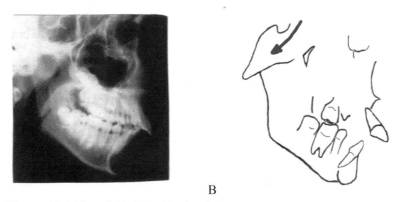

A   B

Figures 15-42A and 15-42B: The head of the condyle is obscured by the dense bone of the cranial base.

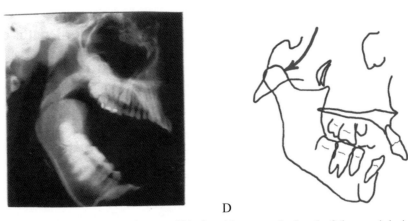

C   D

Figure 15-42C: When the mandible is wide open, the head of the condyle is visible. The mandibular outline of the 15-42B tracing is superimposed on the wide-open image of the mandible (15-42C) and the head (or heads) of the condyle completed as in Figure 15-42D.

11. APPENDIX B.

Mandibular Growth Direction: Forward, Average or Down

Mandibular Growth Direction (MGD) is determined by the line connecting Gnathion at a first age with Gnathion at a second age. The point used does not have to be Gnathion, but whatever point used at the first age is transferred to the second age by superimposing the symphyseal outline at the second age on that of the first and marking Gnathion at exactly the same place. The second tracing is then superimposed over the first, using whatever reference line the investigator prefers, usually, S-Na or B-Na. Gnathion 1 is connected to Gnathion 2 and the angle with its reference line is recorded.

MGD as shown in Figures 15-43, 15-44 and 15-45 is expressed as the anterior angle between MGD and S-Na and also as the anterior angle between MGD and Ba-Na.

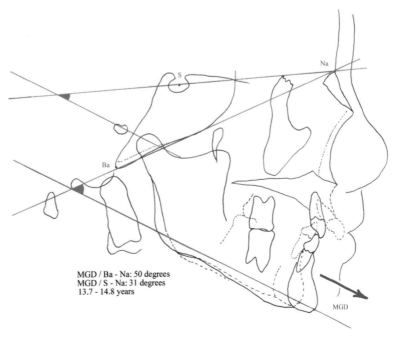

MGD / Ba - Na: 50 degrees
MGD / S - Na: 31 degrees
13.7 - 14.8 years

Figure 15-43: The MGD to S-Na is 31 $^{\circ}$, which is the numerical expression of its forward or horizontal growth direction for the 3.4 years between first and second films.

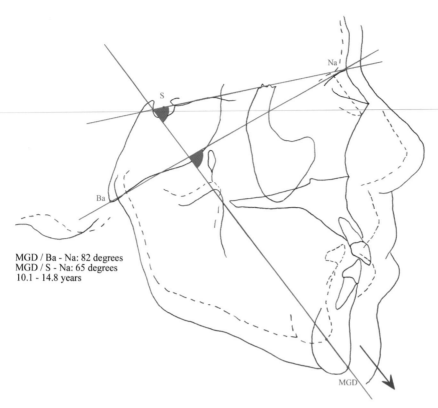

MGD / Ba - Na: 82 degrees
MGD / S - Na: 65 degrees
10.1 - 14.8 years

Figure 15-44: An approximately average MGD of 65° to S-Na.

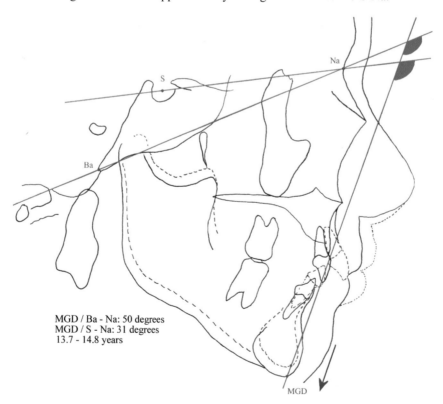

MGD / Ba - Na: 50 degrees
MGD / S - Na: 31 degrees
13.7 - 14.8 years

Figure 15-45: A downward or vertical growth direction for MGD of 117° to S-Na.

Credit:

Images and information courtesy of Acuscape International, Inc. (Glendora, CA) and the founders Dr. William (Bill) Harrell, Jr. (Board Certified Orthodontist, Alexander City, AL) and Dr. David C. Hatcher (Oral & Maxillofacial Radiologist, Sacramento, CA).

12. SUGGESTED READINGS

Athanasiou Athanasios E. (ed). Orthodontic Cephalometry, Mosby-Wolfe, 1995.
This multi-national compendium of cephalometric material has superb illustrations of headfilm landmarks, both photographic and radiographic, followed by comprehensive presentations of almost every aspect of cephalometrics. The material presented is of uniformly high quality and the final chapter provides the average values for the measures used in 22 cephalometric analyses including the Downs, Wits and McNamara.

Jacobson A (ed). Radiographic Cephalometry: From Basics to Videoimaging. Quintessence, 1995.
This handsome volume is illustrated with many excellent photographs, tracings and drawings. Downs', Steiner, Ricketts, Wits and McNamara's analyses are explained in detail with a chapter for each. Templates are provided for Johnston's Template and Jacobson's Proportionate analyses, and five templates are provided to assist in the tracing of the print of a headfilm.

Rakosi, Thomas. An atlas and manual of cephalometric radiography, London: Wolfe Med Pubs. 1982.
This 23-year-old atlas and manual has excellent definitions and descriptions of landmarks.

Fernandez-Riveiro P, Suarez-Quintanilla, Smyth-Chamosa E. Suarez-Cunqueiro M. Linear photogrammetric analysis of the soft tissue facial profile. Am J Orthod Dentofacial orthop;2002;122:59-66.

Ask Us* Am J Orthod Dentofacial orthop; 2002;122:18A-19A.
Tavajohi-Kermani H. Kapur R. Sciote JJ. Tooth agenesis and craniofacial morphology and orthodontic population. Am J Orthod Dentofacial Orthop 2002;122:39-47.

12. REFERENCES

Broadbent BH. A new X-ray technique and its application to orthodontics. Am J Orthodont. 1:45-66, 1931.

Broadbent BH. Cephalometrics. Chapter 15, pp 241-364 in Enlow DH, Hans MG. Essentials of Facial Growth, Saunders, 1998.

Harvold EP. The Activator in Interceptive Orthodontics. Mosby 1974.

Jenkins DH. Analysis of orthodontic deformity employing lateral cephalostatic radiography. Am J Orthodont. 41:442-452, 1955.

Keeling SD, Riolo ML, Martin RE, and TenHave TR. A Multivariate Approach to Analyzing the Relation between Occlusion and Craniofacial Morphology. Amer J Orthod, April 1989;95(4):297-305.

Mair AD, Hunter WS. Mandibular growth direction with conventional Class II non-extraction treatment. Am J Orthod Dentofac Orthop 101:543-9,1992.

McNamara JA, Brudon WL: Orthodontic and Orthopedic Treatment in the Mixed Dentition, Needham Press, 2001.

McNamara JA Jr, Brust EW, and Riolo ML. Soft tissue evaluation of individuals with an ideal occlusion and a well-balanced face, Craniofacial Monograph Series, #28, Esthetics and the Treatment of Facial Form, Center for Human Growth and Development, The University of Michigan, Ann Arbor, Michigan, 1993

Moyers RE, van der Linden FPGM, Riolo ML, McNamara JA. Standards of human occlusal development. Center for Human Growth and Development, Monograph # 5. The University of Michigan, Ann Arbor, Michigan, 1976.

Future Imaging of Orthodontics

Adams, GL, Hatcher, DC, and Miller, AJ. Comparison between traditional two-dimensional cephalometry and a three-dimensional approach, Univer of Ortho, Univer of Calif, San Francisco. Am J Orthod Dentofacial Orthop July 2002:122:117

Bishop P. Size constancy, depth constancy and vertical disparities: a further quantitative interpretation. Biological Cybernetics 1994;71:31-47

Dibbets, JMH, Nolte K. Effect of magnification on lateral cephalometric studies Am J Orthod Dentofacial Orthop 2002;122:196-201

Hatcher D. Diagnostic Imaging. In Davis H, Fonseca R, editors. Reconstruction preprosthetic oral and maxillofacial surgery. Philadelphia: W. B. Saunders; 1995, pp. 86-123.

Hatcher D. Maxillofacial imaging In: McNeill C, editor. Occlusion: Science and practice. Quintessence; 1997, pp. 349-64.

Quintero JC, Trosien A, Hatcher D, Kapila S. Craniofacial imaging in orthodontics: historical perspective, current status and future developments. Angle Orthod 1999; 69:491-506.

Harrell WE, Hatcher DC. In Search of anatomic truth: 3-dimensional digital modeling and the future of orthodontics, (in press) Am J Orthod Dentofacial Orthop - Technobytes section, Sept 2002.

CHAPTER 16

Section I	Section II	Section III	Section IV
1. Developmental, Psychosocial, Behavioral, and Compliance Aspects of Care 2. Prenatal Craniofacial Growth 3. Postnatal Caniofacial Growth 4. Growth of the Craniofacial Skeleton 5. Development of the Dentition and Occlusion	6. Classification and Terminology 7. Etiology of Malocclusion 8. Force Systems and Tissue Response 9. Tissue Engineering in Orthodontics 10. Clinical Epidemiology and Malocclusion	11. Orthodontic Exam and Diagnosis 12. Analysis of Orofacial and Jaw Musculature 13. Analysis of Dentition and Occlusion 14. Dental Dysmorphogenesis 15. Analysis of Orofacial Skeleton 16. Planning Orthodontic Treatment	17. Preadolescent Treatment 18. Adolescent Treatment 19. Adult Treatment 20. Treatment of Patients with Craniofacial Anomalies 21. Retention, Relapse and the Recurrence of Malocclusion 22. The Adverse Effects of Orthodontic Treatment

The Planning and Timing of Orthodontic Treatment

Christopher S. Riolo

James L. Vaden

"Sometimes it is better to be lucky than smart but don't count on it. " Dr. I.M. Aleatory

1. INTRODUCTION

Except in a few instances, malocclusion does not directly impact overall health, but many malocclusions are severe enough to impact function. Some potential consequences to the presence of a malocclusion are: increased tooth wear, aggravation of an existing periodontal problem, exacerbation of temporomandibular joint disorders, difficulty with oral hygiene and perhaps, most significantly, psycho-social consequences (See Chapter 1). It must be remembered that not all patients with a malocclusion want orthodontic intervention, although it obviously would have lasting benefit. Thus, all patients and/or parents should be fully informed of the possible long-term consequences of their malocclusion's correction and their various treatment options.

For the general dentist who is interested in providing orthodontic treatment, screening and case selection are probably the most important aspects of the treatment process. The decision to treat or to refer, as well as the timing of these decisions, can set the stage for a satisfying and successful experience for both the clinician and the patient or lead to frustration and disappointment for both. Dental schools do not have the time or the resources to implement a curriculum necessary to provide the dental student with the clinical experience that allows him or her, as a general dental practitioner, to successfully treat a broad spectrum of orthodontic problems. Additionally, orthodontic "short" courses that are available have a significant limitation: complex malocclusions cannot be treated in a short amount of time and without "in depth" orthodontic knowledge.

The purpose of this chapter is to provide the dental clinician with the information necessary to identify those patients who need orthodontic treatment and either refer them to an orthodontic specialist for treatment or initiate treatment themselves at the appropriate time.

2. SCREENING FOR ORTHODONTIC TREATMENT

It is necessary to perform an initial exam in order to determine whether an orthodontic problem exists. This is the initial screening process. If an orthodontic problem appears to exist, in order to establish a diagnosis and treatment plan, the collection of orthodontic records is needed. Treatment should _not_ begin without a diagnosis, treatment plan, the establishment of treatment goals, and **stopping criteria** (See Chapters 10 and 17).

The purpose of the orthodontic examination is: 1.) to determine if the collection of orthodontic records is justified, and 2.) to gather the information necessary, in conjunction with a set of orthodontic records, to describe the problem and any possible etiologic factors (See Chapter 8). Orthodontic records, in conjunction with the information gathered at the initial exam, are then used to determine an orthodontic diagnosis and treatment plan which includes the timing and tactical options for treatment. Additional information from the general dentist, other dental specialists, speech therapists and/or the patient's physician may also be required in the treatment planning process.

Screening can be defined as the possible identification of unrecognized disease or disorder by the utilization of tests and/or examinations that can be applied rapidly. Screening is a cursory exam only; a positive exam that indicates need for orthodontic treatment requires a more thorough diagnostic examination. The diagnostic exam typically includes medical and dental history review and a careful and complete patient examination. A complete set of orthodontic records minimally includes intra- and extra-oral photographs, panoramic x-ray or full mouth x-rays, lateral cephalometric x-ray, study casts and the appropriate bite registrations. In many instances, these two exams are combined to form the initial new patient exam. In order to ascertain whether or not there is a malocclusion for which there may be an appropriate treatment, three questions must be asked and answered: 1.) Does a problem exist? 2.) What is the problem and its etiology? 3.) What are the available solutions for this problem?

The American Association of Orthodontists recommends an orthodontic screening examination by age 7. The screening may be performed by the general dentist or the patient may be referred directly to the orthodontist for an orthodontic screening exam. If the general dentist performs the screening and is unsure of the proper course of action, a referral to an orthodontic specialist should be made. The orthodontist may opt to do nothing at that time, or he/she may decide it is appropriate to intercept the problem before the emergence of the permanent dentition. It is important that the parents of the patient receive complete information so that they can make an informed decision as to whether they want to pursue interceptive procedures or do nothing. The patient's referring general dentist should be informed of all that transpires between the specialist and the family.

3. MULTIPLE PHASES OF ORTHODONTIC TREATMENT

The orthodontic literature is replete with information regarding early or multiple phases of orthodontic treatment. Most of these published studies should be interpreted with care because the results and conclusions are influenced by factors related to study design, methods employed in the analysis of the data and the opinions and predispositions of the investigators. These studies frequently show that similar quantitative changes can be achieved in a given amount of time. However, while the quantitative changes may be similar, most researchers have also shown a qualitative difference in the results of these treatment tactics. For example, the changes claimed may be said to be exhibited in the maxillary arch versus the mandibular arch or may be said to be expressed in **basal bone** rather than in the dentition or in **alveolar bone**. In addition, not all functional appliances are claimed to influence the dental arches in a similar manner. Some, such as the Herbst or Frankel, are thought to influence both the maxillary and mandibular arches, albeit the putative changes in these arches are expressed differently. Some orthodontists believe that, in some instances, early treatment can minimize the time that fixed appliances are employed in a subsequent phase of treatment by making the problem less severe. On the other hand, several phases of treatment are often complicated, time consuming and frequently more expensive. It may be easier to address selected orthodontic problems at earlier ages due to developmental factors. Interceptive or early orthodontic treatment should be initiated only if the patient and parent choose early treatment, or if doing so will minimize or eliminate a problem and increase the probability that an ideal orthodontic result can be more easily achieved when a second treatment phase is initiated. The answer to the question of whether or not early treatment is indicated depends largely on the problems that need to be solved and probable patient compliance, as well as clinician and patient/parent preferences. Early referral to the orthodontist allows both the dental practitioner and the parents to consider the options and make informed treatment decisions.

An early phase of orthodontic treatment should be initiated to address problems in three main areas: 1.) functional shifts in the three planes of space, 2.) development of the dentition, and 3.) discrepancies in the size and/or shape of the mandible and maxilla and their respective alveolar arches. Some patients may benefit from early or two-phase treatment. Total treatment time, total cost of treatment, and quality of the final orthodontic result should be considered and carefully discussed with the patient prior to initiating early treatment.

4. DEVELOPING A TREATMENT PLAN

4.1 DEFINING TREATMENT GOALS

Treatment goals can be subdivided into:

1.) Ideal treatment,
2.) Compromise treatment,
3.) Treatment to address a specific symptom or target disorder.

The definition of a successful treatment result can vary, depending on the patient's chief complaint, dental history and severity of the dental or skeletal **dysplasia**. Treatment goals are defined and determined by the three factors listed above (chief complaint, severity, and factors from the dental history), not by the ability of the orthodontic provider. Treatment goals are influenced by the orthodontist's concepts of oral health and function. While the patient and his/her family may be primarily concerned with esthetics, if appropriate treatment goals cannot be agreed upon by the orthodontic provider and the patient/parent, a referral to another specialist should be made. If no agreement can be reached, no treatment should be attempted.

Compromise treatment may sometimes be considered when ideal treatment is impossible or impractical. Reasons for considering compromise treatment may be related to periodontal health, occlusal function, stability of the orthodontic result, orthodontic mechanical considerations, as well as patient desires. When compromise treatment is considered for reasons other than the patient's desires, there must be compelling reasons for the orthodontist to render treatment.

4.2 SELECTING TREATMENT TACTICS

Three orthodontic problems are most often treated in the primary or in the mixed dentition. These are:

1.) Obstacles to normal growth and development of the dento-alveolar complex, such as anterior or posterior cross bites with and without a functional shift.
2.) Problems that prevent normal development and function of the occlusion; i.e., tongue thrusts and digit habits.
3.) Problems that have a significant social impact for the patient: severe maxillary protrusion and/or malaligned anterior teeth.

The specific treatment tactics selected to correct the problem are dependent on factors that involve the nature of the problem presented as well as patient compliance. Discussion of specific treatment tactics is beyond the scope of this chapter (See Chapters 17-22).

4.3 CRITERIA FOR TERMINATION OF TREATMENT

There are four reasons for termination of a treatment phase:

1.) Treatment goals have been reached.
2.) Further treatment will not result in attainment of the treatment goal or improvement in the esthetic or functional result.
3.) Unfavorable sequelae such as decay, dental decalcification, periodontal pathology or root resorption that may negatively impact the patient's dental health become apparent.
4.) The parent/patient requests treatment termination.

4.4 RETENTION CONSIDERATIONS

Retention of the orthodontic result should be considered at the treatment planning stage and discussed with the parent and patient (See Chapter 21). Frequently, patient compliance is required in order to maintain the orthodontic result. Orthodontic retention is influenced by many factors which include the type of resultant treatment occlusion, the pre-treatment occlusion and the orthodontic treatment mechanics. Retention may additionally involve a **frenectomy** and/or a circumferential fiberotomy in conjunction with removable retainers, fixed retainers, bonding of teeth and equilibration.

5. TREATMENT PLANNING IN THE PRIMARY DENTITION

5.1 DENTAL CONDITIONS THAT MAY BE TREATED IN THE PRIMARY DENTITION ARE:

1.) Anterior or posterior crossbites: Both anterior and posterior crossbites can be effectively treated in the primary dentition because of the biology of skeletal maturation. Early treatment of **anterior crossbite**s may be especially effective. These problems are sometimes treated with expansion appliances, often in conjunction with a face mask appliance.

2.) Early loss of primary teeth when space loss may result: The loss of a first or a second deciduous molar may allow the mesial migration of the posterior teeth and thereby decrease **available arch length**. On occasion, the distal migration of the anterior teeth takes place. Early loss of a primary second molar nearly always results in the mesial migration of the permanent first molar and often requires space maintenance.

3.) Retained primary incisors or supernumeraries that interfere with the eruption of permanent **incisors:** Anterior supernumeraries or a **mesiodens** can interfere with the development and eruption of the **succedaneous** dentition (Figure 16-1). The decision to surgically remove a supernumerary can be a difficult one. It is important to wait for some development of the permanent dentition before removing a supernumerary. On the other hand, delaying the extraction of supernumeraries too long will most likely lead to space loss and possible displacement and/or impaction of a permanent tooth or teeth.

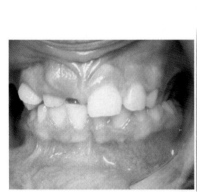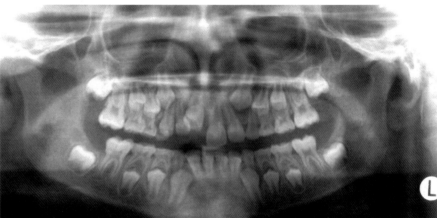

Figure 16-1: Supernumeraries between the maxillary right central and lateral incisors has impeded the eruption of the central incisor.

4.) Ectopic positions of teeth that result in interference with normal occlusal function or development of normal occlusal function: Ectopic teeth can result in functional shifts that interfere with normal growth and development of the dentoalveolar complex (Figure 16-2). Ectopically erupted teeth can also affect the health of the teeth due to traumatic occlusion or degeneration of the supporting dental structures, such as fenestration of the gingiva (See Chapters 5, 13, and 14).

5.) Openbites due to tongue thrusting or digit habits: Openbites caused by complex tongue thrusts or by digit habits should be monitored so that changes to the dental arches are not allowed to become severe. Intervention with habit appliances or with partial fixed appliances may be indicated because many tongue thrusting habits can often be most effectively treated early. This is because neuromuscular behaviors that result from an abnormal oral environment become ingrained as patients mature. Abnormal tooth positional changes that are produced by parafunctional behaviors tend to worsen if left unattended, thus, these problems are often best intercepted when discovered, rather than corrected after they have an opportunity to become fully developed.

6.) Severe malocclusions: Craniofacial anomalies can be associated with severe skeletal **malocclusions** (See Chapter 20). The most common severe primary dentition malocclusion is associated with a **cleft lip** and/or palate. Cleft lip/palate treatment involves complicated and lengthy treatment sequences which frequently employ a team approach. The team approach to the treatment of patients who have craniofacial anomalies, including those with cleft lip and palate, involves a group of specialists and generalists from a variety of dental and medical disciplines.

5.2 CONTRAINDICATIONS TO TREATMENT IN THE PRIMARY DENTITION

1.) There is no treatment available that is likely to have lasting benefit to the patient. This may be due to the fact that the same result can be obtained with treatment at a later time or because the potential for relapse is high.

2.) Social immaturity of the child makes orthodontic treatment impractical: The attitude of the child toward orthodontic treatment may make treatment difficult or impractical (See Chapter 1). Fear of dental impressions and a strong gag reflex are often the most formidable obstacles to initiating an early treatment phase in young children. Allowing patients to familiarize themselves with the dental chair, suction, air/water syringe, cheek retractors, etc., can help alleviate apprehension of the orthodontic experience. It is always more important that the child have a positive dental experience than to successfully complete a specific procedure on a particular day.

6. TREATMENT PLANNING IN THE MIXED DENTITION

The opportunity for interception of a malocclusion is greatest in the mixed (transitional) dentition (See Chapters 17 and 18). Treatment may be initiated in the mixed dentition provided it is likely that there is an advantage in initiating treatment, and that it is likely that the results will be lasting in the permanent dentition. The goal of mixed dentition treatment should be to eliminate or modify problems that may lead to more severe malocclusions in the permanent dentition.

6.1 CONDITIONS THAT SHOULD BE TREATED IN THE MIXED DENTITION

1.) Early loss of primary teeth that may lead to loss of **available arch length**: Early loss of primary teeth can often lead to loss of available arch length. This loss is most commonly manifested by mesial migration of a permanent first molar after the loss of a maxillary or mandibular second deciduous molar. Treatment of this problem may consist of, but is not limited to, the placement of fixed appliances such as a **band** and loop space maintainer, upper and/or lower loop lingual wires, or a transpalatal **arch wire**. This condition may also be addressed with removable appliances that hold or regain space, such as a retainer or a **headgear**. When holding space in one arch, especially with a loop lingual wire, space maintenance in the opposing arch may also be indicated so that a Class II or Class III molar relationship is not exacerbated. For example, preventing mandibular molars from migrating anteriorly may result in exacerbating a Class II dental relationship due to the mesial migration of the maxillary molars. The choice of a space maintenance or space regaining appliance depends upon specific circumstances and child/parent desires. For example, removable appliances require cooperation from the patient, but the treatment fee for some of these removable appliances may be significantly less expensive than it would be for fixed appliances.

2.) Regaining lost space due to **ectopic eruption** and/or early loss of primary teeth: If space is not maintained after the early loss of one or more primary teeth, **arch length** loss can occur. If there is loss of arch length, the clinician must decide to either 1.) regain the lost space, 2.) maintain the remaining space, or 3.) defer treatment in anticipation of extracting permanent teeth later. If the decision is made to regain the space, it is usually best to proceed with treatment as soon as practicable. Regaining space due to the mesial migration of posterior teeth (primarily first permanent molars) is more easily accomplished before the eruption of the second permanent molars. Space loss due to ectopic eruption most commonly involves the maxillary first molars (See Figure 16-2).

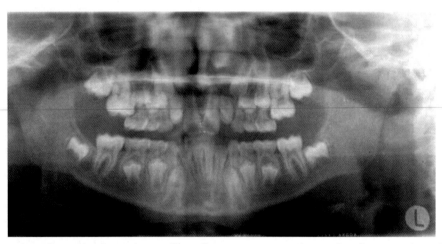

Figure 16-2: Panoramic radiograph of ectopic maxillary first permanent molars and early resorption of the roots of the second deciduous molars.

Ectopic mesial eruption may necessitate the early removal of the second deciduous molars in order to allow full eruption of the permanent first molars before regaining the lost **arch perimeter**.

    3.) Ectopic position of the teeth that results in interference with the function or the development of normal occlusion: (See Section 5.1 number 4.)

    4.) Supernumerary or impacted teeth that interfere with development of dentition: (See Section 5.1 number 3.)

    5.) **Ankylosis** of primary teeth: Ankylosis of a primary tooth may cause impaction of permanent teeth as well as distortion of the alveolus. **Ankylosed** primary teeth should be monitored and extracted if they are causing either of these conditions to occur. The panoramic radiograph in Figure 16-3 shows ankylosis of primary second molars that has resulted in a severe distortion of the alveolus and the impaction of the permanent second premolars.

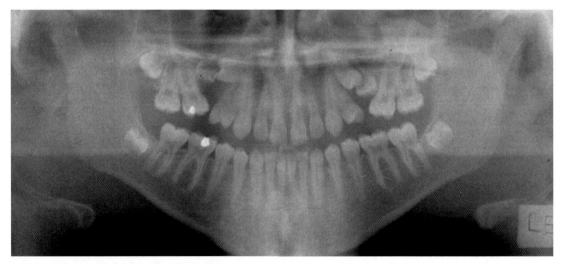

Figure 16-3: Panoramic radiograph of ankylosed maxillary second deciduous molars. The ankylosed primary teeth have resulted in distortion of the alveolus and impaction of the second premolars.

    6.) Crossbites in conjuction with functional shifts: Crossbites may exist for a number of reasons which include a narrow or hypoplastic maxillary arch, excessive width of the mandibular arch or ectopic eruption of teeth. The etiologies of narrow maxillary arches are influenced by both genetic and environmental factors. Some of the environmental factors linked to narrow maxillary arches may include, but are not limited to, breathing obstructions, digit habits, and abnormal tongue function.

6.2 CONDITIONS THAT MAY BE TREATED IN THE MIXED DENTITION

1.) Habits which may lead to malocclusion: There are a number of oral habits that have the potential for deleterious effects on the development of the orofacial structures. These habits include thumb and finger (digit) habits, as well as lip sucking and tongue thrusts. If these problems are not addressed in the primary dentition, they must be addressed in the mixed dentition and not allowed to persist until the permanent dentition is present.

2.) Extreme **labioversion** of the maxillary anterior teeth, especially when **lip incompetence** is present: Extreme labioversion of the maxillary anterior teeth can significantly increase the risk of trauma to these incisors. This is especially true when the overjet is greater than 6 mm in the presence of lip incompetence. Treatment of this condition in the mixed dentition with either fixed or removable appliances is indicated if there is patient and/or parent desire. It must be emphasized during the consultation that mitigation of this problem in the mixed dentition does not preclude further treatment in the permanent dentition.

3.) Extreme skeletal Class II malocclusions: Many severe Class II division 1 or division 2 malocclusions require extended treatment time, particularly if the practitioner employs two stages of treatment. For example, a removable functional appliance or a **headgear** treatment phase may be used to attempt to improve the dental relationship of the first molars sufficiently to minimize the treatment time of a **fixed appliance** phase (See Figure 16-4A through 16-4H).

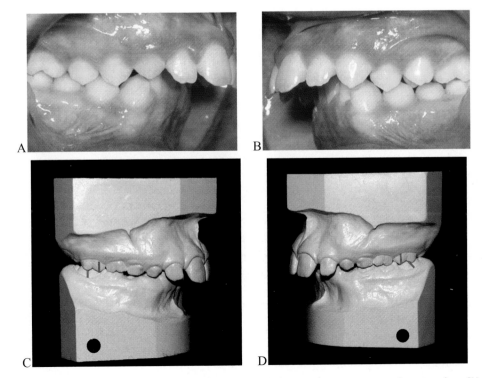

Figure 16-4A-D: A.) and B.) show the right and left intraoral pretreatment photographs. C.), D.) compare the casts on the right and left sides before and after treatment with a cervical facebow.

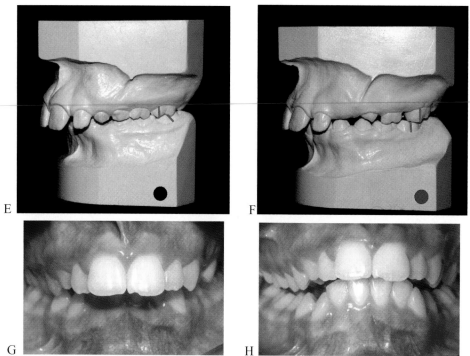

Figure 16-4E-H: E.) and F.) compare the casts on the right and left sides before and after treatment with a cervical facebow. G.) Pretreatment, H.) photo following phase I treatment with the Kloehn headgear. Provided by Dr. Roberto Lima.

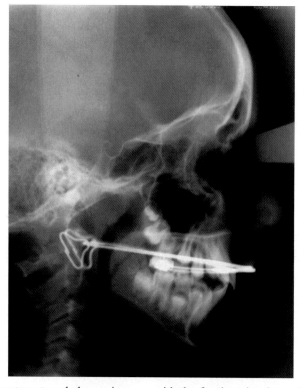

Figure 16-5: Shows the post treatment cephalometric x-ray with the facebow in place. Provided by Dr. Roberto Lima.

For some patients, it is important to minimize the length of the fixed appliance treatment phase due to the risk of adverse sequelae. Common adverse sequelae include decalcification of teeth and hypertrophy of the gingiva. Numerous treatment tactics may be employed to address Class II malocclusions. If a significant Class II correction is required, an extended treatment time may result. Therefore, in order to minimize adverse sequelae such as white spot lesions, an early treatment phase involving a **removable appliance** (functional appliance or face bow) may be desirable. It is unlikely that a spatial change of more than 4mm per year can be achieved with any combination of treatment tactics. The type of treatment that is rendered will be dependent on:

1.) the nature and severity of the malocclusion.
2.) patient/parent desires and anticipated cooperation levels.
3.) the early treatment "philosophy" and/or protocol of the practitioner.

The family must be made aware of the fact that mixed dentition treatment of a severe Class II malocclusion will necessitate two phases of treatment; therefore, the overall treatment time will be of longer duration than a single phase of treatment.

Numerous treatment tactics are currently being utilized to address the severe Class II problem. Most involve some appliance, either removable or fixed, simple or complex, that will "disarticulate" the Class II dental relationship and position the mandible forward. Treatment modalities run the gamut from expansion of the maxillary arch (so that the mandible has to be positioned forward to achieve occlusion) to fixed appliances with Class II elastics on the erupted permanent teeth. In the middle of this spectrum are some of the functional appliances, sometimes used in conjunction with maxillary expansion and/or headgear.

Whatever the approach, the parent/patient must be advised that the result will be dependent on at least two unknowns: 1.) the physiologic response of the patient to the given treatment modality, and 2.) the level of patient cooperation. No matter what type of early treatment is rendered, the goal should be to make the permanent dentition stage of treatment less difficult for the patient and practitioner so that the likelihood of achieving an optimal result is increased.

4.) Dental Class II malocclusions: Space maintenance and eruption guidance can be utilized in the correction of Class II molar relationships. For example, a transpalatal arch on the maxillary first molars, sometimes in conjunction with a headgear, can work to prevent the upper molars from migrating anteriorly into the **leeway space** in an attempt to mitigate a Class II dental relationship.

5.) Space supervision and eruption timing problems: Deficiencies in available space in the dental arch can limit treatment options. Treatment complications due to space deficiencies can be especially problematic in the mandibular arch in patients who exhibit Class II division 2 and Class III malocclusions. Discrepancies in the timing of eruption of the permanent dentition can result in loss of available arch perimeter and increase the risk of impaction of teeth. Additionally, **serial extraction**, which is the removal of selected primary and permanent teeth, can be employed to minimize problems caused by irregularities in eruption timing and by severe arch length tooth size discrepancies. There are a myriad of serial extraction protocols which correspond to specific problems. In general, serial extraction should be avoided unless the practitioner has experience with fixed appliance therapy and is familiar with serial extraction protocols. General indications for serial extractions are listed below. There are, of course, exceptions to every rule and to every generalization. If these indicators are used and the problem has been selected properly, the resulting malocclusion correction should require less time in fixed appliance therapy. The farther one deviates from these guidelines, the more work will be required during fixed appliance orthodontic treatment. Severe problems can occur if one or more of the indicators are ignored.

Indications for serial extractions:

1.) Minimum 5.0 mm of crowding in each dental quadrant
2.) Coincident upper and lower midlines
3.) Bilateral Class I molar relationship
4.) Balanced skeletal pattern in all three planes of space

Complicating factors for serial extractions:

1.) Class III molar relationships
2.) Class II molar relationships
3.) Unbalanced skeletal patterns of any kind (transverse, anterior-posterior or vertical)
4.) Unequal crowding in the maxillary and mandibular arches
5.) Unequal crowding bilaterally in either arch
6.) Midline discrepancies (>2 mm)
7.) Negative overbites or impinging deep bites

6.) Esthetic or functional problems: Esthetic problems may have social consequences that justify treatment in the mixed dentition, even though their correction does not lessen the severity of the malocclusion. Most commonly, these problems are large maxillary midline diastemas, severe malalignment of the maxillary anterior teeth, and/or large overjets with concomitant lip incompetency that may increase the probability of accidental trauma. In addition, malocclusions, which affect speech, impinging overbites that are painful and/or that affect gingival health, and traumatic occlusions may be a concern to the parent and/or patient. These problems should be addressed as directly as possible in the shortest amount of treatment time.

7.) Class III malocclusions: While the use of chin cup therapy to minimize mandibular growth has been found to be of limited utility, expansion and protraction of the maxillary arch can sometimes be quite effective in the right circumstance. Due to the complexities of Class III treatment, minimization of crowding by maintaining available arch length is indicated in the mixed dentition. The elimination of **functional shifts** (especially anterior shifts) is always indicated and, in the case of Class III dental malocclusions, is especially important.

8.) Gross skeletal disharmonies: Gross skeletal disharmonies often result in a combined orthodontic/surgical treatment plan. For some patients, extended treatment in either one or two phases may result in an acceptable compromise without surgical intervention. In other instances an early phase of orthodontic treatment may result in modifying the type or extent of the surgical procedures required to achieve a correction. For example, early expansion of the maxillary arch may result in the need for a surgical procedure in only one jaw versus two jaws in order to achieve the desired orthodontic correction.

7. TREATMENT PLANNING IN THE PERMANENT DENTITION

Any malocclusion can be treated in the **permanent dentition,** although the treatment may be complicated by the absence of an adequate amount of growth. Orthodontic treatment in the adult is often complicated by the presence of deteriorated dental conditions such as missing teeth, prosthodontic restoration and periodontal disease. Many adult malocclusions require complex treatment involving combined orthodontic, periodontic, prosthodontic and oral surgery treatment plans.

8. COMPLICATING FACTORS IN ORTHODONTIC TREATMENT

Complicating factors may necessitate compromised orthodontic treatment results. Experience is required to manage these factors and, in general, referral to an orthodontic specialist is indicated.

8.1 DENTAL FACTORS

Tooth size discrepancies, which are also called "**Bolton discrepancies**" can be a major impediment to achieving an ideal occlusion. Bolton discrepancies often require interproximal reduction and/or cosmetic bonding in order to achieve proper mesiodistal tooth widths for an acceptable esthetic appearance. Dental asymmetries can cause major mechanical complications and may result in compromised treatment results. Other dental complicating factors include missing or impacted teeth.

8.2 SKELETAL FACTORS

Moderate skeletal asymmetries and more severe symmetric skeletal dysplasias can be difficult or impossible to resolve with orthodontic treatment alone. A combination surgical and orthodontic treatment plan may be required if an ideal dental and skeletal result is desired. Often, severe skeletal dysplasias require the use of treatment modalities that require increased patient compliance. The patient compliance factor can reduce the predictability of the final treatment results.

8.3 NEUROMUSCULAR FACTORS

Abnormal tongue posture as well as perioral and facial muscle posture and function during speech, **deglutition** or at rest can effect changes in the dentition and alveolar complex. Tongue thrusting or abnormal facial muscle posture can complicate orthodontic treatment and severely complicate retention of the orthodontic correction. Non-nutritive sucking is defined as the sucking of an object (usually a pacifier) or a digit (usually a thumb or finger) which can cause movement of teeth, as well as affect the growth and development of the alveolar complex. Oral habits are not uncommon among children less than 9 years old and usually are not of great concern in children less than 8 years old. The parents and patient should be informed of possible dental consequences and encouraged to correct the behavior. If significant alveolar changes that threaten to compromise future orthodontic treatment results are apparent, there are a number of fixed appliances that may aid in habit resolution. In general, digit habits can lead to increased overjet, protrusion of the maxillary incisors and constriction of the maxillary arch. Abnormal perioral muscular forces can lead to distortion of the dental alveolar complex, most notably retruded lower incisors. Surprisingly, even relatively severe distortions of the alveolar complex can be corrected orthodontically without the need for surgical intervention.

8.4 PATIENT COOPERATION FACTORS

In order to achieve an excellent orthodontic result, patient cooperation is always required. The patient needs to understand that excessive appliance breakage can negatively impact treatment time and the ultimate orthodontic result. Lack of compliance with the treatment plan, such as failure to wear a **removable appliance**, elastics or headgear will always adversely affect the final orthodontic result. If good oral hygiene is not forthcoming, treatment termination to prevent negative sequelae from affecting the teeth and their supporting structures may be indicated. Time invested in patient education before treatment begins can help reduce non-compliance during orthodontic treatment.

8.5 BIOLOGIC/OTHER FACTORS

Decalcification of the teeth, destruction of alveolar bone due to periodontal disease, and **iatrogenic** problems such as **root resorption** can severely compromise the orthodontist's ability to achieve an ideal orthodontic result. Dental decalcification during treatment is most commonly found between the orthodontic bracket and the gingival margin. Decalcification can be controlled with good oral hygiene, diet modification, use of prescription fluoride rinses/gels by the patient and the application of a fluoride varnish by the dental practitioner. Patients who are at risk for dental decalcification during orthodontic treatment are those who have a history of caries and decalcification.

Iatrogenic root resorption is a less common problem during orthodontic treatment. Screening for root resorption is commonly done half way through treatment by taking a panoramic x-ray. Early termination of orthodontic treatment may be indicated if significant root resorption is found.

Bone loss due to periodontal disease may be a significant problem during orthodontic treatment, though this is a rare occurrence for children. Screening for periodontal disease should be done for all orthodontic patients before the initiation of treatment. For children and adolescents, this usually consists of examining a panoramic radiograph or a full mouth series of periapical radiographs and a **periodontal screening and recording**. Adult patients should be referred to a general dentist or periodontist for a complete periodontal charting before the initiation of orthodontic treatment. A history of periodontal disease is not a strict contraindication for treatment, but no active periodontal disease should exist before or during orthodontic treatment. Patients with a history of periodontal disease should be monitored by their general dentist or periodontist every 3 months while in orthodontic treatment.

9. SUGGESTED READINGS

Andrews LF,: The Six Keys to Normal Occlusion. Am J Orthod 1972; 62:296-309.

O'Brien K., et al., Factors affecting the uptake of orthodontic treatment. Br J Orthod, 1996. 23:331-334.

Bennett E, and Phillips C. Assessment of health-related quality of life for patients with severe skeletal disharmony. Int J Adult Orthod Orthognath Surg, 1999. 14: p. 65-75.

Glover ME. Occlusal therapy and its role in the etiology and treatent of periodontal diseases. Texas Dental Journal, 1988. 105(11): p. 18-22.

Ramfjord, S.P. and M.M. Ash, Jr., Significance of occlusion in the etiology and treatment of early, moderate, and advanced periodontitis. Journal of Periodontology, 1981. 52(9): p. 511-7.

Beck K, Kock G, and Rozier R. Prevalence and risk indicators for periodontal attachment loss in a population of older community-dwelling blacks and whites. J Periodontol, 1990. 60: p. 521-528.

Davies T., et al., The relationship of anterior overjet to plaque and gingivitis in children. Am J Orthod Dentofac Orthop, 1988. 93: 303-309.

Bennett E., et al., Psychometric considerations in the assessment of orthodontic treatment expectations, in Orthodontic treatment: Outcomes and effectiveness, C. Trotman and J.A. McNamara, Editors. 1995, Center for Human Growth and Devolopment, The University of Michigan: Ann Arbor, Michigan.

Riolo ML, Moyers RE, and TenHave TR. Imprecision and Bias in Orthodontic Treatment. Am. J. of Orthod 1988;93:138-142.

Vig K., et al., Developing outcome measures in orthodontics that reflect patient and provider values. Seminars in Orthodontics, 1999. 5: p. 85-95.

Last J. A dictionary of epidemiology, ed. I.E. Association. 1988, New York, New York: Oxford University Press.

Ngan P, and Fields HW. Open bite: a review of etiology and management. Pediatric Dentistry, 1997;19(2): 91-8.

Kotsomitis N, and Freer TJ. Inherited dental anomalies and abnormalities. ASDC Journal of Dentistry for Children, 1997. 64(6): p. 405-8.

Frankel R. The theoretical concept of underlying the treatment with functional correctors. Trans Eur Ortho Soc, 1966: p. 237-252.

Hagg U, and Pancherz H, Dental facial orthopedics in relation to chronological age, growth period and skeletal development: Analysis of 72 male patients with Class II Division I malocclusion, treated with the Herbst appliance. Eur J Ortho, 1988. 10: p. 168-176.

Haas AJ, Rapid palatal expansion: A recommended prerequisite to Class III treatment. Trans Eur Ortho Soc, 1973: p. 311-318.

Wieslander L. Early or late cervical traction therapy in the mixed dentition. Am J Orthod Dentofac Orthop, 1975. 67: p. 432-439.

Hawkins JK. Treatment Planning for the Mixed Dentition Malocclusion- Treatment and Goals. Ann R Aust Coll Dent Surg 1994; 12:160-169.

Lima RMA. Longitudinal Study of Anteroposterior and Vertical Changes in Skeletal Class II Patients Treated with Kloehn Cervical Headgear. The Edward H. Angle Society of Orthodontists. Scottsdale, Arizona. 2002.

McNamara JA, Brudon WL: Orthodontic and Orthopedic Treatment in the Mixed Dentition, Needham Press, 2001.

Section IV
Treatment and Effects

This section considers preadolescent, adolescent and adult treatment and the treatment of patients with craniofacial anomalies. Also considered are retention, relapse, recurrence of malocclusion and the adverse effects of orthodontic treatment.

Chapters:

CHAPTER 17

Preadolescent Orthodontic Treatment and Orthodontic Treatment During Active Stages of Growth and Development

Michael L. Riolo

Colin A. Mayers

William M. Northway

Herein the term **early treatment** means orthodontic therapy during the active stages of craniofacial growth, including that of the dentition. It implies two things: 1.) it may be advantageous to treat some malocclusions during or in anticipation of active growth, and 2.) methods are available for such treatment.

1. UNDERSTANDING ORTHODONTICS DURING GROWTH AND DEVELOPMENT

1.1 RATIONALE

a.) Some malocclusions can be prevented or intercepted. The theory and rationale underlying the concepts associated with each term (prevention and interception) vary and are not generally interchangeable. Each is a useful alternative when properly applied. The clinical problem is when, and to what extent, each option is appropriate. Only a few studies give accurate reports on those malocclusions that can be prevented and/or intercepted. Popovich and Thompson, at the Burlington Orthodontic Research Centre in Canada, demonstrated that while few malocclusions can truly be prevented, roughly 25% can be intercepted. One-fourth is a significant number, and many of these can be intercepted with theory, appliances, and knowledge now readily available to the clinician.

b.) More alternative methods are available for treating patients at a young age. When growth has largely ceased, treatment options are limited to moving teeth or **orthognathic surgery**.

When the patient is young, one may be able to 1.) remove etiologic factors, 2.) enlist natural growth forces, and/or 3.) enhance differential growth and development responses, prior to eruption of most permanent teeth. Though many of the orthopedic appliances in use today look simple, guidance of the developing dentition and growing craniofacial skeleton is a very complicated matter. While the construction of a "growth guidance" appliance may be simple, the applied biology for its implementation is generally more sophisticated and difficult than treatment after puberty. We know more about the biology of tooth movement, which is influenced by bracketed appliances, than we do about the biologic alteration of facial growth, which is the basis of early functional orthopedics. It should be remembered that skeletal growth guidance is only one aspect of the options for early orthodontic treatment available to the clinician.

c.) The clinician can utilize growth better in the young, and there is more growth available. Growth can only be controlled while growth is happening. The earlier one starts treatment, the more total growth one can affect.

1.2 BENEFITS

The following are some of the more compelling reasons for **early treatment**:

1.) The possibility of achieving a better result.
2.) Some forms of treatment can only be done at an early age.
3.) Early treatment of serious deleterious habits is more effective than treatment after years of ingrained habit reinforcement.
4.) There are psychological advantages to early treatment in some children.
5.) Younger patients are often more cooperative and attentive to both parent and clinician.
6.) Many clinicians feel that compromise of quality of treatment result is less apt to be necessary.
7.) If permanent teeth are allowed to erupt into normal positions, the tendency toward relapse will be diminished.

There are two reasons why early treatment may obviate compromise of quality: 1.) it may remove etiologic factors and restore normal growth and development, and 2.) it may reduce the severity of a developmental pattern, making possible easier and more precise tooth positioning in the adolescent.

1.3 DIFFICULTIES

Misperceptions exist about the goals of **early treatment.** Clearly defined goals need to be established in the development of a treatment approach. The removal of primary dental and neuromuscular etiologic factors and the correction of skeletal dysplasias prior to the eruption of the majority of the permanent teeth are two such goals. Typically neither of these factors results in precise positioning of teeth.

Some proponents of **functional jaw orthopedics** have urged the use of this type of appliance by describing deficiencies and misuses of precision bracketed appliances, implying such problems do not occur with their favored systems. But there are negative outcomes present with any appliance. Frequently, these may be related to misperceptions about the goals of treatment, if not the appliance itself.

Improper early treatment can be useless and may be harmful. Just as growth can be directed advantageously, it can also be misdirected. Multiphase treatment may lengthen the chronologic treatment time. Time of treatment is properly measured by tracking the number of hours spent by the dentist with the patient; treatment time should not be measured on the calendar. Multiphase treatment may achieve results with less "chair time" but longer "calendar time". During extended "calendar time" treatment regimes patient cooperation is likely to wane.

The subtleties of early development introduce variability in diagnosis and treatment planning. When growth has diminished, the features of a malocclusion are clearly seen and the diagnosis is more certain. Early diagnosis and treatment planning need to be subject to periodic reassessment. Dynamic diagnosis and treatment "planning" involves an on-going process of evaluating response and adjusting treatment accordingly.

2. GOALS FOR EARLY TREATMENT

The general principles of Diagnosis and Treatment Planning are presented in Section III of this book and Diagnosis in Chapters 11 and 16. A few specific comments are pertinent herein.

2.1 DENTITION AND OCCLUSION

Several tooth size analyses (Mixed Dentition, Bolton, and Sanin-Savara analyses) are useful (see Chapter 13). Since these analyses are static, it is important to realize the possible effects of growth and development on their results. While time and growth do not alter tooth size, they change tooth positions and bony and soft tissue relationships, which are not part of any of the dental analyses. The dentition and occlusion must be analyzed repeatedly during development.

2.2. MUSCULATURE

Clinical analysis of muscular function (See Chapter 12) is generally neither quantitative nor precisely discriminating, making it difficult to appreciate the clinical implications of the enormous variability of facial muscle behavior. Dentists, appreciative of our own ignorance and our need for further knowledge, should not assume that other disciplines are more advanced. Speech scientists, otolaryngologists, and physiotherapists are important resource persons. Therefore, interaction is essential in developing a coordinated, individualized approach for each patient.

2.3 CRANIOFACIAL SKELETON

Some cephalometric procedures fail us when we most need them (i.e., during active growth), but this is no reason to avoid the cephalometric study of every case (See Chapter 15). The question has been asked, "In which case should one take a cephalogram?" It is proper to order radiographs routinely to diagnose caries and to ascertain the presence and normal development of all teeth. In these author's opinions, it is no less important to be assured of normal skeletal growth.

2.4 TREATMENT PLANNING

The essence of **early treatment** planning is proper timing. This involves the integration of several kinds of developmental data applied specifically to one particular patient (See Chapters 4 and 5). Optimal treatment planning is dependent on the earliest possible diagnosis. Orthodontic treatment deferred until **adolescence** may decrease the difficulty of treatment planning, since the permanent dentition is completed and most skeletal growth has ceased, though the delay may also reduce options, complicate treatment, and compromise results.

3. ASSESSMENT OF THE RESULTS OF EARLY TREATMENT

One must take care not to transfer to the younger child concepts of success which are valid and useful in adolescence. Constant re-diagnosis is the theme of clinical assessment during growth, for that "simple **anterior crossbite**" may later prove to have been an early expression of a mild skeletal Class III. One should not just ask "did I succeed or fail?", but "what has improved?", "which features persist?", "which may worsen with time despite my treatment?", etc. The purpose of assessment during multiphase and all **early treatment** is to identify the improvements obtained and to prescribe what is left to do.

3.1 DEFINING A SATISFACTORY RESPONSE

Early treatment may be deemed satisfactory if the following conditions are achieved:

1.) Primary etiologic factors have been removed or are controlled.
2.) Tooth positions and space needs are satisfactory and can be kept there until full eruption of the permanent dentition.
3.) Skeletal deviations originally present have been improved at the rate and extent originally planned and can be controlled until the dentition is completed and skeletal growth has diminished. When evaluating the skeletal response to **early treatment**, it is important to identify significant deviations still present due to those portions of the craniofacial skeleton not affected by the therapy and which have not responded to treatment as well as envisaged. In Chapters 13 and 15 some methods for assessing the response to orthodontic treatment are described.

3.2 WHAT TO DO WHEN EARLY TREATMENT IS UNSATISFACTORY

There is no guarantee that any orthodontic therapy will proceed as planned. Separation of the effects of treatment and changes resulting from growth is a difficult and sophisticated analytic problem not yet completely resolved. When **early treatment** seems to have gone poorly, three plans of action are available: 1.) determine and try a more appropriate treatment; 2.) defer further treatment until a later time; and 3.) refer the patient to a colleague for further treatment. Specific rules are impossible because of the wide variety of cases, treatments, and patient responses; but one dictum is certain, namely, complete diagnostic records prove their worth when treatment progress must be assessed.

4. CLINICAL PROBLEMS AND PROCEDURES

4.1 NUMBER OF TEETH

4.1.1. Congenitally Missing Teeth

By "missing teeth" it is meant those teeth whose germs did not develop sufficiently to allow the **differentiation** of the dental tissues. Congenitally missing teeth numbers 1, 4, 16, 17, 23, 26, and 32 are illustrated in Figure 17-1. Also note the delayed development of teeth numbers 20 and 29, and the ankylosis of teeth numbers K and T.

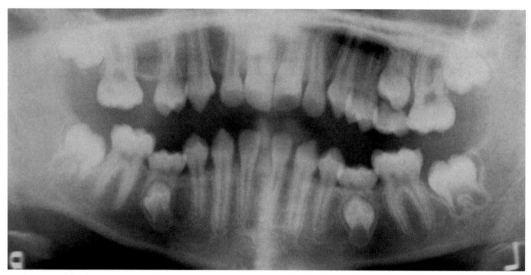

Figure 17-1

a.) Causes – There are three known and agreed upon causes of congenital absence of teeth: See Chapters 5, 7 and 14.

1.) Heredity – There is a familial distribution of congenital absence of teeth, and thus heredity is an etiologic factor of major importance (see Chapters 7, 14); e.g., ectodermal dysplasia – teeth are frequently found to be congenitally missing in conjunction with other clinical manifestations of disturbances in the development of ectodermal tissue (for example, anhidrosis and absence of the hair follicles).
2.) Localized Inflammations or Infections.
3.) Systemic Conditions – Rickets, syphilis, and severe intra-uterine disturbances are claimed by some to lead to the destruction of developing tooth germs.

The relationship between congenital absence of teeth and generalized tooth size diminution should not be forgotten (see Chapter 5). When one tooth is not developing, it is important to measure all of the other teeth to discover any genetic field effects on general tooth size. Peg lateral incisors associated with the congenital absence of teeth is noted in Figure 17-2.

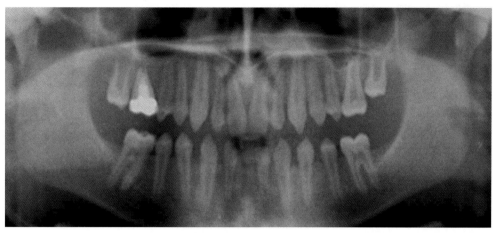

Figure 17-2

It is known that congenital absence of teeth is associated with certain variations in craniofacial morphology, so a cephalometric analysis is required.

4.1.1.2. Diagnosis (See Chapter 11)

4.1.1.3. Treatment

4.1.2. Loss of Permanent Teeth (Trauma, Caries, Agenesis, and Other Causes)

4.1.2.1. Treatment of Loss of Individual Teeth

The loss of fully developed, erupted permanent teeth is a major orthodontic problem. In the anterior region, trauma is the principal cause, whereas caries is largely responsible for early loss of the first permanent molars. Important to an understanding of the effects of loss of permanent teeth is knowledge of physiologic tooth drifting after extraction. The tendency to mesial drifting is more marked in the maxilla and highly age specific in the mandible. When the first permanent molar is lost before the eruption of the second molar, the lower premolars drift toward the distal. Once the premolars erupt into full occlusion, this distal drift is significantly diminished, and the primary movement reducing the space is mesial tipping and migration of the second molar. The actual outcome is significantly influenced by other factors such as the vertical growth pattern of the patient, cusp anatomy, and a multitude of oral, muscular and respiratory dispositions of the individual patient.

4.1.2.1.1. Maxillary Lateral Incisors

– Two courses of treatment are available: 1.) moving the cuspids mesially for use in place of lateral incisors; and 2.) opening space for a prosthesis. The choice is dependent on:

- Age of the patient.
- Conformation of cuspids.
- Position of cuspids.
- Suitability of central incisors and cuspids as abutments.
- Desires of the patient.
- Depth of bite.
- The original occlusion
- The skeletal pattern
- Quality and quantity of bone at the **edentulous** site

Option (1): Moving the cuspids to serve as lateral incisors.

Advantages are:
-   -It is unnecessary to prepare abutment teeth.
-   -There is less chance for maxillary third molars to become impacted.
-   -It is permanent (not necessary to replace at a later date).

Disadvantages are:
-   -Advanced orthodontic skills and fixed appliances are required.
-   -Case selection is more particular than for the prosthetic procedure.
-   -Generally, more time is required.
-   -It is more difficult if the cuspids are completely erupted.
-   -Potential relapse of spacing.
-   -Cuspid guided occlusion is very difficult to achieve.

Follow this procedure if:
-   -The cuspids are unerupted or only partially erupted and appear of normal size and favorable shape.
-   -The central incisors are of normal mesiodistal dimension.
-   -The maxillary molars are already positioned mesially.
-   -There are no contraindications to orthodontic therapy.

Early steps in treatment:
-   -Remove the maxillary primary cuspids, if still present, to hasten the eruption of the maxillary permanent cuspids before the premolars. Removal of bone atop the cuspids sometimes hastens and redirects their eruption path. The central incisors are brought toward the midline and the cuspids are guided to erupt mesially. The premolars and molars should be allowed to move mesially to allow Class II relations in the buccal segments.

-   -Grind the labial surfaces of the cuspids and flatten their incisal edges to simulate lateral incisors. Since the cuspid is thicker labiolingually than a lateral incisor, it is also necessary to reduce the lingual surface significantly to allow the cuspid to be placed more lingually in the line of the arch than is usual. This will also diminish the cuspid eminence by moving the root lingually. It is best to do the reshaping in multiple stages to avoid pulpitis. All of the grinding is followed by polishing and the application of fluoride. Finally, check the new occlusion for occlusal interferences.

    If satisfactory aesthetics have not been obtained by grinding and reshaping of the cuspids alone – this sometimes is seen when the incisal edges are acutely angled – etch the tooth and add a cosmetic bonding material as desired.

Prognosis: This procedure can produce good results. It is indicated when early treatment is possible. Usually much depends upon skillful use of the fixed appliances, since exact placement of roots is necessary for aesthetics and stability. Figure 17-3A illustrates a patient with congenitally missing teeth numbers 4, 7, and 10 and Figure 17-3B illustrates the result after treatment.

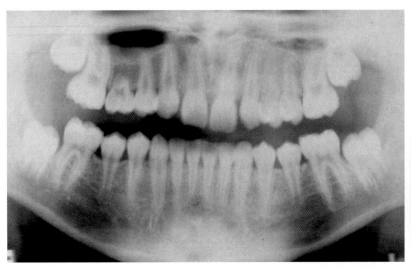

Figure 17-3A

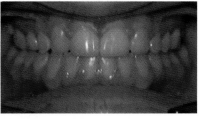

Figure 17-3B

Option (2): Alternative procedure: Opening space for prosthesis

>   Advantages are:
>   -Generally, less movement of teeth is required.
>   -A shorter treatment time is required.
>   -Can be used on the majority of patients.
>   -Increase in number of teeth increases the lip support and thus facial fullness.
>
>   Disadvantages are:
>   -It may be necessary to prepare abutment teeth.
>   -Any bridge typically may have to be redone at a later date.
>   -Aesthetic problems may be difficult; for example, matching shades, hiding gold margins and pontics, though an implant may be an optimal alternative to a bridge(s).
>   -If an implant is chosen, the procedure has to be delayed until skeletal growth is complete. This may require an interim prosthesis, and the alveolus must be monitored for sustained adequacy of width.

Steps in treatment: Preliminary treatment is likely to involve moving the central incisors together and/or moving the lateral segments of the maxillary arch distally. A retainer with a pontic may be worn until the appropriate time for a bridge, a bonded bridge (Figure 17-4), or an implant to be placed.

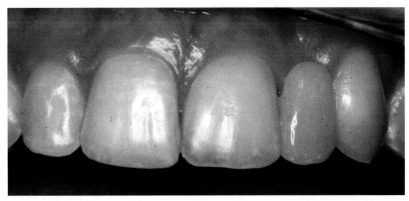

Figure 17-4

4.1.2.1.2. Mandibular Second Premolars

There are at least five alternative procedures for missing second premolars. The following preexisting conditions should be considered when choosing an approach:

-**Angle classification**
-Crowding
-Age at time of recognition
-Alveolar contour
-Developmental status of the third molars

Clinical approaches:

a.) Preserve the primary tooth – this usually requires a reduction in mesiodistal crown width in order to accommodate the rest of the posterior teeth in interdigitation. It is recommended that, following reduction, the polished surface(s) be coated with a sealant to reduce any tendency for caries. Care should be taken to recontour the tooth so as to resemble a broad, well-shaped premolar and minimize food trapping. The flared roots will resorb slightly as spaces are closed, but seldom is this a progressive condition, and the presence of adjacent teeth is nicely tolerated. Of course, there are occlusal schemes and certain cases where the entire width is tolerated, but this often compromises the posterior occlusion and leaves the case in a flush terminal plane occlusion, or worse.

b.) Extract the second primary molar and close the space orthodontically – this plan is especially appealing in crowded cases or those that present in mild Class III configuration. Space closure works better the earlier it is started. There is also advantage in the incorporation of the concept of hemisection, a method developed by Professor Frans PGM van der Linden. Hemisection involves the removal of the distal portion of the second primary molar while leaving the mesial portion in place with a calcium hydroxide treatment. This accomplishes a number of favorable events:

1.) it insures the careful removal of the tooth (too often **alveolar bone** is lost at the time of extraction of the entire tooth – especially if it is **ankylosed**), 2.) less of the alveolus is likely to resorb during the spontaneous closure of a 5mm space than an 11mm space, 3.) the residual mesial portion of the tooth provides an antagonist to the maxillary teeth and prevents the tongue from intervening, and 4.) most significantly in cases with anchorage problems, the mesial portion acts as one more agent preventing the anterior teeth from drifting backward during space closure. Hemisection also reduces the duration of fixed orthodontics necessary for space closure. In most cases, the permanent molar drifts, with slight tipping, toward the mesial; more vertically growing cases experience more forward movement. Figure 17-5A illustrates such a case before treatment, Figures 17-5B-C show an intermediate stage, and Figures 17-5D-E show the case after treatment.

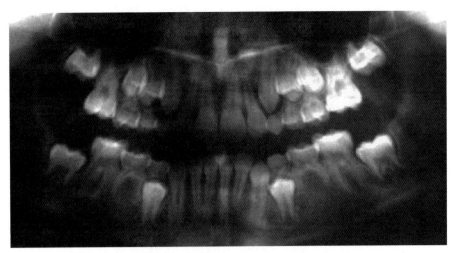

Figure 17-5A

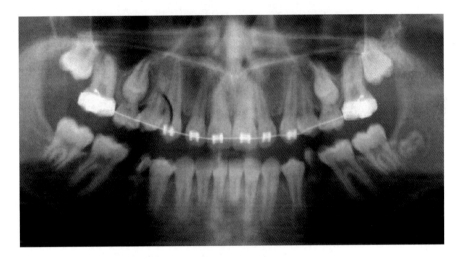

Figure 17-5B

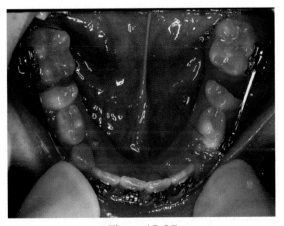

Figure 17-5C

Figure 17-5A,B,C,D,E: Congenitally missing second premolars treated by extracting the second deciduous (primary) molar and closing space orthodontically. (See pages 435-438). Figure 17-5A illustrates a case before treatment, Figures 17-5B-C show an intermediate stage, and Figures 17-5D-E (next page) show the case after treatment.

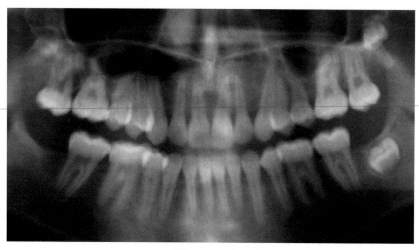

Figure 17-5D

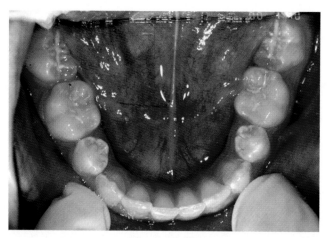

Figure 17-5E

c.) If space closure is not an option and the primary molar cannot be maintained, the next least invasive procedure would be an **autogenous** transplant. Reports confirm long term success of transplanted teeth at above 90%. Often an upper premolar can be sacrificed with no real impact on **anchorage**; and if anchorage is an extreme concern, third molars will often provide excellent replacement for missing lower premolars. Figure 17-6A-D illustrates the stages of treatment utilizing teeth numbers 1 and 16 to replace congenitally missing teeth numbers 20 and 29. This is less expensive than implants and has a similar success rate, when the procedure is provided with care.

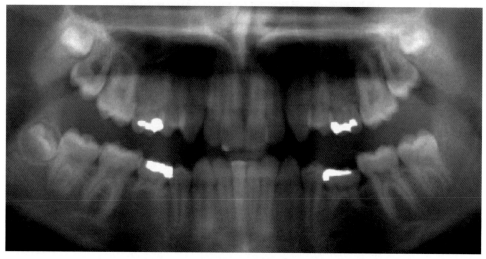

Figure 17-6A

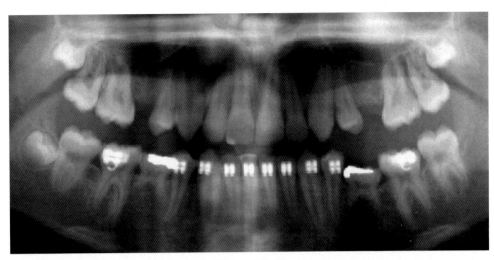

Figure 17-6B

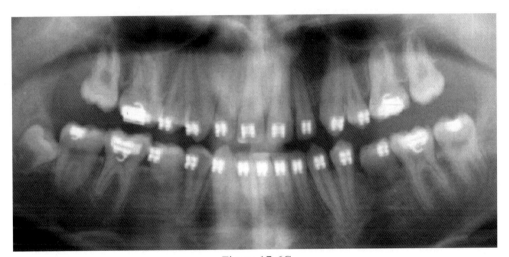

Figure 17-6C

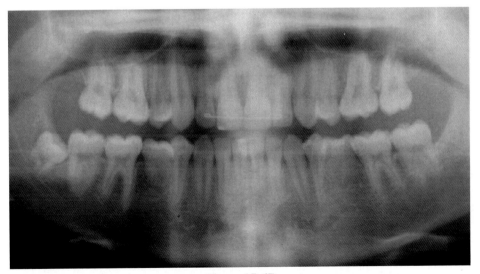

Figure 17-6D

d.) Implants make excellent replacement teeth, but care needs to be taken in protecting the adequacy of the alveolus; and provision must be made to maintain the appropriate amount of space until facial growth is complete. Figures 17-7A-E illustrates the treatment of a case utilizing implants to replace congenitally missing teeth numbers 20, 21, 24, and 29.

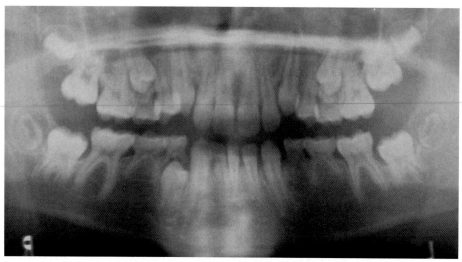

Figure 17-7A

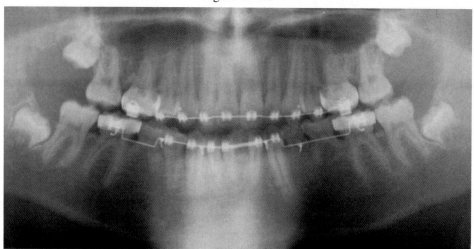

Figure 17-7B

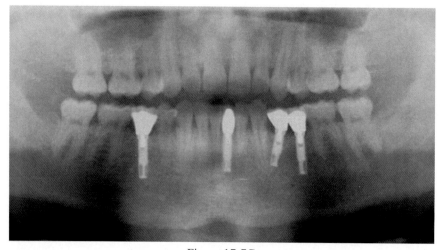

Figure 17-7C

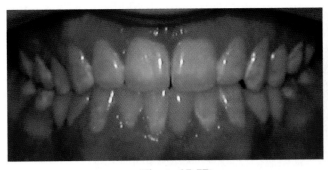

Figure 17-7D

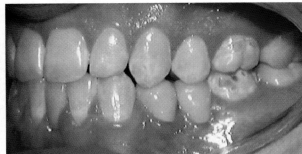

Figure 17-7E

e.) A fixed prosthesis/bridge is another alternative. Like an implant, this procedure should be postponed until adulthood. Unless a bonded bridge is used, pulp chambers need time to shrink so they won't react to the heat generated while preparing the adjacent anchor units. During this growth supervision, the maxillary plane of occlusion should be monitored to guard against hyper-eruption. While a brief course of orthodontic care is likely necessary to align the teeth and parallel the roots, this should not be as lengthy as that which would normally be required to close the space.

4.1.2.1.3. Maxillary Central Incisors

Loss of central incisors is a common problem in young people whose friends' baseball bats and hockey sticks are etiologic agents. An implant was used to replace the traumatic loss of tooth number 9 in Figures 17-8A-C.

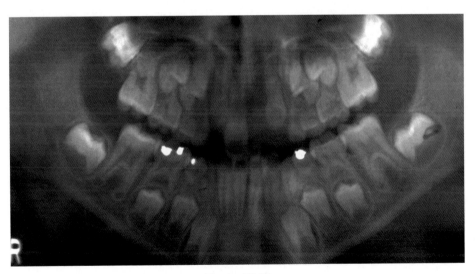

Figure 17-8A

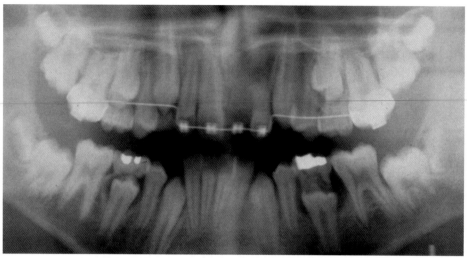

Figure 17-8B

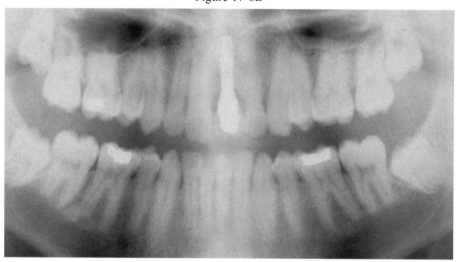

Figure 17-8C

The contralateral central incisor tends to drift across the midline, and the lateral incisor and cuspid on the affected side move mesially. Spacing may occur between the lateral incisor and cuspid or distal to the cuspid. Typically, the lateral segments of the arches do not move mesially until considerable time has elapsed. A prosthetic appliance with a pontic should be placed at once and worn until an age when a permanent restoration can be placed. If drifting has already begun, treatment with an appliance is necessary to regain the lost space and symmetry.

4.1.2.1.4. Maxillary Cuspids

This condition, seen rarely, gives rise to distal tipping of the central and lateral incisors with possible mesial movement of the first premolar. The suggested course of action is to move the premolar distally and the incisors mesially, holding space until an implant can be placed.   In Class II cases, consideration should be given to space closure, converting the premolar into a canine, as discussed above.

4.1.2.1.5. First Premolars

The loss of a first premolar without control of the rest of the occlusion is a difficult situation to handle. The incisors and cuspid drift distally and the posterior teeth tip mesially. Spacing probably will appear in the anterior segment. Only rarely can the dentist tip the remaining teeth back to near-normal positions with simple mechanics; more frequently, a comprehensive appliance is required.

4.1.2.1.6. Second Premolars

The same general considerations apply for the second as for the first premolars.

4.1.2.1.7. First Permanent Molars

Special consideration must be given to the first permanent molars because they often are lost early in life as a result of caries. If the first molar is lost before eruption of the premolars, the premolars may drift into the space left by the first molar. This is especially common in the mandibular arch. When first molars are lost, an increase in the **curve of Spee** usually occurs owing to the change in the axial inclination of the remaining posterior teeth. There also may be a deepening of the bite anteriorly. The result of the loss of one or more first molars at any age typically mandates sophisticated clinical treatment. Immediate steps should be taken to control and direct the drifting of the remaining teeth while a long-term treatment plan is developed.

The loss of one or more first permanent molars requires special, and often complicated, treatment planning. Considerations include:

- The number of molars lost
- The presence and status of the third molars
- The status of all other molars
- The basic malocclusion, other than that associated with the loss of the first molars, particularly the depth of the bite
- The eruptive stage of the premolars and second molars, and
- The skeletal pattern

The combination of concomitant factors and their severity determines their priority of impact. It is difficult to define precise rules of procedure for every combination of variables.

4.1.2.1.8. Mandibular Incisors

The same principles discussed for maxillary incisors apply for lower incisors, but care must be taken immediately to prevent the **extrusion** and/or lingual displacement of the incisors or cuspids adjacent to the site of loss. An acid-etched replacement may suffice until such time that all anterior teeth have normal centric stops and there is no crowding.

4.1.2.2. Multiple Loss of Permanent Teeth

When more than one tooth is lost, many of the same principles apply as for the loss of individual teeth. When teeth are lost simultaneously, as in the case of trauma, there is less immediate drifting of the remaining teeth. No simple rules can be stated, but do not overlook the possibilities of improving the occlusion with orthodontic treatment before inserting a prosthesis. Multiple and sequential loss of teeth in adults is a common problem requiring orthodontic attention prior to reconstructive dentistry (see Chapter 17).

4.1.3. Supernumerary Teeth

Supernumerary teeth are encountered less frequently than congenitally missing teeth. Their role in the etiology of malocclusion is presented in Chapter 7.

4.1.3.1. Diagnosis

This is based on radiographic findings and on careful measurement of the teeth in question. If it is noted that an erupting tooth varies in size, shape, eruption sequence or positioning from the contralateral tooth, a thorough radiographic evaluation should be done to check for the possibility of the tooth being a supernumerary. Similarly, a radiographic evaluation should be done if a tooth's eruption is delayed significantly from the contralateral side. A common example might be a case where one maxillary central incisor and both maxillary laterals are erupting without clinical evidence of the eruption of the other central incisor. Occlusal view radiographs are especially helpful in locating and diagnosing supernumerary teeth (see Chapters 13 and 14).

4.1.3.2. Treatment

1.) In the Primary Dentition – Supernumeraries are encountered only rarely in the primary dentition. They can present as well-formed supplemental teeth or in the form of a fused tooth. A good rule to follow is to leave them in place unless they are causing some form of malocclusion or malfunction, for example, a **functional crossbite** because of tooth interference.

2.) Teeth with Abnormal Crowns – These teeth only rarely can have functional use in the mouth. Often they are placed so that the normal teeth must change their course of eruption. Figures 17-9 A-C illustrate the presence of a supernumerary tooth in the midline which has caused tooth number 8 to erupt toward the distal.

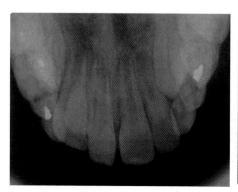

Figure 17-9A

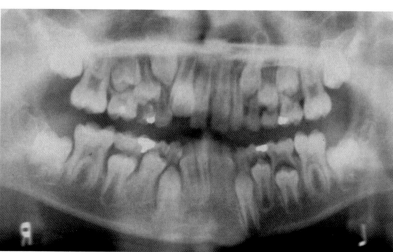

Figure 17-9B

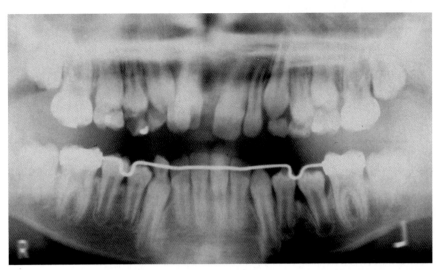

Figure 17-9C

If this is the case, remove the supernumerary teeth, taking care not to harm the follicles of the other teeth. If the supernumerary teeth can do no harm, they may be left in position until a later time. They follow no set pattern of eruption, so they must be observed at regular intervals, and removed eventually.

4.1.3.2.3. Supplemental Teeth of Normal Size and Shape

Maxillary lateral incisors are the teeth seen most frequently in this category, as illustrated in Figures 17-10A and B with supernumerary tooth number 7, although supplemental maxillary central incisors are observed as well.

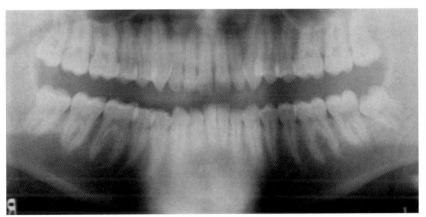

Figure 17-10A

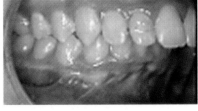

Figure 17-10B

Rarely is the size of the crown of a supernumerary tooth exactly that of the normal teeth. If the problem is unilateral, measure all three teeth; that is, the two normal teeth and the supernumerary tooth. The mesiodistal diameter of two of the teeth will be found to be most nearly the same. The odd-sized tooth can be considered the accessory tooth. There are instances in which the supernumerary tooth is of good formation and in better position to remain in the arch than the normal tooth.

4.1.3.2.4. Supernumerary Teeth Showing Variations in Size and Shape

These teeth should be removed as soon as it is possible to do so without damaging nearby normal teeth.

4.1.3.3. Discussion

Early diagnosis and observation will enable one to decide on the timing of treatment. The supernumerary tooth is seldom a major orthodontic problem if it is dealt with early in the development of the dentition.

4.2 VARIATIONS IN SIZE AND SHAPE OF TEETH

Variation is typical in nature, and teeth are no exception. Malalignment of teeth frequently is an expression of a disharmony between the size of teeth and the dimensions of the **basal arch** (Figure 17-11). There are practical limitations to the extent that the bony arches can be changed to accommodate large teeth. We are particularly restricted in altering the mandibular **arch perimeter** and width, both of which nearly always decrease with time.

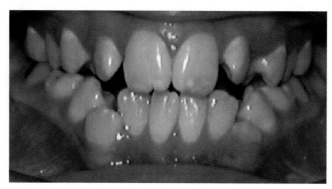

Figure 17-11

Cephalometrics may provide information concerning variations in the pattern of growth and dimensions of the facial skeleton. Biologically there is a rather high correlation between the widths of all teeth. This fact makes it possible to measure certain erupted permanent teeth and to predict, with some reliability and **validity**, the sizes of the teeth not yet erupted, a procedure explained in Chapter 13. The determination of whether teeth will fit into a given arch is one of the most problematic of all orthodontic diagnostic decisions. But to try to make the decision without even knowing the size of the teeth is to handicap oneself unnecessarily.

4.2.1. Diagnosis

A Boley gauge may be used to measure teeth, although its large size makes it less handy in the mouth. Record the measurements of the teeth as part of the written examination record. Additional help with measurement may also be obtained from the other occlusal diagnostic procedures described in Chapter 11. Position of the teeth within the facial skeleton is learned from the cephalogram. Leighton and Hunter have shown that crowded mandibular arches are more likely to be found in faces with steeper mandibular and occlusal planes, a shorter posterior face height, and a shorter mandibular corpus. How positions may be altered to relieve crowding is often a matter of clinical analysis. Certain cephalometric analyses are useful to estimate the best positions of the teeth to fit the skeletal profile and provide the most aesthetic lip outline (See Chapters 11 and 16). Occasionally there will be asymmetry of crown sizes, a finding complicating the achievement of good occlusion. The Sanin-Savara and Bolton analyses (See Chapter 13) are invaluable in this instance.

4.2.2. Large Teeth (Macrodontia)

The term "large teeth" is relative, for teeth that are large for one dental arch may not be large for another. The problem of teeth that are too large for their arch (or is it an arch too small for the teeth?) is discussed later under Space Management (Section 4.4.1). In reading the section on space management, pay particular attention to the sections on space supervision.

4.2.3. Small Teeth (Microdontia)

Always measure the teeth to make sure that the problem is truly one of tooth size. Small teeth usually result in generalized spacing, whereas functional problems such as various sucking or tongue habits, or diastemas related to tissue attachments, are more likely to result in more localized spacing problems.

Orthodontic therapy frequently is contraindicated in cases of generalized small teeth because tongue and lip habits often return the teeth to their original positions after the spaces have been closed. Many times patients are best left alone unless the aesthetics are unusually poor, in which case crowns or laminates may be used or the teeth may be built up by cosmetic bonding. In other instances, the arch may be consolidated and bridgework placed.

4.2.4. Anomalies of Crown Shape

Developmental anomalies showing alteration in coronal conformation are seen in all of the permanent teeth. The teeth affected most frequently are maxillary lateral incisors, mandibular second premolars, and the third molars.

4.2.4.1. Maxillary Lateral Incisors

The term "peg lateral" is applied when only the middle lobe of the tooth calcifies. Treatment is determined by two factors: 1.) the age at which the condition is discovered; and 2.) the size, shape and position of the malformed crown and root.

If the crown and root of the lateral incisor are such that the placement of a crown is not advisable, the tooth might be extracted. If the condition has been noted prior to eruption of the cuspids, proceed as in the case of congenitally missing lateral incisors. When the condition presents after eruption of cuspids, an implant or bridge to replace the lateral incisor may be considered instead of orthodontics.

If the "peg lateral" incisor has a normal root and sufficient crown for the preparation of a satisfactory crown, this type of prosthesis is favored. Alternatively, the "peg lateral" incisor may be built up with composite during or after orthodontic therapy. Care must be taken to preserve sufficient space in the arch to insert a restoration of proper mesiodistal width. An acrylic plate often is of use in opening space or for centering the tooth in the space between the central incisor and the cuspid. Banding several anterior teeth and the first molars will permit the use of a labial archwire to open spaces with coils. It also makes possible accurate placement of each tooth and provides better root angulation. Figure 17-12A illustrates a patient with congenitally missing tooth number 7, peg tooth number 10, and tooth number 8 is narrower than tooth number 9. Figure 17-12B is after orthodontic treatment, noting that a temporary veneer had been placed on tooth number 10 for treatment purposes. Figure 17-12C is with veneers on teeth numbers 8, 9, and 10 and Figure 17-12D shows an acrylic plate with a pontic for tooth number 7.

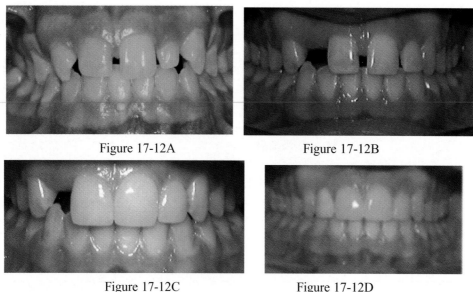

<table>
<tr><td>Figure 17-12A</td><td>Figure 17-12B</td></tr>
<tr><td>Figure 17-12C</td><td>Figure 17-12D</td></tr>
</table>

4.2.4.2. Mandibular Second Premolars

This tooth frequently is seen with two lingual cusps. The tooth is thus wider mesiodistally, and the extra cusp is of little concern. When such a tooth is seen in the radiograph before its eruption, you may wish to take steps to ensure that a bit more space is available in the arch. Abnormal ovoid or "egg-shaped" crowns also are observed as seen in Figure 17-13A, and are difficult to place in a satisfactory intercuspation as seen in Figure 17-13B with the resulting mild Class II molar relationship.

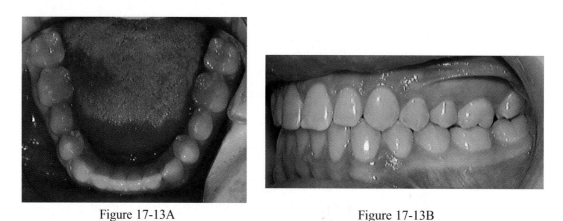

Figure 17-13A   Figure 17-13B

4.2.4.3. Miscellaneous Anomalies of Shape

Other anomalies of coronal shape may be observed. Each anomaly presents a separate problem requiring special treatment.

4.3 SPACING OF TEETH

4.3.1. Localized Spacing

4.3.1.1 Etiology

Localized spacing may be a result of many causes other than variations of normal spacing. Treatment is highly individualized, but knowledge of the general principles of etiology and diagnosis is helpful.

Problems in localized spacing and in excessive spacing at one or a few contact points usually are attributable to 1.) missing teeth, 2.) undue retention of primary teeth, or 3.) a deleterious sucking habit.

4.3.1.1.1. Missing Teeth

Congenitally Missing Teeth – This problem may cause localized spacing, but it may be seen in more than one spot because adjacent teeth often drift into the space (Figure 17-14).

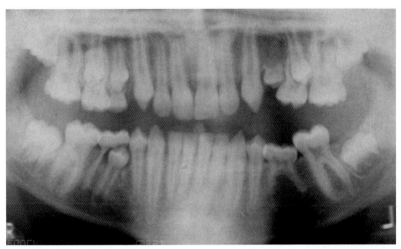

Figure 17-14

Unerupted Teeth – Sometimes a tooth is impacted or remains unerupted. The spacing problem is then localized, and the plan of treatment is determined by the chances of bringing the tooth into its normal relationship (Figure 17-15).

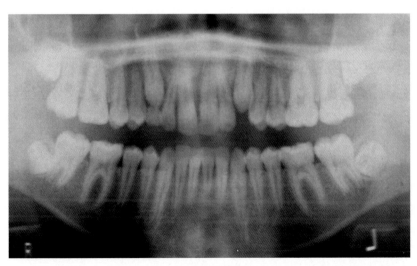

Figure 17-15

Loss of Permanent Teeth – This matter is discussed in section 4.1.2, Loss of Permanent Teeth.

4.3.1.1.2. Undue Retention of Primary Teeth

Belated loss of primary teeth may force the erupting permanent teeth into undesirable positions. Later, when the primary tooth is exfoliated, a space results. This sequence of events is seen most frequently in the maxillary cuspid region.

4.3.1.1.3. Sucking Habits

The patient's sucking habits may cause a localized spacing of the teeth. Read Chapters 7 and 11 to help understand this problem and plan its treatment.

4.3.1.2. Spacing Between Maxillary Central Incisors

One of the malocclusions of most concern to patients is **diastema** between the maxillary central incisors. Excessive spacing in such a prominent place in the dentition is generally felt to be unsightly, although it does little to reduce masticatory efficiency. Treatment of this disorder is solely for cosmetic and psychological effects.

Data in the *Handbook of Orthodontics*, 1988, 4th Ed., R. E. Moyers, Chapter 13, pg. 357, suggest that too much emphasis has been placed on the labium frenum and too little on structures and development at the midline. It also is of interest that, in a series of patients studied by Moyers, nearly one-fourth was developing normally, though the patients' chief complaint concerned existing tooth spacing.

4.3.1.2.1 Examination and differential diagnosis

See *Handbook of Orthodontics*, 4th Ed., 1988, R. E. Moyers, Chapter 15, pg. 357.

4.3.1.2.2. Supernumerary Teeth at the Midline

The diagnosis of this condition is based solely on radiographic studies unless the supernumerary tooth has erupted. A supernumerary tooth is a condition likely to cause an increase in the space between the maxillary central incisors as seen in Figure 17-16. This is discussed in Section 4.1.3 of this chapter, Supernumerary Teeth.

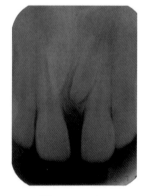

Figure 17-16

4.3.1.2.3. Congenitally Missing Lateral Incisors

Treatment of this condition is discussed in this chapter in Section 4.1.1, Congenitally Missing Teeth. Figure 17-17 illustrates a typical midline diastema associated with the congenital absence of lateral incisors.

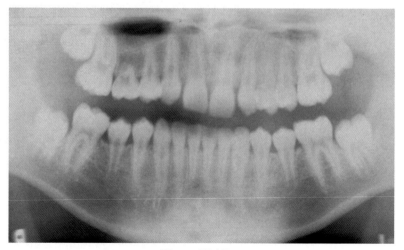

Figure 17-17

4.3.1.2.4. Enlarged Labium Frenum

Diagnosis – The enlarged or malposed labium frenum may be diagnosed by observation alone or by lifting the lip (Figure 17-18).

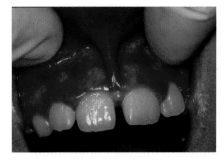

Figure 17-18

However, it is impossible to detect all enlarged or malposed frena in this manner. The final diagnosis must be based on a radiograph. The normal osseous septum between the maxillary central incisors is V-shaped and bisected by the **intermaxillary** suture, which sometimes is not visible in the radiograph. When the labial frenum inserts on the palatal side of the septum, the fibers of the frenum run across the bone, rounding it over so that the septum is shaped like a spade (See Figure 17-19A-B). On occasion, a shallow trough is seen. Even when the fibers insert so deeply as not to cause blanching when the lip is displaced, the condition may be diagnosed in the radiograph. Another consideration is that, when the free gingival margin is elevated while pulling on the lip, a potential problem for the long-term periodontal contour can exist.

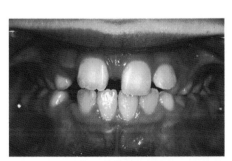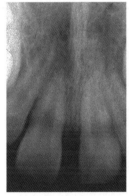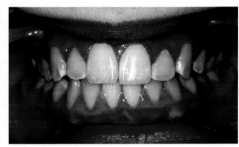

Figure 17-19A   Figure 17-19B   Figure 17-19C

Treatment

Treatment consists of bringing the incisors together <u>before</u> excising the frenum. The incisors may be bracketed, a short wire ligated into place and the teeth pulled together by ligatures or light elastics. After the central incisors have come into juxtaposition, excise the frenum and maintain the **orthodontic appliance** in position while healing is taking place. Care must be taken during the surgery to avoid a deficient papilla. The scar tissue formed will help in retention. If excision is undertaken before orthodontic movement, the teeth must be moved through the newly formed scar tissue. In either case, retention is recommended. Figure 17-19C illustrates the result after treatment.

4.3.1.2.5. Imperfect Fusion at the Midline

The midline is a common site of development faults, such as epithelial rests and inclusion cysts. The condition may be related to imperfect fusion at the midline, for histological study of the tissue included within such osseous bifurcations has shown connective and epithelial tissue. A wide variety of forms will be observed, all of which must be differentiated from the normal suture. A distinctly W-shaped osseous septum may be associated with this condition, as well as a circumscribed irregular ovoid area. The separation of the osseous septum may be shallow or continue well into the alveolar process.

Treatment — One should proceed exactly as they would for a malposed or enlarged labial frenum except that the included tissue, rather than the frenum, must be excised.

4.3.1.2.6. Spacing as Part of Normal Growth

The central incisors erupt with a space between them (see Figure 17-20A). This space is diminished when the lateral incisors erupt and may finally be closed by the wedging of the erupting cuspids. In the absence of abnormal midline structures or gross variations in tooth size, it can be assumed that the midline space will close naturally (Figure 17-20B).

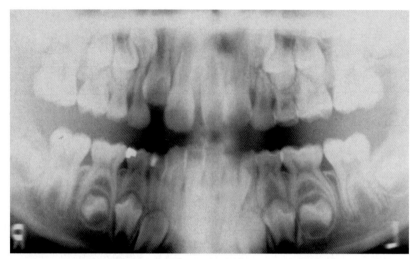

Figure 17-20A

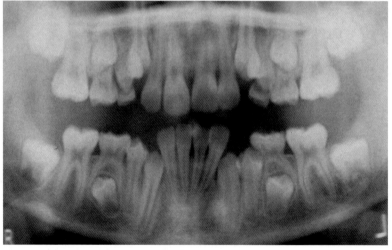

Figure 17-20B

4.3.2. Generalized Spacing

Any of several etiologic factors may be involved in generalized spacing of the teeth. It is important to ascertain the presence of true generalized spacing. More frequently, a localized spacing problem is encountered.

4.3.2.1. Small Teeth

If the teeth are small for the size of the **alveolar arch** that includes them, generalized spacing may result. If the teeth, when measured, are very small and there are no other apparent causative factors, the size of the teeth alone may be at fault. Such a condition is uncommon. The best treatment may be by means of buildup with composite, crowns, or consolidation of the arch and placement of bridges or implants. Whether measures such as a series of crowns is to be undertaken is an individual matter, dependent on the wishes of the patient and his/her perception of the cosmetic problem. Some problems of spacing due to small teeth may best be left alone, though it may be difficult to convince your patient that this course of action is appropriate.

4.3.2.2. Large Tongue (**Macroglossia)**

Another rather rare cause of generalized spacing is an unduly large tongue. Diagnosis is made by careful examination of the tongue when extended as well as at rest. The lateral edges of the tongue, when it is too large for the alveolar arch, usually display scalloping where the tongue rests against the lingual surfaces of the teeth, although this feature is not diagnostic. Treatment is contraindicated unless gross malocclusion is present, in which case a wedge of tissue may be excised from the tongue (Figure 17-21).

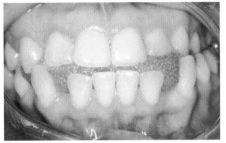

Figure 17-21

4.3.2.3 Sucking Habits

Sucking habits may cause rather generalized spacing of the teeth, although they are more likely to cause a localized spacing of the maxillary anterior teeth. See Chapters 7 and 11 for a discussion of digital sucking and Chapters 1 and 11 for suggested therapy in thumb sucking and tongue thrusting (see Figure 18-10 and 7-15). Figure 17-21A and B are illustrations of a self-reported tongue sucker.

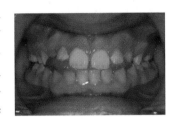

Figure 17-21A

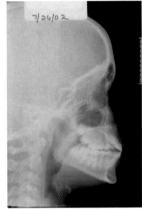

Figure 17-21B

4.3.2.4. Abnormal Tongue Posture

Abnormal tongue posture may also cause generalized spacing (see Chapters 7 and 16). The prognosis is dependent on the reason for the atypical postural position. Endogenous protracted postures are most intractable, while those associated with nasorespiratory dysfunction (e.g., mouth breathing) often are correctable when normal respiratory function returns. Tongue-thrust may also create generalized spacing (See Chapters 7 and 11).

4.4 PROBLEMS SINGULAR TO THE TRANSITIONAL DENTITION

4.4.1. Space Management

4.4.1.1. General Considerations

Space management is a general term that includes four subdivisions: space maintenance, space regaining, space supervision, and gross discrepancies. All problems in space management fall into one of the four categories. The differential diagnosis among them is determined primarily by the Mixed Dentition Analysis (see Chapter 13), but other predispositions to crowding must not be overlooked. Crowded mandibular arches have been shown to be associated with steep mandibular and occlusal lines, short posterior face height, short mandibular corpus, lingual inclination of incisors, and mesially inclined molars. Further, the lower incisors and **symphysis** are less protrusive in crowded cases.

4.4.1.2. Maintenance of Arch Perimeter

Space maintenance is typically undertaken when the following conditions are present: 1.) loss of one or more primary teeth; 2.) optimally, no loss of arch perimeter; and 3.) a favorable Mixed Dentition Analysis prediction.

The problem of maintenance of arch perimeter is not peculiar to the mixed dentition, for the arch perimeter is likely to shorten quickly at any time following the loss of either a primary or a permanent tooth, and arch perimeter continues to diminish gradually throughout life. However, certain difficulties in the mixed dentition are so singular as to require separate techniques and separate discussion. Here, the explanation will be confined to problems of perimeter maintenance, which may appear in a normally developing dentition as a result of caries or unwanted loss of teeth.

It is important to separate space maintenance cases from 1.) space regaining and 2.) space supervision.

4.4.1.2.1. Caries of Primary Teeth

The most frequent cause of arch perimeter loss in the mixed dentition is caries of the primary molars. A carious lesion on the distal surface of the second primary molar, in particular, allows the first permanent molar to move mesially. The first step in maintaining arch perimeters is to preserve intact the size of the primary molar crowns. A most important preventive orthodontic appliance is a proper restoration in a primary molar. In Chapter 7, the role of caries in the etiology of malocclusion is discussed. Research affirms the etiologic role of caries in many space management malocclusions.

4.4.1.2.2. Loss of Individual Primary Teeth

Generally, it is necessary to place space maintainers when a posterior primary tooth has been lost (Figure 17-22A-B). Note that even though the lost left first primary molar space has been maintained, the band and loop maintainer are poorly adapted (Figure 17-22B). Often, the effect of the tooth loss on the total **arch length** is not noticed. A space maintainer to hold space after the loss of a single tooth should generally be placed if the following conditions are present: 1.) the permanent successor is present and developing normally; 2.) the arch length has not been shortened; 3.) the space from which the tooth has been lost has not diminished; 4.) the molar or cuspid interdigitation has not been affected by the loss; and 5.) there is a favorable Mixed Dentition Analysis prediction. Typically, there is no reason to insert a space maintainer if the permanent successor is absent, nor should one maintain 4 mm of space for a tooth known to be 7 mm in width. The type of space maintainer to be used depends on the site of the loss, the patient/parent preference and the operator's skill.

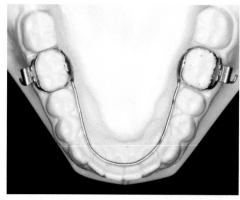
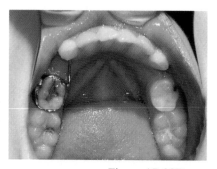

Figure 17-22A   Figure 17-22B

4.4.1.2.2.1. Primary incisors

Primary incisors may be lost prematurely as a result of trauma. Multiple loss of incisors from caries is also seen. Space maintainers are not necessary in treatment; however, this is not a rigid rule. Before the permanent teeth have developed sufficiently to maintain the dimensions of the arch, the loss of a primary incisor can result in rapid closure of space. In the case of premature loss of primary incisors, make a record cast and occlusal radiographs for diagnosis and study. Space maintainers for primary incisors are less apt to be needed if the primary tooth has been lost after the child is 4 years of age.

4.4.1.2.2.2. Primary cuspids

Although the primary cuspids may be removed prematurely because of caries, the eruption of crowded permanent incisors is a more frequent cause of their premature loss, and can often be unilateral, leading to asymmetries. It is not uncommon for lower lateral incisors to initially erupt lingually of their proper alignment, and to roll out toward the labial with further development and as the primary incisors exfoliate. In the crowded case, the lateral incisor will be even more likely to erupt lingually. As it makes its labial movement, it can provide pressure to the root of the primary cuspid, which can result in resorption of the root and premature exfoliation, particularly if the cuspid cannot move labially or distally (Figure 17-23). Unilateral loss of a mandibular primary cuspid poses a special problem since the dental midline can quickly be displaced. Such resultant unilateral drifting of teeth complicates arch integrity and jeopardizes its symmetry. Extraction at this time removes some of the anchorage in the anterior part of the mouth; all of the lower anterior teeth tip lingually, and, as they do, a worsening in the level of the **attached gingiva** on the facial surfaces has been observed. (Reference: Powell, R.N. and McEniery, T.M., "A longitudinal study of isolated gingival recession in the mandibular incisor region," J. Clinical Perio., 1982, 357-364). Further, this lingual tipping of the incisors will most likely need to be regained at a later date. Such an adverse side-effect is worsened in vertical growers and those with such exaggerated overjets that they have lower lip trapping. The most conservative approach is to place a well fitted lower lingual arch (LLA) prior to extracting the contralateral cuspid. This LLA should be adjustable and anchored on the permanent molars.

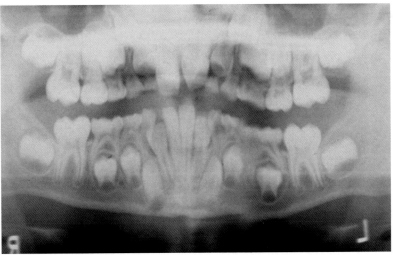

Figure 17-23

Following the loss of primary cuspids, the mandibular perimeter may shorten from the front, since the lips may tip the permanent incisors lingually, causing them to lose their occlusal stops and increasing the overjet and the overbite. As a result, the erupting mandibular permanent cuspids may move anteriorly across the roots of the lateral incisors, finally emerging in **labioversion**. If other posterior teeth also move anteriorly, it is more difficult to correct the cuspid's malposition. Such cuspid malposition is best averted by prevention of lingual tipping of the incisors. A lower lingual arch is a useful tool to support the incisors from tipping lingually (Figure 17-24).

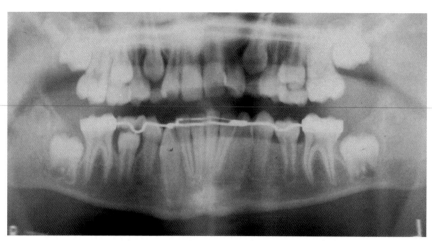

Figure 17-24

In the maxillary arch, the problem of loss of a primary cuspid is similar, although the typical sequence of eruption and the permanent cuspid's position increases its chances to move labially out of the ideal **arch form**. The upper arch is more apt to shorten posteriorly, but it is also easier to produce distal orthodontic movement of the first permanent molar to provide added or regained room in the arch for better placement of cuspids and premolars.

   Primary molars - Premature loss of primary molars has long been associated with space loss and eruptive difficulties, especially when the second primary molar has been affected. The concept that the first primary molar loss is not so deleterious has been fostered by limitations in measurement techniques. When the second primary molar is lost prematurely (in the maxilla or the mandible), either as a singular event or in conjunction with the premature loss of the first primary molar, the first permanent molar will migrate toward the mesial. Likewise, the eventual eruptive position of the permanent cuspid moves toward the distal. Both of these events reduce the amount of space available for the accommodation of the permanent cuspid and bicuspids. The extent to which space is lost will determine whether the teeth eventually erupt crowded or if the amount of crowding will actually result in the impaction of a tooth, most often the second bicuspid.

Loss of the mandibular first primary molar is typically followed by a more mesial migration of the permanent molar than occurs in the maxilla. It appears that the upper second primary molar is a better anchor against mesial migration than the mandibular second primary molar. In both arches, the eventual eruptive position of the cuspid tends to migrate markedly more toward the mesial than when the second primary molar is lost. The net loss in the lower **arch circumference** averages about 2.8 mm, which usually translates into crowding in the affected quadrant. In the maxilla, the premature loss of the first primary molar provokes an interesting phenomenon: the first bicuspid erupts prematurely, usually repositioning toward the mesial, in front of the second primary molar. (The slight distal force that this places on the second primary molar might play a role in the improved **anchorage** in the maxilla, compared to the mandible.) The result is that there is a suffi-cient reduction in space available for the permanent cuspid, and it predictably erupts out toward the labial. In a study examining 13 consecutive cases of premature loss of the maxillary first primary molar, 11 experienced "blocking out" of the permanent cuspid; one of the remaining cases had microdontia (Reference: Northway, JADA, 131, Dec. 2000, 1711-20).

4.4.1.2.2.3. Multiple Loss of Primary Teeth

Usually, when several primary teeth are lost, the arch perimeter is shortened before intervention occurs and thus regaining, not maintenance, is indicated. Sometimes it will be necessary to extract more than one primary tooth at the same appointment. If this is necessary, it is best to insert the appliance the very day the teeth are removed. Typically, a lingual archwire space-maintainer is used through the mixed dentition. This is a dynamic, rapidly changing period of development unsuited to the application of a static prosthetic approach. The design of any appliance depends on the individual situation. Several suggestions will be found in Chapter 11.

4.4.1.2.2.4. Mesial Drift of Permanent Molars

In some cases, space can be lost just from drift that occurs in certain individuals. **Mesial drift** of the first permanent molars generally involves a mixture of three separate kinds of tooth movements, namely, mesial crown tipping, rotation, and **translation**. There are distinct differences in the mode of mesial movement between the upper and lower first permanent molars. These differences are caused by variations in root number and form, crown shape, in occlusal relationships, and the position of other permanent teeth, particularly the maxillary second permanent molar. The age at the time of loss of the root of the primary second molar, especially as it relates to the sequence and status of eruption of the adjacent teeth, is predictive of the response in terms of rate and amount of space loss and the impact that it has on the opposing occlusion. In cases where the roots have been maintained following the loss of a severely destroyed primary crown, the root system has had a profound effect in slowing the rate of arch circumference reduction. The roots should not be left if they are infected and might cause purulence and abscessing of adjacent structures. This type of inflammation can cause serious problems for the **succedaneous** tooth.

When the second primary molar is lost, the tipping of the permanent molar causes the distobuccal cusp to become more prominent occlusally. Because of the large lingual root of the maxillary first permanent molar, rotation of the crown also is seen with mesial tipping, the distobuccal cusp becoming more prominent buccally as well. When the second primary molar is lost prior to the eruption of the first permanent molar, translation of the first permanent molar during its eruption may be seen.

Mandibular first permanent molars display mesial tipping, crown rotation, and translation as well, but they are more likely to show lingual tipping during mesial movement. The lingual tipping is caused by the absence of a lingual root and the fact that occlusal function occurs buccally to the center of mass of the lower molar, a condition aggravated as the first molar drifts mesially. Figure 17-25 clearly illustrates the differences in mesial drifting of mandibular (Figure 17-25A) and maxillary (Figure 17-25B) first permanent molars.

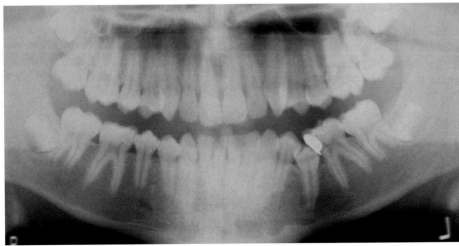

Figure 17-25A

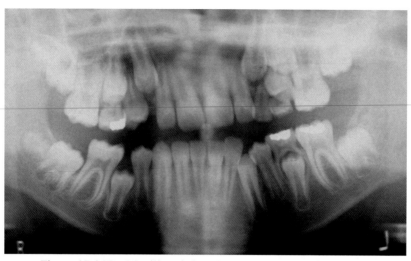

Figure 17-25B: Maxillary left and mandibular right space loss.

When the second primary molar is lost, space maintenance should be employed until the full eruption of the second bicuspid and the second molar. If at all possible, space maintainers should be designed to use the permanent molars as anchor teeth (Figure 17-22A). The often used "**band** and loop" is actually highly ineffectual due to the ability of primary teeth to drift and the response when the adjacent teeth loosen and exfoliate. Before inserting any appliance to maintain the second primary molar space, one must determine whether or not space has already been lost, which generally dictates space regaining prior to space maintaining procedures. If the extraction of a second primary molar is anticipated, it would be wise to have the placement of a space maintainer readied for insertion at the extraction appointment, if not before, to maximize the effect of reducing space loss. In some cases where space has already been lost, or further crowding is anticipated, it may be appropriate to incorporate the eventual extraction of permanent teeth into the treatment plan.

1.) Distal Movement of First Permanent Molars – The basic tooth movement necessary in space regaining is distal movement of first permanent molars, which must be the reverse of the movements that have occurred as the teeth drifted mesially. The selection of which space-regaining appliance to use is dependent on whether tipping, rotation, translation, or combinations of these movements are required to place the first permanent molar in its normal position.

4.4.1.3. Regaining Space in the Arch Perimeter

Space regaining means that all of the following conditions are present: 1.) one or more primary teeth have been lost; 2.) some space in the arch has been lost to mesial drift of the first permanent molar; and 3.) a Mixed Dentition Analysis shows that if one could regain the space that was lost, there would be adequate room for all the teeth and the normal mixed dentition space.

Correction of arch perimeter loss should take place where the loss has occurred. Note the molar relationship, cuspid interdigitation, and overjet, since they provide the key to the site of the shortening.

After locating where the arch has shortened, determine, by means of a Mixed Dentition Analysis (described in Chapter 13), the exact amount of space that must be regained and the most logical tooth movements to recover that space. Usually, some distal movement of first permanent molars is necessary. Figure 17-26 illustrates one of several appliances available for this purpose, although it is easier to regain space before the second molars are erupted.

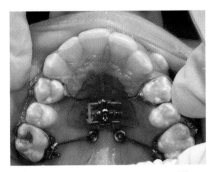 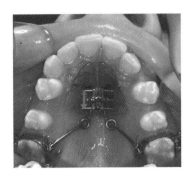

Figure 17-26

4.4.1.4. Space Supervision

Space supervision is the term applied when, according to a Mixed Dentition Analysis, it is doubtful that, without a treatment intervention, there will be room for all the teeth. The prognosis for space supervision is always guarded, whereas the prognosis for regaining space and for space maintenance is usually good. Space supervision cases will better pass through the mixed dentition with clinical guidance than they will without guidance. Space supervision should not be undertaken without patient cooperation and parental understanding that it is an optional early treatment approach and that the patient will likely need later comprehensive care.

Space supervision has several basic principles: 1.) generally, space supervision is not begun until the mandibular cuspid and first premolar show approximately one-quarter to one-third of the root formed, 2.) primary teeth may need to be extracted serially to provide an eruption sequence of cuspid, first premolar, and second premolar in the mandible and of first premolar, cuspid, and second premolar in the maxilla, 3.) an effort is made to keep the mandibular teeth erupting well ahead of the maxillary; and 4.) typically, clinicians take care that a **late mesial shift** of the maxillary and mandibular first permanent molars does not occur. Specific space supervision protocols exist for:

  1.) Mesial step (Class I) protocol
  2.) Flush terminal plane (end-to-end) protocol
  3.) Distal step (Class II) protocol
For details, see Chapter 15 in the *Handbook of Orthodontics* by R. E. Moyers, 4th Ed., 1988.

4.4.1.5. Gross Discrepancy Problems

Gross discrepancy problems are those in which there is a great and significant difference between the sizes of all the permanent teeth and the space available for them within the alveolar arch perimeter. Gross discrepancy problems ordinarily cannot be diagnosed until the early mixed dentition, as no clinically useful correlation has been shown to exist between the size of the primary teeth and those of the permanent dentition.

The difference between space supervision cases and gross discrepancy problems is largely one of strategy. In space supervision, the goal is to squeeze all permanent teeth into what obviously is minimal or deficient space. In the gross discrepancy problem, it is accepted at the start that insufficient space is available and therefore extraction of permanent teeth is necessary.

  1.) Diagnosis – A meticulous Mixed Dentition Analysis is necessary (See Chapter 13); however, it must be remembered that the skeletal pattern has a significant effect on the alignment of teeth within the dental arch.

2.) General Rules – No dentist should extract permanent teeth as a part of orthodontic therapy unless he/she has the technical skills to correct all the sequelae of those extractions. Extraction itself provides space, only some of which may be absorbed by spontaneous alignment of crowded teeth. The remaining space closure and alignment of teeth is critical to a case's success. Nearly every case in which permanent teeth are extracted requires comprehensive appliance therapy to close the remaining spaces, parallel the roots, establish a proper occlusal plane, and correct the **intercuspation**. Figure 17-27 illustrates an example of a patient having all four 1st premolars extracted with no orthodontic treatment.

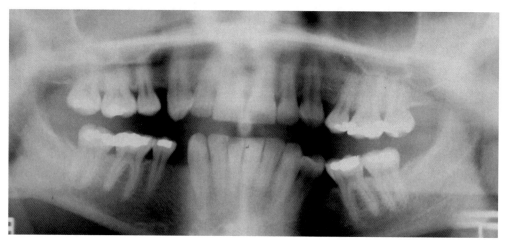

Figure 17-27

A few general rules for clinicians provide insurance against involvement in unwanted complications. The following were suggested by Eisner. When a case satisfies the requirements of all the rules, it may be treated by a **serial extraction** protocol.

-Rule 1: There should be a Class I molar relationship bilaterally.
-Rule 2: The facial skeleton should be balanced anteroposteriorly, vertically, and transversely.
-Rule 3: The discrepancy should be at least 5 – 7 mm in all four quadrants.
-Rule 4: The dental midlines should coincide.
-Rule 5: There should be neither an open bite nor a deep bite.

Few discrepancy cases will meet all the requirements of these rules, and the more a case deviates from them the more difficult it will be to treat.

The removal of all four second permanent molars in cases has recently been enthusiastically revived and advocated, although it is not recommended as a routine treatment for gross discrepancy problems. Second molar extraction is an old strategy with specific utility. The procedure has special problems. The removal of second permanent molars, when indicated, may be part of adolescent gross discrepancy treatment. It must be noted that there is a significantly different response of maxillary third molars to second molar extractions than there is for mandibular third molars. Mandibular third molars rarely attain satisfactory positions after second molar extractions without an additional period of comprehensive orthodontics,

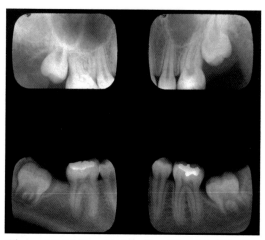

Figure 17-28 Provided by Dr. Allen Moffitt (See Reading List).

sometimes including subsequent treatment several years after the extractions. Figure 17-28 illustrates this concern.

4.4.2. Difficulties in Eruption

4.4.2.1. Alterations in Sequence of Eruption

Certain variations in the order of eruption of the teeth have been shown to be symptomatic of certain malocclusions. It is true that a more normal sequence of eruption provides the best chance for maintaining the arch perimeter intact. A serious problem occurs in clinical situations when the second permanent molar erupts ahead of any cuspids or premolars. If noted early, a holding arch will prevent premature shortening of the arch perimeter.

4.4.2.1.1. Premature Eruption of Individual Teeth

Permanent teeth may erupt unusually early if the primary predecessor has lost a considerable amount of bone from around its roots; e.g., periapical lesions may result in extensive bone resorption via early loss of the primary tooth and the inflammatory response in the region. All of these conditions hasten the arrival of the permanent tooth.

4.4.2.1.2. Delayed Eruption of Individual Teeth

Individual teeth may be delayed in eruption because of retarded tooth development (Figure 17-29A, idiopathic failure to erupt (Figure 17-29B) or premature loss of the primary predecessor. When a primary tooth is removed prior to the initiation of root formation of the permanent successor, and hence the start of its eruption, bone may reform occlusal to the permanent tooth before eruptive movements can begin; thus, eruption actually is delayed by the premature loss of the primary tooth. A critical factor is the amount of root formation of the permanent tooth at the time of loss of its predecessor.

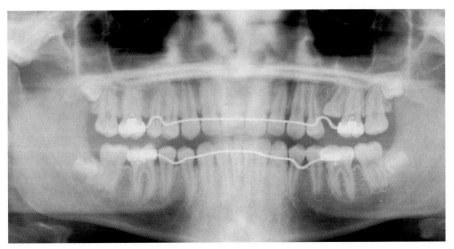
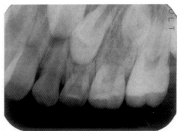

Figure 17-29A

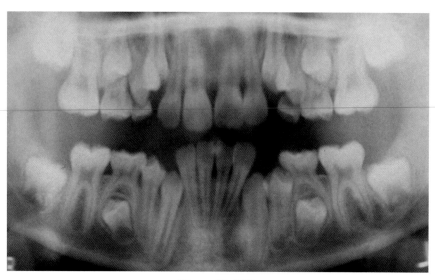

Figure 17-29B

The maxillary and mandibular second premolars are the teeth most likely to develop in a manner disharmonious with adjacent teeth, and thus their eruptive development must be watched more carefully (see Chapters 13 and 14). Unduly retained primary second molars or their root fragments may be obstructive impediments to eruption.

Idiopathic failure to erupt is also seen and is difficult to diagnose before the failure occurs. It is usually difficult to treat. All such cases in delayed eruption need to be differentiated from **ankylosed** permanent teeth and watched carefully.

4.4.2.2. Ectopic Eruption of Teeth

Ectopia means out of the normal position, or misplaced. Any tooth may be in ectopia during eruption, although some are more frequently so than others. Only those teeth in which ectopic eruptions most often are a clinical problem will be dealt with here.

4.4.2.2.1. Maxillary First Permanent Molar

The following, in combination, usually account for the abnormality.

1.) The teeth in ectopia are significantly larger than normal.
2.) The maxillary first permanent molar is erupting at an abnormal angle, indicating that the tooth germ probably was abnormally placed.
3.) The maxillary length (depth) is shorter, and tuberosity growth may lag significantly.
4.) The morphology of the distal surface of the maxillary second primary molar and of the mesial surface of the maxillary first permanent molar are ideally suited for locking of the latter tooth during its eruption.
5.) The distal root of the second primary molar is oriented sufficiently to the distal that it deflects the permanent molar more toward the mesial, causing it to become caught at the cervix of the primary tooth. Resorption of root, and eventually the distal aspect of the primary molar, is initiated and may proceed unless the permanent tooth becomes freed (Figure 17-30). Frequently, ectopia of the maxillary first permanent molar is bilateral. When it is unilateral, excessive tooth width is not as important an etiologic factor as the misplacement of the developing tooth germ.

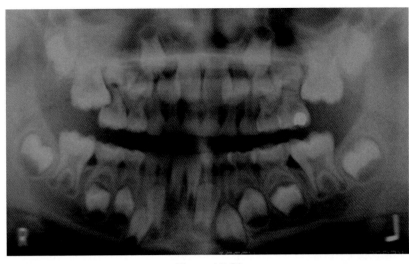

Figure 17-30

4.4.2.2.2. Maxillary Cuspids

Maxillary cuspids may develop ectopically, in which case they may become impacted (See Section 4.4.2.4, Impaction of Teeth). Cuspids also are forced into **ectopic eruption** when there is insufficient space in the arch (see Section 4.4.1, Space Management).

4.4.2.2.3. Mandibular Incisors

Only rarely are the mandibular incisors in ectopic eruption, although the lateral incisor frequently is thought to be. When an incisor in the lower arch is or seems to be in ectopia, the condition is most likely caused by the prolonged retention of a primary predecessor or excessively large permanent teeth. Mandibular lateral incisors normally erupt lingually to their final position. However, they soon are moved into the line of the arch by the tongue unless there is insufficient room for them. Figures 17-31A-C illustrates the ectopic eruption of the mandibular right lateral incisor and its subsequent position after a first phase of treatment.

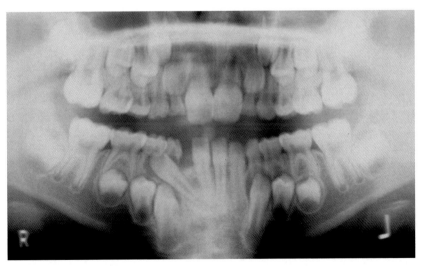

Figure 17–31A

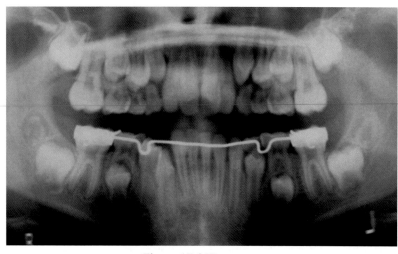

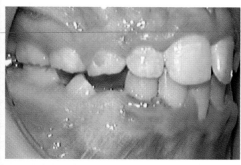

Figure 17-31B   Figure 17-31C

4.4.2.2.4. Other Teeth

Although any tooth may erupt ectopically due to local causes, the most serious ectopias are those in which the tooth germ itself forms ectopically.

When planning treatment, always keep in mind three objectives: 1.) Placement of the tooth in its normal position; 2.) retention of a favorable sequence of eruption; and 3.) maintenance of arch perimeter.

4.4.2.3. Transposition of Teeth

Transposition of teeth is a rare but clinically difficult developmental anomaly and almost invariably involves the permanent cuspid. Transpositions may occur in either jaw and may be unilateral or bilateral. In the maxilla, three times as many transpositions are reported with the first premolar as with the lateral incisor (Figure 17-32). Almost all mandibular transpositions are with the lateral incisor (Figure 17-33A-B).

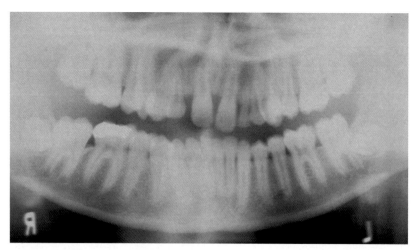

Figure 17-32

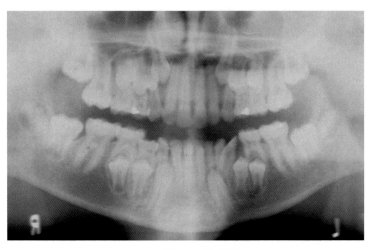

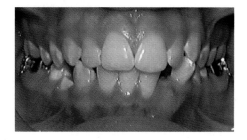

| Figure 17-33A | Figure 17-33B |

4.4.2.3.1. Etiology

The causes of all transpositions are not well understood, although retained primary cuspids are the best documented single etiologic factor. Transpositions are frequently found in conjunction with other dental anomalies such as dental **agenesis** and malformation of dental shapes (especially peg-shaped maxillary lateral incisors). They present as disturbances in eruptive positioning and developmental order as a consequence of genetic disturbance (see Chapter 7).

In treating these cases, early diagnosis and subsequent timing of treatment is critical. When treating the canine-first premolar transposition (nearly 70% of diagnosed transpositions), the early extraction of the primary canine is critical. It is also theoretically possible that there may be an actual transposition on the **anlage** of the teeth.

4.4.2.3.2 Diagnosis

Diagnosis consists of two steps: 1.) identification and 2.) classification into incomplete or complete transposition. Incomplete transpositions display crown misplacement only; complete transpositions involve the whole tooth. Incomplete transpositions left unattended may develop into complete, or nearly complete, transpositions. Radiographs taken at several angulations and careful palpation of the roots are essential to diagnosis and treatment planning. Do not delay a diagnosis and concomitant treatment plan for these cases. Superior results are achieved when correcting these early as teeth can be brought through the alveolar bone rather than out and around an adjacent tooth.

4.4.2.3.3. Treatment

Early recognition makes possible a change in the eruptive path of the permanent cuspid by removal of the retained primary tooth, opening space in the arch, surgical uncovering of the transposed permanent tooth, and its orthodontic placement into position.

When the cuspid is completely transposed, treatment to correct arch positions is far more difficult. Leaving the teeth transposed is then sometimes a prudent alternative.

4.4.2.4. Impaction of Teeth

Impactions are teeth so closely wedged in the alveolar bone they are unable to erupt. Unfortunate common misusage applies the term to any tooth that does not erupt.

Although there are hereditary patterns leading to impacted teeth, the etiologic factors of most concern are malposed tooth germs, prolonged retention of primary teeth, localized pathologic lesions, and shortening of the length of the arch.

Any tooth can be impacted, but the teeth involved most frequently are the mandibular third molar, maxillary cuspid, maxillary third molar, mandibular and maxillary second premolars, and maxillary central incisor, in that order. The cause varies greatly with the tooth.

4.4.2.4.1. Diagnosis

Impaction is diagnosed most frequently and easily when a tooth is long delayed in erupting past its normal dental developmental timing. Routine early radiographs are invaluable. Impacted teeth may or may not be in ectopia. Maxillary cuspids, for example, frequently are; mandibular second premolars seldom are. It is important to observe in each case whether the impacted tooth is also misplaced.

4.4.2.4.2. Mandibular third molars

The clinical implications of third molar development and incisal crowding are discussed more thoroughly in Chapters 13 and 21, since **adolescence** is the age at which their prophylactic removal has been advocated. Two important questions are as yet incompletely answered: 1.) Does the eruption of lower third molars cause incisal crowding? and 2.) How does one predict the eruptive positioning of lower third molars? Although eruption of this tooth often is indicted as a primary cause of anterior crowding, one should remember that, even if its eruption is a factor, it cannot exert any effect until the patient is about 16 to 18 years of age. Many problems in lower incisor crowding appear before this time. See Chapter 21 for discussions of current views on the role of mandibular third molars in incisor alignment.

4.4.2.4.3. Maxillary Cuspids

This tooth may be simply impacted, as sometimes happens when the primary cuspid fails to resorb, or the permanent cuspid may be impacted ectopically. Figure 17-34: a maxillary cuspid impacted but not ectopic, and Figure 17-35: a maxillary cuspid both impacted and ectopic.

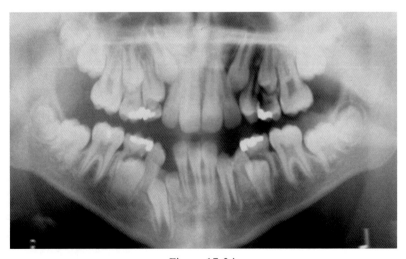

Figure 17-34

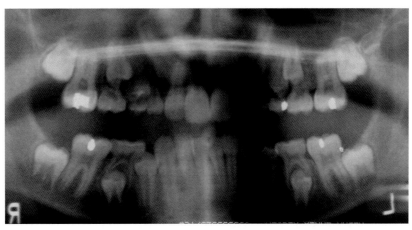

Figure 17-35

4.4.2.4.4. Mandibular and Maxillary Second Premolars

The impaction of these teeth is largely a matter of loss of arch perimeter (Figure 17-36A). They will erupt spontaneously only if the molars are moved distally before the root length of the premolars is too advanced. After their roots are formed, they will no longer erupt spontaneously and traction may need to be applied. Figures 17-36B-C illustrate the treatment result after regaining space and bringing tooth number 20 into arch alignment.

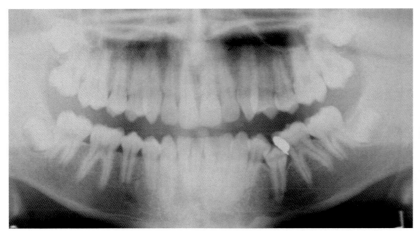

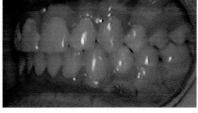

Figure 17-36A   Figure 17-36B

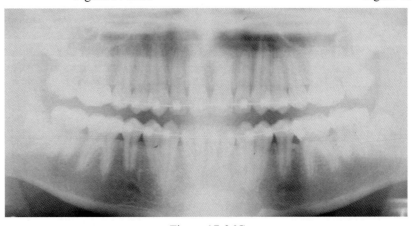

Figure 17-36C

4.4.2.4.5. Second Molars

Mandibular second molars may be impacted or severely malposed (Figure 17-37). One may be caught under the crown of the first molar and become more firmly locked in place if the first molar is uprighted or moved distally in mixed dentition space management.

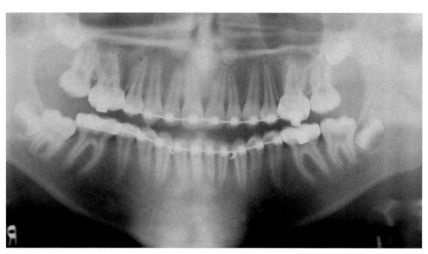

Figure 17-37

When teeth are impacted, the following treatment planning principles should be held in mind: remove interferences to eruption before root formation is completed, hold sufficient space in the arch, and bring appliance forces to bear in a gentle manner.

4.4.2.5. Ankylosed Primary Teeth

Occasionally, a primary molar fails to maintain itself at the level of occlusion (Figure 17-38). This condition has been erroneously called "submergence". Great variations are seen, and although many are of no practical significance, it is not unusual to see a primary molar buried beneath the cervical of adjacent teeth and partially covered by soft tissue. Investigators believe that most "submerged" teeth are **ankylosed** to the alveolar process. Treatment is generally planned as if all such primary molars were ankylosed. When a primary molar becomes ankylosed, there is a localized arrest of eruption and alveolar growth for that tooth; adjacent teeth then proceed to greater occlusal heights. First permanent molars tip mesially over the crown of ankylosed second primary molars.

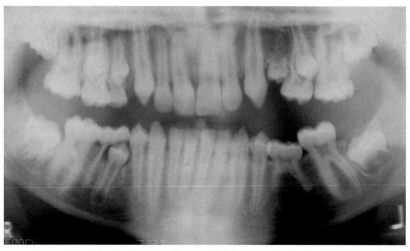

Figure 17-38

In treatment, four situations must be avoided: 1.) loss of **arch length**, 2.) extrusion of teeth in the opposite arch, 3.) interference with the eruption of succeeding permanent teeth, and 4.) loss of alveolar bone during less than judicious extraction, which is the primary factor in the reduction of vertical alveolar bone height.

4.4.2.6. Ankylosed Permanent Teeth

First molars and second molars are the permanent teeth most apt to become **ankylosed** (Figure 17-39). When an ankylosed permanent molar is retained into adulthood, the effects can be devastating, since local vertical alveolar growth has been inhibited. Three courses of action are available: 1.) loosening and repositioning the tooth with forceps; 2.) extraction; and 3.) replacement with implant or transplant. Routine success with the loosening method should not be expected even when a complete **orthodontic appliance** retains the tooth. Figures 17-39A-C illustrate the problem of ankylosed tooth number 30. Tooth number 30 was extracted and Figure 17-39D shows the patient prepared for an implant after orthodontic treatment.

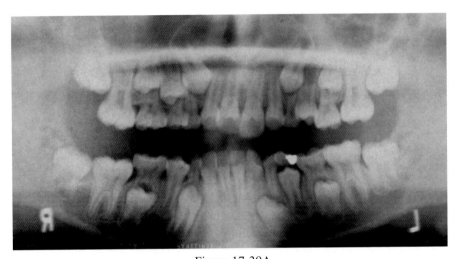

Figure 17-39A

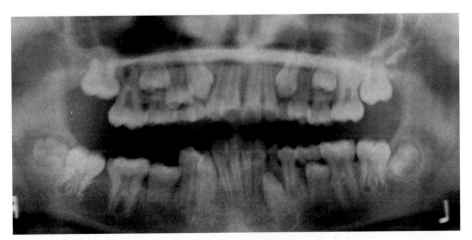

Figure 17-39B

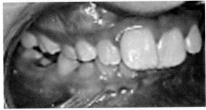

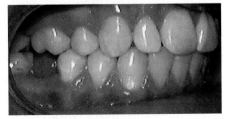

Figure 17-39C   Figure 17-39D

4.5 LATERAL MALRELATIONSHIPS OF DENTAL ARCHES

Failure of the two dental arches to occlude normally in lateral relationship, known as lateral or **posterior crossbite**, may be due to localized problems of tooth position or alveolar growth, or to gross transverse disharmony between the maxilla and the mandible. This condition is common to mouth-breathers and children with persistent oral habits such as thumb and finger sucking. It is also a predictable finding among individuals with vertical growth patterns. It generally presents an inadequate palatal vault and fails to allow favorable positioning of the tongue during rest. It may involve one or more teeth in the lateral segments, and it may be unilateral or bilateral. Regardless of the cause or the severity of the malocclusion, some neuromuscular adjustment of the mandible must occur to provide satisfactory function. Crossbites may originate in the dentition and alveolar process, the craniofacial skeleton, the temporomandibular musculature, or combinations of any of these (See Chapter 7). The importance of lateral malrelationships in the etiology of some temporomandibular disorders must not be overlooked.

4.5.1. Differential Diagnosis

The principal concern of the examiner is to localize precisely where the primary problem lies. Is it confined to the maxilla? Mandible? Both?

4.5.1.1. Transverse Dental Malrelationships

Dental crossbite involving only the localized tipping of a tooth or teeth initially causes little effect on the size or shape of the **basal bone** (Figure 17-40). Usually there is an anterior and/or posterior lateral bite shift present. Typically, the midlines coincide when the jaws are apart and diverge as the teeth come into occlusion. This case shows the opposite, which is due to the fact that the anterior teeth are shifted from normal midline position. Some of the teeth in crossbite will not be centered buccolingually in the alveolar process; therefore, the most important single diagnostic point is to identify the localized asymmetry in the **dentoalveolar arch**.

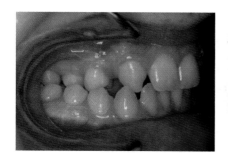 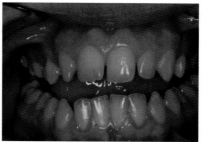 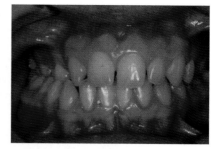

Figure 17-40

4.5.1.2. Muscular or Functional Malrelationships

"Neuromuscular crossbites" display functional adjustment to tooth interferences. They are similar to dental crossbites except that neuromuscular adjustment is more significant than the malpositioning of teeth. A functional analysis of the occlusal relationship provides both the differential diagnosis and identification of the tooth interferences (See Chapter 11). There is no clear-cut differentiation between dental and neuromuscular types of crossbite except, perhaps, in the treatment. In the former (dental), teeth must be moved; in the latter (neuromuscular), occlusal repositioning may be gained by correction of orthopedic jaw relations or by equilibration, of which the second permits reflex changes in mandibular positioning. The pure neuromuscular type is seen most often in young children. Both dental and neuromuscular types require occlusal and muscular adjustments to complete their correction. Although many neuromuscular crossbites in the deciduous dentition are corrected solely with occlusal equilibration, this approach is frequently a failure.

4.5.1.3. Osseous or Skeletal Dysplasia (**Skeletal Crossbite**)

Aberrations in bony growth and/or morphology may give rise to crossbites in two ways: 1.) asymmetric growth of the maxilla or mandible and 2.) lack of agreement in the basic widths of the maxilla and mandible.

Asymmetric growth of the maxilla or mandible may be the result of inherited growth patterns, trauma which impedes the normal growth on the affected side, or a long-standing functional mandibular displacement. Crossbites due to asymmetric bony growth are most difficult to treat, particularly when the condition has advanced unattended for many years. The teeth are moved to provide the best possible occlusion in the circumstances, the maxilla is made wider by a palatal separating appliance, or, in extreme cases, orthognathic surgery is necessary at a later date.

Lack of harmony between the maxillary and mandibular widths usually is due to a bilaterally contracted maxilla. In such cases, muscles usually shift the mandible to one side to acquire a sufficient occlusal contact for maximal intercuspation (Figure 17-41).

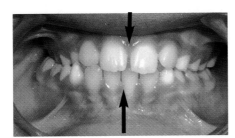 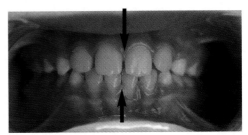

Figure 17-41

A more severe condition is that in which the mandibular denture occludes completely within the maxillary arch. When this mediolateral problem is combined with a skeletal Class II malocclusion, it produces one of the most severe of all malocclusions. In mandibular hypertrophy and prognathism, the mandible is excessively wide for the maxilla as well as unduly long; therefore, a mediolateral occlusal problem exists in addition to the Class III malocclusion.

Study carefully the closure pattern of the mandible, noting at which stage of closure lateral deviations occur. When the lateral shifting occurs late in closure, it usually is the result of dental interferences.

If the deviation of the midlines of the lower and upper face increases throughout opening, the primary fault is likely to be skeletal asymmetry. In cases of bilaterally symmetric dental arches in each jaw with one arch grossly wider than the other, the patient may demonstrate several different closure paths and several occlusal relationships. A posteroanterior cephalogram is desirable in all but the most obvious and simple of the neuromuscular and dental types of posterior crossbite.

4.5.2. Treatment

There is sound clinical research to support the earliest possible treatment of all posterior crossbites (see Suggested Readings).

4.5.2.1. Dental Crossbite (Individual Teeth)

Case Analysis – Rarely is one tooth alone tipped. In most cases, its antagonist in the opposite arch is out of position also. Thus, the maxillary first molar may be tipped lingually and the mandibular first molar is tipped slightly buccally, so both teeth must be moved.

Always measure the amount of space into which the tooth is to be moved. Many individually malposed teeth are wider than the space available for them in the arch. If such is the case, that space must be increased before the crossbite can be corrected.

4.5.2.2. Dentoalveolar Contraction and/or Crossbite

Crossbites in this category usually involve several posterior teeth.

Case Analysis – It is important to learn how much of the condition is due to actual dentoalveolar contraction and how much to neuromuscular adaptive positioning of the mandible (See Chapter 12). The greater the neuromuscular component involved in a case is, the better the prognosis for a stable result.

If the midlines are together when the patient occludes in his or her accustomed position, there usually is very little muscular adaptation, and the case is purely one of narrowing of the maxillary alveolar arch.

If the midlines are not together when the patient occludes in his or her accustomed position, some functional adaptation probably has taken place.

4.5.2.3. Gross Disharmony Between Osseous Bases

Case Analysis – These cases are of two types: one in which the maxilla is relatively narrow and one with excessive maxillary width and/or mandibular narrowness. In either case, the basic problem may be complicated by a skeletal Class II or Class III morphology. Sometimes the cast analysis alone makes obvious where the primary problem lies, but a posteroanterior cephalogram is still a necessity. If a Class II relationship is present, it is important to complete the Class II cephalometric analysis to localize the anteroposterior **dysplasia**. Often the treatment of the mediolateral osseous disharmony is but the first step in a complicated treatment of skeletal Class II morphology. Whatever the condition, early analysis and treatment are advantageous, since this condition is more difficult to handle when growth is near completion. A series of articulated casts mounted with a facebow transfer and functional wax bite may aid in both the cast and cephalometric analysis. Careful evaluation of the cephalograms, mounted models, and **freeway space** may be useful when correction utilizing vertical development of the alveolar process is contemplated.

4.6 CLASS II (DISTOCLUSION, POSTNORMAL OCCLUSION)

The term "Class II" is a generalization which groups together malocclusions of widely varying morphologies. Class II is a common severe malocclusion. When combined with serious space management problems, it becomes a very difficult malocclusion to treat. In Class II, secondary features of the malocclusion are important to the treatment plan. Vertical skeletal dysplasia, muscle dysfunctions, and space for alignment of teeth are frequent complicating factors in Class II.

The following pages constitute a brief outline and are not intended in any way to suggest that Class II malocclusions should be treated routinely in general practice. However, since Class II is the most common severe malocclusion, every dentist must have a correct understanding and perspective for whether a patient should be treated or referred.

4.6.1. Differential Diagnosis

4.6.1.1. Skeletal Morphology

Because of the immense variability within Class II, it is impossible to treat all cases alike. Differential diagnosis is the basis for differential treatment. Therefore, diagnosis includes identification of the discriminating Class II features of the individual case to be treated. A cephalometric analysis is a necessity when diagnosing and planning treatment of Class II malocclusions, and it should facilitate the development of individualized treatment plans though localization and identification of the anatomic regions at fault.

4.6.1.2. Dental and Occlusal Malpositions

The dental aspects of Class II are largely adaptations to the skeletal and muscular pattern, although they may exist alone to such an extent as to produce Class II dental relationships in a balanced facial skeleton. The dental features must be studied in a cephalogram (See Chapter 15) and dental casts (see Chapter 13), as well as in the patient. Occlusal plane malrelationships and vertical dentoalveolar abnormalities often are adaptations to the total skeletal dysplasia.

4.6.1.3. **Arch Form**

In Class II, the maxillary arch is more likely to be narrow and elongated and thus disharmonious with the mandibular **arch form**. Since coordination of the arches is an early and important part of Class II treatment, identification of arch form disharmonies is essential.

4.6.1.4. Neuromuscular ("Functional") Features

The neuromuscular features seen at diagnosis often seem to be largely adaptive to the skeleton and tooth positions typical of Class II malocclusion. The establishment of normal neuromuscular function at the earliest possible time has often been the primary goal of early treatment. Lip positions imposed by the facial skeleton may cause increased labioversion and/or linguoversion of the maxillary and/or mandibular incisors, and they may not be in accordance with each other. Since the lips and tongue must affect an anterior seal during swallowing and in the production of certain speech sounds, their efforts to do so in the presence of a skeletal dysplasia often result in some aggravation of the incisal relationships.

Functional mandibular retraction is a common feature of Class II malocclusion in the primary and mixed dentitions. Other common neuromuscular factors which may accompany the Class II state are mouth-breathing and abnormal tongue activities. Study Chapter 12, Analysis of the **Orofacial** and Jaw Musculature, and Chapter 13, Analysis of the Dentition and Occlusion, to understand and identify the neuromuscular features of Class II problems.

4.6.2. General Strategies for Class II Treatment

Strategy is planning. In this instance, it includes planning how to cope with a Class II malocclusion. Since there are many complicated aspects to Class II malocclusion, a variety of clinical strategies have been developed through the years.

Some of the strategies listed are more appropriate for some Class II types than others. The time at which Class II treatment is begun is critical, and the strategies which can be employed depend on the age of the patient.

  a.) Differential Restraint and Control of Skeletal Growth – The use of extra-oral traction to inhibit maxillary development is a frequent method of treatment for some types of Class II malocclusions.
  b.) Differential Promotion of Skeletal Growth – Some types within Class II are characterized by mandibular deficiency. Clinicians employ functional appliances to attempt to improve or promote mandibular growth and affect the size and shape of the mandible and timing of growth. Figure 17-42 illustrates one example of many types of functional appliances.

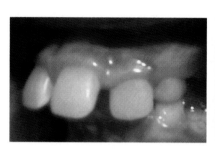 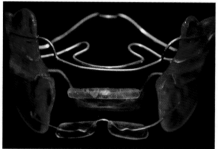 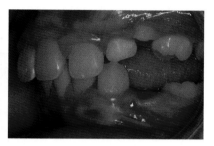

Figure 17-42

c.) **Guidance of Eruption** and Alveolar Development – Malpositions of permanent teeth may be the result of skeletal dysplasia, or the teeth may have been guided into malpositions by the abnormal functioning of lips and tongue. During eruptive development the alveolar process must adapt to the skeletal dysplasia which characterizes Class II, often resulting in greater alveolar height anteriorly than posteriorly, narrowed maxillary **alveolar arches**, and other effects. The clinician may prevent excessive alveolar maldevelopment by guiding and altering the eruption of the teeth and purposely controlling alveolar growth; the permanent teeth often can be guided to better positions during eruption than they would have achieved untreated.

d.) Movement of Teeth and Alveolar Processes – One of the most common strategies of orthodontic treatment is that of moving teeth to reshape the alveolar processes and provide better occlusion. Such tooth movements and alveolar changes are also used to camouflage serious skeletal dysplasias, particularly when skeletal growth is largely completed.

e.) Translation of Parts During Growth – It is possible during growth to change the relationship of skeletal parts. A common procedure illustrates this point. Because a narrow maxilla is frequently found in Class II malocclusions, it is possible to use palate-widening devices, which physically orthopedically separate the mid-palatal suture, moving the halves of the maxilla apart. The space created at the midline of the maxilla fills in with bone, and maxillary and mandibular growth then proceeds more normally than it otherwise would have done, and a more normal and anterior neuromuscular occlusal position is possible.

f.) Training of Muscles – Abnormal muscle function is a frequent and important aspect of the Class II malocclusion and is often a prominent etiologic factor in its development. One of the primary purposes of functional appliances is to optimize the reflex activities of the facial and jaw muscles. Today, myotherapy is infrequently employed as a separate entity from the orthodontic appliance itself.

g.) Surgical Translation of Parts – On occasion the skeletal dysplasia is so severe that orthodontic treatment alone cannot correct the problem, and orthognathic surgery is then employed in conjunction with orthodontic treatment. Such surgical procedures are usually carried out after growth is essentially completed (See Chapter 19).

Because control of unfavorable growth is a prominent feature of Class II strategy, it is obvious that the methods employed for early treatment are different than those used during **adolescence**, when skeletal growth is waning, and adulthood, when growth is mostly completed.

4.6.3. Tactics for Class II Therapy

Strategy is planning; **tactics** involve management and execution. In orthodontic treatment, **tactics** means the use of orthodontic appliances, although this term also includes removal of etiologic factors and myotherapy.

4.6.3.1. **Functional Appliances** (Functional Jaw Orthopedic Appliances)

Functional appliances are employed to alter the neuromuscular environment of the developing dentition and masticatory muscles. They are also used to disarticulate teeth, to promote mandibular growth, guide the eruption of the permanent teeth, and differentially control alveolar development, among other things.

4.6.3.2. **Orthopedic Devices**

In orthodontic usage the word "orthopedic" presents the idea of physically promoting changes in the shape or position of the craniofacial skeleton.

4.6.3.2.1. **Extra-oral Traction** to the Dentition

Extra-oral forces may be applied to control the position of the maxillary dentition, to restrain or promote maxillary corpus growth, or to move the maxillary teeth mesially or distally. Vertical dentoalveolar development can also be affected. Similar extra-oral traction appliances are sometimes employed to move mandibular teeth as well.

4.6.3.2.2. **Extra-oral Traction** to the Chin

Extra-oral forces are applied vertically by means of a chin cup to diminish the development of anterior face height, a feature of Class II malocclusions with vertical overdevelopment.

4.6.3.2.3. **Palatal Widening**

Palatal widening appliances are used to translate the maxillary halves physically in order to improve their positions and affect subsequent growth of the skeleton and teeth.

4.6.3.3. **Bracketed Appliances**

Banded and bonded orthodontic appliances are commonly used to improve the positions of teeth and to reshape the alveolar processes (coordinate the arches).

4.6.3.4. **Muscle Training**

Myotherapy is an adjunctive treatment tactic in Class II therapy involving a retraining of the way the orofacial musculature works. It should not be forgotten that functional appliances are providers of myotherapy.

4.6.3.5. **Orthognathic Surgery**

Orthognathic surgery offers immediate translation of parts of the severely dysgnathic craniofacial skeleton. Orthognathic surgical procedures have become highly developed and are an important part of orthodontic treatment for severe skeletal Class II problems, but their use is generally limited to near adulthood and adulthood (See Chapter 19).

4.6.4. Rationale for Early Class II Treatment

4.6.4.1. Skeletal Morphology

A goal of early Class II skeletal treatment is to achieve a more favorable skeletal morphology prior to the complete eruption of the permanent dentition. Therapy aims at restraint of midface growth, promotion of mandibular growth, widening of the maxilla, control of dentoalveolar adaptation, or planned combinations of these strategies. The approach is based more on the particular details of the patient's own skeletal morphology than the appliance. In **adolescence**, it is difficult to compensate for the vertical skeletal aspects of Class II with tooth movements. They may be improved in earlier years by controlling the basal skeletal growth and by differential management of the alveolar processes and occlusal plane.

Since there are distinct sexual differences in the timing of the pubescent growth spurt and in the cessation of craniofacial growth (See Chapters 11 and 15), the rationale for skeletal Class II therapy varies with gender: females generally are treated earlier. The tendency in males for craniofacial growth to continue past the second decade of life is a complicating factor, irrespective of the time treatment was begun. Logic and the same clinical research evidence support the use of early skeletal Class II treatment, since achieving a balanced skeletal profile prior to the eruption of most permanent teeth minimizes the need for tooth movements.

4.6.4.2. Dental and Occlusal Aspects

The first of the dental aims of early Class II treatment is to obtain normal molar and incisal relationships and establish normal occlusal function prior to the eruption of the cuspids, premolars, and second permanent molars. If these aims are achieved in concert with skeletal correction, the arrival of the remaining teeth usually results in good occlusal function and an occlusal plane better related to the profile. Early reduction of excessive labioversion of incisors creates functional incisal stops, helping to control the occlusal plane. It also reduces the chances of their accidental fracture and improves aesthetics and lip function.

In Class II there often is disharmony between the upper and lower arch forms. A second dental aim is widening the maxillary arch form, thereby aiding incisal retraction, improving occlusal function, easing anteroposterior skeletal correction and improving occlusal relations.

Distinct sexual differences exist in the eruption of teeth and in the amount of space available for alignment of teeth. Teeth erupt earlier in females and generally have less space for alignment due to smaller arches.

Exact protocols for early treatment of the dental features of Class II malocclusion include the following points differentially according to skeletal features: 1.) distal rotation, tipping, and movement of the maxillary molars to correct the Class II molar relationship, a procedure that may open the bite and lengthen the maxillary arch perimeter, 2.) restraint of the maxillary dentition while the midface grows forward, thus changing the relative position of the maxillary dentition to its base, 3.) retraction and intrusion of maxillary incisors reducing the **dentoalveolar protrusion**, producing normal incisor function, and improving lip and tongue movements, and 4.) control of the mandibular arch perimeter and fitting of the mandibular incisors to the skeletal profile, **functional occlusal plane**, and maxillary incisors.

4.6.4.3. Neuromuscular Features

Early treatment of the neuromuscular aspects of Class II malocclusion is undertaken to establish a normal neuromuscular environment that will aid function and growth and neither aggravate nor distort the developing skeletal pattern. Such therapy often consists of control of deleterious habits and treatment of the skeletal and dental features in order that normal neuromuscular function can dominate. Sometimes, in the primary dentition, the neuromuscular pattern is the dominant Class II theme, for example, nasorespiratory or airway problems, a faulty oral posture, or sucking habits.

The aims for treating the neuromuscular features of Class II in the mixed dentition are similar; however, the permanent molars and incisors must be corrected. In Class II malocclusions without severe skeletal features, correction of the dental symptoms alone may restore near-normal function of the neuromusculature. In other cases, primarily those with a severe skeletal pattern, it is much harder to achieve adaptation and conditioning of the muscles, and myotherapy may be a useful part of the therapy. In such cases, this will need to be continued throughout the retention period. This point underlies the rationale for the use of functional jaw orthopedic appliances as retainers in some cases, as these appliances aid in skeletal, dental, and neuromuscular correction. The establishment of normal neuromuscular function at the earliest possible age is one of the most important steps in treatment of Class II malocclusions.

4.6.5. Planning Differential Early Treatment of Class II malocclusion

Most Class II malocclusions are first seen by the family dentist or pediatric dentist. This brief outline of Class II treatment is provided to give a general background and an understanding of the principles involved. It will aid in 1.) the recognition and grouping of cases according to their significant differences, 2.) the concept of referring or treating as soon as the problem is recognized, 3.) providing explanations to the parents and patients, and 4.) being able to work as a team member with a specialist who might be treating the case. It is also intended to be of benefit in the selection of cases for treatment and in the recognition of the more difficult problems.

In the United States of America there has been an enthusiastic interest in Class II treatment by the non-orthodontic specialist. This enthusiasm has been prompted largely by the promotion of appliances often without sufficient accompanying teaching of diagnosis and craniofacial growth.

No pretense of depth is intended but only a brief, correct orientation toward standard clinical practice for the correction of Class II malocclusion. It is presented primarily as an orderly introduction to the various concepts and strategies employed in treatment of various Class II problems.

Thus we have defined clinical Class II types for several reasons:

-To group cases with similar needs for ease in planning strategies and tactics.

-To locate the site(s) of skeletal imbalance

-To estimate the effects of growth on the present imbalanced form. (Growth alone will not correct a Class II problem; it often exacerbates the problem.)

-To determine the appropriate treatment for the special needs of a particular case. Many treatments may improve a characteristic disorder, but which is optimal? (See 1981 article for details of differential diagnosis of Class II cases. Also, see Handbook of Orthodontics, 4th Ed., 1988, Yearbook Medical Publishers, by R. E. Moyers and M. L. Riolo. Also, see Chapter 15 of Handbook for more details on tactics.)

4.7 CLASS III, MESIOCLUSION, AND PSEUDO CLASS III

Three rather distinct types of malocclusion may all appear to be mesioclusions. True Angle Class III, or mesioclusion, is a skeletal dysplasia involving mandibular hypertrophy, marked shortening of the midface, or a combination of these two. The pseudo-, or apparent, Class III is a positional malrelationship; a reflex functional mandibular protraction in Figures 17-43A-E. A third condition, simple **linguoversion** of one or more maxillary anterior teeth, is an abnormal axial inclination of maxillary incisors with no real Class III features. It will be noted that the first condition is a problem of skeletal morphology and osseous growth, the second an acquired muscular reflex, and the third a problem in dental positioning. In all three conditions, the maxillary anterior teeth are behind the mandibular teeth, but only the first two present with the mandibular molars ahead of their normal position. The third condition, linguoversion of maxillary anterior teeth, is a Class I malocclusion discussed later in this chapter. The first two are discussed together here for clarification of the differential diagnosis.

4.7.1. Differential Diagnosis

4.7.1.1 Patient Examination

The differentiation of true and pseudomesioclusion requires a precise examination of the patient for the following items.

4.7.1.2. Profile

Study the profile carefully for evidence of the effects of the skeletal dysplasia on the soft tissues and facial musculature. The lip relationship during occlusion and mandibular posture is particularly revealing, for the profile improves as the mandible drops from occlusal contact relationship to the postural position only for the pseudo-Class III patient. In Figures 17-43A you see the extraoral photos that demonstrate the short lower face height and overclosed Class III profile; Figure 17-43B the intraoral photos that demonstrate the anterior crossbite and deep overbite; Figure17-43C demonstrates the phase I post-treatment facial photos with a short lower face height; Figure 17-43D with the expanded upper arch during which three of the anterior teeth corrected to a normal relationship; Figure 17-43E illustrates four anterior teeth in a normalized relationship.

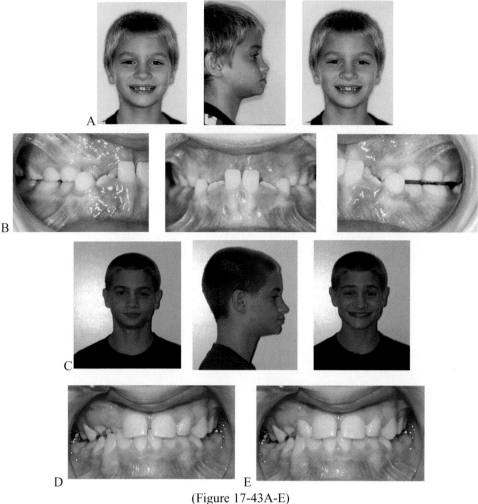

(Figure 17-43A-E)

Skeletal Class III cases are less likely to have a functional shift during closure. Translation of the mandible forward in pseudomesioclusion can be confirmed by gently placing the fingertips over the temporomandibular joint during opening and closure.

4.7.1.3. Molar Relationship

Note the relative positions of the first molars both in occlusion and in the postural position.

-True Class III – A distinct Class III relationship persists in both positions.

-Pseudo Class III – There is apt to be a shift from a Class I to a Class III relationship as the mandible closes. Manipulate the mandible posteriorly to ascertain if it is possible to assume a more normal relationship with the maxilla. Read carefully the section on crossbites, for pure pseudomesioclusions are in reality **anterior crossbites** sometimes involving maxillary narrowness plus an occlusally prompted forward positioning of the mandible. Mild cases of skeletal Class III may have a functional element, particularly in young children; therefore, the cephalometric analysis is critical.

b.) Cephalometric Analysis – The purposes of the cephalometric analysis (see Chapter 15) are: 1.) to separate pseudo from true Class III malocclusions, 2.) to identify the specific morphologic features of any skeletal dysplasia, since discriminate characteristics determine the specific strategies and tactics of treatment, and 3.) to ascertain the relative importance of skeletal and functional features when they are combined. The cephalometric analysis, more than any other single diagnostic procedure, aids in determining the timing of treatment and indicates the choice of appliances.

Obtain lateral cephalograms in the usual occlusal (intercuspal) and postural positions, as well as the posteroanterior view.

1.) Profile Analysis, Skeletal – The Profile Analysis (See Chapters 11 and 15) enables one to localize skeletal and dentoalveolar contributions to the Class III profile.

2.) Vertical Analysis – The Vertical Analysis is often critical in skeletal Class III since it reveals dentoalveolar adaptations to the basic skeletal pattern.

4.7.1.4. Pseudo Class III

The pseudo Class III shows normal values for the Basic Morphologic Analysis, when one has discounted the functional mandibular translation. This may be done by taking a lateral cephalogram with the mandible held in the retruded contact position by a bite registration *in situ*. Mildly deficient values for the maxillary dentoalveolar unit distance may be seen in the profile analysis, and the maxillary incisors may be more upright than normal. The vertical analysis will be normal.

4.7.1.5. Skeletal Class III

There are three basic categories of skeletal Class III malocclusion: midface deficiency, **mandibular prognathism**, and a combination of the two.

4.7.1.6. Midface Deficiency

Patients with Class III midface deficiency display a Class III maxillo-mandibular relationship, a diminished **cranial base** – maxilla value and normal cranial base – mandible values. The profile analysis usually shows shortened maxillary skeletal unit and maxillary dentoalveolar unit distances. The mandibular skeletal unit distance is near normal, but the mandibular dentoalveolar unit distance may be slightly above normal. A midface deficiency can be treated with facemask protraction and Class I forces from the facemask to the hooks on an upper fixed appliance (Figure 17-44).

4.7.1.7. Mandibular Prognathism

Patients with mandibular prognathism show a Class III maxillo-mandibular relationship, and excessive cranial base – mandible dimension both horizontally and vertically, and may show a diminished cranial base angle. Both the mandibular skeletal unit distance and mandibular dentoalveolar unit distance are excessive. In severe cases, the maxillary dentoalveolar unit distance may also be excessive as the maxillary teeth tip labially to obtain function with the mandibular incisors, which have been carried forward by the excessive mandibular length. A vertical analysis is critical in mandibular prognathism. Anterior face height is usually excessive when compared with posterior face height, particularly in the lower anterior third of the face. Mandibular prognathism is sometimes seen without excessive anterior face height (i.e., the mandibular border is not steeply positioned).

4.7.1.8. Midface Deficiency and Mandibular Prognathism

Some patients show a combination of mild midface deficiency and mild mandibular prognathism, for which treatment differs from that required by either the pure midface deficiency or mandibular prognathism. The prognosis usually is not as poor as for the serious mandibular prognathism.

4.7.2. General Strategies for Early Treatment

Treatment strategies for the three types of Class III malocclusion are quite clear and different. For pseudo-Class III, one's aim is to obtain normal dental and occlusal relationships by prompting a normal neuromuscular environment for a normally developing craniofacial skeleton. Cases of skeletal Class III with midface deficiency require midface orthopedic traction to promote maxillary growth forward to match a more normally placed mandible. Patients with mandibular prognathism must have the excessive growth redirected when practical. Cases combining the features of midface deficiency and mandibular prognathism require combined strategies.

4.7.3. Rationale for Early Treatment

Some research evidence shows that it is possible to alter and redirect the growth of the craniofacial skeleton in early Class III conditions.

4.7.4. Tactics for Early Treatment

4.7.4.1. Pseudo-Class III

Figure 17-44

In the early dentition, the patient sometimes can be treated by equilibration or by the use of a **removable appliance** (Figure 17-44A). The removable appliance acts as an extension of the lower incisal edges, contacting the lingual surfaces of the maxillary anterior teeth. On closing, the mandible is forced to be retruded, and the maxillary anterior teeth, if they are tipped lingually, will be moved labially. The bevel of the appliance should be ground very carefully so that all teeth contact evenly and the load is well distributed to avoid trauma. Another option is the use of a maxillary removable appliance with a posterior bite plane to open the bite and finger springs to the teeth in need of crossbite correction (Figure 17-44B). If marked improvement is not seen quickly, the case should be reassessed, for the original diagnosis probably was erroneous or the patient is not wearing the appliance full time. This appliance has limited use, but in selected cases it is advantageous.

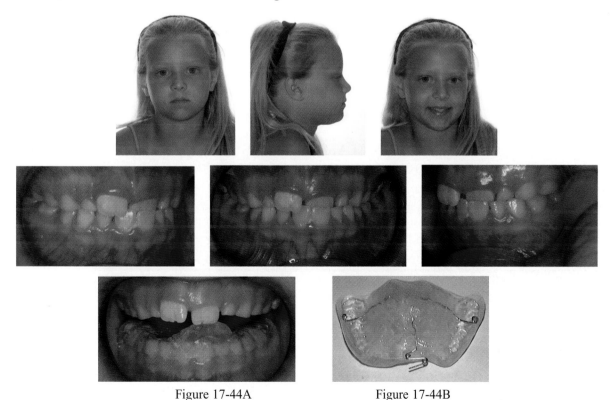

Figure 17-44A   Figure 17-44B

4.7.4.2. Midface Deficiency

Even mild midface deficiency should be diagnosed in the primary or very early mixed dentition.

Treatment is typically indicated at that time also. Frequently, maxillary palatal expansion with or without facemask protraction is indicated. Immediately after the maxillary midline suture has been fractured during orthopedic expansion, the maxilla is also amenable to forward movement if a sufficient force is rendered. The facemask is capable of delivering such a forward movement and there are some less bulky intraoral appliances that can have a similar effect. This proves to be very effective for the mild midface deficiencies. Placing braces on the lower arch for heavy Class III mechanics is not viable, since the few mandibular teeth that are present would respond by tipping toward the lingual. It is debatable as to whether or not early treatment is recommended in the severe skeletal Class III. In many cases, worsening the compensatory changes at an early age increases the pre-surgical orthodontic need later.

4.7.4.3. Mandibular Prognathism

Patients with mandibular prognathism require appliance therapy that is quite different from that used for midface deficiency. Graber has reported that chin cup treatment utilizing heavy extraoral traction rotates the mandible posteriorly, decreases the **gonial angle**, restricts vertical condylar growth, and causes the corpus of the maxilla to rotate slightly clockwise. The result is an improvement in the A – B relationship of the skeletal profile and change in the articular angle and in the orientation of the ramus to the cranial base. Woodside reports success with functional appliances – showing similar effects horizontally but transferring some of the expected mandibular horizontal growth in a more vertical direction. With either chin cup or **activator** therapy the dentoalveolar development is altered both vertically and horizontally in order that alveolar process adaptations may help mask the skeletal dysplasia. The more significant the mandibular prognathism, the poorer the prognosis and the more likely the patient is headed toward an orthognathic surgical treatment plan; therefore, caution should be used in any early treatment.

4.7.4.4. Midface Deficiency and Mandibular Prognathism

Skeletal Class III patients showing both midface deficiency and mandibular prognathism may be improved by face mask therapy, and in the mandible by either chin cup or functional appliance therapy. Devices which combine chin cup traction and midface protraction are appropriate for some cases.

4.8 LABIOVERSION OF MAXILLARY INCISORS (EXCESSIVE OVERJET) WITH CLASS I MOLAR RELATIONSHIP

This condition seems similar to a Class II **maxillary dentoalveolar protrusion** malocclusion, since the anterior teeth of the maxilla are in labioversion; the maxillary posterior teeth, however, remain in near Class I occlusion. There is a good facial skeletal morphology, otherwise a greater Class II molar relationship would have resulted. The cause may have been a thumb- or finger-sucking habit, so the condition may be accompanied by a dentoalveolar open bite and maxillary narrowness (See Figure 18-9) It also is found with a deep overbite due to overeruption of the maxillary and mandibular incisors.

4.8.1. Diagnosis

This condition must be carefully differentiated from a skeletal Class II, Division I malocclusion in which the lower teeth may have drifted forward, causing anterior crowding yet maintaining a Class I molar relationship.

4.8.2. Treatment

If there is an active tongue-thrust, abnormal tongue posture, or finger-sucking habit, generally the first step in treatment is to attempt to differentially diagnose and correct the habit. It is noted that it may be easier to correct some habits such as finger habits than other habits such as primary tongue thrusts or tongue posture problems, which may be extremely difficult to correct.

4.9 ANTERIOR CROSSBITES, SIMPLE

Simple anterior crossbites are dental malocclusions resulting from abnormal axial inclinations of maxillary anterior teeth. They must be clearly differentiated from mesioclusions, which they may seem to resemble. The simple anterior crossbite has many other names (e.g., "locked-in" incisors and "scissors bite"). The use of the word "simple" implies that some anterior crossbites are more complicated, and they are, particularly those which accompany a Class III malocclusion or are part of a skeletal deep bite. Not all anterior crossbites are "simple"!

4.9.1. Diagnosis

The molar relationship should be noted carefully in the postural **rest position** and in occlusion. If a Class II or Class III relationship is seen at either position, the problem is not a simple anterior crossbite, for the latter is solely a matter of lingually tipped maxillary anterior teeth, without serious disruption of the molar relationship. A cephalometric analysis is always needed. Simple anterior crossbites may involve one or more teeth.

4.9.2 Treatment

4.9.2.1. Single Tooth

A single anterior tooth in crossbite may be brought into alignment easily, provided there is space in the arch for it. If there is not, space must be created before tipping the offending tooth labially. When there is sufficient space, the tooth may be brought directly into line.

An acrylic inclined plane, shown in Figure 17-45A, is effective. It must be adjusted carefully and not left in place unduly long (View Figure 17-44A for pretreatment photos).

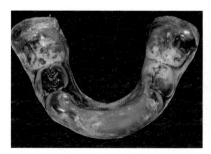 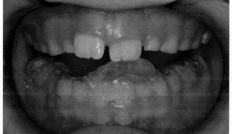 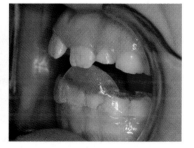

Figure 17-45A

4.9.2.2. Several Teeth

Treatment of several teeth in crossbite requires the observance of the same fundamentals needed for a single tooth. Lingual archwires with auxiliary springs are effective. Labial archwires and banded anterior teeth are also excellent. The inclined plane appliance is sometimes recommended. While an aid in "jumping the bite," the inclined plane alone would be inefficient for a complete correction. Further, the act of flaring teeth by putting them into traumatic occlusion, as the inclined plane does, can be hazardous to the periodontium. An acrylic posterior bite plane with finger springs as seen in Figure 17-

46A may be used for a single incisor or a few incisors in need of crossbite correction. Figures 17-46B and C shows the successful treatment with this type of appliance.

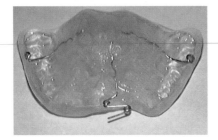
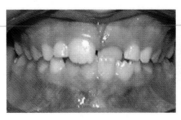
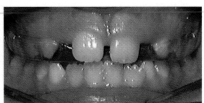

Figure 17-46A   Figure 17-46B   Figure 17-46C

4.10 BIMAXILLARY PROTRUSIONS

4.10.1. Bimaxillary Prognathism

Bimaxillary prognathism must be differentiated from **bimaxillary dental protrusion**.

Bimaxillary prognathism is a skeletal problem in which both maxilla and mandible have a relationship more forward than normal with respect to the cranium and cranial base. In true bimaxillary prognathism, both the maxilla and the mandible are forward with respect to the **anterior cranial base**, and the axial inclinations of the teeth are nearer normal than in bimaxillary dental protrusion. There are distinct ethnic variations in the normal position and size of both the maxilla and mandible. Typically, African-Americans of North America have a normal maxillo-mandibular skeletal relationship which, by North American Caucasian standards, might be termed "bimaxillary prognathism" (See Chapter 13). The same may be true for other ethnic groups.

Because bimaxillary prognathism is a problem in the basic morphology and growth pattern of the bony skeleton, interception is not a very satisfactory strategy. A common mistake is made when the basic skeletal morphology is not recognized and attempts are made to impose a dentoalveolar profile, which proves to be too "flat" on the overall facial profile with both the maxilla and mandible abnormally forward. Lip and soft tissue adaptation then may be not as pleasing as anticipated.

4.10.2. Bimaxillary Dental Protrusion

Bimaxillary dental protrusion is **procumbency** of both dentitions on the bony bases and must be discriminated from bimaxillary prognathism. There may be familial tendencies, as in bimaxillary prognathism, but bimaxillary dental protrusion can also arise from mesial drifting of the teeth in both arches. The condition also is seen when larger than normal teeth are found in conjunction with normal or smaller than normal osseous bases. Bimaxillary dental protrusion may not be treated very effectively at an early age.

4.11 OPEN BITE

4.11.1. Definition

Open bite is the failure of a tooth or teeth to meet antagonists in the opposite arch (See Figure 18-9). During the normal course of eruption, it is expected that the teeth and their supportive alveolar bone will develop until occlusal antagonists are met. Any interference with the normal course of eruption and alveolar development may result in an open bite. The causes of open bite generally may be grouped under four headings (see Chapter 7): 1.) disturbances in the eruption of the teeth and alveolar growth, for example, ankylosed primary molars, 2.) mechanical interference with eruption and alveolar growth, such as a finger-sucking habit or lip and tongue posture, 3.) constricted maxilla, and 4.) vertical skeletal dysplasia. The last, though seen less frequently, is a quite different and much more difficult problem.

Unfortunately, there are two current definitions of open bite. Throughout this book, the term "open bite" means the lack of functional antagonistic teeth. This definition is not only functionally correct, it is more pragmatic.

4.11.2. Diagnosis

The definition of open bite is, in a sense, the diagnosis, but to plan treatment one needs to learn the etiology and to localize precisely the extent of the inadequate vertical development. We may divide open bites into 1.) simple open bites, those confined to the teeth and alveolar process; and 2.) complex open bites, those based on primary vertical skeletal dysplasia – the so-called "skeletal open bites" – which are more varied and much more difficult to treat.

When vertical cephalometric analyses (See Chapter 15) reveal no abnormal measurements and the sole problem is the failure of some teeth to erupt into occlusion, the condition is termed simple open bite.

When a vertical cephalometric analysis reveals disharmonies in the skeletal components of anterior face height (e.g., very short upper face height, or total anterior face height disproportionately long relative to the total posterior face height), dentoalveolar vertical development sometimes cannot cope with the skeletal morphology well enough to guarantee anterior functional occlusal stops. This disorder is termed complex or a skeletal open bite. In a simple open bite alveolar adaptation cannot or does not take place; in a complex open bite alveolar adaptation does take place, but it cannot be sustained.

4.11.3. Treatment

4.11.3.1 **Anterior Open Bite**, Simple

When studying **anterior open bites** before treatment, take care to note the relationship of the osseous bases to the dentition. Preoccupation with the dentoalveolar aspects of the open bite may lead one to overlook a more basic skeletal problem. Always suspect a habit of some sort when an open bite is first seen, since the majority of simple anterior open bites are caused by digital sucking habits or abnormal tongue posture. If, during eruption, the teeth repeatedly encounter a finger, thumb, or tongue, eruption is impeded and an open bite results.

In young children, treatment generally consists of controlling the habit, which alone may be sufficient to permit the teeth to erupt to normal positions. Retention, after treatment, of any malocclusion due to a sucking habit is almost impossible unless the habit is overcome completely and normal lip and tongue function are restored.

Often the best way to break the habit is to correct the open bite itself. This is certainly true for a simple **tongue thrust** that is maintaining an open bite created by an earlier sucking habit.

4.11.3.2. Posterior Open Bite, Simple

Open bites in the posterior region are rare in young children and usually result from a lack of vertical alveolar development, either ankylosed primary molars or "idiopathic failure to erupt". Lateral "tongue-thrusts" are largely tongue postures adaptive to an open bite resulting from another cause. A common example illustrates the point. Ankylosed primary molars result in a localized cessation of alveolar development, creating a **posterior open bite**. The tongue must spread laterally to seal the open bite space during reflex swallowing. When the primary teeth are removed, the tongue's continued lateral swallowing movements may impede the eruption of the premolars.

Primary failure of secondary teeth to erupt may also be the cause of a localized open bite that may be present either anteriorly or posteriorly. The tooth at fault may also affect neighboring teeth. It is important to establish which tooth is at fault before exacerbating the problem by moving unaffected teeth in the direction of the affected tooth.

4.11.3.3. Complex or Skeletal Open Bite

Complex or skeletal open bite is a symptom of a variety of serious skeletal dysplasias including such varied morphologies as Class II, vertical type 1 (steep **mandibular plane** or excessive anterior total face height), mandibular prognathism, and several of the craniofacial syndromes (e.g., Downs' Syndrome). The most frequently encountered skeletal open bite is that with an upward tipped palatal plane and inadequate development of anterior upper face height (see Suggested Reading List, Moyers, et al., 1981). Skeletal contributions to open bite are often overlooked in young children, which is unfortunate, since the later they are discovered the more difficult the treatment. One reason early or incipient skeletal open bite is unnoticed is the insensitivity of many cephalometric analyses to any but the most gross vertical dysplasias.

A few clinical guidelines and principles are helpful.

- The earliest possible diagnosis is essential because the condition is not self-correcting and usually worsens with time.
- Removal of all possible etiologic factors as soon as diagnosed is important. Consultation with the pediatrician or otolaryngologist may be important. When referring the patient to the physician, send along the cephalogram and a summary of your cephalometric findings. When you document the case well, understanding and cooperation is usually assured.
- Since these cases may be very difficult and require prolonged and varied appliance therapy, they challenge the experience and skills of the best orthodontists.

4.12 DEEP BITE (EXCESSIVE OVERBITE OR VERTICAL OVERLAP)

4.12.1. Definition

A wide range of incisal overlap is seen with normal posterior occlusal relations. Depth of bite becomes a defined clinical problem when occlusal or temporomandibular function is, or may become, impaired and when facial aesthetics is harmed. The depth of bite must be related to the health of the soft and supporting structures, temporomandibular function, and may affect future dental and skeletal growth. Incisors in labioversion may seem to have normal overbite, but their correction by simple tipping may produce a deeper bite. Therefore, deep bite as a clinical problem is not defined in terms of millimeters but in light of future changes of aesthetics and function.

Closed bite (excessive overbite resulting from loss of posterior teeth), only rarely seen in young children, must not be confused with deep bite.

4.12.2. Diagnosis

The factors contributing to excessive overbite vary with the type of occlusion. Their determination is the most important step in diagnosis. Excessive overbite is not to be viewed as an isolated entity. It must be seen as a part of the total malocclusion. In good occlusions, the amount of overbite is determined largely by dental factors, that is, crown length, root angulation, and tooth position. In Class I malocclusion the depth of bite is controlled by dental factors, for example, length of the crowns of the incisors, elevation of the maxillary first molars, and the angle between the long axes of the central incisors as well as by skeletal features. However, in Class II relationships, the skeletal morphology dominates dental features. Diminished anterior lower face height and shortened ramus height, in particular, dominate the dental factors mentioned above. Consequently, depth of bite is usually more difficult to correct and retain in Class II than in Class I malocclusion. Cast analysis alone or observations based solely on the occlusal position are insufficient. A proper cephalometric analysis and determination of the interocclusal freeway space are necessary.

The amount of freeway space is a critical factor in prognosis (See Chapters 11, 12, 13 and 15). When there is a larger than normal distance between the postural and the intercuspal (usual occlusal) position, greater opportunities exist for correction by guiding vertical alveolar development. Study the freeway space carefully (an MPI may be appropriate in some cases) (refer to Chapter 11).

A detailed vertical cephalometric analysis is required (see Chapter 14), but many cephalometric analyses do not discriminate vertical details well. Proper treatment planning depends on specific localization of skeletal contributions to the deep bite.

4.12.3. Treatment

When an excessive overbite is seen in the primary dentition, it is likely to have a skeletal basis. **Activator** type appliances may be used to direct differential alveolar growth, reduce the interocclusal distance, and improve skeletal morphology.

If the overbite seems excessive in the mixed dentition when there is a Class I molar relationship and normal skeletal morphology, it usually is due to one or more of the following related factors:

-Overdevelopment vertically of the incisal regions,
-Inadequate elevation of the maxillary first molars (i.e., the **anatomic crown** of the molar has not erupted to its full **clinical crown** height).
-Failure to recognize a normal stage of development. The overbite is greater just after eruption of the permanent incisors and decreases with eruption of the posterior teeth.

None of these factors requires heroic orthodontic treatment. Eruption of the first molars can be aided by appliance therapy and the incisors depressed as necessary. Appliances may help, too, if the curve of Spee is excessive. The functional jaw orthopedic appliances are suited to direct vertical skeletal development and to control adaptive alveolar growth in Class I deep bite as well as Class II deep bite disorders.

With a Class II molar relationship, treatment of overbite should be directed to the total Class II problem. Understanding of the different vertical types within Class II helps one in planning therapy. The choice of appliances is largely determined by the type of Class II malocclusion, but functional appliances are advantageous for early treatment of deep bites with retruded shorter mandibles. The more severe the skeletal aspects of the deep bite, the more there is to be gained by early treatment.

4.13 CRANIOFACIAL MALFORMATIONS

Although gross craniofacial deformities appear rarely, each instance poses enormous problems in clinical management for the surgeon and orthodontist (see chapters 2 and 20). Babies with severe congenital malformations require immediate surgical, medical, and dental attention of a very specialized nature. Troubled parents turn instinctively to the family pediatrician and dentist for advice. Ordinarily, abnormalities are not the responsibility of the family dentist, but the dentist has the obligation to send the parent to a craniofacial anomalies center (sometimes called a **cleft palate** team or center), for the team approach is essential for these children. Center teams are made up of clinicians from many fields sharing research and treatment responsibilities and individualizing the therapy for each child. Surgeons, speech therapists, pediatric dentists, orthodontists, psychologists, and prosthodontists are all involved in planning the combined treatment. However, the speech therapist and orthodontist will spend the most time in corrective work and guiding the development of more difficult cases.

The most common of the serious congenital deformities is that of cleft lip and/or palate, which occurs in approximately one in 700 North American white children (See Chapters 2 and 20).

It is the responsibility of every family dentist to be thoroughly acquainted with a craniofacial anomaly or cleft palate team long before the need for their services arises. In this way, when advice is sought, the answer is prompt and authoritative.

4.14 TEMPOROMANDIBULAR DYSFUNCTION

4.14.1. Definition

There is increasing evidence that some of the signs and symptoms associated with temporomandibular dysfunction in adults are first seen in young children (see Suggested Readings, and Chapters 11 and 12) and that certain occlusal disorders in childhood predispose to later temporomandibular dysfunction. Accordingly, it is proper to consider temporomandibular dysfunction as an important potential aspect of the development of malocclusion.

5. SUGGESTED READINGS

Understanding Preadolescent Treatment

Baumrind S, Korn EL, Isaacscon RJ, et al: Quantative analysis of the orthodontic and orthopedic effects of maxillary traction. Am J Orthod Dentofacial Orthop 1983; 84;442-465.

Billiet T, Pauw G, Dermaut L: Location of center of resistance of the upper dentition and the nasomaxillary complex. An experimental study. Eur J Orthod 2001; 23:263-273.

Bjerklinn K: Follow-up control of patients with unilateral posterior cross-bite treated with expansion plates or the quad-helix appliance. J Orofac Orthop 200; 61(2):112-124.

Hamilton DC: Very early and early treatment and growth modification utilizing orthopedic/functional concepts. Monograph, 1999.

Hasler R, Ingervall B: The effect of a maxillary lip bumper on tooth positions. Eur J Orthod 2000; 22 (February):25-32.

Klocke A, Drmeddent, Nanda RS, Ghosh J: Muscle activity with the mandibular lip bumper. Am J Orthod Dentofacial Orthop 2000; 117:384-390.

McNamara JA Jr, Brust EW, Riolo ML: Soft tissue evaluation of individuals with an ideal occlusion and a well-balanced face. Esthetics and the Treatment of Facial Form. Center for Human Growth and Development, University of Michigan 1993; 115-146.

Moyers R, van der Linden FPGM, Riolo ML, McNamara JA: Standards of Human Occlusal Development. University of Mich 1974. Center for Human Growth and Development, University of Michigan.

Nanda SK: The Development Basis of Occlusion and Malocclusion. Quintessence Publishing Co., Inc. 1983.

Pinto, Ary Santos, et al: Morphological and positional asymmetries of young children with functional unilateral posterior crossbite. Am J Orthod Dentofacial Orthop 2001; 120:513-520.

Proffit WR, Fields HW. Orthodontic treatment planning: limitations, controversies and special problems. In: Contemporary orthodontics. 3rd ed. St. Louis: Mosby; 2000:271.

Robertsson, Stefan, Mohlin, Bengt; The congenitally missing upper lateral incisor. A retrospective study of orthodontic space closure versus restorative treatment. Eur J Orthod 2000; 22:697-710.

Riolo ML, et al: Facial soft tissue changes during adolescence. Craniofacial Growth During Adolescence. Monograph #20, Center for Human Growth and Development, The University of Michgan, Ann Arbor, Michigan 1986.

Riolo ML, TenHave TR: The effect of different kinds of appliance therapy on the facial soft-tissue profile. Science and Clinical Judgement in Orthodontics. Center for Human Growth and Development, University of Mich 1985; 163-179.

Riolo, M.L., Moyers, R.E., TenHave, T.R., Mayers, C., "Facial Soft Tissue Changes During Adolescence", in Craniofacial Growth During Adolescence, Mongraph #20, Craniofacial Growth Series, Center for Human Growth and Development, The University of Michigan, Ann Arbor, Michigan, 1987

Riolo ML, Ten Have T: The effect of different kinds of appliance therapy on the soft tissue profile, in Vig PS, Ribbens KA (eds), Science and Clinical Judgement in Orthodontics, monograph 19. Craniofacial Growth Series, Ann Arbor, Mich, Center for Human Growth and Development, University of Michigan, 1984.

Riolo ML, Mayers CA, Xianglon Z: The relationship between changing craniofacial growth theories and orthodontic treatment. Craniofacial Growth Theory and Orthodontic Treatment. Center for Human Growth and Development, University of Mich 1989; 187-206.

Riolo ML, Ten Have T: The effect of different kinds of appliances therapy on the soft tissue profile, in Vig PS, Ribbens KA (eds), Science and Clinical Judgement in Orthodontics, monograph 19. Craniofacial Growth Series, Center for Human Growth and Development, University of Michigan, Ann Arbor, Mich.

Warren, John J., et al; Effects of oral habits' duration on dental characteristics in the primary dentition. JADA 2001; 132:1685-1694.

Sato K, Mito T, Mitani H: An accurate method of predicting mandibular growth potential based on bone maturity. Am J Orthop Dentofac 2001; 120:280-286.

Spillane LM, McNamara JA Jr: Maxillary adaptation to expansion in the mixed dentition. Semin Orthod 1995;1(3):76-87.

Thilander B, Rönning O: Introduction to Orthodontics. Langerblads, Karlshamn, Sweden 1995.

Warren, John J., et al; Effects of oral habits' duration on dental characteristics in the primary dentition. JADA 2001; 132:1685-1694.

Potential Goals in Adolescent Treatment

Berger JL, et al: Photographic analysis of facial changes associated with maxillary expansion. Am J Orthod Dentofacial Orthop 1999; 116:563-571.

Potential Goals in Adolescent Treatment

Berger JL, et al: Photographic analysis of facial changes associated with maxillary expansion. Am J Orthod Dentofacial Orthop 1999; 116:563-571.

Clinical Problems and Procedures

Ahsmore JL, et al: A 3-dimensional analysis of molar movement during headgear treatment. Am J Orthod Dentofacial Orthop 2001; 121:18-30.

Baccett T, et al: Treatment and posttreatment craniofacial changes after rapid maxillary expansion and facemask therapy. Am J Orthod Dentofacial Orthop 2000; 118:404412.

Bierderman W: The Problem of the ankylosed tooth. Den Clin North Am 1968; pp 409-424.

Basciftce FA, Karaman AI: Effects of a modified acrylic bonded rapid maxillary expansion appliance and vertical chin cap on dentofacial structures. Angle Orthod 2002; 72(1):61-71.

Bilodeau JE: Class III nonsurgical treatment: A case report. Am J Orthop Dentofac 2000; 118:560-566.

Boyd RL: Clinical assessment of injuries in orthodontic movement of impacted teeth. Am J Orthod Dentofacial Orthop 1982; 82:478-486.

Cameron CG, Franchi L, Baccetti T and Mcnamara JA. Long-term effects of rapid maxillary expansion: a posteroanterior cephalometric evaluation. Am J Orthop Dentofac 2002;121:129-135.

Ciambotti C, et al: A comparison of dental and dentoalveolar changes between rapid palatal expansion and nickel-titanium palatal expansion appliances. Am J Orthop Dentofac 2001; 119:11-20.

Czochrowska EM, Stenvik A. Bjercke B, and Zackrisson BU. Outcome of tooth transplantation: survival and success rates 17-41 years post treatment. Am J Orthop Dentofac 2002;121:110-9.

Dale JG: Guidance of occlusion: serial extraction. In Graber TM, Swain BF (eds), Orthodontics, Current Principles and Techniques, St Louis, CV Mosby, 1985.

Deguchi T, et al: Craniofacial features of patients with Class III abnormalities: Growth-related changes and effects of short-term and long-term chincup therapy. Am J Orthop Dentofac 2002; 121:84-92.

Dahan JS, Lelong O, Celant S: Oral perception in tongue thrust and other oral habits: Am J Orthop Dentofac 2000; 118:385-391.

Dahan JS, Lelong O Celant S, Leysen V: Oral perception in tongue thrust and other oral habits. Am J Orthop Dentofac 2000. 118:385-391.

Færøvig E, Zachrisson BU: Effects of mandibular incisor extraction on anterior occlusion in adults with Class III malocclusion and reduced overbite. Am J Orthop Dentofac 1999; 115:113-124.

Ghafari J, Shofer FS, Jacobsson-Hunt U, Markowitz DL, Laster LL: Headgear versus functional regulator in early treatment of Class II, division 1 malocclusion: a randomized clinical trial. Am J Orthod Dentofacial Orthop 1998; 113(1):51-61.

Gianelly A. Leeway space and the resolution of crowding in the mixed dentition Semin Orthod 1995;1:188-94.

Holm U: Problems of compensative extraction in cases with loss of first permanent molars. Trans Eur Orthod Soc 1970; pp 409-427.

Hotokezaka H, et al: Severe Dental Open Bite Malocclusion with Tongue Reduction after Orthodonic Treatment. Angle Orthod 2001; 71 (3):228-236.

Jacobson A, Evans WG, Preson CB, et al: Mandibular prognathism. Am J Orthop Dentofac 1974; 66:140-171.

Kajiyama K, Murakami T, Suzuki A: Evaluation of the modified maxillary protractor applied to Class III with retruded maxilla in early mixed dentition. Am J Orthop Dentofac 2000; 118:549-558.

Kapust AJ, Sinclair PM, Turley PK. Cephalometric effects of face mask/expansion therapy in Class III children: a comparison of three age groups. Am J Orthop Dentofac 1998; 113:204-12.

Kim, J.C. et al: Cephalometric variables as predictors of Class II treatment outcome. Am J Orthod 2000; 118:636-640.

King GJ, Wheeler TT, McGorray Sp, Aiosa LS, Bloom RM, Taylor MG. Orthodontists' perceptions of the impact of phase 1 treatment for Class II malocclusion on phase 2 needs. J Dent Res 1999;78:1745-53.

Kusnoto J, et al: Orthodontic correction of transverse arch asymmetries. Am J Orthod Dentofacial Orthop 2002; 121:38-44.

Little RM, Wallen TR, Riedel RA: Stability and relapse of mandibular anterior alignment-first premolar extraction cases treated by traditional edgewise orthodontics. Am J Orthod Dentofacial Orthop 1982; 80:349-365.

Lima RMA: Longitudinal study of anteroposterior and vertical changes in skeletal Class II patients treated with Kloehn cervical headgear. Midwest component Edward H. Angle Society of Orthod. Jan 2002 submitted and accepted for publication Angle Orthodontist, July 2002.

Mason C, Papadakou P, Roberts GJ: The radiographic localization of impacted maxillary canines: A comparison of methods. Eur J Orthod 2001; 23(February):25-34.

McLain JB, Profitt WR, Davenport RH: Adjunctive orthodontic therapy in the treatment of juvenile periodontics: report of a case and review of the literature. Am J Orthod Dentofacial Orthop 1983; 83:290-298: The effect of palatal expansion therapy on the periodontal supporting tissues. Am J Orthop Dentofac 1982; 81:12-21.

McNamara JA, Brudon WL: Orthodontic and Orthopedic Treatment in the Mixed Dentition, Needham Press, 2001.

McNeil RW, Joondeph DR: Congenitally absent maxillary lateral incisors: treatment planning considerations. Angle Orthod 1973; 43:24-29.

Miyawaki S, et al: Eruption speed and rate of angulation change of a cyst-associated mandibular second premolar after marsupialization of a dentigerous cyst. Am J Orthod 1999; 116:578-584.

Moffitt, AO. Eruption and function of maxillary third molars after extraction of second molars. The Angle Orthod. 1998;68(2):147-152.

Moyers RE, Riolo ML, Guire KE, et al: Differential diagnosis of Class II malocclusions. Part1. Facial types associated with Class II malocclusions. Am J Orthop Dentofac 1980; 78:477-494.

Northway WM. Anteroposterior arch dimension changes in French Canadian children: a study of the effects of dental caries and premature extractions. Master's Thesis: Universite de Montreal. 1977.

Northway WM. Wainright R, Demirjian A. Effects of premature loss of deciduous molars. Angle Orthod. 1984;54:295-329.

Northway WM, Wainright R. D E Space - a realistic measure of changes in arch morphology: space loss due to unattended caries. J Dent Res 1980;59:1577-1580.

Northway WM. The not-so-harmless primary first molar extraction. JADA Dec 2000; 131:1711-1720.

Ngan P, Yiu C: Evaluation of treatment and posttreatment changes of protraction facemask treatment using the PAR index: Am J Orthop Dentofac 2000; 118;414-420.

NIH Consensus Development Conference for Removal of Third Molars. J Oral Surg 1980; 3:235-236.

Thilander B, Skagius S: Orthodontic sequelae of extraction of permanent first molars: a longitudinal study. Trans Eur Orthod Soc 1970; pp 429-442.

Toroglu MS, Uzel E, Kayalioglu M, Uzel I. Asymmetric maxillary expansion (AMEX) appliance for treatment of the unilateral posterior crossbite. Am J Orthop Dentofac Dentofacial Orthop 2002;122:164-173.

Vanarsdall RL, Corn H: Soft-tissue management of labially positioned unerupted teeth. Am J Orthod Dentofacial Orthop 1977; 72(1):53-64.

Von Bremen J, Pancherz H: Efficiency of early and late Class II Division 1 treatment. Am J Orthop Dentofac 2002; 121:31-36.

Wheeler TT. et al: Effectiveness of early treatment of Class II malocclusion. Am J Orthop Dentofac 2001; 121:9-16.

Woods MG. Mandibular arch dimensional and positional changes in late mixed-dentition Class I and II treatment. Am J Orthod Dentofacial Orthop 200;122:180-188.

Wilhelm BM, et al; A comparison of cranial base growth in Class I and Class II skeletal patterns. Am J Orthod Dentofacial Orthop 2001; 119:401-418.

CHAPTER 18

Adolescent Treatment

Thomas J. Cangialosi
Estella S. Efstratiadis

1. INTRODUCTION

ORTHODONTIC TREATMENT DURING ADOLESCENCE

Adolescence is generally defined as the period of physical and psychological development from the onset of puberty to maturity. In effect it is a transitional period of development between childhood and adulthood. It is during this period that most patients with malocclusions and dentofacial deformities are comprehensively treated. The reasons for this are the following: Once the permanent dentition has erupted, it usually becomes obvious to the dentist, the patient and the parents that a problem exists which most likely will not improve with further dentofacial growth and development. In addition, it is during **adolescence** that most children become conscious of their appearance and want to see it improved.

There are scientific as well as clinical reasons which indicate that this may be the best time to initiate treatment. For instance, successful orthodontic treatment of **Class II malocclusion** depends in large part on initiating treatment in conjunction with a mandibular growth spurt in a favorable direction. Rapid palatal sutural expansion may also be achieved more easily before connective tissue ossification, and patients with mild to moderate Class III malocclusions may be candidates for maxillary protraction during this period. Judicious use of the "E" space from the exchange of the primary second molars and second premolars may also change a treatment decision from extraction to nonextraction in borderline crowded or **bimaxillary protrusion** patients.

In this chapter, treatment of the various types of malocclusions frequently encountered during **adolescence** will be discussed separately and in detail.

2. SAGITTAL INTERJAW RELATIONSHIPS

Most malocclusions are often described in the **sagittal plane** as is evidenced by the **Angle classification**, which addresses only the relationship of the maxillary to the mandibular teeth. However, occlusion is a dynamic, three dimensional biological entity. Therefore, malocclusion should be described in the sagittal, vertical and transverse dimensions both dentally and skeletally.

2.1 Class II Division I Malocclusion

The common features of this malocclusion are: mandibular molars in **distoclusion**, canines in a Class II relationship, proclined maxillary incisors with a marked excessive overjet relationship. In addition, there may be crowding or spacing of anterior and/or posterior teeth, the overbite relationship may be normal, deep or there may be an **anterior open bite**, and there could be a transverse discrepancy which is manifested by a **posterior crossbite** relation of one or several teeth in a posterior segment. This could result in a mandibular lateral shift which may complicate treatment procedures.

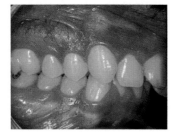 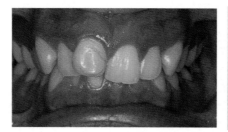 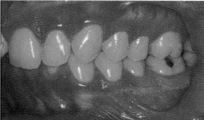

Figure 18-1: Class ll Division 1 Malocclusion.

As stated previously, a malocclusion may be either dental or skeletal in nature or a combination of both. Therefore, it is possible for the dental relationship to be Class II while the sagittal skeletal relationship of the maxilla to the mandible is normal both in an anterior-posterior and vertical direction. Likewise, a Class I dental relationship may exist with a Class II skeletal pattern. It is obvious that those malocclusions with severe skeletal discrepancies are the most difficult to treat and have the poorest prognosis regarding the treatment result and stability.

2.1.1. Class II Division I Malocclusion with Normal Skeletal Pattern

In the case of a Class II malocclusion with normal sagittal and vertical skeletal relationships, orthodontic tooth movement combined with mandibular growth which is normal in magnitude and direction will usually suffice to establish a Class I occlusion and a harmonious facial appearance. This may be accomplished by maintaining the position of the maxillary molars (relative distalization) or actively distalizing them while the mandibular dentition is carried downward and forward as the mandible grows in the proper direction toward its normal position. Some additional correction of the Class II molar relationship may be obtained by orthodontic mesial movement of the mandibular molars. During orthodontic treatment extrusion of both the maxillary and mandibular posterior teeth typically occurs in conjunction with vertical development of the alveolar processes. This posterior vertical development is helpful in correction of deep anterior overbite relationships, and may be enhanced using either fixed or functional appliances in treatment.

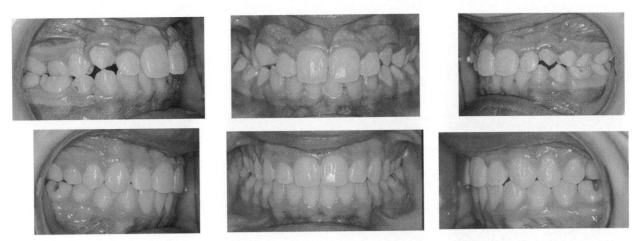

Figure 18-2: Class II Division 1 Malocclusion. The top row demonstrates pretreatment. Bottom, post-treatment.

2.1.2. Class II, Division I – Malocclusion with Skeletal Discrepancy

When a Class II, Division I malocclusion is the result of a sagittal inter-jaw discrepancy, orthodontic tooth movement alone will seldom suffice to correct the existing Class II dental relationship. This type of malocclusion is the result of an imbalance between the maxilla and mandible which would be caused by one or a combination of the following:

1.) **Maxillary protrusion**
2.) **Maxillary hyperplasia**
3.) **Mandibular retrusion**
4.) **Mandibular hypoplasia**

When evaluating patients with Class II malocclusion cephalometrically, the ANB angle is generally higher than normal. In patients with a skeletal Class II relationship, the ANB angle often exceeds 5 or 6 degrees.

In the presence of one of the above conditions in the adolescent dentition, orthopedic forces, either extra-oral or intra-oral, should be utilized to inhibit forward growth of the maxilla while allowing the mandible to express its greatest potential for forward development.

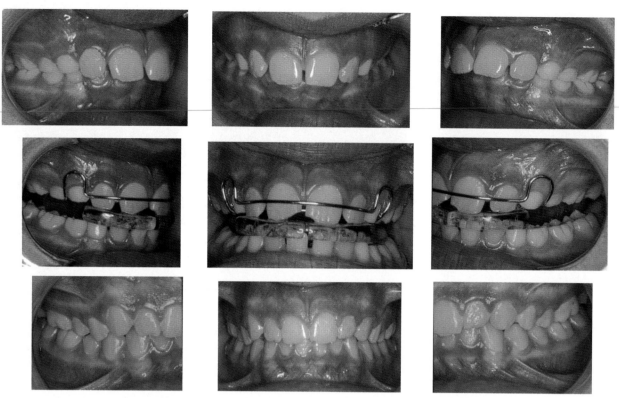

Figure 18-3: Class II malocclusion treated with functional appliance.

It is also important to assess the patient's vertical skeletal pattern when deciding the direction of extra-oral force application in correction of the Class II malocclusion. In the case of a skeletal deep overbite **(hypodivergent)** pattern, vertical (extrusive) force application may be applied in conjunction with dis-talization of the maxillary dentition and mesialization of the mandibular dentition. However, if the Class II malocclusion is characterized by an open-bite **(hyperdivergent)** pattern, application of verti-cal extrusive forces in the posterior segments of the maxillary and mandibular arches are contraindicat-ed, since these forces would tend to worsen the open-bite pattern.

In the treatment of Class II malocclusions with skeletal discrepancies, the patient's skeletal pattern both vertically and horizontally will determine, or have a substantial effect on, the prognosis for the success-ful outcome of treatment. In general, those patients who exhibit a forward direction of mandibular growth, in conjunction with appropriate orthopedic and orthodontic force applications, will have the more favorable prognosis. A favorable treatment outcome is also dependent upon patient cooperation in wearing certain treatment aids such as functional appliances, **bite plates**, extraoral force appliances and class ll elastics. In those cases where the skeletal discrepancy is extreme or patient cooperation is deficient, it may be necessary to mask the malocclusion by the extraction of permanent teeth or by **maxillofacial** surgery when growth is complete.

2.2 CLASS II DIVISION 2 MALOCCLUSION

The Class II Division 2 malocclusion is characterized by all or some of the following conditions.

1. Retroclined (lingual axial inclination) maxillary central and sometimes lateral incisors.
2. Flaring of the maxillary lateral incisors or canines
3. Deep and scissor-like anterior overbite approaching or exceeding 100%.
4. **Hypodivergent skeletal pattern**. (low mandibular plane angle).

5. Frequently a normal sagittal interjaw relationship of the maxilla and mandible. (The ANB angle is many times in the normal range).
6. A well developed chin.
7. A short lower anterior face height.

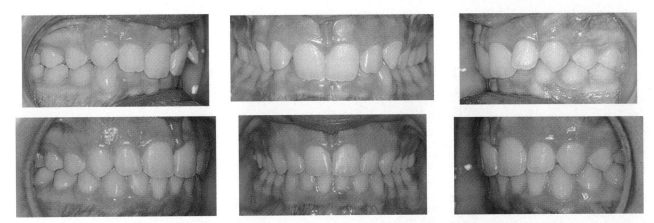

Figure 18-4: Class II Division 2 Malocclusion pre-treatment and post-treatment.

In this type of malocclusion, the extraction of permanent teeth should be avoided, if at all possible, since extraction therapy tends to deepen the already severe overbite condition. The traditional method of treating this malocclusion is to procline the maxillary incisors, converting the malocclusion to a Class II division 1, and then apply mechanics to distalize the maxillary arch with emphasis on extrusive mechanics to open the bite, increase lower face height and improve the facial soft tissue profile.

Careful attention should also be given to the vertical relationship of the maxillary incisors to the upper lip. Bite opening is generally achieved by a combination of some **extrusion** of posterior teeth and some intrusion of anterior teeth. The anterior teeth should be intruded until they are in a good relationship with the upper lip (approximately 1 mm of dental display at rest). This may be accomplished with fixed appliances by the use of intrusion arch wires, which move the incisors in an apical direction.

2.3 CLASS III MALOCCLUSION

Class III malocclusion may be categorized as either pseudo Class III or true Class III malocclusion. The pseudo Class III is generally caused by an anterior mandibular shift due to premature occlusal contacts. This malocclusion may be treated successfully by the application of orthodontic forces directed at eliminating the prematurities and mandibular shift. Patients with pseudo Class III malocclusions will present with an **anterior crossbite** but will be able to bring their anterior teeth into an edge-to-edge relationship when requested. In order to get a true determination of the sagittal jaw relationship, the lateral cephalometric radiograph should be taken with the mandible in its most retruded position. Measurement of the sagittal jaw relationship will generally show that the skeletal pattern in these cases tends to be a Class I relationship. Patients with true skeletal Class III malocclusion will usually have ANB angles which are below normal and frequently with negative values (e.g., ANB –2 degrees or less). In general, mechanics used to treat this type of malocclusion should focus on opening the bite to clear the occlusion, protraction of the maxillary anterior teeth, and retraction of mandibular anterior teeth, which will allow the mandible to assume a more normal posterior position. The prognosis for treatment outcome and stability for this type of malocclusion is excellent. The true Class III malocclusion involves a skeletal discrepancy in which the mandible is in a **mesioclusion** in relation to the maxilla. The degree of difficulty in treatment depends on the severity of the skeletal discrepancy. As in the Class II malocclusion, extremes in vertical dimension (**divergency**) add to the difficulty in the treatment of Class III malocclusion.

If the Class III skeletal pattern is mild to moderate in degree with a relatively normal vertical relationship, the malocclusion may be treated during **adolescence** with fixed orthodontic appliances and the application of Class III **intermaxillary mechanics**. In some patients, extraction of permanent teeth, usually maxillary second premolars and mandibular first premolars, may be required depending on the severity of crowding present.

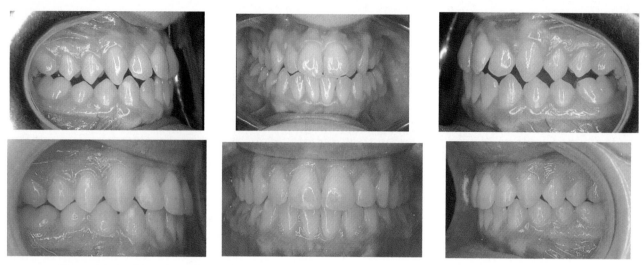

Figure 18-5: Class III Malocclusion (non-extraction treatment), pre-treatment and post-treatment.

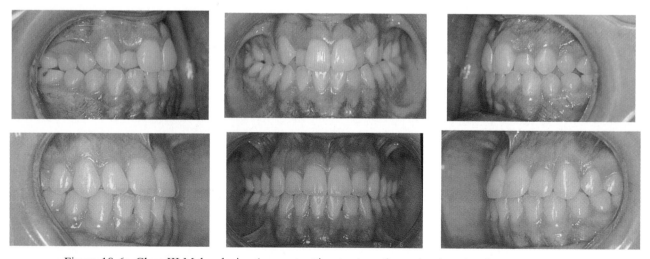

Figure 18-6: Class III Malocclusion (non-extraction treatment), pre-treatment and postreatment.

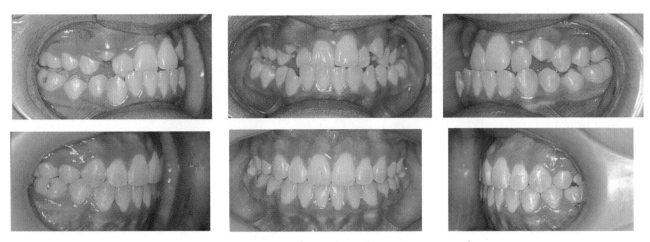

Figure 18-7: Class III Malocclusion (extraction treatment), pre-treatment and post-treatment.

In more severe cases, orthodontic forces may be applied to protract the maxilla and/or the maxillary dentition. These forces are generally applied by the use of a **face mask** appliance in conjunction with rapid maxillary expansion. The reason for the use of rapid maxillary expansion is that it has been shown that the maxilla moves slightly forward and downward during this procedure, and it is thought that disruption of the circummaxillary sutures may also facilitate forward movement of the maxilla. When the maxillo-mandibular relationship is sufficiently improved, fixed orthodontic appliances are placed to complete treatment. When treatment is complete, it is extremely important to closely supervise the retention phase until it can be determined that growth is complete. If the Class III skeletal relationship is very severe and/or complicated by severe vertical discrepancy, the malocclusion will require a combination of orthodontic treatment and **orthognathic surgery**. The surgical phase of treatment should be completed only after it has been determined that craniofacial growth is complete in order to prevent relapse due to an unfavorable growth pattern.

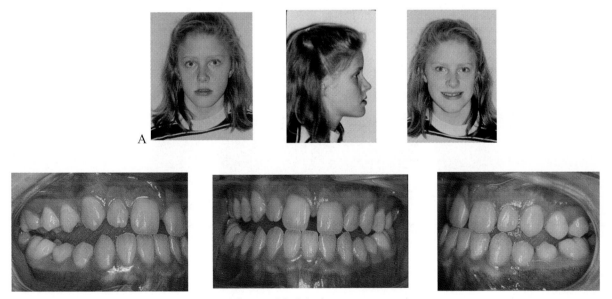

Figure 18-8A (see next page)

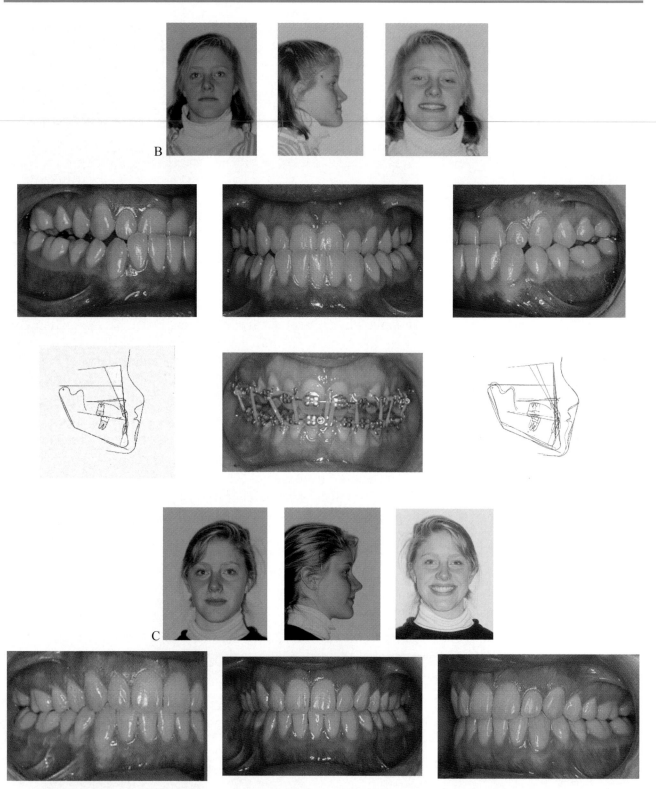

Figure 18-8: Results of Orthognathic Surgery for a Class III Malocclusion. A.) Class III malocclusion and lateral open bite at 12 years of age. B.) Class III malocclusion at 15 years of age. C.) Results of orthognathic surgery and orthodontics.

3. VERTICAL PLANE MALOCCLUSION

As mentioned earlier, a developmental disturbance of the occlusion frequently affects more than one plane. However, the abnormality may be more severe in one plane and it may actually characterize the malocclusion. For example, a malocclusion may be referred to as a "**deep bite malocclusion**" or an "**open bite**" malocclusion. Indeed, a vertical dental discrepancy contributes greatly to the severity of a malocclusion and to the degree of difficulty in its treatment. Moreover, if the vertical plane discrepancy is associated with the patient's skeletal pattern in addition to the dental discrepancy, the severity of the malocclusion and degree of difficulty in treatment increases considerably. Severe skeletal vertical discrepancy will also worsen the prognosis for treatment outcomes and posttreatment stability.

When evaluating these patients, cephalometric measurements which describe divergency of the denture bases are used. These may include the following: **Sella-Nasion to Mandibular Plane (SN-GoGn)**, **Palatal Plane to Mandibular Plane (PP-GoGn)**, **Palatal Plane to Sella-Nasion (SN-PP)** and **the gonial angle** (the angle formed by the **posterior border of the ramus** and the lower border of the body of the mandible. Measurements which are more than two standard deviations higher than normal would indicate that a skeletal discrepancy exists.

3.1 **ANTERIOR OPEN BITE** MALOCCLUSION

When the maxillary incisors do not overlap the mandibular incisors (e.g., there is a space between them), the condition is referred to as **anterior openbite** and may be dental or skeletal in nature. Determination of the etiology of the openbite is critical to its successful treatment (See Chapter 7).

In the case of a dental openbite, the etiologic factor is usually a habit such as **thumbsucking** or persistent **tongue thrust**. Cephalometric values are generally close to normal. In treating this type of malocclusion, elimination or control of the habit is essential. Patient counseling in conjunction with a habit breaking appliance such as a **tongue crib** and fixed orthodontic appliances may lead to successful treatment. While controlling the habit, orthodontic forces should be directed toward preventing extrusion of posterior teeth while allowing extrusion of maxillary and mandibular incisors to their correct vertical relationship to lip position. Depending upon upper incisor to lip position, some maxillary posterior intrusion may also be necessary.

In patients with skeletal open bite there is generally excessive vertical growth of the posterior dentoalveolar complex. These patients will exhibit a steep or hyperdivergent mandibular plane and a longer than normal anterior face height. In some instances the maxilla may also be rotated upward in a counterclockwise direction. If the skeletal discrepancy is mild to moderate, prevention of extrusion or actual intrusion of maxillary posterior teeth will be desirable to help in closing the bite. This may be accomplished with the use of a **high-pull extraoral force appliance** and/or a posterior bite block appliance. Care must be exercised not to overextrude the anterior teeth, since in skeletal openbite they may already be extruded beyond normal. If the skeletal discrepancy is moderate to severe, a combination of orthodontics and orthognathic surgery may be required to intrude or impact the maxillary posterior segments in order to close the bite anteriorly. Patients with anterior openbite, whether dental or skeletal, will exhibit a tongue thrust when swallowing. Stability of the final treatment result cannot be achieved unless the habit is eliminated or controlled. Long term retention with an appliance which has a tongue crib is recommended.

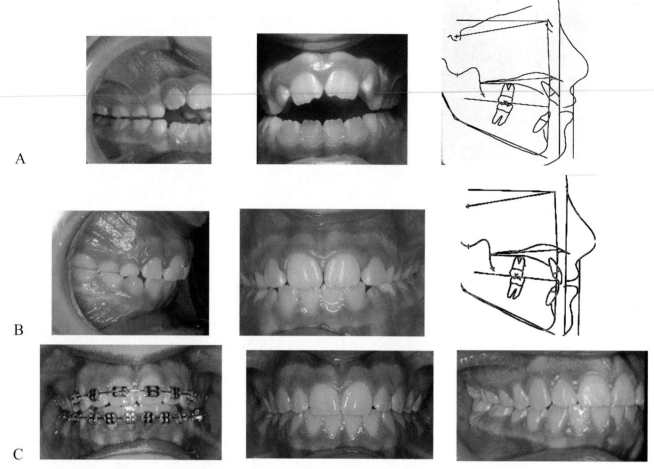

Figure 18-9: Anterior Open Bite in Mixed Dentition. A) pre-treatment, B) after first phase of treatment with expansion and habit appliance, and C) final phase of treatment with fixed appliances.

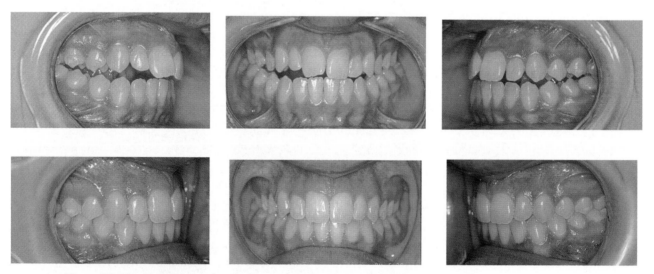

Figure 18-10: Open bite malocclusion, pre-treatment and post-treatment

3.2 DEEP OVERBITE MALOCCLUSION

When the maxillary incisors overlap the mandibular incisors by an excessive amount, this condition is referred to as a deep overbite. Generally, a normal overbite relationship would be approximately 1 to 3 mm. In extreme cases of deep overbite, the mandibular incisors may be in contact with the palatal mucosa. This is referred to as an "impinging" overbite. Deep overbite may be caused by overeruption of the anterior teeth (maxillary, mandibular or both), or by inadequate development of the posterior dento-alveolar complex.

As with openbite, deep overbite malocclusions may have both dental and skeletal components. Cephalometrically, angles of divergency are generally lower than normal. Measurements which are greater than two standard deviations below normal indicate that the deep overbite is skeletal in nature and the prognosis for treatment and stability is guarded. This type of malocclusion is best treated during **adolescence**, since principles of growth modification may be successfully applied during this period of active growth. For example, the use of a removable appliance with an anterior bite plane or a **functional appliance** will disocclude the posterior teeth to allow vertical development of the dentoalveolar structures, which will reduce the anterior overbite. Fixed orthodontic appliances to level the dental arches by intrusion of incisors and extrusion of molars and premolars will also help reduce the overbite. The use of **intermaxillary elastic force**, either Class II or III, will also help to extrude posterior teeth.

If the deep bite is due in part to a skeletal discrepancy, long term retention with a **removable appliance** with an anterior bite plane should be used. In cases of extreme skeletal discrepancy, orthognathic surgery may be required after growth is complete.

4. CLASS I MALOCCLUSION

A Class I malocclusion may be characterized by a normal anterior-posterior relationship of the dental arches to each other, which may be termed **"neutroclusion"**. In these patients, the mandible and the maxilla are generally considered to be in a normal antero-posterior relationship to each other as indicated by a normal value of the ANB angle (approximately 2 degrees).

While molars and canines are in a Class I relationship, other problems may exist either within each arch individually or between the dental arches.

Some of the problems which may exist are:

1. Crowding and/or rotations of teeth.
2. Spacing of anterior and/or posterior teeth.
3. Moderate to severe deep overbite.
4. Moderate to severe openbite.
5. Moderate to severe overjet.
6. Flaring of maxillary and mandibular anterior teeth.
7. Anterior or posterior crossbites of one or more teeth.

Class I malocclusion is the most common malocclusion and, since in most cases it does not involve a skeletal discrepancy, its treatment outcome is generally successful and predictable. In most instances, fixed appliances should be used to treat these cases.

In a Class I crowded malocclusion, a decision must be made as to whether the dental arches can be aligned and leveled with or without the extraction of permanent teeth. This decision is made based on the severity of crowding and the axial and spatial relationships of the anterior teeth. In general, if there is 5 or more millimeters of crowding in the mandibular arch, extractions may be necessary. If space analysis reveals 8 mm or more of **arch length discrepancy**, **anchorage** consideration will be very important. Enough space must be provided to uncrowd the teeth and possibly upright and retract them to a more normal axial and spatial relationship so that lip competence may be attained.

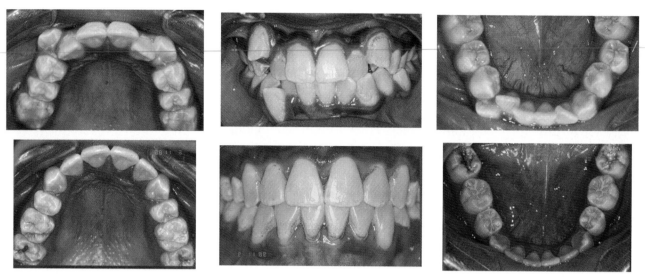

Figure 18-11: Class I crowded malocclusion treated with extractions.

In cases where the primary second molars are still present and there is some mandibular crowding, it may be possible to use the "E" or **leeway space**, which is approximately 2 mm. per side, to resolve some of it.   The leeway space in the maxillary arch is approximately 1mm. per side. If the maxillary and mandibular molars are in a cusp to cusp (flush terminal plane) relationship, some distalization of the maxillary molars while the mandibular molars are held in position will provide additional space in the maxillary arch and create a Class I molar relationship. Use of the leeway space with some lateral and anterior expansion (flaring) of the maxillary arch may allow a case to be treated without extraction of permanent teeth.

5. TRANSVERSE DISCREPANCY

Transverse discrepancies are most frequently manifested as crossbites of the posterior maxillary and mandibular dental arches. The crossbite relationship of the maxillary **dental arch** to the mandibular dental arch may be unilateral or bilateral. It may be a lingual or buccal relationship. It may also be skeletal or dental in nature. In a **lingual crossbite**, the buccal cusps of the maxillary posterior teeth occlude inside the buccal cusps of the mandibular teeth. In a **buccal crossbite**, the lingual cusps of the maxillary posterior teeth occlude buccal to the buccal cusps of the mandibular posterior teeth.

Dental crossbites are usually the result of an abnormal bucco-lingual axial inclination of the posterior teeth. A unilateral crossbite may be the result of a lateral mandibular shift in response to a constricted maxillary dental arch or, more rarely, a true unilateral maxillary asymmetry and constriction (see Chapters 13 and 17).

This type of crossbite may be treated by the use of a fixed or removable expansion appliance which will tip the teeth into their proper axial relationships. Another method for treating this type of crossbite involves banding the posterior teeth and using cross elastics to attain reciprocal movement of the teeth in both arches to correct the crossbite.

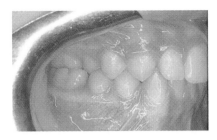
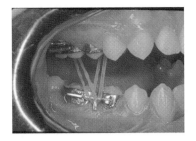
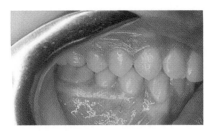

Figure 18-12: Simple Crossbite Malocclusion. Views of the pre-treatment, treatment and post-treatment.

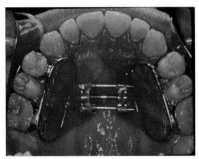

If the crossbite is due to a skeletal malrelationship between the maxilla and mandible with the teeth in normal axial relations, orthodontic treatment aimed at tipping the teeth to mask the skeletal malrelationship may cause them to be flared excessively. This may be unstable and could compromise periodontal health. In this instance where the maxilla is narrow in relation to the mandible, a lateral mandibular shift is often present and rapid palatal expansion is generally required. In this type of expansion, a special appliance is constructed which will exert orthopedic force to the two halves of the palate and cause opening of the midpalatal suture. This appliance utilizes a jack screw which is either attached to **bands** on the maxillary first molars and first premolars or may be bonded directly to the teeth.

Figure 18-13: Rapid Palatal Expansion Appliance.

In most instances, rapid palatal expansion of the maxillary arch can be completed in two to three weeks from the beginning of activation of the appliance. Each activation of the screw provides 0.25 mm of expansion. The patient or family member is instructed to activate it once in the morning and once in the evening so that expansion occurs at the rate of 0.5 mm per day. After completion of the expansion, the appliance should remain in place for a minimum of four months while reossification of the midpalatal suture area takes place.

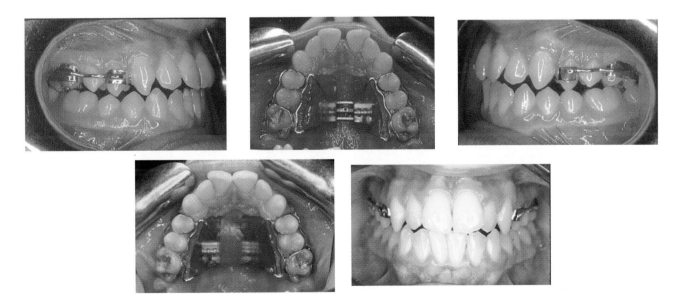

Figure 18-14: Rapid Palatal Expansion Appliance in active treatment and rapid palatal expansion appliance (retention).

Posterior buccal crossbites are extremely difficult to treat. If the mandibular teeth are inclined lingually, it may be possible to correct the crossbite utilizing **arch wires** and cross elastics. If the buccal crossbite is bilateral (referred to as Brodies's syndrome), it may require surgical intervention.

Facial asymmetry may be the result of a **functional crossbite** due to constriction of the maxillary dental arch and shift of the mandible to one side to achieve adequate occlusal contact, or to a skeletal dysplasia, due to overgrowth of one side of the mandible. Trauma of the mandibular **condyle** at a young age may disturb the normal mandibular growth and result in facial asymmetry. These patients present malocclusions characterized by crossbites. A combination of orthodontic treatment and orthognathic surgery is the most predictable treatment for most of these conditions. Treatment with functional appliances in young children may help to guide the growth and development of the mandible and the associated musculature.

6. DENTAL ANOMALIES

6.1 IMPACTIONS

Sometimes permanent teeth are not able to erupt into their proper position in the dental arch. This may be due to several factors, including lack of adequate space in the arch, ectopic eruptive path or lack of sufficient eruptive force. The latter condition is referred to as primary failure of eruption. In each of these instances, the teeth involved remain embedded in bone and generally require surgical exposure of the crowns and redirection of the path of eruption by means of orthodontically directed forces.

In the case of maxillary and particularly mandibular third molars, impaction is generally a result of insufficient space in the arch or poor eruptive path. In most cases of impacted third molars, the treatment of choice is generally extraction. Other than third molars, the teeth most commonly impacted are the maxillary canines; however, the maxillary incisors and second premolars, mandibular second premolars and canines are also frequently impacted (See Chapters 5 and 13). In the case of maxillary incisors, impaction may be due to the presence of a supernumerary tooth which lies palatal to the roots of the permanent incisors. This tooth is referred to as a **mesiodens**. In order for the permanent incisor to be brought into the arch, it is necessary for the mesiodens to be extracted and for gentle orthodontic force to be applied to the impacted tooth. Preferably, this should be done prior to completion of root formation of the impacted tooth.

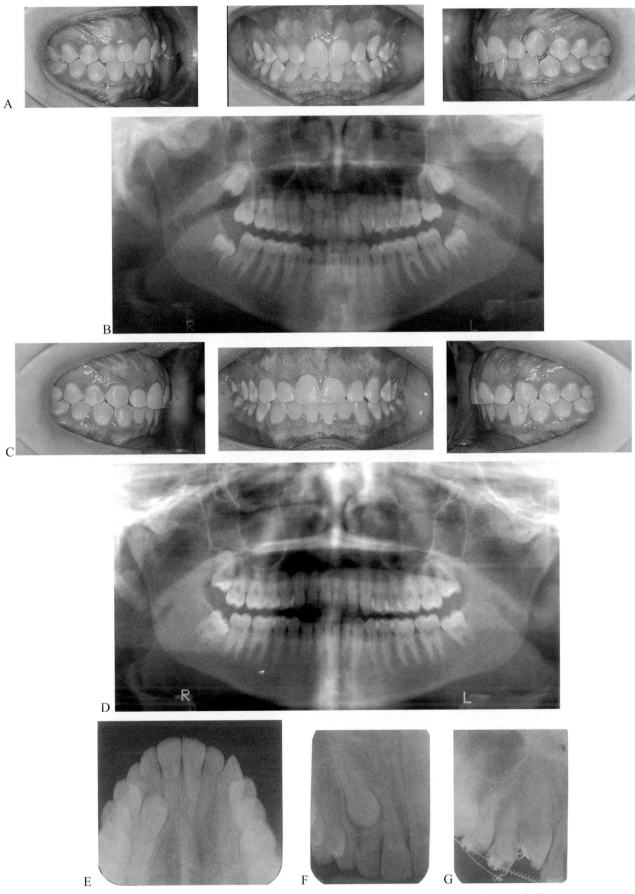

Figure 18-15: Treatment of an impacted right maxillary canine. A.) Pre-treatment intra-orals B.) panorex, C.) post-treatment intraorals, D.) panorex, E.) pre-treatment occlusal radiograph, F.) pre-treatment periapical radiograph and G.) mid-treatment periapical radiograph.

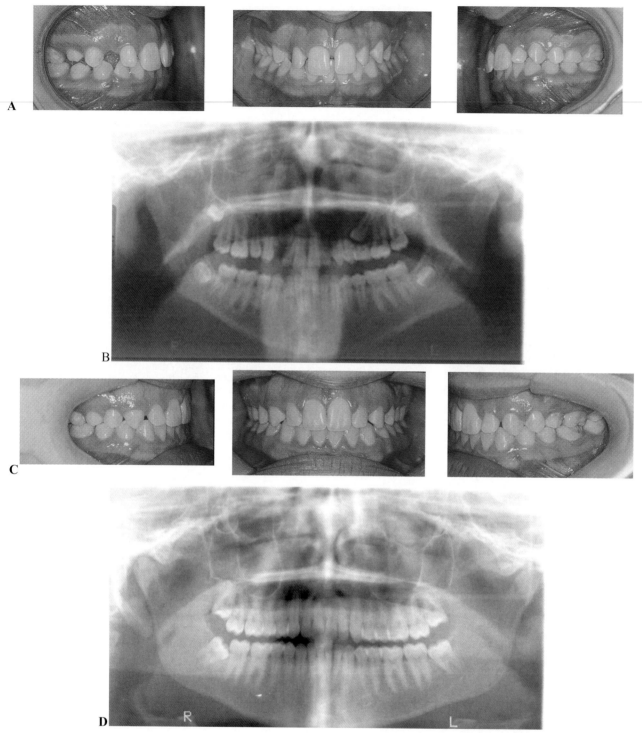

Figure 18-16: Malocclusion with maxillary right canine and left second premolar. A.) Pre-treatment intraorals, B.) Pre-treatment panorex, C.) Post-treatment intraorals, D.) Post-treatment panorex.

6.2 MISSING, ATYPICAL AND/OR TRANSPOSED TEETH

The treatment of any malocclusion may be complicated by missing teeth, whether congenital or extracted, or by atypical, malsized, malformed or fractured teeth. These cases often require creative treatment planning and communication with the patient's general dentist and the orthodontist and other dental specialists in order to achieve a functional and esthetic outcome.

Frequently, a decision must be made regarding whether a missing maxillary lateral incisor should be replaced or whether the canine should be moved next to the central incisor and reshaped. In either case, some tooth movement is often required either in order to open space to accommodate a pontic or implant or close space between the central incisor and the canine.

In these cases, tooth size discrepancies existing between the maxillary and mandibular anterior teeth will commonly require some orthodontic adjustment in order to establish a good overbite and overjet relationship. Whenever possible, it is preferable to maintain or move the maxillary canines into a Class I relationship for the best function and esthetic result.

Another commonly missing tooth is the second premolar, either maxillary or mandibular. Again, a decision will have to be made as to whether it would be better to close the space orthodontically or to adjust the space for a restorative procedure. This decision may be based on whether or not there is sufficient space in the **dental arch** and whether there is a necessity to extract other permanent teeth. It is often necessary to do a **diagnostic set-up** of the teeth to determine the best functional and esthetic result.

Occasionally a tooth will erupt in a transposed position. A common transposition is for the maxillary canine to erupt between the first and second premolars. This occurrence can cause tooth size problems between the maxillary and mandibular anterior teeth as well as occlusal interferences. When the teeth are fully erupted it is extremely difficult and often impossible to move the transposed teeth to their correct position. Transposed teeth may have to be altered in shape and size, either by judicious grinding or by prosthetic means. For example, if a premolar is in the canine position, the lingual cusp may have to be altered to prevent a balancing interference.

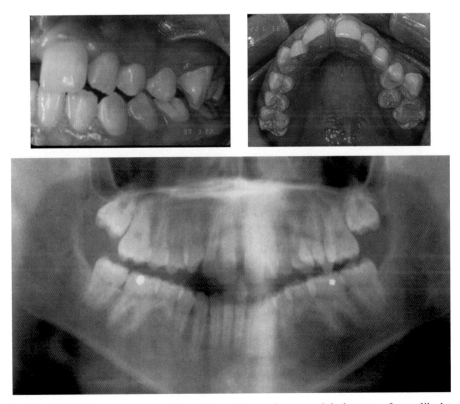

Figure 18-17: Transposed maxillary left canine and congential absence of mandibular second premolars.

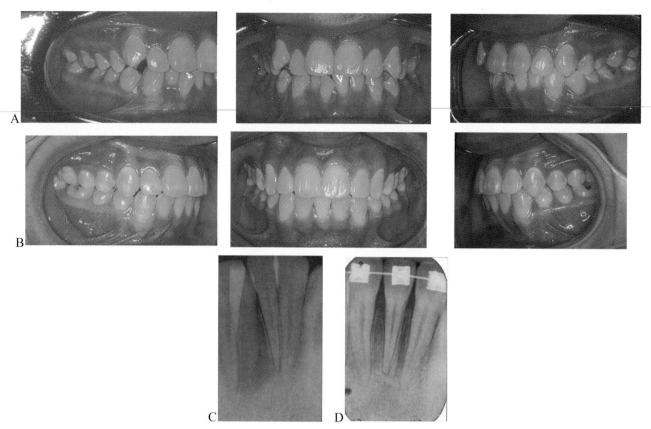

Figure 18-18: Malocclusion with fractured mandibular right central incisor. A.) Pre-treatment intraorals, B.) Post-treatment intraorals, C.) Pre-treatment periapical, D.) Mid-treatment periapical.

7. SUGGESTED READINGS

Bishara SE. Facial and dental changes in adolescents and their clinical implications. Angle Orthod 2000;70(6.):471-83 70:471-483.

Vig KW, Fields HW. Facial growth and management of orthodontic problems. Pediatr.Clin.North Am 2000.Oct.;47.(5.):1085-123. 47:1085-1123.

Kluemper GT, Beeman CS, Hicks EP. Early orthodontic treatment: what are the imperatives? J Am Dent Assoc 2000 May.;131(5):613-620.

Boyd RL. Enhancing the value of orthodontic treatment: incorporating effective preventive dentistry into treatment. AM J Orthod Dentofacial Orthop 2000 May;117(5):601-603.

Albert E. Considerations and treatments to erupt impacted teeth. J.Gen.Orthod 1998; 9:13-27.

Boecler PR, Riolo ML, Keeling SD, and TenHave TR. Skeletal changes associated with extraoral appliance therapy: An evaluation of 200 consecutively treated cases. The Angle Orthodontist 1989; 59:263-270.

Moorrees CF. Thoughts on the early treatment of Class II malocclusion. Clin Orthod Res 1998;1:97-101.

Peck S, Peck L, Kataja M. Mandibular lateral incisor-canine transposition, concomitant dental anomalies, and genetic control. Angle.Orthod 1998;68:455-466.

Vig KW. Nasal obstruction and facial growth: the strength of evidence for clinical assumptions. Am J Orthod Dentofacial Orthop 1998;113:603-611.

Stratford NM. Orthodontic treatment using functional appliances. J Ir Dent.Assoc 1997;43:110-116.

Moore RN. Principles of dentofacial orthopedics. Semin Orthod 1997;3:212-221.

Champagne M. The anterior open bite problem (infraclusion). J Gen Orthod 1995;6:5-10.

Alcazaren AB. Discovery of displaced canines among adolescents in the mid-section of the maxillary and mandibular apical areas and their management. J Philipp Dent Assoc 1996;48:5-10.

Sadowsky PL. Craniofacial growth and the timing of treatment. Am J Orthod Dentofacial Orthop 1998;113:19-23.

Ngan P, Hu AM, Fields HW. Treatment of Class III problems begins with differential diagnosis of anterior crossbites. Pediat Dent 1997;19:386-395.

Barton S, Cook PA. Predicting functional appliance treatment outcome in Class II malocclusions—a review. Am J Orthod Dentofacial Orthop 1997;112:282-286.

Delaire J. Maxillary development revisited: relevance to the orthopaedic treatment of Class III malocclusions. Eur J Orthod 1997;19:289-311.

Shroff B, Siegel SM, Feldman S, Siegel SC. Combined orthodontic and prosthetic therapy. Special considerations. Dent Clin North Am 1996;40:911-943.

Prahl-Andersen B, Fischer CE. Management of developmental asymmetrical facial growth. Semin Orthod 1996;2:64-83.

Nanda RS, Ghosh J. Facial soft tissue harmony and growth in orthodontic treatment. Semin Orthod 1995;1:67-81.

Bishara SE. Impacted maxillary canines: a review. Am J Orthod Dentofacial Orthop. 1992;101:159-171.

Moorrees CF. Growth and development in orthodontics. Curr Opin Dent 1991;1:609-621.

Riolo, M.L., Moyers, R.E., TenHave, T.R., Mayers, C., "Facial Soft Tissue Changes During Adolescence", in Craniofacial Growth During Adolescence, Mongraph #20, Craniofacial Growth Series, Center for Human Growth and Development, The University of Michigan, Ann Arbor, Michigan, 1987.

Nielsen IL. Vertical malocclusions: etiology, development, diagnosis and some aspects of treatment. Angle Orthod 1991;61:247-260.

Fields HW, Sinclair PM. Dentofacial growth and development. ASDC J Dent Child 1990;57:46-55.

Toroglu MS, Uzel E, Kayalioglu M, Uzel I. Asymmetric maxillary expansion (AMEX) appliance for treatment of the unilateral posterior crossbite. Am J Orthod Dentofacial Orthop 2002;122:164-173.

CHAPTER 19

Section I	Section II	Section III	Section IV
1. Developmental, Psychosocial, Behavioral, and Compliance Aspects of Care 2. Prenatal Craniofacial Growth 3. Postnatal Caniofacial Growth 4. Growth of the Craniofacial Skeleton 5. Development of the Dentition and Occlusion	6. Classification and Terminology 7. Etiology of Malocclusion 8. Force Systems and Tissue Response 9. Tissue Engineering in Orthodontics 10. Clinical Epidemiology and Malocclusion	11. Orthodontic Exam and Diagnosis 12. Analysis of Orofacial and Jaw Musculature 13. Analysis of Dentition and Occlusion 14. Dental Dysmorphogenesis 15. Analysis of Orofacial Skeleton 16. Planning Orthodontic Treatment	17. Preadolescent Treatment 18. Adolescent Treatment 19. Adult Treatment 20. Treatment of Patients with Craniofacial Anomalies 21. Retention, Relapse and the Recurrence of Malocclusion 22. The Adverse Effects of Orthodontic Treatment

Adult Orthodontic Treatment
Valmy Pangrazio-Kulbersh

I. INTRODUCTION

Increased awareness of the importance and benefits of a healthy and esthetically pleasant dentition, psychological well being, self-image and social success are motivating adults to seek orthodontic treatment more so now than in the past. It is interesting to note that in the past 20 years the number of adult patients over 30 years old seeking orthodontic treatment increased by 35%, totaling about 20% of the orthodontic patients in private practices. The dental professionals are also becoming more knowledgeable about the possibilities of adult tooth movement to facilitate the restoration of function and health to the components of the stomathognathic system. General dentists are the major source of referrals (65%), followed by these specialists: oral surgeons (15%), periodontists (6%), and prosthodontists (2%). The rest of the patients are self-referred.

Interdisciplinary treatment is becoming more important as the number of referrals increase from the general practitioners and other dental specialists. With the advent of new dental procedures which could correct malaligned teeth with restorations such as bonding, veneers or crowns in a much shorter time, the demand for adult orthodontic care appears to be decreasing. The alignment of the teeth and improvement of esthetics can be accomplished over a much shorter period of time and without the need for orthodontic appliances, utilizing what is known as esthetic restorations and procedures.

The dentist should give careful consideration to these procedures, since most of them are designed for esthetic purposes only and will not improve the function or health of the dentition. Proper diagnosis and careful evaluation of the alignment of the teeth, the health of the periodontal tissues, occlusal and skeletal relationships as well as the health and function of the temporomandibular joints should be considered before commencing an irreversible procedure which does not address the factors mentioned above.

2. DIFFERENCES BETWEEN ADULT AND ADOLESCENT TREATMENT

The information gained through the treatment of adolescents can be applied for orthodontic intervention in adults; however, major differences exist between these two groups. These differences are: 1.) **Adult orthodontic treatment** is usually initiated by the dentist to obtain occlusal harmony. 2.) There is no advantage or deleterious effect of growth on treatment. 3.) Periodontal disease is present in 80-90% of adult patients. 4.) Large numbers of adult patients have mutilated dentitions. 5.) Due to a change in occlusal scheme and occlusal loading, tooth mobility is increased in the presence of occlusal trauma. 6.) Lack of long-term stability requires a different approach to retention. 7.) Increased dysfunction of the temporomandibular joint requires a careful approach to the change in occlusal scheme. 8.) Due to the compromised crown to root ratio, the utilization of differential force systems and segmental orthodontic mechanics is indicated. 9.) The adult patient is more concerned with esthetics; therefore, the utilization of less conspicuous orthodontic appliances should be considered (ceramic brackets, lingual braces, removable appliances). 10.) The motivation for treatment is also different between adults and adolescents. Adults seek treatment because of a strong desire for esthetic change or under the suggestion of their dentist to improve their function or facilitate restoration of broken down dentition. Careful consideration should be given to the reasons why the adult is seeking orthodontic treatment, since the satisfaction with the end result will depend on their initial expectations and motivations. The patient that seeks treatment to improve function and dental alignment is more likely to have a better psychological response than a patient whose motivation comes from others or is expecting an impact on others by their perceived change in their physical appearance. The understanding of the differences between adult and adolescent treatment is necessary to reduce the risks of adverse treatment effects that can occur when improper treatment modalities or theories are used.

3. GOALS OF ADULT ORTHODONTIC TREATMENT

3.1 OBJECTIVES OF TREATMENT

As with any orthodontic treatment, the goals of adult orthodontic therapy are the achievement of improved function, stability and esthetics through the establishment of the six keys to normal occlusion whenever possible. Unfortunately, due to the differences already cited in the adult, the attainment of all the components of the **6 keys to normal occlusion** is often not possible. Therefore, another set of goals should be considered beside the ones that strictly dictate the **intercuspation** of the dental units. These added sets of objectives are: elimination of occlusal interferences and trauma to reduce tooth mobility and promote periodontal healing, obtain better bone and gingival architecture to improve tooth/periodontal tissue relationships, establish proper tooth position and improve the plane of occlusion for prosthetic replacement, achieve harmony between teeth and TMJ function and address the patient's chief concern, which is improvement of dental and facial esthetics.

3.2 CONTRAINDICATIONS FOR TREATMENT

Despite the large number of patients that can benefit from orthodontic treatment, certain contraindications must be considered. The presence of advanced local and/or systemic disease, such as metabolic or endocrine disorders, could adversely affect tooth movement and predispose the patient to tooth loss. Patients with excessive generalized vertical and/or horizontal bone loss as well as poor crown to root ratio and significant **root resorption** and where orthodontic tooth movement will not improve the bone level should not undergo orthodontic treatment. Since orthodontic appliances increase the changes for retention of plaque and concomitant gingival inflammation which could adversely affect tooth movement, patient motivation for the maintenance of excellent oral hygiene and cooperation with the instructions given by the orthodontists to produce the desired treatment result in the shortest possible period of time is essential. The orthodontist should also very carefully evaluate the stability and retention needs of the patient before embarking on adult tooth movement. If the patient does not want to consider the fact that permanent retention and long-term management is needed to maintain the results, treatment should not be initiated.

4. INTERRELATIONSHIPS BETWEEN ADULT ORTHODONTICS AND PERIODONTICS

Before considering adult orthodontics it is necessary to understand the interrelationship between periodontics and adult orthodontics. Recent advances in basic science related to periodontal biology and clinical trials on prevention and treatment of periodontal disease, as well as recent advances in orthodontic treatment due to the improvements of materials like bracket systems, wire composition, bonding agents, etc., have changed many treatment concepts in periodontics and orthodontics.

It is well known that cell mobilization and conversion of **collagen** fibers is slower in adults. Hyalinized areas are formed more easily on the pressure side of an orthodontically moved tooth, thus preventing tooth migration. Once the hyalinized zone is removed by **undermining resorption**, tooth movement occurs and regeneration and reorganization of the periodontal ligament takes place. When inflammation is present in the periodontal tissues, the PDL regeneration does not occur and periodontal tissue breakdown follows. Hence, the elimination and control of inflammation before and throughout orthodontic treatment is imperative to ensure the health of the supporting tissues during and after adult orthodontic therapy. In order to avoid the formation of hyalinized zones, light forces (20 to 30 grams) should be utilized for tooth movement according to Proffit and Melsen. Clinical studies carried out by Boyd have demonstrated that with plaque control, teeth with reduced periodontal support can undergo tooth movement without compromising their periodontal situation. Furthermore, studies by Ingber and Krall have demonstrated reduction of probing and pocket depth in orthodontically moved teeth in adults.

According to Dorfman and Kennedy, a minimal band of **attached gingiva** can be maintained during orthodontic treatment in the absence of inflammation and trauma. A free gingival graft is recommended when the amount of attached gingiva is minimum and the tooth is to be moved labially. If tooth movement is confined to the alveolar support, no harmful effect on the surrounding tissues is to be expected, according to Wennstrom. Trossello and Gianelly found that adults had an increased prevalence of root resorption after orthodontic treatment. Thus, it appears that apart from root resorption, adult orthodontic tooth movement has minimal detrimental effect on the periodontal tissues short or long-term when gingival inflammation is controlled.

5. INTERRELATIONSHIPS BETWEEN ADULT ORTHODONTICS AND PERIODONTAL THERAPY

It is recommended that adult orthodontic tooth movement be preceded by periodontal therapy to eliminate the inflammation that rapidly deteriorates the periodontium. Scaling, root planing, open flap debridement procedures and gingival grafting should be done before orthodontic treatment. Osseous surgery is to be postponed until after orthodontic treatment. The bone architecture will change with tooth movement, and possibly less bone recontouring will be necessary after tooth movement.

If successful treatment results are to be expected, plaque and inflammation control should be done not only before but throughout orthodontic therapy.

Table 19-1:

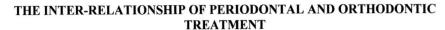

THE INTER-RELATIONSHIP OF PERIODONTAL AND ORTHODONTIC TREATMENT

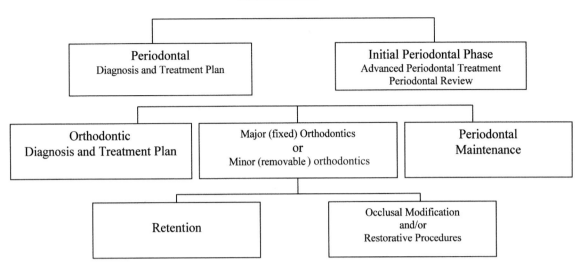

6. TREATMENT PLANNING CONSIDERATIONS FOR THE ADULT PATIENT

Treatment planning for all orthodontic patients includes establishing a set of specific objectives for each individual. The establishment of specific treatment goals allows the orthodontist to design the appropriate **mechanotherapy** to accomplish the objectives set forth. Due to the complexities associated with adult treatment, it is imperative that proper diagnosis and treatment planning is completed before starting treatment. Furthermore, because of the need for the involvement from other areas of dentistry to completely restore function, interdisciplinary treatment planning should be considered. Coordinating orthodontic treatment with other therapies is mandatory.

6.1 ORTHODONTIC RECORDS

The diagnosis and treatment planning should arise from careful clinical examination of the patient as well as from the evaluation of orthodontic records. The orthodontic records should include: facial (frontal and profile) photographs, a frontal smile photo is also recommended since it allows the professional to evaluate the amount of gingival display and integrate its modification as part of the treatment plan, if required. Also, it provides the practitioner with a visualization of any midline deviation problems. The radiographs required are: lateral cephalogram, frontal cephalogram specially indicated in patients whose facial analysis suggested the presence of **facial asymmetry**, panoramic x-ray and a full set of periapical radiographs to evaluate the periodontal status as well as the anatomy of the roots. Models mounted in **centric relation** (CR) on a semi-adjustable articulator is essential to properly diagnose the occlusal problems of an adult patient. The presence of occlusal interferences creates an occurrence of muscle pattern which could guide the mandible into a false occlusal relation (CO-CR discrepancy). Detection of any **centric occlusion-centric relation** (CO-CR) disharmony is essential to avoid suprises due to misdiagnosis and improper treatment planning. Roth has suggested that even in the absence of obvious signs or symptoms of temporomandibular joint (TMJ) dysfunction, adult patients, and specifically those with mutilated dentitions, should undergo **splint** therapy to eliminate muscle splinting and to avoid treatment planning from a false mandibular position.

6.2 SEQUENCE OF ADULT TREATMENT

Once the diagnosis and treatment plan have been established, a treatment sequence should be considered as follows:

1.) Emergency relief of pain.
This step, in many instances, will precede the gathering of orthodontic records and follow-up diagnosis.

2.) Therapy of soft tissue lesions.
   a.) Hygiene instructions
   b.) Scaling and root planing
   c.) Correction of inadequate restoration
   d.) Root resection and endodontic treatment

3.) Treatment of the lesions of the attachment.
   a.) Flap surgery and root planing
   b.) Guided tissue regeneration
   c.) **Autogenous** keratinized mucosal or connective tissue grafts
   d.) Orthodontic therapy
   e.) **Occlusal adjustment**
   f.) **Myofunctional** therapy

4.) Provisional stabilization and retention
5.) Reevaluation for further therapy, i. e., extraction of non-restorable teeth
6.) Completion of periodontal treatment.
7.) Final occlusal adjustment
8.) Restorative prosthetic dentistry
9.) Continued periodontal care

7. TREATMENT OPTIONS

Limited Tooth Movement and Comprehensive Orthodontic Treatment.

Several factors must be taken into consideration when deciding the approach to tooth movement in an adult patient. The first decision that the dentist must undertake is related to the severity of the malocclusion. The decision must be made as to whether the movement of teeth is within the scope of limited tooth movement, or if the malocclusion is so severe that comprehensive orthodontic mechanics must be applied.

7.1 LIMITED TREATMENT

Limited tooth movement is carried out either with removable or partial fixed orthodontic appliances and is aimed at specific and limited goals. In most instances, limited tooth movement is considered as an adjunct to the overall treatment of the adult.

The specific problems that can benefit from limited tooth movement are:

a.) Pre-prosthetic repositioning

Molar uprighting: to 1.) improve parallelism of the abutments, improve pontic space or create space for implant replacement of missing teeth, and 2.) **Forced eruption** to facilitate preparation of the root for crown placement.

b.) Correction of dental alignment
1.) crowding and rotations, 2.) spacing, 3.) crossbite

Limited tooth movement can improve esthetics and facilitate periodontal therapy.

7.1.1. Pre-prosthetic repositioning

7.1.1.1. Molar Uprighting

This is one of the most common reasons for orthodontic treatment in adults. The lower first molars appear to be the teeth that are most frequently missing. As the result of loss in arch integrity, several adverse effects can occur, such as: mesial tipping of the second and/or third molars, distal drifting of the bicuspids, extrusion of the opponent tooth, altered gingival form, infrabony defect mesial to the tipped tooth due to abnormal occlusal loading, malaligned marginal ridges, opening of the contact points with concomitant food impaction and posterior bite collapse.

Besides inadequate parallelism of the abutments, the clinicians are faced with other problems before the replacement of the missing molar, such as: excessive preparation of the abutments with potential need for endodontic treatment, inadequate pontic space, abnormal loading of the bridge, and excessive osseous surgery for the elimination of the infrabony defects. Most of these problems can be eliminated by orthodontically repositioning the teeth neighboring the extraction site.

A thorough evaluation of the occlusion and the skeletal characteristics of the patient is indicated. Molar uprighting is best accomplished by means of limited tooth movement when an acceptable occlusion is present. **Acceptable occlusion** can be defined as one in which there is a local dental malposition without a significant skeletal dysplasia and which exhibits anterior disclusion and cuspid guidance.

An assessment of the vertical dimension is also very important. Patients with dolichocephalic faces (high mandibular plane angle) are not good candidates for molar uprighting procedures which involve distalization of the crowns. This type of tooth movement will further increase the vertical dimension and have a tendency to open the bite due to the posterior repositioning of the crown and **extrusion** of the tooth caused by the orthodontic mechanics.

Appliance Selection

Before selecting an appliance for molar uprighting, one must consider certain options in tooth movement.

a.) Uprighting by distal crown movement.
b.) Uprighting by mesial root movement.
c.) Mesial movement of the bicuspids.
d.) Space closure.
e.) Retention.

Another important treatment consideration is the disposition of the third molar. In many instances, the presence of an antagonist and the occlusion will dictate the fate of the third molar. Also, the demands for anchorage should be part of the overall appliance design selection.

7.1.1.1.1. Distal Crown Movement

Orthodontic procedure for uprighting by distal crown movement:

When only a single tooth is to be uprighted, the clinician has the option of choosing between a removable or fixed orthodontic appliance. When a **removable appliance** with a finger spring mesial to the tooth to be uprighted is used, this appliance will only have limited control of tooth movement, and just distal crown tipping will occur without vertical and/or transverse control. Because of this limitation, as well as the dependence on patient cooperation, removable appliances are not very widely prescribed.

Partial fixed orthodontic appliances are more effective in controlling tooth movement in three planes of space and are capable of delivering more controlled forces to the teeth involved. Direct bonded brackets should be attached to the anchoring teeth (premolars and canine); the molar should carry a double buccal tube which will lodge the main **arch wire** and auxiliary spring when necessary. A lingual cuspid-to-cuspid retainer wire should be used to increase anchorage, as well as to prevent buccal displacement of the anchoring units or the lingual movement which could occur, especially when the molar needs to be torqued buccally. The initial leveling takes place with a very light and flexible wire which could be engaged in the brackets and tubes without permanent deformation.

The selection of the size, configuration and alloy composition will depend on the alignment of the anchoring teeth and severity of the mesial tipping. Generally, a light rectangular wire like a 17 x 25 braided stainless steel, a nickel titanium (niti) or a heat activated copper niti can be used during the initial leveling stage. The addition of a T-loop to a stainless steel wire makes the wire flexible enough to be inserted into the tube of the tipped molar. This configuration is indicated when the bicuspids and cuspids are in good alignment. The distal portion of the T-loop could be activated by bending it gingivally to continue with the distal tooth movement. As the uprighting movement takes place, occlusal adjustment should be performed at each visit (4-6 week intervals) to reduce trauma from occlusion, excessive tooth mobility and pain and to promote healing of the supporting tissues. After the initial leveling, a stiffer wire may be needed to complete the uprighting, or the utilization of an auxiliary spring may be indicated to continue with the desired tooth movement. The auxiliary uprighting spring is attached mesially to the main arch wire between the bicuspids without resting on the second bicuspid bracket and is inserted into the gingivally positioned auxiliary tube of the molar attachment. It should be activated 10 mm gingivally to the main arch wire. After the uprighting has been accomplished, a final rigid rectangular wire is used for stabilization if necessary (Figure 19-1).

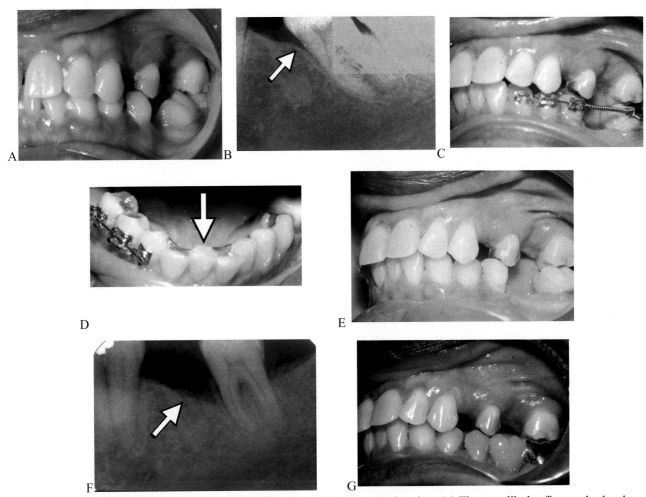

Figure 19-1: Unilateral uprighting of a severely tipped mandibular second molar. A.) The mandibular first molar has been lost and the second and third molars tipped mesially. B.) Note the change in bone architecture and vertical bony defect developed mesial to the second molar. The third molar was extracted due to the lack of an antagonist tooth. C.) Partial orthodontic appliances were placed on the cuspid, first and second bicuspids and second molar. An open coil spring was used to distalize and upright the second molar. D.) A Cuspid-to-cuspid lingual retainer was used to prevent the mesial displacement of the anchoring units (cuspid and bucuspid) E.) Final molar position after uprighting F. Note the bone recontouring and filling in of the vertical bony defect. G.) Final restoration in place.

When the second and third molars are to be uprighted, the same orthodontic procedure as described before can be utilized. The main tube of the double buccal attachment on the second molar is converted into an open bracket by removing the cap so that the main arch wire can be more easily inserted into the third molar tube. Instead of a T-loop, a box loop is more effective in these cases. Since the anchorage demands are increased when uprighting two molars, a lingual fixed cuspid-to-cuspid retainer should always be used. Removable appliances are not indicated in these instances (Figure 19-2).

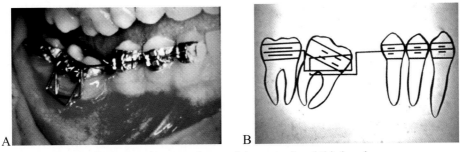

Figure 19-2: Box loop used to upright second and third molars.

7.1.1.1.2. **Molar Uprighting by Mesial Root Movement**

When it is not desirable to increase the length of the **edentulous** span, the orthodontic mechanotherapy should be altered to transmit the forces to the roots as well as the crowns. Cinching the wire distally will produce mesial root movement if the wire is prevented from sliding backwards. To accomplish this, the initial leveling wire should be stopped against the mesial of the cuspid bracket and distal to the molar tube. If an uprighting auxiliary spring is used, the portion of the spring that is anchored to the main arch wire should be positioned so that it rests against the mesial of the bracket of the first bicuspid and the posterior portion is tied back through the helical loop around the hook of the second molar tube. The cuspid, first and second bicuspids should all be ligated together to resist the reciprocal force generated by the spring, which will tend to distalize the bicuspids and prevent transmission of the force to the molar root. This setup also requires careful consideration of the anchorage demands.

7.1.1.1.3. **Mesial Movements of the Bicuspids**

When the bicuspids have drifted distally and there are interproximal spaces between them and the cuspids, the utilization of an open coil spring is indicated to reposition these teeth mesially and obtain closure of the contact points. The open coil spring (push coil) should be cut longer (half the width of the bracket) than the edentulous space in order to deliver the desired 100 grams of force. The distal portion of the wire should protrude slightly beyond the molar tube in order to allow for the distal drift of the molar. It is important to remember that at each appointment (4-6 week intervals), the tooth or teeth undergoing uprighting should be scaled and root planed and occlusal adjustments should be performed to decrease inflammation, trauma from occlusion, excessive tooth mobility and discomfort (Figure 19-3).

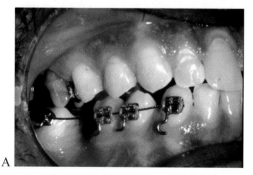 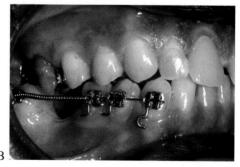

A   B

Figure 19-3: Compressed open coil spring used to move the second molar distally and first and second bicuspids mesially to close the contact points. A.) Initial leveling wire. B.) Open coil in place

7.1.1.1.4. **Complete space closure of the extraction site**

This procedure should not be accomplished with segmental orthodontic mechanics due to the significant demands for increased anchorage. When space closure is indicated, comprehensive orthodontic treatment should be considered (Figure 19-4).

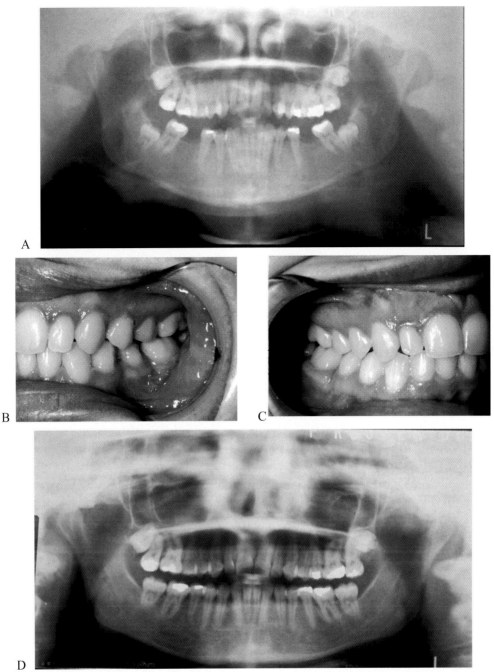

Figure 19-4: Bilateral loss of the first molars with impaction of the third molars. A.) Panorex before treatment. Full orthodontic mechano-therapy was used to correct the alignment of the teeth, move the second molars mesially and allow for eruption of the third molars. B.) and C.) Occlusion after treatment D.) Post-treatment Panorex. Note complete closure of extraction sites maintaining the molars in an uprighted position with good root parallelism.

7.1.1.1.5. **Retention**

The uprighted teeth should be retained in place until the placement of the prosthetic device. If the abutments have restorations or are to be prepared for crowns for the attachment of the pontic, an intracoronal stabilization bar could be used. If implants are to be used, then the brackets with a rigid finishing wire, usually a .019 x .025 stainless steel wire, are left in place passively until the time for placement of the restoration. The preparation for a bridge should start when the periapical radiograph indicates the reappearance of the **lamina dura** of the **alveolar bone** around the uprighted tooth. This usually takes place 8-12 weeks after the tooth has reached its final position.

7.1.2. Forced Eruption

Forced eruption is defined as the orthodontic movement of a tooth in the coronal direction through the application of continuous forces to cause changes in the architecture of the soft tissue and bone. This procedure facilitates the conservative management of non-restorable teeth when caries, trauma or periodontal disease makes the traditional restorative approach impossible.

The maintenance of the **"biologic width"** is imperative in the restoration of a tooth that has been destroyed near the level of the alveolar crest. Forced eruption helps in restoring the biologic width, making possible the placement of the restoration away from the functional epithelial attachment, thus preventing periodontal inflammation and breakdown. To maintain a healthy periodontium, 3 mm to 4 mm of tooth length is needed from the alveolar crest to the coronal extention of the remaining tooth structure.

When making the decision for a forced eruption procedure, the practitioner has to evaluate the health of the pulpal tissue. Forced eruption of vital teeth should be accomplished with slow, light forces (2-3 mm over a 4-month period) to avoid damage to the pulp and root. This slow coronal movement of the tooth will elicit new bone formation in the coronal direction. When this newly formed bone interferes with the placement of the restoration, then crown lengthening with osseous surgery is indicated. Because the gingival contours follow the bone remodeling, even in the cases where osseous surgery is necessary, the overall esthetic soft tissue result is excellent. Endodontically treated teeth can be extruded more rapidly with the application of heavier forces. The coronal movement of the tooth under this condition occurs with less bone remodeling, and in some cases may even obviate the need for osseous recontouring, especially when the tooth movement is done in conjunction with a **circumferential sulcus fiberotomy** before and weekly during tooth movement. Severance of the supracrestal fibers has the advantage of allowing more rapid tooth movement and eliminates the tensile stress on the alveolar bone, thus preventing crestal bone deposition. This allows for more direct inspection of the extruded sound tooth structure without excessive gingival overlay, as well as aiding in the prevention of relapse of the extruded tooth.

Forced eruption can also be successfully used to treat 1 or 2 wall infrabony pockets by leveling the vertical bony defect as new bone is formed when the tooth moves coronally. In order for this to occur, light continuous forces should be used. Periodic scaling, root planing and occlusal reduction is necessary to eliminate inflammation and occlusal trauma that could prevent bone healing.

The practitioner should be aware that restorative procedures after forced eruption require careful consideration, since a smaller diameter of root is exposed. Preparation of the surface will require modification to allow for healthy blending of the restoration with the gingival margins. It is important to realize that the restoration will have a larger taper from the incisal edge to the gingival margin due to the dimension of the root surface. Careful attention should be paid to avoid over-contouring the restoration and interfering with gingival health (Figure 19-5).

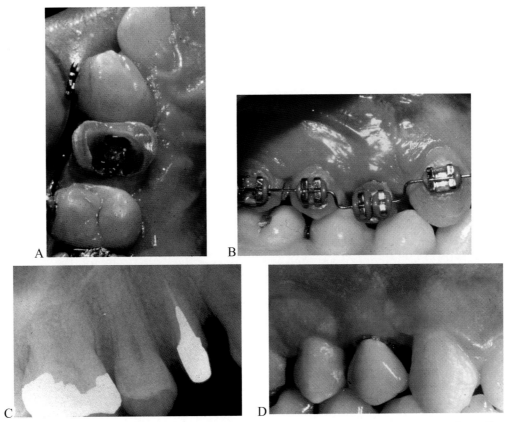

Figure 19-5: Forced eruption. A.) Severely decayed first bicuspid B.) Partial orthodontic appliance with occlusally stepped wire to extrude tooth. Occlusal reduction is needed to create space for extrusion. C.) Extruded tooth. Note reestablishment of biologic width. D.) Final restoration.

7.1.2.1. Appliance Selection

Partial fixed orthodontic appliances are most effective and allow for better control of forces and tooth movement in the three planes of space. Orthodontic brackets can be directly bonded to the mesial and distal teeth adjacent to the one to be erupted. The bracket on the tooth to be erupted should be offset gingivally. An initial rigid wire (.019 x .025 stainless steel, or SS) should be used to prevent the movement of the anchoring teeth.

An elastomeric module (elastic chain or thread) is then run from the tooth to be extruded to the archwire and replaced at 3-4 week intervals to accomplish the extrusion. As the tooth moves coronally stiffer wires can be used to accomplish the final tooth movement. In some instances, an occlusal step in the wire is necessary in order to further erupt the tooth if the initial position of the bracket was not sufficient to accomplish the total amount of root exposure required for the restoration. A T-loop design can also be considered. A .017 x .025 SS wire can be used with T-loops mesial and distal to the tooth to be erupted, eliminating the need for elastomeric use.

7.1.2.2. Retention

The arrangement of the principal fibers of the periodontal ligament occurs after 8 to 9 weeks of tooth movement. The supracrestal fibers do not reattach in the same fashion and remain stretched even after a retention period of 2-3 months. The supracrestal fibers do not account for relapse of forced erupted teeth, since those fibers are either resected during the procedure with the circumferential sulcus fiberotomy or during the periodontal osseous surgery done prior to the placement of the restoration. The periods of stabilization can vary from 2-6 weeks. The healing of the periodontal tissues will dictate the time of placement of the final restoration. No retention is necessary afterward. The ultimate success of this procedure depends on the establishment of an acceptable crown to root ratio, periodontal health and placement of an esthetic restoration.

This technique should be offered to patients along with crown lengthening and extraction and placement of an implant. Even when considering placement of an implant to replace the decayed tooth, crown lengthening could be used to improve the bone and gingival margins and to obtain better esthetic results.

7.1.3. Correction of Dental Alignment

Probably one of the main reasons why adult patients seek orthodontic therapy is for the correction of esthethically unpleasant alignment of anterior teeth. Beside the esthetic factor, the correction of malposed teeth aid in the maintenance of periodontal health through the facilitation of hygiene, more favorable distribution of occlusal forces, and avoidance of food impaction. Therefore, the correction of crowding, spacing, rotation, crossbites, and tipped teeth is not only indicated for esthetic reasons but to facilitate restorative procedures and maintain oral health.

7.1.3.1. Correction of crowding and rotations

Crowding and rotations are the expression of tooth size/**arch length** discrepancies, and therefore require the creation of spaces in the dental arches for their correction. The spacing necessary for this correction can be obtained through flaring of the anterior teeth, transverse expansion of the dental arches, interproximal stripping or extractions.

7.1.3.1.1. Appliance Selection

The correction of minor anterior or posterior crowding and rotations can be accomplished with segmental orthodontic mechanics. Before selecting the appliance, the practitioner should have a clear idea of the space required for the correction. If the correction of the crowding can be done increasing the arch length through flaring of the incisors without compromising the preservation of the overjet and incisal guidance, and without placing them in an unstable position over the **basal bone**, then brackets are bonded to the molars. Molars are considered the anchoring teeth for the incisors and cuspids to be realigned. An initial light .016 niti wire is placed and retied at 4-6 week intervals until the wire is fully engaged in the brackets and all crowding and rotations are resolved. The wire should be cinched back distal to the molar tubes to avoid disengagement and excessive flaring of the incisors. After the initial leveling has been completed with round wires, then a rectangular finishing wire is used (.017 x .025 or .019 x .025 niti) to detail tooth position.

When the correction of crowding requires the creation of space, interproximal enamel reduction is indicated. Approximately ½ mm of enamel can be removed at the mesial and distal surfaces of the upper incisors to a total of 4-5mm. Due to the smaller mesio-distal dimension of the lower incisors, less space can be gained in the lower anterior region. When interproximal stripping is considered for the correction of anterior crowding, a diagnostic set-up is indicated to evaluate the space requirements and ultimate alignment. The mechonotherapy is similar to the one described above (Figure 19-6). After the alignment has been completed, the teeth should be retained in position for about 6 months, either with a fixed cuspid-to-cuspid lingual retainer or a removable Hawley or invisible clear plastic retainer.

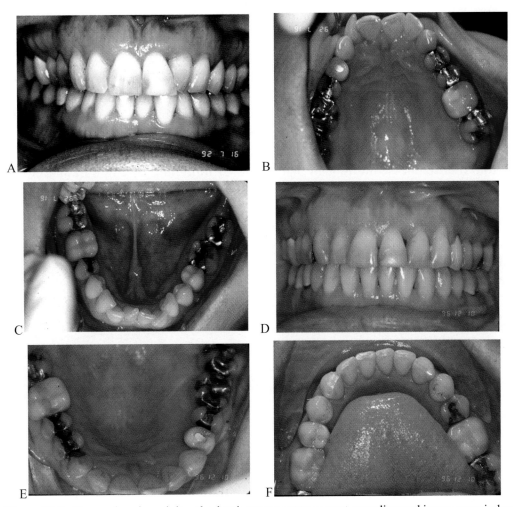

Figure 19-6: Comprehensive adult orthodontic treatment to correct crowding and improve periodontal health. A.), B.) and C.) Pre-treatment intraoral views showing the amount of upper and lower crowding and constriction of the dentoalveolar arches. D.), E.) and F.) Post-treatment intraoral photography. Note the change in arch form, which contributed to the correction of the crowding in conjunction with interproximal stripping to reduce the mesio-distal crown width of the posterior teeth at the expense of the amalgam restorations and reshaping of the upper and lower incisors.

7.1.3.2. **Correction of Anterior Spacing**

One of the most sought-after treatment procedures by adults is the closure of an anterior maxillary midline **diastema** to restore an esthetic smile. The etiologic factors involved in the production of excessive interdental spacing in the anterior region of the maxillary and/or mandibular arches are: Arch length/**tooth size discrepancy** (congenital), loss of teeth, presence of CO-CR discrepancy due to a premature posterior contact that forces the mandible to shift anteriorly (producing the flaring of a maxillary tooth or teeth), periodontal disease, abnormal labial frenum or abnormal interseptal bone architecture, presence of supernumerary teeth and habits like **tongue thrust**, nail biting, etc. The recognition and elimination of the etiologic factors is essential in order to institute the appropriate mechanotherapy.

7.1.3.2.1. **Appliance Selection**

Partial fixed **orthodontic appliance** consisting of brackets bonded to the anterior teeth and first molars is the appliance of choice in most cases. The space closure can be obtained with <u>elastomeric modules</u> (elastic chains) around an .018 SS arch wire placed after the initial light leveling wire. If the teeth are flared, the arch wire can be stopped short with a helical loop and tied back with an "O ring" elastic to retract the incisors during space closure. In the absence of an overjet, complete closure of an anterior diastema may not be possible, and space redistribution is recommended to facilitate the placement of esthetic restorations to fill in the spaces and to complete the treatment. This same consideration applies to those cases where there is a Bolton tooth size discrepancy. When the anterior spacing results from shifting caused by tooth loss, careful consideration should be given to the type of restoration to be used on the missing tooth. If implants are to be considered, the generalized spacing should be closed with a compressed push coil spring to open the space for the implant and the roots should parallel the extraction site to avoid interference with implant placement. A minimum of 6 mm of space is necessary at the root level for safe implant placement for a maxillary lateral incisor (Figure19-7).

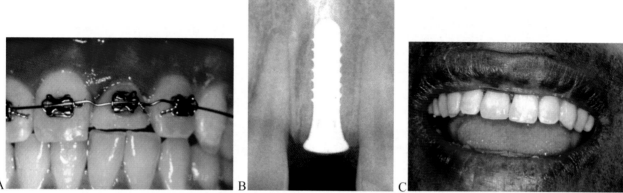

Figure 19-7: A.) Upper 2x4 appliance to align anterior teeth and obtain root parellism. B.) Implant placed, note position of roots and adequate space for implant. C.) Final restoration.

If the tooth movement requires only tipping to close the spaces, a Hawley retainer with finger springs can also be used to close and redistribute spaces. When the cause of the diastema is a prominent labial frenum, the **frenectomy** should be performed after the space closure and prior to the removal of the orthodontic appliance. The scar tissue formed would help maintain the space closed. The maintenance of the space closure is very difficult in some instances, therefore, a lingual fixed retainer is recommended to stabilize the results (Figure 19-8).

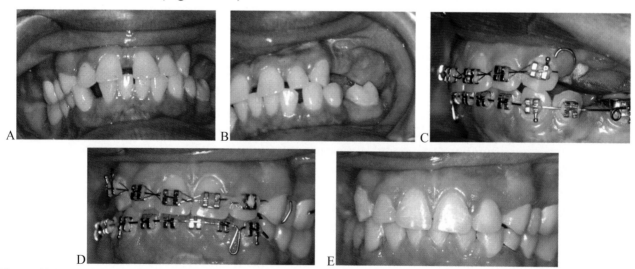

Figure 19-8: Partial orthodontic treatment to realign the upper and lower anterior teeth. A.) Pre-treatment occlusion. Note the generalized spacing and diastema in the upper and lower arches. B.) Buccal view of the occlusion. Note the supra eruption of the lower left first molar. C.) Partial orthodontic appliances placed in the upper and lower arches. Note the helical loop mesial to the lower left first molar used for uprighting it. A modified maxillary Hawley appliance with posterior bite block on the left side was used to support the lower first molar and prevent further eruption. D.) The upper diastema was closed with an elastomeric chain. The lower spacing was closed with a loop incorporated in the arch wire. E.) Final occlusion.

7.1.3.3. **Correction of Crossbites**

The **correction of crossbites** by means of limited orthodontic treatment mechanics is confined to dental movements only, therefore, only crossbites of dental origin can be corrected with partial orthodontic treatment. Crossbites can exist in either the anterior and/or posterior region of the arches and can be either a local problem or the manifestation of a more complicated general malocclusion (skeletal problem). The careful use of diagnostic records will help elucidate the nature of the problem and facilitate the institution of the appropriate mechanotherapy. From the orthodontic records one must determine: a.) space availability for tooth movement b.) presence of functional shift c.) angle classification d.) width of the maxilla to the mandible e.) type of tooth movement required for the correction of the cross bite (tipping versus **bodily movement**).

7.1.3.3.1. **Appliance Selection**

The correction of a single tooth **anterior crossbite**, when only tipping movement is necessary for tooth alignment, can be easily accomplished with a modified Hawley retainer with a mattress spring adapted to the lingual surface of the incisor and activated every 4-6 weeks to produce the desired tooth movement (Figure 19-9).

In cases where there is a deep bite (more than 50%), a bite plane should be incorporated posteriorly in the appliance to open the bite anteriorly and allow for labial tooth movement. As soon as the bite is "jumped", the posterior **bite plate** is removed and the overbite present will maintain the labial repositioning of the tooth and help in the retention of the correction.

When the anterior crossbite involves multiple teeth, a partial fixed orthodontic appliance is recommended for the correction of **linguoversion**s. An upper and/or lower 2x4 or 2x6 appliance is placed to flare the upper incisors and/or retract the lower incisors. The initial arch wires are light for leveling and stopped long ½ mm distal to the mesial portion of the molar tube so that when the wire is engaged in the tubes, it will be slightly forward of the anterior brackets. This will produce extra tension on the teeth and help with the tipping. When the lower incisors are to be retracted, the wire is stopped short 2 to 3 mm mesial to the molar tube and is tied back to the hook of the tube with an elastomeric module. This will produce the retrusive force needed for lingual tipping of the lower anteriors.   The utilization of compressed open coil springs placed on the buccal segments will also produce the forces necessary for the forward displacement of the maxillary anterior teeth (Figure 19-10).

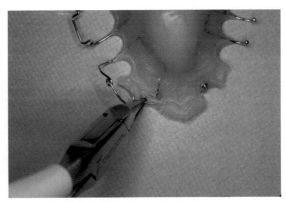

Figure 19-9:   Modified Hawley retainer with mattress spring used to correct a single tooth crossbite.

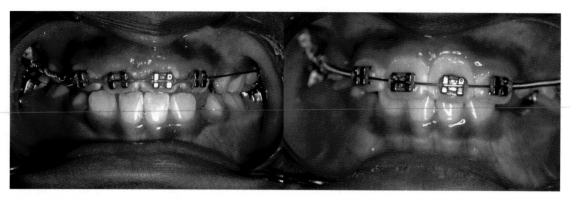

Figure 19-10 : Upper 2x4 appliance with open coil springs used to correct the linguo-version of the maxillary incisors.

The correction of a **posterior crossbite** is limited to the movement of a single tooth in a quadrant. This also is best accomplished with a **fixed appliance**. The utilization of a crisscross elastic has been advocated for the correction of a crossbite in the molar region. Caution should be used when this technique is utilized, since the elastic exerts a vertical force that will extrude the molars and cause traumatic occlusion after the correction (Figure 19-11).

The successful retention of the correction is accomplished through the establishment of the appropriate overbite. When a whole segment is in crossbite, then one must suspect the presence of a skeletal problem which should be handled in the adult through surgically assisted palatal expansion, or, if the problem is in the anterior quadrant, through surgical maxillary advancement, mandibular set-back or combination of the above (Figure 19-12).

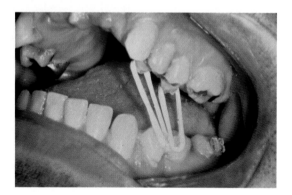

Figure 19-11: Cross elastics to correct posterior dental cross bites.

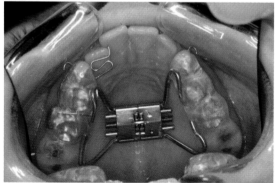

Figure 19-12: Bonded acrylic palatal expander used to correct skeletal cross bites.

7.2 COMPREHENSIVE ADULT ORTHODONTIC THERAPY

The **comprehensive orthodontic mechanotherapy** for the adult patient is based on the same principles of tooth movement and mechanics as in the adolescent patient. Nonetheless, there are some aspects of adult treatment that differ from the treatment of younger patients. These factors include a lack of growth availability, which forces the clinician to correct a dento-skeletal problem with more extensive tooth movement. This affects the roots and periodontal support adversely; therefore, consideration for **orthognathic surgery** is at hand. The malocclusion in adults is well established and there are less chances for modification of **arch form** and length. This could affect the stability of the treatment, therefore, the need for long-term retention should be considered.

7.2.1. **Stages of Treatment**

The stages of comprehensive treatment in the adult is the same as that of younger patients and includes: 1.) **setting up anchorage**, 2.) leveling and alignment, 3.) space closure, 4.) **releveling**, 5.) finishing, and 6.) retention.

7.2.1.1. **Setting up Anchorage**

The anchorage demands are dictated by the amount of crowding, the need for space to level the **curve of Spee** and the amount of incisor **proclination**. When extraction of bicuspids or other teeth is necessary, one must determine if the space closure is to occur from distal movement of the anterior teeth, (maximum anchorage requirement), mesial movement of the posterior teeth (minimum anchorage requirement) or combination of the above (moderate anchorage requirement). The preservation of anchorage, when necessary, can be accomplished through the utilization of a transpalatal arch, Nance holding arch in the maxilla or a lingual arch in the mandible. Another possibility includes modified Hawley removable plates.

7.2.1.2. **Leveling and Alignment**

After the anchorage requirement has been established, the leveling process can be started with the utilization of nickel titanium or copper niti wires, which will deliver light continuous forces to elicit tooth movement without discomfort and excessive extrusion of the posterior teeth. The utilization of the new alloys in orthodontics has facilitated the mechanics for adult orthodontic therapy.

In many instances, specifically in periodontally compromised dentitions, the need for segmental leveling mechanics should be considered to level a deep curve of Spee by intrusion of the incisors. This would prevent excessive extrusion of the periodontally compromised anchorage units and avoid clockwise rotation of the mandible with concomitant increase in the vertical dimension. In patients with edentulous spaces it is important to support the teeth in the opposite arch utilizing a modified Hawley appliance with bite blocks contacting the teeth in the opposite arch. This will prevent their extrusion during leveling and will maintain the vertical space for the replacement of the missing dental units without the need for excessive recontouring of the teeth in the opposing arch to obtain an appropriate occlusal plane.

7.2.1.3. **Space Closure**

The space closure of newly created extraction sites is done again with light continuous forces and taking into account the anchorage demands for the particular case. The utilization of power elastic modules (elastic chains) or niti coils is preferable in adults to the incorporation of closing loops in the main arch wire. It is easier to deliver more continuous light forces when niti coils or elastic chains are used, and they do not impair on the esthetics as much as the loops do. The closure of old extraction sites is more challenging, and in many instances it is very difficult or impossible due to the loss of alveolar bone, collapse of the buccal and lingual cortical plates and possible presence of periodontal defects that could contraindicate the movement of teeth into the space. The practitioner should carefully evaluate each situation to best determine the appropriate plan of action.

7.2.1.4. **Releveling**

This is usually necessary after space closure to establish a good plane of occlusion. The same mechanics used during the initial leveling process applies at this stage.

7.2.1.5. **Finishing**

In order to finalize tooth position in each arch, rectangular wires should be used. The utilization of .017 x .025 or .019 x .025 niti wires of .017 x .025 or .019 x .025 braided stainless steel wires can aid in controlling torque as well as settling of the bite. During this stage, short intermaxillary elastics may be necessary to detail the occlusion.

7.2.1.6. **Retention**

The retention stage in **adult orthodontic treatment** should be planned very judiciously, since it is more likely that long periods of stabilization will be required. The permanent splinting of periodontally compromised teeth is recommended utilizing soft passive wires bonded lingually on the teeth to be stabilized. A thin plastic invisible retainer offers increased esthetics and comfort, easy hygiene and protection against parafunctional habits. In cases where partially edentulous spaces exist, the utilization of the modified Hawley retainer is indicated, with the addition of bite blocks in the edentulous areas to prevent extrusion of the opposing teeth and migration of the neighboring teeth into the space. The restoration of the dentition should be done between 3 to 6 months after the removal of the fixed orthodontic appliances. Delaying the replacement of missing teeth can cause the loss of the alignment obtained with the orthodontic treatment.

The ultimate goal of comprehensive **adult orthodontic treatment** should be the attainment of the six keys to normal occlusion whenever possible to restore health and harmony to the different components of the stomatognathic system.

7.3 **ORTHOGNATHIC SURGERY**

Correction of Severe Dentoskeletal Discrepancies with Orthodontics and Orthognathic Surgery.

The adult patient with a severe dentoskeletal deformity in any of the three planes of space is a candidate for combined orthodontic and surgical treatment. The advancement of the surgical procedures and techniques has made possible the correction of deforming dentoskeletal malocclusions with better and more predictable results. The utilization of **rigid fixation**, which stabilizes the jaw, has made the treatment more acceptable to patients, and at the same time increased the stability of the newly repositioned skeletal bases.

7.3.1. Indications

The indications for surgery is determined by the age of the patient or lack of available growth to modify the dento-skeletal bases and by the degree of severity of the skeletal discrepancy. Proffit has established an "envelope of discrepancy" which states the limits of orthodontic and growth modification, as well as when surgery should be considered.

The effect of extensive tooth movement on the soft tissue profile should also be considered. Significant retraction of the incisors to compensate and correct a Class II malocclusion caused by mandibular ret-

rognathia, for example, will impact unfavorably on the facial esthethic of the patient. Most of the patients that seek orthognathic surgery expect an improvement of facial esthetics. Since esthetic improvement appears to be one of the major reasons why adult patients are willing to undergo surgical treatment, the goals should include not only improvement of function and stability of the results but also a positive psychological effect brought about by the improvement of facial appearance. Psychological evaluation is recommended prior to the initiation of treatment to screen those individuals that could possibly be affected negatively by the treatment outcome and create a problem for the practitioner and themselves.

Besides the severity of the skeletal deformity and psychological profile, other factors that should be considered when treatment planning for surgery are functional and anatomical limitations, patient cooperation and length of treatment.

Severely periodontally involved teeth and/or thin alveolar bone in the palate and **symphysis** will contraindicate extensive tooth movement. Furthermore, if the patient does not want to spend 3 or more years in treatment to camouflage the skeletal disharmony, surgery should be the treatment of choice.

7.3.2. Sequence of Treatment

An active preparatory orthodontic phase precedes the surgical treatment. During this phase, all dental compensations for the skeletal disharmony are removed in order to maximize the surgical movement of the skeletal bases. This preparatory orthodontic phase could take a minimum of 6 months and could be as long as 24 months, depending on the complexity of the case. Cases requiring extractions and orthodontic closure of the extraction sites will have longer pre-surgical orthodontics than those requiring only leveling and alignment for dental decompensation. Once the teeth have been positioned over the basal bone independently in each arch, the patient is ready for surgery.

Heavy rectangular wires should be in place prior to surgery to aid in stability during the post-surgical healing period. Post-surgical orthodontics follow the surgery, and should last 3 to 6 months. Longer post-surgical orthodontic treatment is usually an indication of surgical failure.

The role of the orthodontist is to coordinate the upper and lower dental arches to facilitate the surgeon's job. The coordination of the skeletal bases is done by the surgeon during the actual surgery.

7.3.3. Orthodontic Considerations

The aim of pre-surgical orthodontics is to decompensate the occlusion and position the teeth correctly over the basal bone. It is important to make the patient aware that the malocclusion will become more obvious during the pre-surgical orthodontics due to the elimination of the dental compensation that is present when the jaw bases are not well related to each other.

The horizontal and vertical position of the upper and lower incisors will determine the degree of the anterior movement of the mandible and will influence vertical dimension as well as the lip support and overall esthethic outcome. Therefore, the extraction patterns and leveling considerations will be different in surgical cases than in those to be treated by orthodontic treatment alone. Orthodontic expansion of the dental arches is contraindicated in pre-surgical orthodontics to avoid periodontal problems and to prevent instability.

7.3.4. **Surgical Techniques**

The most common surgical techniques utilized today for the correction of skeletal deformities are:
a.) the Lefort I maxillary osteotomy, which is used modify the position of the maxilla either anteriorly
or posteriorly as well as superiorly or inferiorly. The maxilla could also be split in 2 or 3 segments to
modify its transverse dimension, b.) the bilateral sagittal split ramus osteotomy to either set the
mandible back or advance it, and c.) segmental alveolar procedures for the correction of more localized problems. Genioplasties are commonly done to enhance the esthetic results. In complex cases, a
combination of these techniques is necessary to obtain ideal results.

Rigid fixation has made the surgical techniques more stable and more comfortable for the patients. The
success of orthognathic surgery is based on the understanding of the basic orthodontic and surgical
principles, communication between the patient, orthodontist, surgeon and all the other practitioners
involved in the final restoration of function, esthetics and psychological well being of the patient
(Figure 19-13).

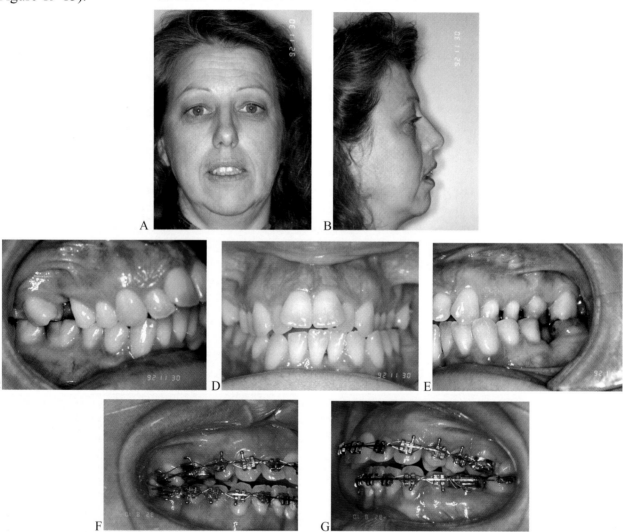

Figure 19-13 A-G - See legend on next page.

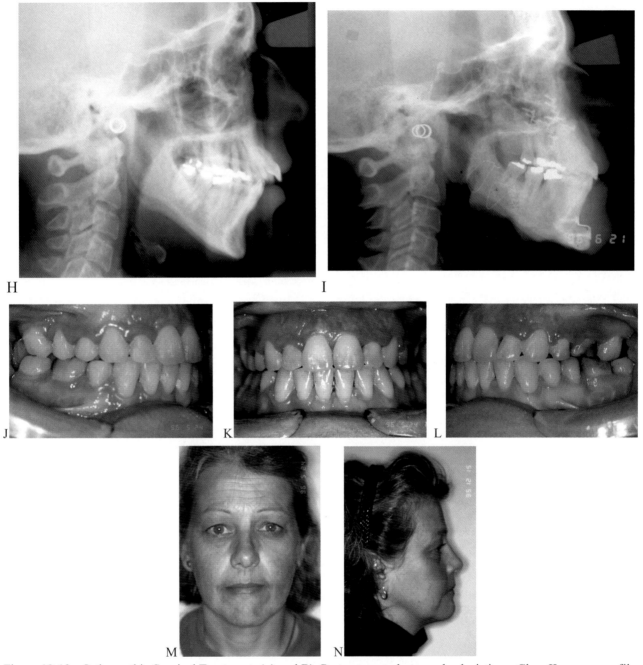

Figure 19-13: Orthognathic Surgical Treatment A.) and B). Pretreatment photographs depicting a Class II convex profile, increased vertical dimension, lip incompetence and facial asymmetry with the chin deviated toward the left side. C.) and D.) and E.) Pretreatment occlusion. Note the maxillary constriction, upper and lower crowding, open bite, mandibular dental midline deviation to the left. F.) and G.) Pre-surgical orthodontic preparation, which required the extraction of the lower right and upper left first bicuspids to correct the crowding and align the dentition. Note the complete closure of the molar and bicuspid extraction sites and the degree of the malocclusion prior to surgery. H.) and I.) Pre- and post-treatment cephalograms showing the severity of the skeletal discrepancy and its correction by Lefort I maxillary osteotomy to impact and widen the maxilla in conjunction with sagittal split ramus osteotomy and genioplasty to advance the mandible and chin. J.) K.) and L.) Post-treatment occlusion. M.) and N.) Post-treatment facial photographs.

8. SUGGESTED READINGS

Kuhlberg, Andrew; Glynn, Ellen: Treatment Planning Considerations For the Adult Patients. Dental Clinics of North America. Vol. 41, No. 1, 1997

Matthews, David P.; Kokich, Vincent G.: Managing Treatment of the Orthodontic Patient with Periodontal Problems. Seminars in Orthodontics. Vol. 3, No. 1, 1997

Roberts, Eugene W.; Hartsfield Jr, James K.: Primary Management of Congenital and Acquired Compensated Malocclusions: Diagnosis, Etiology and Treatment Planning. IDA Journal. Summer 1996

Ong, Mariane A.; Wang, Hom-Lay; Smith, Frederick N.: Interrelationship Between Periodontics and Adult Orthodontics. Journal of Clinical Periodontology. Vol. 25 1998

Zachrisson, Bjorn U.: Clinical Implications of recent Orthodontic – Periodontic Research Findings. Seminar in Orthodontics. Vol. 2, No. 1 1996

Polson, Alen; Caton, Jack; Polson, Anne P.; Nyman, Sture; Novak, John; Reed, Brian: Periodontal Response After Tooth Movement into Infrabony Defects. Journal of Periodontology. Vol. 55 No. 4 April 1984

Melsen, B.; Agerback, N: Eriksen, J; Terp, S.: New Attachment Through Periodontal Treatment and Orthodontic Intrusion. American Journal Orthod. Dentofacial Orthop. Vol. 94, No. 2, 1988

Melsen, B.; Agerback, N.; Markenstane, G.: Intrusion of Incisors in Adult Patients with Bone Loss. American Journal Orthod. Dentofacial Orthop. Vol. 96, No. 3, 1989

Wennstrom, Jan L.; Stokland, Birgitta L.; Nyman, Sture; Thilander, Birgit: Periodontal Tissue Response to Orthodontic Movement of Teeth With Infrabony Pockets. American Journal Orthod. Dentofacial Orthop. Vol. 103, No. 4, 1993

Nevins, Myron; Wise, Roger: The use of Orthodontic Therapy to Alter Infrabony Pockets. Part II. The International J. Of Periodontics and Rest. Dent. Vol. 10, No. 3, 1990

Artun, Jon; Urbye, K.: The Effect of Orthodontic Treatment on Periodontal Bone Support in Patients with Advanced Loss of Marginal Periodontium. American Journal Orthod. Dentofacial Orthop. Vol. 93, No. 2, 1988

Geiger, Arnold M.: Mucogingival Problems and the Movement of Mandibular Incisors: A Clinical Review. American Journal of Orthodontics. Vol. 78, No. 5, 1980.

Wehrbein, Heinrich; Bauer, Waltraud; Diedrich, Peter: Mandibular Incisors, Alveolar Bone and Symphysis After Orthodontic Treatment. A Retrospective Study. American Journal Orthod. Dentofacial Orthop. Vol. 110, No. 3, 1996

Duncan, Warwick: Realignment of Periodontally Affected Maxillary Teeth. A Periodontist's Perspective. Part I: Treatment Rationale and Methodology. New Zealand Dental Journal. Vol. 93, 1997

Beckett, Heather A; Evans, Robert D.: The Interface Between Orthodontics and Restorative Dentistry in the Management of Anterior Tooth Surface Loss. British Journal of Orthodontics. Vol. 21, No. 3, 1994

Harfin, Julia: Adult Orthodontic Treatment. Buenos Aries, 1999 Ed. Med. Panamericana.

Tulloch, F.C.: Uprighting Molars as an Adjunct to Restorative and Periodontal Treatment in Adults. British J. Orthod. Vol. 9, 1982.

Roberts, W.W.; Chacker, F.M.; Burstone, C.J.: A Segmental Approach to mandibular molar uprighting. American Journal of Dent Orthop. Vol. 81, no. 3, 1982

Pontonero, Roberto; Celenza, Frank; Ricci, Gianno; Carnevale, G.: Rapid Extrusion with Fiber Reseccion: A Combined Orthodontic – Periodontic Treatment Modality. International Journal of Periodontics and Restorative Dentistry. Vol. 5, 1987.

Stevens, Barry; Levine, Robert A.: Forced Eruption: A Multidisciplinary Approach for Form, Function and Biologic Predictability. Compendium Cont. Ed. Dent. Vol. 19, No. 10, 1998

Boyd, R.L.; Leggott, P.J.; Quin, R.S.: Periodontal Implications of Orthodontic Treatment in Adults with Reduced or Normal Periodontal Tissues Versus Those of Adolescents. American Journal Orthod. Dentofacial Orthop. Vol. 96, No. 3,1989

Sheridan, J.J.; Ledoux, P.M.: Air Rotor Shipping and Proximal Sealants. J. Clinical Orthodontics Vol. 23, 1989

Spears, F.M.; Matthews, D.M.; Kokich V.: Interdisciplinary Management of Single Tooth Implants. Seminar in Orthodontics. Vol. 3, 1997

Hom, Barney; Turley, Patrick: The Effects of Space Closure of the Mandibular First Molar Area in Adults. Am. J. Orthod. Vol. 85, No. 6, 1984

Phillips, C.; Bennett, M.E.; Broader, H.L.: Dentofacial Disharmony: Psychological Status of Patients Seeking a Treatment Consultation. Angle Ortho. Vol. 68, 1998

Kiyak, H.A.; Bell, R.: Psychological Considerations in Surgery and Orthodontics. In Proffit and White. Surgical Orthod. Treatment. Chapter 3, St. Louis 1991, Mosby

Miguel, J.A.; Turvey, T.A., Phillips, C.; Proffit, W.R.: Long Term Stability of Two Jaw Surgery for Treatment of Mandibular Deficiency and Vertical Maxillary Excess. Int. J. Adult Ortho. Orthognath. Surg. Vol. 19, 1995.

Ackerman, J.L.; Proffit W.R.: Communications in Orthodontic Treatment Planning: Bioethical and Informed Consent Issues. Angle Orthod. Vol. 65, 1985

Gottlieb, E.L.; Nelson, A.H.; Vogels, D.S.: 1990 J.C.O. Study of Orthod. Diagnosis and Treatment Procedures. Results and Trends. J. Clin. Orthod. Vol. 24, 1991

Patient Census Survey Results. Bulletin. Am. Assoc. Ortho. Vol. 15, No. 4, 1997

Chay SH, Rabie ABM. Repositioning of the the the gingival margin by extrusion. Am J Orthod Dentofacial orthop 2002;122 (1):95-102.

Stellzig-Eisenhauer A. Lux CJ. Schuster G. Treatment decision in adult patients with Class III malocclusion: orthodotic therapy or orthognathic surgery? Am J Orthod Dentofacial Orthop 2002;122(1):27-38.

Jacobson R, Sarver DM. The predictability of maxillary repositioning in LeFort I orthognathic surgery. Am J Orthod Dentofacial Orthop 2002;122:142-154.

Hiller ME. Nonsurgical correction of Class III open bite malocclusion in an adult patient. Am J Orthod Dentofacial Orthop 2002;122:210-216.

CHAPTER 20

Treatment of Patients with Craniofacial Anomalies

Bailey N. Jacobson
Ronald S. Jacobson

1. INTRODUCTION

Your dental training and experience will be mostly based on an understanding of what is "normal." If experience teaches us anything, it is that perfection is realistically unattainable when dealing, as you will every day, with imperfect creatures. In spite of that, however, perfection is what we will aim toward as we try to reach our "ideal" goal.

In order to even approach these "ideal" goals, we must have a patient with a potential for what we could call "normal growth and development." A potentially "normal" relationship of the skeletal bases. A potentially "normal" relationship of the hard and soft tissues. A "normal" amount of facial symmetry. A "normal" relation between surrounding muscular force and the supporting structures. Favorable influence of **Wolf's Law** during growth, that form would predictably follow function.

The simplest of all realities is that you will be able to treat a patient only to the maximum of his or her potential.

Young patients usually present predictability and symmetry. A patient born with single or multiple **congenital anomalies** presents just the opposite. For these patients there are few set rules and procedures. No patient will require greater imagination, innovation and patience. Within each type of anomaly there are a multitude of variations, each presenting a different magnitude and difficulty of treatment need, from the minor to the impossible. In most cases, "ideal" must be immediately compromised to thoughts of "maximum improvement." And, the more severe and complex the anomaly, the more difficult it is to gain acceptable improvement.

Orofacial and **craniofacial** patients, young or old, and the clinician must have realistic expectations. There is no question that they would like to function and look "normal" in a "normal" society. For some of them, that goal would be unattainable. From birth to early adulthood, and sometimes later, their habilitation can require a multitude and constancy of procedures, including dental, and a huge financial and time commitment on the part of the family. It is not surprising that some of these patients and their parents become tired, frustrated and, at times, even uncooperative. But, overall, an attitude of pervading hope, patience, understanding and gratitude for team treatment efforts is expressed. It is extremely important that these young people do not get the feeling that their treatment is going on forever, with no end in sight. Treatment should be planned with a definite GOAL in mind and conducted within a definite time frame. As an example, the orthodontist must accomplish as much as possible within a year in a first phase of treatment, not allowing a first phase to melt unnoticed into a second phase. The patient will definitely notice, and the result may be a precipitous drop in rapport and cooperation as the patient becomes more frustrated and disheartened.

The main thrust of this chapter shall be strategies for treatment: the dental implications of each of the orofacial and craniofacial anomalies described. The purpose of the following paragraphs is to offer enough insight into the treatment of patients born with the more common orofacial and craniofacial anomalies to allow you to make that treatment of these very special patients a comfortable part of your everyday dental life.

2. THE TEAM CONCEPT

The concept of team care of our patients, whether orofacial and craniofacial or not, has become part of the daily routine. The problem is diagnosed and the patient's program of care is treatment planned before any treatment begins. Many times they require only one professional's expertise, but there are times when others with special talents need to be brought in, in the proper order, in order to effectively complete the total plan of treatment. For no patient is this more necessary than in one born with an orofacial or craniofacial anomaly. The dentist is only one part of the overall effort in treatment of these patients. Your treatment must always fit into a logical sequence of treatment events, coordinated with the other members of the patient's treatment "team." A group of practitioners is not necessarily a "team." A true treatment team was defined years ago as "a close, cooperative, democratic, multiprofessional union devoted to a common purpose — the best treatment for the fundamental needs of the individual."   The benefits of team care for the patient with a craniofacial anomaly are now well recognized around the world, offering an environment for communication, cooperation and coordination of effort.

2.1 THE MEMBERS OF THE TEAM

The Craniofacial Habilitation Team should include the following specialists: primary care physician, plastic surgeon, dentist/orthodontist/prosthodontist, speech-language pathologist and otolaryngologist/audiologist with possible addition of a psychologist, geneticist, social worker, nurse practitioner, oral surgeon, neurosurgeon and neurologist.

2.2 THE DENTIST ON THE TEAM

The goal of the dentist/orthodontist/prosthodontist on the team is "to allow the patient to obtain optimal **maxillofacial** development, acceptable occlusion and appearance with objective diagnostic records and treatment criteria established, as needed, to promote the following:

A healthy oral environment, including **periodontium** and supporting tissues.

A maximum functional and esthetic occlusion, one that will adhere to orthodontic norms antero-posteriorly and laterally (i.e., Class I relationship and no crossbite).

A skeletal relationship of supporting alveoli and basal bones in keeping with a normal postural relationship for both entities, in conjunction with a maxillofacial surgeon, if necessary.

A skeletal relationship that will serve as an underlying support for esthetic draping of soft tissue, in conjunction with a maxillofacial surgeon, if necessary.

A dental relationship that will enhance normal speech.

To provide treatment to support the other disciplines involved (i.e., pre-surgical and post-surgical treatment to aid and enhance the surgical care)."

Remember, these are the dental goals, the "ideal". It's immediately obvious that it will require the help of other disciplines to allow the dentist to even approach these goals with our orofacial and craniofacial patients. One of the largest limiting factors has to be the severity of the patient's anomaly. Usually, the more severe, the more the limitations, and the more the probable compromise.

Is it necessary to become a member of a team before participating in the treatment of a patient? Absolutely not. A team can function purely in a consultative way. They can make an evaluation of the patient's needs and then suggest where and when dental treatment can fit into the overall picture. They can put you in touch with the patient's other health professionals and you can learn the patient's other needs and how to help enhance the quality of the overall treatment result.

The kind of **multidisciplinary** treatment usually needed by a patient born with a congenital birth defect can represent an immense financial commitment on the part of the family. Many of these families fall under the protective umbrella of state or governmental agencies that have agreed to help them face the financial burden. If dental treatment is necessary because of a congenital anomaly, it may well be subsidized by an agency of this kind, and contacting the social worker on the team or the patient's case worker will usually supply the necessary information for the dentist's participation in the program.

3. THE PATIENT WITH A CLEFT OF THE LIP AND PALATE

3.1 ETIOLOGY

Though other theories have been advanced, the most accepted theory is that some time between the 4th and 12th week of intrauterine development of the fetus, some disturbance causes a failure of mesodermal penetration and **fusion** of the developing processes of the maxilla. The maxillary, nasomedial and nasolateral processes may make contact but, without fusion, will then separate and displace as the fetus develops. The earlier the disturbance, the more severe the resulting cleft. Partial fusion will result in an "incomplete" cleft. The three processes usually join and fuse to create the intact nose and **primary and secondary palate**.

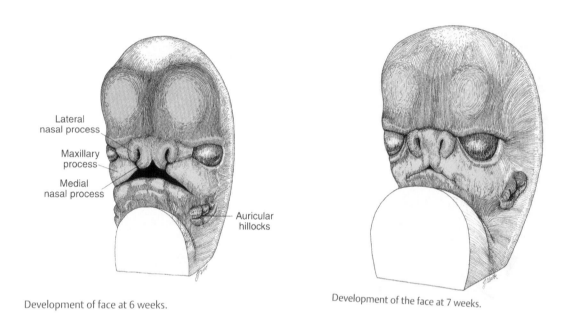

Development of face at 6 weeks.

Development of the face at 7 weeks.

Lateral nasal process

Maxillary process

Medial nasal process

Auricular hillocks

Figure 20-1: Embryology of the palate and the maxillofacial region (Avery).

Each of the processes carries with it cartilage, bone, connective tissue, muscle, nerves and blood vessels. The nasolateral process forms the lateral portion of the nose. The fusion of the two nasomedial processes centrally and with the maxillary processes laterally form the medial portions of the nose, the lip, the **primary palate** (anterior to the **incisive foramen**) and the secondary palate (posterior to the incisive foramen). At approximately 7 weeks, the palatal shelves are developing vertically with the tongue interposed. Then, the tongue drops and the shelves swing up or re-direct their growth horizontally and grow toward each other, to meet and fuse from anterior to posterior. (For greater detail, See Chapter 2).

3.2 INCIDENCE

The occurrence of **cleft lip** and palate does not know the bounds of social class of the family, the seasons of the year or the age of the parents. It happens in approximately one out of seven hundred fifty live births. In the general population that means that the average family has approximately .13% chance of having a baby with this congenital defect. It has been estimated that, in the United States, there are approximately 250,000 cleft lip and palate individuals under the age of 21 years. That sounds like a large number, but, when spread across the face of this nation, means that the chance that you will add some of these patients to your practice is rather slim, unless you are part of a team whose expertise attracts larger numbers of them for treatment.

Many feel that at this number is low because there is under-reporting of the occurrence of the clefts by unsophisticated hospital staff, who are the first to see the baby during and after birth. The records of the hospitals and local agencies that add to the statistics are just not accurate or complete. In the turmoil of the birth day, it is not unreasonable to consider that many of the more subtle defects may escape detection. These delivery room notations are passed to the birth record and hence to the local and state agencies that record the birth and, if the notations are incomplete, so are the incidence statistics. Many defects are not found until later and never make it into the incidence statistics. Considerable effort is being made to rectify this problem.

This is the most frequent of the orofacial and craniofacial anomalies that you will encounter, and the involvement of the dentist and dental specialist has reached an all-time high as the importance of the teeth to all facets of this patient's habilitation becomes appreciated.

When cleft lip and palate occurs, approximately 60-80% of the children will be male and 60% of the clefts will be unilateral, on the left side. In approximately one-third of the cases there is a family history, indicating genetic influence. Other suggested causes can be mutated genes, aberrations of the chromosomes or, least frequently, environmental agents to which the mother is exposed during the 4th to 12th week of pregnancy that may interfere with the development of the fetus. At this point in time there is great reluctance on the part of the medical and dental community to prescribe drugs of any kind for an expectant mother because of the fear that the fetus may be affected in any way, unless the risk to the mother is greater than the risk to the fetus.

If one of the parents is affected, the chance that their child will be affected is about 4%, which is about 40 times the frequency in the general population. If an affected parent already has a child with a cleft, the chance that the next child will be affected as well jumps to about 17%.

3.3 CLASSIFICATION

Since collaboration and communication between members of the treating team is so important in the coordination of the treatment plan for these patients, some means of describing the patient's defect is necessary. Rather than making lengthy written or oral descriptions of the patient's problem, many classification systems have been proposed and used to date, starting as early as 1922, but none of which has been accepted universally. One of the oldest systems, introduced by Veau in 1931 is quite simplistic; it has its shortcomings but is still commonly used around the world. At least it offers a rather graphic view of the types of cleft possible and can introduce us to the subject. There are basically five common types of cleft of the lip and palate, as seen in Figure 20-2.

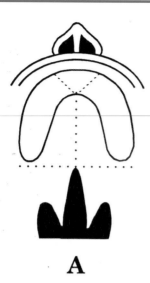

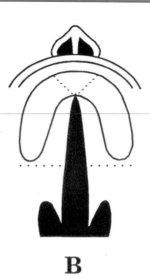

Figure 20-2A: Diagram of a cleft of the soft palate only. Veau Class I — Cleft of the soft palate only. This cleft extends from the posterior tip of the soft palate (**uvula**) to the posterior border of the hard palate. This type of cleft has little dental implication, but may have varying effects on speech.

Figure 20-2B: Diagram of a cleft of the hard and soft palates only. Veau Class II — Cleft of the **hard** and **soft palates** only. This cleft extends from the posterior tip of the uvula to the incisive foramen at the junction between the hard palate and alveolus. This is also the division between the secondary (posterior) and primary (anterior) palates. This type of cleft has some dental implication, with possible maxillary constriction due to palatal scarring from surgical closure.

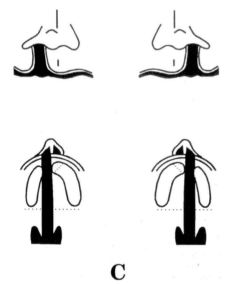

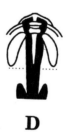

Figure 20-2C: Diagram of a complete right or left unilateral cleft of the lip and palate. Veau Class III -- Right or left unilateral cleft of the lip and palate. This cleft extends from the posterior tip of the uvula, past the incisive foramen and through the **alveolar ridge** to the base of the nostril (alar base) on the affected side. This type of cleft has many dental implications.

Figure 20-2D: Diagram of a complete bilateral cleft of the lip and palate. Veau Class IV -- Bilateral cleft of the lip and palate. This cleft extends from the posterior tip of the uvula, past the incisive foramen, dividing both right and left around the premaxilla and through the **alveolar ridge** to the alar base of the nose on both sides. This type of cleft has the greatest dental and speech implications.

Veau Class V -- Cleft of the lip only. A rather unusual cleft which extends just from the anterior of the alveolus, through the lip to the alar base of the nose. The alveolus may be affected as well by "submucous clefting," a notching seen in the intact **alveolar ridge**. This may also affect the developing anterior teeth.

Recognizing the fact that Veau's classification failed to provide any real detail about an individual patient's cleft configuration, many attempts have been made over the years to improve detailing. A committee of the American **Cleft Palate**/Craniofacial Association developed an extremely sophisticated system, but perhaps the most useful one was developed by Kernahan in 1958. It is called the "Striped Y" and is very widely used at this time. It is an easy schematic system which not only allows quick and accurate description of the cleft, but also makes it possible to note any bridges of tissue across the cleft. Clefts are called "**complete**" if there is total separation of the tissue parts and "**incomplete**" if there is a tissue bridge located anywhere along the cleft.

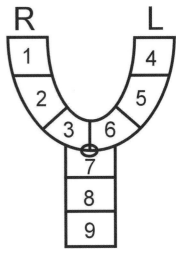

Figure 20-3

The "Striped Y" schematically divides the maxillary structures based on embryological development into anterior and posterior parts, using the incisive foramen as the point of division.

In Figure 20-3, numbers 1 and 4 represent the right and left nostril and base of the nose; Numbers 2 and 5, the right and left lip; and Numbers 3 and 6, the right and left alveolar ridges. Then, the Incisive Foramen separates the anterior (primary) and posterior (secondary) palates. Number 7 is the anterior portion of the **hard palate**; 8 is the posterior portion of the hard palate; and number 9 is the soft palate. **Complete cleft** areas are striped and incomplete areas, where there is a tissue bridge, are shaded.

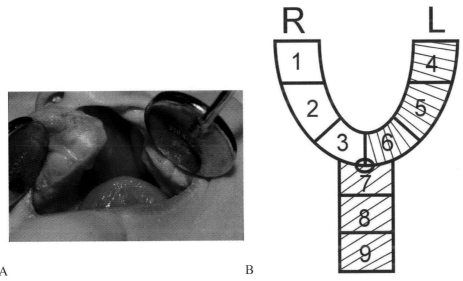

A   B

Figure 20-4A, B: A unilateral complete left cleft of the lip and palate and the corresponding Striped-Y schematic (Kernahan, 1958).

. . . .

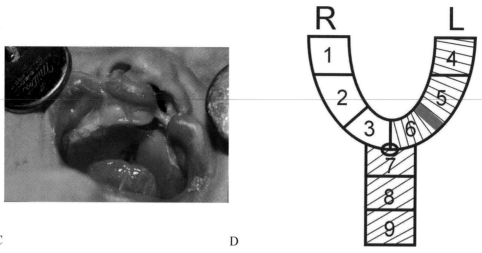

C   D

Figure 20-4C, D: An **incomplete** unilateral left cleft of the lip and palate and the corresponding Striped-Y schematic.

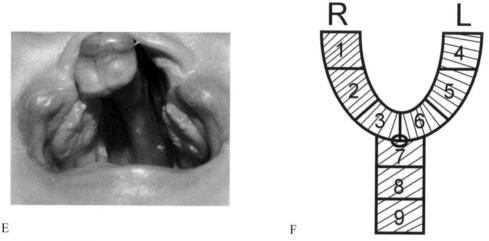

E   F

Figure 20-4E, F: A complete bilateral cleft of the lip and palate and the corresponding Striped-Y schematic.

Figure 20-4 A, B, C, D, E, and F shows examples of three cleft lip and palate infants on the left and their schematics on the right. Note on the bilateral cleft lip and palate infant, the view all the way to the superior surface of the nasal chamber from each side of the **vomer** (the base of the nasal septum), the turbinates in the lateral walls of the nasal chamber, the divided hard and soft palates, the lateral alveolar segments, the anteriorly displaced **premaxillary segment**, the short **philtrum of the lip** and **columella of the nose** and the flattened nostrils.

General dental and orthodontic implications will be discussed as the chapter proceeds but, generally speaking, and not surprisingly, the more extensive the cleft deformity, the more difficult the treatment of the patient. The more severe the cleft, the more the potential effect of surgical interventions on growth and development, of displacement and possible deficiency of tissues (including the teeth), of departure from expected treatment responses and of potential for compromised treatment results.

3.4 ASSOCIATED PROBLEMS

As these infants develop, it will become apparent that there are problems that will be encountered that are specifically associated with the fact that they have been born with a visible congenital birth defect (See Chapter 1). Along with possible additional medical problems brought on by secondary defects (i.e., respiratory or cardiac), these problems may include feeding, emotional and psychosocial, speech, hearing, breathing, growth and dental.

3.4.1. Feeding

Problems for the infant will be discussed in the section on placement of the early maxillary orthopedic appliance. As the child's dentition develops, the efficiency of chewing will depend greatly on the degree of malocclusion and the number of teeth maintained. Though the compensatory mechanism is great, it may not be able to overcome many missing teeth or severe tooth malposition, and this will help determine the timing for orthodontic intervention. Typically, the greatest problems will be malalignment of the upper incisors and maxillary arch constriction with buccal segment, and possibly anterior, crossbite. These will usually be treated first in the mixed dentition.

3.4.2. Emotional and Psychosocial

The family begins dealing with emotional problems the moment the parents find out that their infant has been born with a congenital birth defect, especially one as immediately visible and shocking as a **complete cleft** of the lip and palate. There is immediate disappointment, sometimes coupled with guilt, followed by concerns about why it happened, whether it could happen again, whether the family will be able to afford the needed care and, finally, what the future may hold for them and their child. These reactions can often be intensified if the quality of the marriage is not good. Resignation and acceptance usually follows quickly, and then we most often find an intense desire on the part of the parents to know everything about the congenital anomaly, what are the plans for treatment, in what sequence and what they can do to help. It's important that the team provide this information in abundance. The greater the parent's knowledge and involvement, the greater the chance for success of the treatment. Of course, as the child grows, their emotional development will be tied to the parental attitude and action. The concerned and involved parent watches their child's emotional and social development carefully, usually feeling that the presence of the congenital defect has affected both, and even their school work. These feelings are often confirmed by members of the treating team, also relating it to compliance. The fact that many of these patients are under almost constant treatment of one kind or another from birth on can definitely have impact on their attitude toward our treatment, their motivation and their cooperation potential. Though psychological development of these patients has broad effect on the success of treatment, it has, in the past, not had a high priority for finite study.

One of the reasons for the trend toward early corrective surgical intervention is to aid in the child's development of a good self image, which is extremely important (See Chapter 1). "Attractiveness" conveys a much more positive social image, bringing with it enhanced perception by society of brightness, kindness, likeableness and success, even to the point of deserving higher salaries. Children are aware of differences very early, and 10 year old cleft lip and palate children are more inhibited than their peers. Parents and teachers usually expect less of unattractive children.

3.4.3. Speech

Basically, the effectiveness of speech is determined by two factors: the ability of the soft palate to move freely, directing the flow of air between the mouth and the nose and the movement of the tongue in and around the teeth to articulate the sounds. In the cleft lip and palate patient, both factors may be compromised.

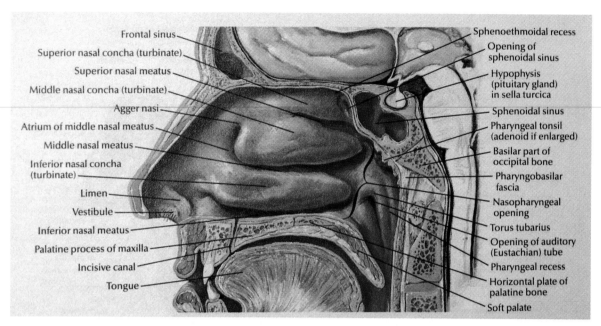

Figure 20-5: Illustration of structures affecting speech and breathing.

The soft palate may suffer different amounts of immobility, depending on the amount of scarring from the surgical palate closure and the final configuration of the musculature governing its movement. Many sounds, such as "p", require the complete separation of the nasal and oral cavities with a build up of pressure in the mouth. This is accomplished by the soft palate raising itself, moving posteriorly and creating an air-tight seal between it and the lateral and posterior walls of the **nasopharynx**. If this is impossible (**velo-pharyngeal** inadequacy) air escapes through the nose during this **plosive** sound, and the patient is "**hypernasal**." This characterizes typical "cleft palate speech." The adenoid pad in the developing cleft palate child helps the immobile soft palate by keeping the posterior wall of the pharyngeal wall forward, making it easier to reach. Of course, this is reason to avoid adenoidectomy in these children if at all possible. The very inadequate soft palate is sometimes surgically attached to the posterior pharyngeal wall (the "**pharyngeal flap**"), leaving ports laterally for the control of air, or a prosthetic **obturator** may be necessary. As dentists, we cannot control the function of the soft palate, but we certainly can see to it that the dentition remains intact and as well aligned as possible, thereby influencing articulation. Maxillary arch constriction, poorly related upper and lower arches, malaligned teeth, **edentulous** spaces and **supernumerary teeth** may certainly have an adverse effect on articulation of sounds. Initial surgical closure of the palate is recommended before the age of 12 months so that, before active speech development, the soft palate can be intact to minimize the development of compensatory articulatory movements.

3.4.4. Hearing

This may stem from some associated developmental anomaly, but more often it arises from poor function of the Eustachian tubes, or simply the fact that the tubes are more exposed to bacteria and food because of the open cleft. These conditions may cause repeated middle ear infections and a gradual loss of hearing. The loss may be detected early when the child continues to raise the volume on the family television set but, unfortunately, often goes undetected until the child enters school.

3.4.5. Breathing

Typically, the cleft lip and palate patient will suffer from partial blockage of the nasal airway, either because of narrowing associated with a constricted maxillary arch, deviation of the nasal septum or placement of a **pharyngeal flap**. This constriction of air flow usually causes chronic mouth breathing with its increased activity of the **perioral muscles**, and may tend to intensify the narrowing of the arches. Growth and maxillary expansion may improve the nasal airflow, but the mouth breathing habit may persist for years.

3.4.6. Growth and Development

The consensus of thought today seems to be that growth and development may be influenced by both genetic and environmental factors (See Chaper 1). Certainly, a child born with a cleft of the lip and palate may be affected by both.

Studies have found that the repaired cleft lip and palate patient will show a deficiency in the growth and development of the maxilla not only antero-posteriorly and vertically, but in the area and width of the palatal tissue, as well. The key word is "repaired." Unoperated cleft lip and palate patients have shown that the maxilla has great capacity for growth in all directions. The needed surgical repair of the lip and palate changes that, introducing scarring, which may be binding and restrictive to the normal downward and forward growth of the maxilla. Vargervik found in the bilateral cleft the premaxillary segment grew at only one-half the pace of her non-cleft controls, and that mandibular growth did not differ. She concluded, therefore, that in the bilateral cleft lip and palate patient with the prominent premaxilla, surgical premaxillary recession should not be necessary because the normally growing mandible should match maxillary position by age 12. She

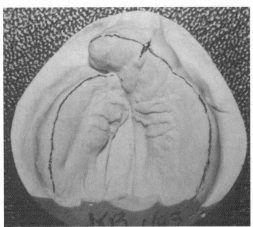

Figure. 20-6: Collapsed maxillary alveolar segments, the smaller, lateral segment being trapped behind the premaxillary segment.

also concluded that the forward growth of the maxilla, and even alveolar growth are directly affected by the amount of scarring of the lip and palate, disagreeing that there must be vertical maxillary deficiency. If the tongue position is low because of maxillary constriction, the result can be increased maxillary alveolar height causing a steeper **mandibular plane** and a more retruded chin position. If the maxillary alveolar segments are allowed to collapse, they may become trapped behind the premaxillary segment. Subtelny has noted that this may cause delayed tooth eruption and alveolar growth in the area of the cleft, and that "one may assume that unlocking the alveolar segments may relieve the bony maxillary segments of their impaction and enhance the possibility of more normal maxillary growth, partially incident to providing better support for the upper lip." Rather than waiting for later "unlocking," we believe that prevention is more the answer, using an early maxillary appliance to control the segment alignment after lip closure, as will be described in more detail later, and placing an early **autogenous alveolar bone** graft to try to stabilize and maintain that bony relation in an attempt to prevent bony collapse and "locking." It has been found that this primary graft does NOT have any deleterious effect of its own on maxillary growth. It may, on the other hand, help avoid the segment impaction's restrictive effect on maxillary growth, maintain the width of the floor of the nasal cavity improving nasal air flow, prevent severe skeletal maxillary arch constriction and associated low tongue position with all its potential effects and add symmetry to facial form and appearance. The incidence of **dental crossbite** may not be different with this early approach, but those are usually easily corrected by tooth movement alone, as we will discuss later. The potential for overall general growth of these patients has also been studied. Bowers, et al., found in their sample that the cleft lip and palate children were significantly shorter, with the males thinner, than their non-cleft controls. This lack of overall potential may also affect the size of the teeth in the developing dentition.

3.5 GENERAL DENTAL PROBLEMS AND TREATMENT

As a general rule, the greater the cleft defect the greater the impact on the development and position of the **primary** and **permanent dentitions**. The teeth most often serve as the hub around which other treatment for these patients revolves, bearing heavily on the success of surgery, speech and, of course, final esthetics and function of the dentition. The primary responsibility of the family dentist or pediatric dentist is to maintain the health of the teeth and supporting structures. This may require considerable patience, understanding, imagination and innovation on the part of the dentist.

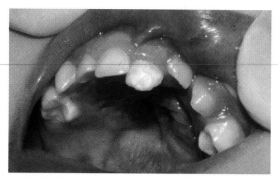

Figure 20-7: Ectopic eruption of the teeth adjacent to the cleft site.

Dental treatment for the cleft lip and palate patient begins with the eruption of the primary teeth. Hopefully, the parents have been counseled very early about the importance of the dentition. In most parts of the United States, fluoride in the water should be naturally increasing the child's resistance to caries and potential tooth loss, but the parents must be made to understand that the wrong diet and lack of oral hygiene can easily overcome the benefits of fluoride. Putting the baby to bed with a bottle should be especially discouraged because of the potential for "bottle caries" and the virtual destruction of the primary teeth as they begin to erupt. As we see the babies on regular recall visits, the parents must also be prepared for several possibilities. First, probable **ectopic eruption** of the upper anterior teeth, especially those adjacent to the cleft site.

The primary central incisor next to the cleft usually erupts inclined lingually and toward the cleft with an extra wide diastema between the central incisors. Next for the possibility that the lateral incisor in the cleft site(s) may be congenitally missing, may have anomalous form or may erupt palatally. If a primary alveolar bone graft had been placed, the primary lateral incisor may erupt right into the graft site.

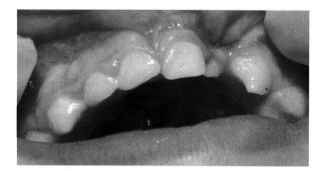

Figure 20-8A: Primary lateral incisor erupting into alveolar graft site.

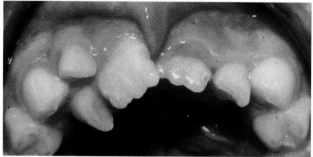

Figure 20-8B: Supernumerary erupted in cleft site.

Next, the possibility that there could be extra teeth (**supernumeraries**) erupting in or near the cleft site. As discussed later, supernumerary teeth are quite common in the cleft lip and palate patient. Last, the "bite" may need attention when the baby gets a little older. Because of the bending and molding of the alveolar segments under the influence of the surgically closed lip, or because of the tightness of the surgically closed lip, the upper anterior teeth may erupt lingually and into crossbite, as might the primary canines.

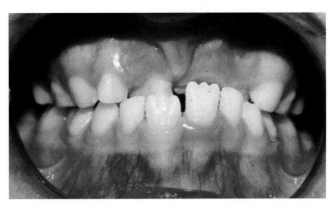

Figure 20-9: Eruption into crossbite of lingually inclined upper anterior teeth.

Even though corrective treatment will not be undertaken until much later, the parents can be prepared for the problem. The baby may posture the mandible forward and occlude in **anterior crossbite** because of the tooth interference, and assurance that this is probably a tooth problem as opposed to a skeletal problem is important. It is most common for the parents to ask for a projection of the dental problems and possible treatment from infancy all the way to young adulthood so they can have a sense of what may lie ahead.

The parents are encouraged to take the child to the dentist for the first visit as soon as the primary teeth have erupted. Of course, in the meantime, the child's teeth should be regularly brushed. Remember, these young children have been under almost constant medical attention since birth and, by the time they reach your office, may be quite disenchanted with the world of health professionals in general. Here is where patience will be needed. It seems only logical that if the first visits to the dentist are very early, where needed work should be quite minimal, the resultant rapport would be better than if the first visit was later when their first introduction to dentistry could be the restoration of a carious lesion. Ideally, the early visit should involve only an examination; a few rides up and down in the chair, light prophylaxis and the patient can be placed on recall. By the time the patient is four years old there will have been several visits, and the first full mouth radiographs may be taken at that time for caries detection and determination of the number and position of the developing permanent teeth. As the child continues to grow and the permanent dentition begins to make its entrance, there are some specific problems that may be presented because of the presence of the cleft.

3.5.1. Nasal Congestion

As has been discussed previously, these patients will probably be primarily mouth breathers because of the associated reduction of the nasal airflow by deviation of the nasal septum or constriction of the nasal passages. Obligate mouth breathing usually brings with it the fear that work in the mouth may interfere with that breathing, and the patient may be quite concerned. This may mean that use of a rubber dam may be limited and only with sizeable air holes, and that cotton rolls should be clamped into place. Work may have to be limited to one small area at a time in order to keep the patient comfortable.

3.5.2. Tautness of the Lips

The use of cotton rolls for work on the upper anteriors may be impossible because of the lack of **gingivo-labial sulcus**. Surgical repair and revision of the upper lip may result in a very tight lip, which seems bound down to the gingiva of the premaxillary area. This seems more prevalent in a bilateral cleft and may not only cause excessive pressure on the upper anteriors, but also may make the upper lip rather immobile, making access difficult. This difficulty is not only experienced by the dentist, but by the patient as well and may make adequate brushing of the teeth quite difficult. The use of miniature sized mirrors and pediatric sized toothbrushes may help. If this condition is quite severe, surgical deepening of the sulcus may be possible.

3.5.3. Radiographic Problems

Upper periapical films will be most difficult because of the variations encountered in the shape of the palatal vault of the operated cleft palate patients. The palatal vault may be very shallow and flat or very high, narrow and constricted and may vary in different palatal areas on the same patient. Tube angulations must be placed perpendicular to the plane of each film instead of using predetermined angulations for best results though, because of the great difference between tooth angulations and palate and film angulations, root length accuracy is not predictable. Because of mouth breathing, fast film is best used. A good panoramic film has the advantage of being able to provide a great deal of information with a completely extraoral approach. It may lack finite detail about the anterior roots and periodontal ligament spaces and interproximal caries, but has much greater range for the identification of missing or ectopic teeth and evaluation of the integrity of the temporomandibular joints. It can then be supplemented by anterior periapicals and bitewings, limiting the number of periapicals needed.

3.5.4. Anesthesia

It is extremely important that the patient be as comfortable as possible during treatment. These patients will probably be more fearful and will probably require more treatment than the usual dental patient. Their dentition is critical to the success of their overall habilitation and this usually requires many visits and constant surveillance by their dentist. Fear of discomfort, as with any patient, can delay and complicate their treatment. The use of topical and local anesthetics will be necessary and many of these patients, because of their dental phobias and extent of needed repair, will require general anesthesia. Accomplishing profound local anesthesia of the upper anteriors may not be easy. The cleft and its subsequent surgical repair result in considerable variation of the innervations to the area, especially in the bilateral cleft. In the bilateral cleft, the nasopalatine nerve innervates the area alone, so profound anesthesia is possible only by infiltrating high in the incisive canal. The unilateral cleft would have some anterior superior alveolar innervation to the area, as well.

3.5.5. Tooth Formation and Eruption

We have already discussed that children with cleft lip and palate seem to demonstrate a reduced overall growth potential. The crowns of the primary and permanent dentitions develop all through infancy and childhood and their sizes may be affected by this reduced general growth. Werner and Harris found that their unilateral and bilateral cleft palate samples show significantly reduced mesiodistal diameters of the teeth compared to their controls, and agreed that "size reduction throughout the permanent dentition argues for attenuation of overall growth potential of individuals with cleft lip and palate rather than for the cleft being an isolated, unassociated defect." Along with some diminution in size, significant delay in timing of eruption and **asymmetrical** development has also been found.

3.5.6. **Malocclusion**

The most common dental problem exhibited by the cleft lip and palate patients is malocclusion. The effects of the cleft are superimposed on whatever malocclusion would have occurred through growth and development. The cleft itself, or the scarring from needed surgeries, can create an imbalance between maxillary and mandibular growth; the greater the imbalance, the greater the malocclusion.

With growth imbalance comes muscular imbalance, and **Wolf's Law** dictates that form shall follow function. Both primary and permanent dentitions are affected. Most usually there is crossbite, either anterior or posterior, or both. There are usually also rotations and displacement of the upper incisors, especially those adjacent to the cleft site. The orthodontic implications will be discussed later.

3.5.7. Caries

Because of the importance of the teeth to a person's habilitation, this has perhaps the greatest dental implication to the patient with cleft lip and palate. Though early study showed similar incidence of caries between cleft and non-cleft populations, it has more recently been shown that a cleft palate population shows a statistically significant increase in caries, mostly on the proximal surfaces. Establishment of early contact with the cleft palate child and regular visits with good preventive maintenance programs and diet control can only help reduce the risk to the integrity of the teeth and supporting tissues. Adding to that, systemic fluoride and topical fluoride applications at least twice each year can reduce the rate of caries by 70%. Occlusal pit protection by placement of sealants can reduce the incidence of occlusal caries by 80-100%.

3.5.8. The Supporting Tissues

Poor oral hygiene or reduced **vestibular space**, which makes access to many areas for cleaning and tissue massage difficult, was found to be responsible for increased marginal gingivitis and an increased annual loss of **attached gingiva** in cleft palate patients. Bragger, et al., studied the progression of periodontal disease over an 8-year period in 52 adult patients with cleft lip, ridge and palate. The rate of progression over the entire 8 year period was not statistically different at the cleft and control sites, but " the cumulative periodontal destruction at 26-28 years of age was statistically significant and more pronounced at cleft sites, as revealed by greater probing pocket depth and loss of clinical attachment." They found radiographic evaluation of **alveolar crestal bony heights** unreliable, and that "at age 18-20 years of age, the patients demonstrated poor oral hygiene, generalized plaque accumulation and signs of gingival inflammation, as well as beginning periodontal disease documented as loss of clinical attachment and radiographically assessed loss of alveolar bone height." The fact that the prominent causative factor was high plaque accumulation points again to the reversibility of the situation by early establishment of a strong preventive maintenance program and regular recall visits and prophylaxis.

3.5.9. **Dental Hypoplasia**

This is the most common dental defect found in the cleft lip and palate patient, particularly involving the anterior teeth immediately adjacent to the cleft site. The crowns may be discolored or pitted and malformed, possibly with enlarged cingula or marginal ridges and excessively curved labial surfaces. If the tooth adjacent to the cleft is a lateral incisor, often the crown is quite small and conical in shape. Usually the root development and form is adequate, however, and if the teeth can be preserved they can most often be useful. In the young patient, these central and lateral incisors should be saved until after orthodontic treatment. If a bone graft has been placed in the cleft site, these teeth can often be moved to a good esthetic and functional position, and then the permanent restoration by crowning, veneering or esthetic bonding can be accomplished.

3.5.10. **Congenital Absence**

Approximately half of the cleft lip and palate population will have congenital absence of the permanent lateral incisor on the side of the cleft. The primary dentition is most often intact, though the teeth next to the cleft may be displaced, with supernumeraries appearing more often than congenital absence. The incidence of congenital absence of second premolars in the general population is 6.6%, whereas in the cleft palate population it can range from 24-50%, with maxillary second premolars most often affected. With the potential of delayed development of the teeth, definite diagnosis of **agenesis** of the second premolars should be delayed until 8 or 9 years of age.

If there is congenital absence of a primary tooth, usually the lateral incisor, no treatment should be necessary. There may be migration of the primary central incisors toward the cleft site, but this should not create a functional problem.

Congenital absence of the permanent lateral incisor in the cleft site(s) could have impact on speech articulation, but most certainly has impact on dental and facial esthetics. Missing anterior teeth for more than a short time can have a psychological effect on the child with regard to a lessening of their self-image, and should be avoided, if possible. Certainly the fact of the congenital absence will be noted radiographically with the first set of full mouth periapicals or panoramic x-ray and, if the central incisors are not in need of early orthodontic treatment for alignment, a removable palatal appliance with one or two teeth attached in the early mixed dentition can make all the difference in the world for the child. If early orthodontic intervention is necessary, the tooth can be placed on the retainer. Later, in the treatment planning for the comprehensive orthodontic treatment, the fate of the space for the lateral incisor(s) can be determined, depending on the magnitude and nature of the rest of the developing malocclusion. If there is a choice between leaving the space open for eventual bridgework, implant or closing the space and placing the canine in the lateral incisor position, it is usually best to leave the space open. First, that leaves the canine in the best functioning position for occlusion and second, the prosthetic lateral incisor replacement usually gives the best esthetic result, which is most important to the patient.

If it is determined radiographically that there is congenital absence of one or more second premolars, care should be taken that the natural space maintainers, the second primary molars, be preserved if at all possible. If one is lost prematurely, unilateral or bilateral space maintainers should be placed as soon as possible to prevent tipping of the adjacent permanent teeth and **iatrogenic** space loss, which may unnecessarily complicate an already difficult orthodontic diagnosis and treatment plan.

3.5.11. **Supernumerary Teeth**

These occur as much as 21% more often in patients with cleft lip and palate, especially in those with complete unilateral and bilateral clefts. This is especially true in the area of the lateral incisor near the cleft site, and may happen because the occurrence of the cleft may also create a fold in both the embryonic **dental lamina** and attached tooth germ. These teeth may be found in both the primary and permanent dentitions either radiographically or erupting in or near the cleft site. Since these teeth bring additional alveolar bone with them as they erupt, if they are not directly in the path of future surgery, do not interfere with articulation in speech, do not cause the patient discomfort and are not carious, they can be maintained indefinitely. It is even possible, in the instance where the lateral incisor on the side of the cleft is congenitally absent, that a supernumerary in the area, if it has a large enough root, can be moved into the lateral incisor position and later crowned or bonded as a natural substitution.

3.5.12. **Ectopic Eruption**

One in every four cleft lip and palate children will have ectopic eruption of an upper first permanent molar. This may cause early loss of the second primary molar, continued mesial eruption of the first molar and loss of space for the developing second premolar. The problem should be identified as early as possible. It may show radiographically, or by late emergence of one first molar when compared to its counterpart, or by **extrusion** of the second primary molar causing tenderness of the tooth with interference in the occlusion and an open bite, or by emergence of only the distal cusps of the first molar. If resorption of the distal root of the second primary molar is minimal, attempt should be made to change the eruption direction of the first permanent molar and maintain the second primary molar. The resorbed area on the second primary molar root can be seen as a tunnel that extends from buccal to lingual. Some infiltration of local anesthetic will usually allow a .025 brass wire to be passed through this "tunnel" and tightened around the contact between the two teeth, imparting a distal force to the upper first permanent molar.

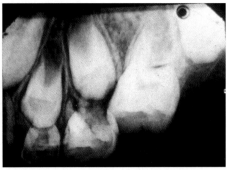

Figure 20-10: Ectopic eruption of the upper first molar, causing partial resorption of the roots of the second primary molar.

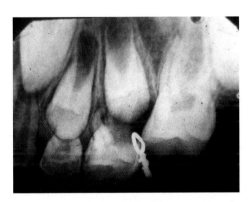

Figure 20-11: Placement of brass separating wire to tip back the ectopic first molar. The second primary molar is supported mesially by the rest of the primary teeth and, since the first permanent molar has no distal support, reactivating the brass every 10 days or so can tip the first permanent molar distally and allow it to erupt into its normal position (See Chapter 17, ectopy).

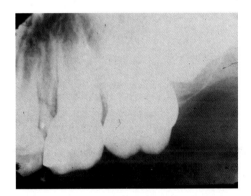

Figure 20-12: Improved eruption of the first molar, preserving the integrity of the second primary molar. Even though the distal root of the second primary molar may have been compromised by the earlier resorption, it is usually stable enough to hold space for the erupting second premolar.

If early loss of the second primary molar cannot be avoided, space maintenance should be employed as soon as the first molar erupts with the space to be later regained as part of comprehensive orthodontic treatment, or limited orthodontic treatment instituted early, space regained and then maintained until the eruption of the blocked out second premolar.

Of course, ectopic eruption of the anterior teeth near the cleft site is quite common. Primary or permanent lateral incisors can erupt far lingually into the cleft site and the central incisors are usually displaced and rotated toward the cleft. Primary tooth ectopic eruption, unless it is involved in crossbite and functional interference with the occlusion, is usually not treated. Permanent tooth ectopic eruption is usually corrected during a first phase of orthodontic treatment.

3.5.13. Other Dental Abnormalities

Some conditions, which may be found less frequently, are:

3.5.13.1. "Saw Tooth" Incisal Edges on the Anterior Teeth.

The only treatment usually necessary is the shaping of the incisal edges to enhance esthetics.

3.5.13.2. Enlarged Mammelons

Cusp-like elevations separated by distinct grooves, which usually extend onto the labial surfaces and may be pitted. Sealant to prevent caries early and bonding or crowning as soon as feasible to enhance esthetics is the treatment of choice.

3.5.13.3. "T" Shaped Upper Lateral Incisors

A large lingual tubercle connected to the incisal edge by a ridge. Sealant should be placed to protect the lingual pits from caries as a good preventive measure and equilibration done as early as possible to eliminate the occlusal interference.

3.5.13.4. Malformation of Upper or Lower First Primary Molars

This requires no treatment.

3.5.13.5. Missing Cusps or Accessory Cusps

Most common are three-cusped upper second primary molars or upper first permanent molars. This requires no treatment. Lower first premolars may have a very small lingual cusp, or an extra one. Lower second premolars may have an accessory buccal cusp. No treatment is indicated.

3.5.13.6. Paralabial Tubercles

Extra elevations on the labial surface resembling cusps. Depending on the possibility that a pulp chamber may also be present, treatment may require flattening by equilibration or bonding or crowning to enhance esthetics, if needed. Exposure of an accessory pulp chamber might require endodontic treatment of the tooth, as well.

3.5.13.7. Mobile or "Free Floating" Premaxilla

In the bilateral cleft of the lip and palate where no alveolar bone graft has been placed, the premaxillary segment may have considerable lateral movement. The quality of the teeth in the premaxillary segment may be poor in length of root and texture of the enamel, and this premaxillary mobility may create problems during operative and prosthetic procedures and during orthodontic treatment. This movement is eliminated by placement of a primary or secondary alveolar bone graft.

IMAGINATION AND INNOVATION

The maintenance of dental health of the cleft lip and palate patient may be the axis around which their entire habilitation revolves. The dentist works as part of a team, not being responsible for the entire plan of treatment for that patient, but often needing imagination and innovation to accomplish the dental tasks that will impact on the successes of the other members of the team, and subsequently the success of the overall treatment of the patient. Certainly cosmetic dentistry will enhance the result of the surgeon.

Special preparation of the teeth may be necessary to support speech appliances, such as an obturator to cover a small opening (**oro-nasal fistula**) in the palate, which allows the unwanted escape of air during speaking. There may be instances where, if there is severe maxillary constriction, the remaining upper teeth must be crowned with built-in retention for the placement of a complete onlay denture to restore the tooth and facial balance.

As the patient's dentist, you should be in communication with the other members of the team, find out their needs and do whatever you can, often with imagination and innovation, to see that they are met. This is the only way you can share in the satisfaction of meeting the ultimate challenge.

3.6 STRATEGIES FOR COORDINATING DENTAL AND SURGICAL TREATMENT

3.6.1. Infant Treatment: Early Maxillary Orthopedics

As a dentist functioning with a **craniofacial** habilitation team, there is no question that your youngest patient will be the one born with a cleft of the lip and palate. Every team will want its members to be involved as early as possible in the business of developing a plan of treatment, maximizing the potential for intercepting and reducing the severity of later problems; those of general growth and development, dental development and speech development. The overriding objective of developing this plan should be to get as close to long term "normal" development in all these areas as possible. The same **bias** we have in treatment of any of our patients -- get as close to an ideal result as possible. Shoot for 100%, remembering that any patient can be treated only to the maximum of their potential. If we aim for the ideal, the individual patient's inherent limitations, whether they are in growth and development, deficiency of tissue or cooperation, will set the level of our potential for successes in function, esthetics and stability of the results. This is true whether the patient is afflicted with a congenital defect or not. Do not automatically set compromised goals. Aim as high as possible. The patient deserves the effort.

Typically, when a child is born with a cleft of the lip and palate the obstetrician or administrative staff of the hospital will notify the pediatrician, who will make referral to the nearest craniofacial team or, in the absence of a formal team, to the plastic surgeon. The family dentist, pediatric dentist or orthodontist will be contacted soon thereafter.

STARTING TIME

The first thoughts of exerting control over the situation occur when the extent of the defect is identified. Remember, the more extensive the cleft, the greater the dental implications. A cleft of the palate only, with an intact alveolar ridge, lip and nasal base, will usually not require early intervention. This cleft may not even be identified at birth, and can sometimes not be discovered for some time afterward. However, if the alveolar ridge is involved in the cleft, not only will the identification usually be immediate, so will the intervention.

Why? It's as simple as Wolf's Law that FORM FOLLOWS FUNCTION. When the cleft results in separation of the parts of the maxilla, the bony segments lose the usual influence of the musculature. Not only is the usual muscular influence absent, but it may be **aberrant** because of the displaced attachments and actually move the segments farther apart. In the usual complete unilateral cleft, the larger alveolar segment containing the attached premaxillary segment is displaced anteriorly and superiorly, resulting in a large space between the two parts of the maxillary alveolus.

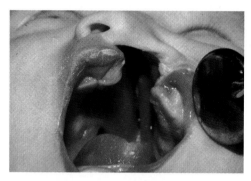 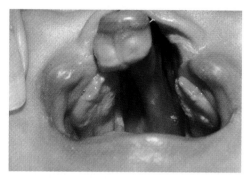

Figure 20-13: The complete unilateral cleft of the lip and palate with displacement of the larger premaxillary segment anteriorly and superiorly

Figure 20-14: The complete bilateral cleft of the lip and palate with free, mobile and anteriorly displaced premaxilla

In the bilateral cleft, the premaxilla is free and mobile, possibly deviated to one side or the other and attached to the "stalk" of the vomer, usually considerably anterior to the smaller lateral segments.

What happens when the musculature of the lip is attached and continuity is established? Muscular pressure is introduced and, according to Wolf's Law, the segments will respond to the pressure by moving.

Uncontrolled, too often the segments will collapse medially very rapidly, allowing the palatal width to decrease excessively, locking the smaller segment(s) behind the premaxillary segment and serving as precursor to later buccal segment collapse and **skeletal crossbite**(s). The crossbite is termed skeletal because the alveolar segment itself is medial in position, and the teeth have no choice but to erupt far in lingual position, as well. It has also been found that segments locked in this position may affect the magnitude of the anterior growth potential of the lateral segment(s). Controlled segment movement at this point can help minimize that collapse.

A small appliance can be made, passively in most cases, to maintain the palatal width in the buccal segments, stabilize the smaller lateral segment(s) and allow controlled movement of the larger segment in the unilateral cleft patient or the premaxillary segment in the bilateral cleft patient to achieve and maintain better **arch form**.

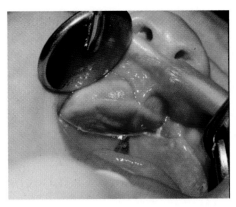 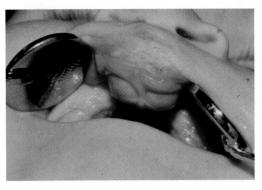

Figure 20-15A: Ideal alignment of the maxillary segments in the complete unilateral cleft of the lip and palate.

Figure 20-15B: Ideal aligment of the maxillary segments in the complete bilateral cleft of the lip and palate.

This view is contrary to those who feel that the smaller segment(s) is actually retropositioned and should be moved forward instead of allowing the larger segment to rotate backward. As an option, the segments can then be stabilized, as we do at Children's Memorial Hospital in Chicago, with the placement of a primary, autogenous alveolar bone graft.

McNeil, in 1950, first presented the concept of controlling segment alignment with an active role for an appliance. His mode of treatment, involving sectioning and repositioning of the segments on study casts, was difficult and tedious, with constant concern about appliance retention and the infant's safety.

Why not let the pressure of the lip closure do the work? Keep the appliance passive and build one with predictable and strong retention, reducing cause for concern. Hence, the introduction of the "Combination Maxillary Orthopedic Appliance" in 1964.   A detailed alginate impression yields a study cast with great detail and an appliance without external wings or ties, the main retention garnered from the undercut areas in the medial portion of the cleft, mostly the nasal surface of the separated palatal shelves. "Combination" in two ways: because it is made of both soft and hard acrylics and because it can be made either passive or active for maxillary expansion, when needed.

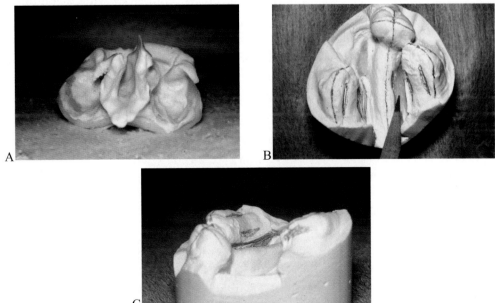

Figure 20-16A-C: A.) Posterior view of a detailed maxillary alginate impression. B.) A detailed maxillary study cast of a complete bilateral cleft of the lip and palate showing areas of undercut. C.) A view of the study cast showing the most important undercut for retention of the appliance, between the palatal shelf and the inferior turbinate.

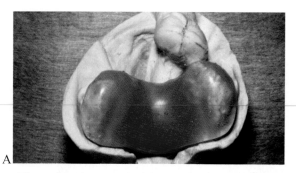
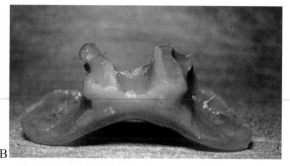

Figure 20-17 A, B: A). The "combination" maxillary infant orthopedic appliance. B.) Posterior view of the appliance showing the soft acrylic extending nasally into the undercut areas.

Aside from controlling the movement of the segments after surgical closure of the lip, other benefits of this passive appliance are possible. These are: improvement in feeding, prevention of abnormal tongue posture development, reduction in incidence of food aspiration, normalizing the air flow by early separation of the oral and nasal spaces, increased protection of the openings of the **Eustacian tubes** from food impaction and subsequent infection and early parental involvement. The retention of the appliance also allows the placement of a nasal extension to try to improve the form of the alar base on the cleft side(s) before the surgical closure of the lip.

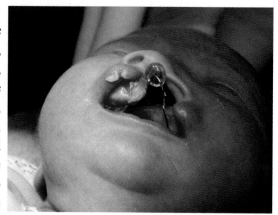

Figure 20-18: An appliance in place with a nasal extension to attempt to improve the shape of the alar cartilage before surgical lip closure.

The parents have counseling on early feeding with a member of our team support staff, then the placement of the appliance somewhat changes the situation. There is now a bridge of plastic across the previously wide-open palatal cleft. Part of the palatal cleft has been obturated. Not enough to allow the infant to be able to create the negative intraoral pressure necessary for suckling, but enough to provide a medial shelf against which the nipple can be exercised. Up to this time, the baby may have required a special "premie" nipple or a regular nipple with a large cross-cut in order to be able to feed adequately. Many parents will also use a plastic bottle with a smaller crosscut nipple so that a slight squeezing of the bottle can control the flow of formula. By whatever means, the formula flow, because of the lack of suckling capability, has been fast and the parents will say that the baby requires frequent "burping" because of the amount of air swallowed with the formula. Some also are sure that the baby has frequent cramping from the swallowed air. Though many feel that a child can be adequately fed without an early appliance, our clinical experience has been that, at least at this stage in the very young infant, feeding improves. It seems that, because of the simulated hard palate provided by the appliance, less formula is lost through the nose. Many of the parents can stop using the plastic bottle to force the flow and can go to a smaller crosscut on the nipple. They can now place the nipple in the center of the infant's mouth instead of having to move laterally, and many find that the ease of feeding improves and the amount of air swallowed, and the cramping, lessens. This may be because, with the appliance in place, the child itself can better control the flow. Part of the natural suckling response is the movement of the mandible that compresses the nipple. Negative pressure (vacuum) is not possible because of the open posterior palate, but natural mandibular movement is there and when the nipple is compressed against the appliance, the crosscut opens and the formula flows. When the compression is released, the formula stops, giving the infant a chance to swallow without choking.

After the appliance fits to satisfaction, the parents are instructed to remove and clean it once every week to 10 days, to be patient as the baby will usually need some time to adjust and to call if they have any problems or questions. Lip surgery is usually scheduled soon after appliance placement.

The parent is instructed to leave the appliance in place for two weeks following the closure of the lip so as not to disturb the surgical site, and the baby is reappointed to the office at that time, when the appliance is removed and cleaned. Trimming will begin to allow segment movement, if necessary. The displaced larger segment in the unilateral cleft or premaxillary segment in the bilateral cleft will move downward, backward and laterally to start closing the space between the segments, and appliance trimming is limited to the area just behind these segments to allow for controlled "bending" and repositioning until segment contact is made.

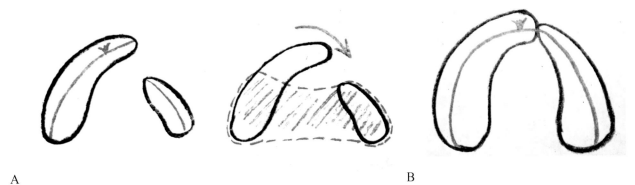

A   B

Figure 20-19A and B: A.) Diagram showing placement of the maxillary orthopedic appliance to help stabilize the buccal segments while the premaxillary segment "molds" to improved position. B.) The schematic ideal arch alignment.

In this bilateral cleft lip and palate patient, three days after the appliance was placed the lip was surgically closed in one step. The baby was seen by us two weeks later for appliance cleaning and re-insertion, then it was left in place full time, removed only every 10 days or so by the parents for cleaning. Approximately four weeks after lip closure a great deal of premaxillary repositioning is evident when compared to the initial alignment.

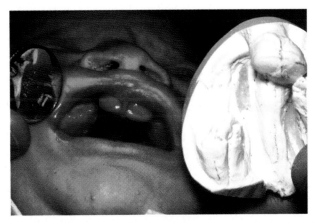

Figure 20-20: On right, initial study cast of complete bilateral cleft of the lip and palate
and on left, arch alignment improvement approximately 4 weeks post-surgical lip closure.

Except for some trimming of the anterior edge of the appliance behind the moving premaxilla, the appliance is unchanged, the stability and retention is still good and there is no evidence of tissue irritation beneath the appliance. By approximately four months after lip closure there has been dramatic arch alignment. This has been accomplished primarily by maintenance of the **arch width** by the passive appliance, and adjustment and reorientation of the premaxillary segment in response to pressure from the newly established muscular band of the now continuous lip. The original appliance is still in place, although the anterior portions of the lateral maxillary segments by now have been completely freed of acrylic cover, allowing the premaxillary segment to move to complete contact with the lateral segments.

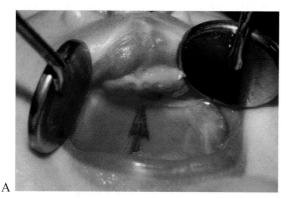
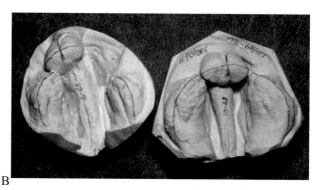

A   B

Figure 20-21A and B: A.) Patient in Figure 20-20 after approximately 4 months post-lip surgery. B.) Study casts showing initial (on left) and arch form just before alveolar graft placement, "molding" occurring due to pressure from newly closed lip.

If the primary alveolar bone graft is desired, segment contact is a definite prerequisite. This is so the surgical undermining of tissue, and any possible long-term effects, can be minimized when the graft is placed. If the appliance has been trimmed over the first few months and the segments do not achieve contact, the appliance is usually removed to allow for some medial movement of the lateral segments. If there is still an inherent lack of tissue and contact is still not made, our team will forego placement of a primary graft and look to the secondary graft procedure, timed either to the eruption of the lateral incisor or to the canine, if the lateral incisor is congenitally absent.

If, after segment contact is accomplished, a primary alveolar bone graft is placed, the appliance plays an important part in the stabilization of the graft area, which occurs within two months of graft placement. The appliance is then continued, mainly as an aid in feeding, until shortly before the palate is surgically closed, usually before 12 months of age.

STOPPING TIME

Two to three weeks before surgical closure of the palate, the appliance is removed to allow the palatal tissue to recover from any surface irritation caused by appliance contact. Tissue tolerance is surprisingly good and, within a few days, the palatal tissue is firm and strong and ready for palatal surgery. The infants are used to feeding with the appliance and don't like being without it but, by this time, they are big and aggressive enough to recover quickly and, as long as the parents are warned ahead of time, there is usually no problem.

Most of our infants will wear the same appliance from birth to just before palatal closure. How is this possible? Because the retention areas are medial, the appliance is extended initially just one millimeter or so over the crest of the ridge. The infant grows laterally, right out of the appliance. By the time the appliance is discontinued, the lateral borders are not at the crests of the alveolus, but considerably medially. When the appliance is removed prior to palate surgery, its outline will remain depressed in the soft tissue for a short time. After the palate is surgically closed, the infant is placed on recall by the team and monitoring of the development of the dentition begins.

There may be a need for variations from the basic appliance. First, if the maxillary segments are collapsed initially, a rare occurrence, there may be the need for expansion of the segments before the lip is surgically closed to allow for proper alignment of the segments. The retention of the appliance is usually good enough that a spring tension jack screw may be added to it and the segments slowly moved apart to allow room for the alignment.

Second, as mentioned previously, a rather new innovation is the addition of a nasal extension from the appliance (See Figure 20-18) before the lip closure surgery, or presurgical taping to try to reshape the alar cartilage, which is usually quite flat. Many surgeons feel that this makes for better post-surgical alar shape and symmetry. Also, if the nasal tip is supported while the premaxillary area moves posteriorly either during pre-surgical taping or after lip surgery, it is hoped that the **columella of the nose** can be lengthened, again enhancing the final nasal form and symmetry.

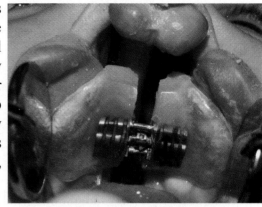

Figure 20-22: Patient with spring-tension jackscrew appliance to gain expansion prior to surgical lip closure to allow for better placement of the premaxillary segment.

To review, our overall objective for this early phase of treatment have not been to try to prevent the occurrence of anterior or lateral crossbites in these patients, but to reduce their severity. We differentiate between DENTAL crossbite, where the affected maxillary teeth are lingually inclined and SKELETAL crossbite, where the entire lateral segment(s) may be medially displaced. Later orthodontic correction of these dental crossbites involving tooth movement only (and primarily easy tipping movement) should be much less involved than that of the skeletal type, which could involve surgical expansion of the segments. Rapid Maxillary Expansion (RME) of the segments is not advised because most surgical closures of the palate result in a tissue bridge across the palatal void which, if the buccal segments are rapidly moved away from each other, may stretch and tear, resulting in oro-nasal fistulae (palatal opening between the oral and nasal cavities) which can be extremely difficult, if not impossible, to repair.

3.6.2. The Bone Graft

Of all of the facets of treatment of the cleft lip and palate patient, none have stimulated the discussion and controversy over the years as has the timing and placement of an alveolar bone graft. The controversy, unfortunately born and bred from the comparison of the proverbial apples and oranges and the difficulty of conducting real, controlled studies, will probably never be completely resolved.

A broad view of the current thinking seems to indicate that, around the world, there is agreement that placement of an alveolar bone graft at some point is definitely encouraged. There is also agreement that the graft should be placed with a minimum of undermining of surrounding tissue, in order to minimize the potential secondary effects on growth. About the timing and the source of donor bone, there is not general agreement. Keller and Jackson describe the advantages of alveolar graft placement as providing bone through which teeth can erupt, improvement in dental and gingival health "because osseous support and keratinized gingiva are provided to the teeth on either side of the cleft", stabilization of the premaxilla in bilateral clefts, more efficient use of fixed dental prosthesis, separation of the oral and nasal cavities by closure of the alveolar fistula, improvement in hypernasality (escape of air through the nose during speech) by closure of the alveolar cleft, improved symmetry of the alar base and maxilla by only grafting, creation of a nostril sill and nasal spine, raising of the nasal floor to the level of the non-cleft side, improvement of nasal septum position and nasal function and, in edentulous patients, allowing for "simultaneous or delayed placement of titanium osseo-integrated implants, which initially stabilize the graft and later function as bone anchorage for a dental prosthesis." The potential for the use of implants was also discussed by Turvey.

There are generally three windows of opportunity regarding the timing of alveolar bone grafting: First, within the first year of life (Primary); Second, at about the time of eruption of the upper permanent lateral incisors (Secondary); and, Third, at about the time of eruption of the upper permanent canines (Secondary).

3.6.2.1. The **Primary Autogenous Alveolar Bone Graft**

This is the graft that is placed some time before the patient's first birthday. Rib is usually preferred as the donor site for this early graft. It is usually quite easily and quickly obtained on an infant, with low morbidity. Approximately one inch of intact rib is removed sub-periosteally, re-forming rapidly, leaving a very small scar and little discomfort for the child. After the alveolus graft bed is prepared, our surgeons section the rib longitudinally, half reduced to bone chips and the other half kept intact. Undermining of tissue is minimal. The bone chips are packed sub-periosteally between the exposed segments of the maxilla in the graft bed and the intact half is placed as is only onto the labial surface of the alveolus. As time goes by, this rib undergoes resorption and re-mineralization and serves as a matrix for the "bridge" of alveolar bone between the maxillary segments.

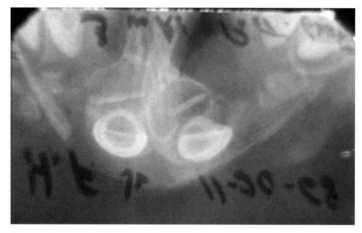

Figure 20-23: Radiograph showing placement of bilateral alveolar bone grafts using split rib segment.

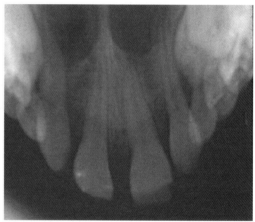

Figure 20-24: Radiograph showing eruption of permanent lateral incisors into bilateral alveolar bone graft sites.

It is our experience that this early grafted autogenous bone will withstand the development of the primary and permanent dentition around it, and will encourage the developing anterior teeth to erupt into the graft site. Also, recent studies have found that primary graft placement does not affect midfacial growth and development.

3.6.2.2. The **Secondary Autogenous Alveolar Bone Graft**

The great majority of treating teams time the placement of the alveolar bone graft to the stage of development of the dentition. Secondary grafts may be timed just before the eruption of the permanent upper lateral incisor in the cleft area (if it is present) at approximately 7 years of age, or to the permanent upper canine eruption at around 11 years of age. This timing is thought to have less potential effect on maxillary growth because of the later placement and that it provides more resultant bone to encourage tooth migration into the cleft site. Some feel that the teeth should be moved into the graft site within two months of graft placement or the grafted bone may resorb. Interestingly, El Deeb found that, though they showed no discoloration, **root resorption** or other radiographic evidence of pathology, 31% of the canines in his study that erupted into the graft site did not respond to pulp testing. The teeth adjacent to the bone graft were unaffected.

For the secondary graft, there are a few more choices for the donor bone. Because the child is much larger, access is improved and iliac crest, calvarial bone and tibial bone seem favored at this time.

3.6.3. Documentation and Diagnosis

When ready to embark on some kind of dental treatment for the patient born with a cleft of the lip and/or palate, the first step is the gathering, documentation and evaluation of all possible information about the patient relevant to the needed treatment. This is especially true of needed orthodontic treatment, which involves not only the dentition but the surrounding soft and hard tissue, as well. That information will usually be retrieved from the following sources:

3.6.3.1. Pertinent Medical and Dental Histories

Now is the time for gathering or updating past medical and dental information about the patient. Along with the information we need on all patients, we want to add questions like: What is the name and location of the patient's plastic surgeon and speech therapist? What are the associated anomalies and what has been their treatment? Is the patient on any medication at this time? Are there any other general medical problems that may impact on treatment? Does the patient anticipate any surgery in the near future? Does the patient experience any **myofascial** pain? Have there been any temporomandibular joint problems and/or treatment? What previous surgeries have been performed and has an alveolar bone graft been placed? What was the source of the graft (rib, iliac crest, tibia or calvarial bone)? Has there been any trauma to the dentition, especially the upper anteriors (fracture, repair), that might cause concern for **ankylosis**? Does the patient suffer from allergies or nasal blockage that might cause mouth breathing?   Do any other members of the family have a cleft of the lip and/or palate? When was the last team evaluation, if there is one seeing the patient, and what is their plan for future treatment?

3.6.3.2. Complete Clinical Evaluation

This may be your first face-to-face contact with the patient, and the time to start establishing the rapport that will be critical to the success of your treatment. Concentrate on the patient, not on the parents. Discuss what you see first with the patient, then with the parent. Make the patient feel like he or she is the important one; that the treatment is theirs and the result is theirs and that, without their help, the result cannot be as successful. You are usually speaking to a young adolescent who is very aware, very interested and very concerned about what is happening. Perhaps somewhat apprehensive and perhaps somewhat unmotivated to embark on another treatment, but who wants to be the focus of your attention and who can be quite offended if they are not.

Find out their chief concern. What do they hope to accomplish with treatment? Is their concern primarily esthetic? Do they have speech or chewing problems? Try to get a sense of their alertness and general attitude. An adolescent does not mask a lack of motivation, frustration or outright hostility well. This, obviously, bears directly on cooperation potential. What is their general stature and size for their age group? This might give some insight into growth potential. Listen to their speech. Do they speak precisely or does your (untrained) ear note something unusual, possibly indicating some tongue postural or speech articulation problem. **Aberrant** muscular activity can have its effect later on, especially during the retention phase of the orthodontic result. Are there any thumb or finger habits still present?

Evaluate their face while you're conversing: The facial profile as to its convexity, lip balance and chin form and frontally, especially regarding symmetry. The severity of asymmetry of the face during function and that on a static photograph can be quite different. You will be treating the one that is functioning. What is the relation between the upper incisors and the face during function? How much gingival display is there when they smile? Is the premaxillary area quite prominent or displaced? Palpate the temporomandibular joints as they open and close to detect any clicking, **crepitus** or discomfort. Measure the maximum opening with a millimeter ruler and note any deviation in mandibular movement on opening and closing.

Classify the malocclusion and note the presence of any cross bites. Map the position of any remaining primary teeth, supernumerary teeth or congenitally missing teeth, as well as the degree of overbite and overjet. What about any hypoplastic crowns, misshapen or undersized crowns (most usually pegged upper lateral incisors), **ankylosed** primary teeth or ectopically erupted teeth? Is there any lateral functional shifting because of the cross bite? Watch the midline between the upper and lower incisors as they speak the words "Mississippi" or "sixty-six", them move to occlusion. If the midline of the lower incisors is centered to the face after speaking then moves laterally to occlusion the problem is usually functional interference. If the midline is off to the face after speech AND in occlusion, the problem is probably structural or skeletal (collapse of the maxillary segment).

What is the level of oral hygiene and the general gingival condition? Is there considerable plaque accumulation and marginal gingivitis? Are there areas, especially the teeth adjacent to the cleft, of gingival recession? Evaluate arch form and symmetry, and note the amount of crowding or spacing of the teeth. Look at palatal form and density of scarring. Are there any openings in the palate (oro-nasal fistulae)? If you're taking an upper impression, you may have to place Vaseline gauze over the opening to prevent impression material from entering and becoming trapped in the nasal chamber.

This is your chance to dynamically evaluate the patient and establish the fact to him or her that you are friendly, gentle, and considerate and that they'll be in good hands. Make the most of it. For general dental examination and needed treatment, this, along with a good panorex or set of full mouth radiographs, may be as far as you have to go in record gathering before you can make the needed decisions. If the treatment is orthodontic, much more is needed.

3.6.3.3. Oriented Facial Photographs

This starts the gathering of "formal" orthodontic records. The orthodontist must accurately document the existing problem from all aspects to provide the information needed to establish the treatment plan, and to be able to coordinate it with the rest of the team's treatment protocol for this patient.

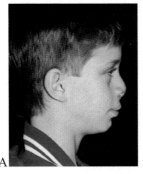
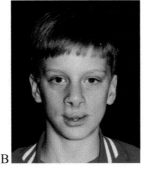
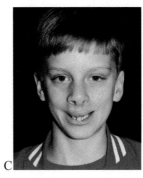

Figure 20-25A, B, and C: A.) Oriented lateral initial facial photograph of a patient with complete bilateral cleft of the lip and palate. B.) Oriented frontal facial photograph. C.) Oriented frontal smile photograph. Note displacement of the premaxillary segment and the upper central incisors inferiorly and to the right.

With the patient standing in front of a blank, contrasting wall, both lateral and frontal color photographs are taken. Proper positioning of the patient's head is important to provide the capability of later comparison. In the lateral view, the patient's head is oriented so that the plane from the **tragus of the ear** to the **infraorbital ridge** is parallel to the floor. Depending on the preference of the operator, the lips may either be in "repose" or in light contact. The surgeons seem to prefer the "repose" position for computer prediction. If you feel there is the possibility of a surgical mandibular advancement for this patient (rare for a cleft lip and palate patient) an additional photo can be taken in this position with the mandible advanced to show the potential esthetic change in facial profile. The frontal photograph is taken with the plane connecting the two infraorbital ridges parallel to the floor for proper orientation.

To assure the same head size on the lateral and frontal facial prints, the lens should be at fixed focal distance for both and the single lens reflex camera moved in and out to focus. For the digital camera, the computer can probably do the cropping.

3.6.3.4. Intraoral Photographs

Intraoral photographs are used to document the lateral and anterior views of the dentition in occlusion. This, in color, will also show plaque accumulation, tissue tone and color, hypoplastic crowns and other tooth color or decalcification problems prior to orthodontic treatment.

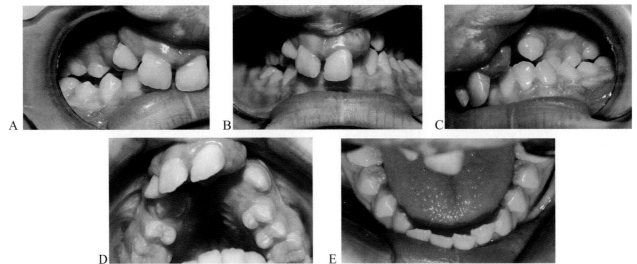

Figure 20-26 A, B, C, D, E: A.) Right lateral view of the dentition in occlusion. Note buccal segment crossbite. B). Patient in Figure 20-25 with frontal view of the dentition in occlusion. Note midline discrepancy. C.) Left lateral view of the dentition in occlusion. Note buccal segment crossbite. D.) Maxillary occlusal view of the dentition. Note poor arch form and maxillary constriction. E.) Mandibular occlusal view of the dentition. Note good arch form.

3.6.3.5. Full Mouth Periapical Radiographs

This series will accurately detail:
>   --the presence of any active carious lesions and previous placement of restorations. This can be one good indication of the patient's caries susceptibility and what can be expected after placement of a **fixed orthodontic appliance**.
>   --the integrity of the roots and possible predisposition to root resorption during orthodontic treatment.
>   --the integrity of the **supporting bone**, including periodontal ligament spaces, crestal bone heights and periodontal pocket formation.   Coordination with the periodontal probing record would be even more helpful.
>   --the presence and position of unerupted teeth. This would identify most congenitally absent, impacted or ectopically erupting teeth.
>   --the presence and location of supernumerary teeth.
>   --confirmation of ankylosis (submersion) of retained primary teeth.
>   --confirmation of the presence and evaluation of the size of an alveolar bone graft.

3.6.3.6. Panoramic Radiograph

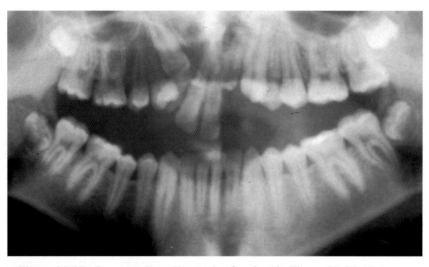

Figure 20-27: **Panoramic radiograph** of patient in Figure 20-25. Note maxillary right canine and left lateral incisor hidden by premaxillary position.

This view is very useful in confirming everything seen on the full mouth periapical radiographs, plus
>   --allowing evaluation of the form and symmetry of the condyles and fossae.
>   --identifying abnormalities in the surrounding areas, such as deviation of the nasal septum.
>   --offering a better view for detecting and locating possible pathology (cysts, tumors, etc.), supernumeraries or ectopically erupting teeth.
>   --usually gives a better view for evaluation of the presence, location and eruption potential of the developing third molars.

3.6.3.7. Lateral and Antero-Posterior Cephalometric Radiographs

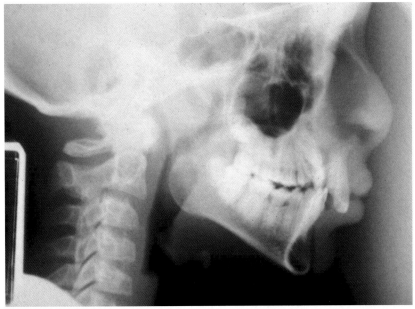

Figure 20-28: Oriented lateral cephalometric radiograph of patient in Figure 20-25.
Note antero-posterior discrepancy between upper and lower anterior segments.

Cephalometric radiographs and their evaluation are invaluable in developing a sense of the spatial relations between the maxilla and the mandible and between the individual jaws and their associated teeth. The numerical relations between these entities, when related to the norms, will allow the orthodontist to determine whether the problem is skeletal or dental in origin (or both), where the insult is centered and whether treatment can affect any change in that area. Also, what the real **procumbency** is of the teeth in relation to their basal bones and which direction the teeth must be moved to improve that relationship. Computer prediction software can be used to ascertain whether surgical changes will be necessary as well as tooth changes to accomplish the best and most stable result, and quantify the magnitude and direction of those surgical changes.

The number and analyses of cephalometric radiographs that are available are too numerous to mention. Each offers an interpretation of the same basic information, and it is up to each practitioner to select the combination of numbers, from whatever source, that will offer the most meaningful evaluation of the relations of both the hard and soft tissues for treatment planning.

3.6.3.8 Study Casts

In our record taking protocol, we usually reserve this procedure for last, as it usually stresses the patient more than the others. Taking the other records first gives us more time to work with the patient and try to relax them. Cleft lip and palate patients are probably more sensitive about oral treatment than most due to of the simple fact that, because of problems with nasal breathing they may be obligate mouth breathers, and they are most uncomfortable when that avenue is even partially blocked. To that end, as with infants, we try to make the impression taking process as fast as possible. An upper and lower impression may be taken utilizing color-coded alginate material (Orthogel by Rocky Mountain Company) which allows withdrawal of a high quality impression in 30 seconds, or less.

The formal, trimmed and polished study casts will serve as a completely accurate initial record. On them measurements may be made to determine tooth size discrepancies or exact **arch length** adequacy or inadequacy. Model surgery may be performed to project new tooth and bony positions in an effort to select the best treatment plan.

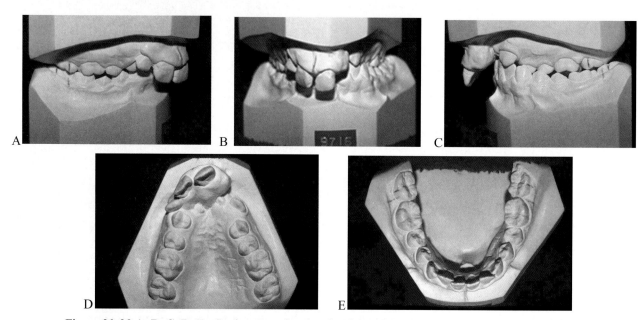

Figure 20-29 A, B, C, D, E: Study casts of patient in Figure 20-25. A.) Right buccal segment. B.) Front view. C.) Left buccal segment. D.) Maxillary occlusal view. E.) Mandibular occlusal view.

3.6.4. Setting of Goals, Team Coordination and Treatment Planning

Any dental or orthodontic treatment of a patient with a craniofacial anomaly is not a unilateral affair. This is especially true with the cleft lip and palate patient. Now that the formal initial records have been taken, the first thing that should be done is that communication should be made with the plastic surgeon. A copy of the initial panoramic and cephalometric radiographs, along with the diagnostic tracing and cephalometric evaluation would be helpful. Let the surgeon know that the patient is now ready for orthodontic treatment and that you would like to coordinate it with the future surgical plans, both in approach and in timing. The surgeon usually serves as the hub around which the team revolves and is usually aware of planned treatment by other members of the team.   General dental treatment, the maximizing of the health of the teeth and surrounding tissues, is paramount and of highest priority. The orthodontic treatment is important, but should be placed in the appropriate sequence of events. Without contact with the team at this time, the orthodontist may embark on a treatment plan that is totally contradictory to future surgical plans and the orthodontic treatment may have to be repeated or the needed surgery changed. Either way, the patient suffers needlessly, not only in possible extra treatment, but also in possible reduction of the function or esthetics of the result.

We feel that the goals for orthodontic treatment should have a strong emphasis on the esthetic result. This does not mean, of course, that the functional result is unimportant, but a beautifully functioning result that is unaesthetic will leave a very unhappy patient and family. A bright and symmetrical smile is very important to the patient's self image and to the evaluation of that patient by our society. The more secure that patient is about the projection of their smile, the better the overall facial appearance and, inevitably, the better the acceptance and ultimate chance for success of the patient. Simplistic, perhaps, but true.

It has been said before that the more severe the cleft, the more difficult it is to get a good, esthetic and functional result. It is obvious that all cleft palate patients cannot be served by one treatment plan, but there are many things that they may have in common. For one example, the relation of the upper incisors to the upper lip and to the face bear heavily on the symmetry and esthetics of the result, no matter what the type of cleft. One of the reasons that the placement of an alveolar bone graft, before or during the orthodontic treatment, is so beneficial is that it removes the bony void of the cleft, providing alveolus into which teeth may erupt or be moved to allow the upper incisors to be centered in the face.

Orthodontic problems for the cleft lip and palate patient can begin very early in the primary dentition with the ectopic eruption of the first maxillary anterior tooth and extend through the mixed dentition and into the permanent dentition. Since the family dentist and orthodontist are part of the team that is watching and evaluating the overall development of the child, these problems will be noted immediately, and the question arises early as to whether the developing problem will require immediate treatment. It would not be difficult to allow these patients to be involved in orthodontic treatment from the time the first problem arises to the time the last problem has been corrected, but it is CRITICAL that this be avoided. Treatment phases should be limited in number and allotted specific time. There should be a definite goal, a definite beginning and a definite end to a phase of treatment, with as long a span of time as possible in between. The most critical orthodontic treatment for these patients will be the comprehensive phase in the full permanent dentition, and the more orthodontic treatment that has occurred before that phase, the worse will be the patient's attitude, the less will be their motivation and cooperation potential and the more compromised will be the final, and most important, result.

3.6.4.1. The Primary Dentition

As was discussed previously, the primary dentition of the cleft lip and palate patient will definitely be affected by the insult of the cleft, primarily to the maxillary dentition and secondarily to the mandibular. The question will be whether the departures from "normal" development will require intervention and, unless there is some profound functional reason, most would say no.

The problems of ectopic eruption, congenital absence or a supernumerary tooth may allow or cause displacement in the position of other primary teeth, but usually no profound functional interference. Articulation in speech is usually not affected. The supernumerary will likely be in the area of the cleft and carries alveolar bone with it. It can usually be left alone, unless it is in direct line of some planned surgery, until much later. This is mainly to preserve the bone and prevent the possibility of an oro-nasal defect that may be created by removal.

The problem most likely to tempt the orthodontist to treatment will be maxillary constriction and crossbite, and the possibility to treat will be directly tied to the "readiness" of the patient and the potential for cooperation.

It has been suggested that, in the patient where a bone graft has not yet been placed, maxillary expansion in the primary dentition can move the unfused maxillary segments as well, also widening the base of the nasal chamber, and removing any potential loss of normal maxillary growth caused by "impaction" of the bony segments. This chapter's authors feel that by placement of an early maxillary alveolar bone graft to attach the segments while they are in good alignment, the "impaction" of the lateral maxillary segments may be minimized or avoided, converting the **"skeletal" crossbite** of collapsed maxillary segments into a "dental" crossbite of teeth only, which can be better treated as part of a first phase of treatment in the mixed dentition. Typically, the "dental" crossbite will present the anterior or buccal teeth in lingual inclination, which can be readily corrected by simply tipping them labially and buccally to the proper axial inclination.

If there is major skeletal segment collapse the teeth may be more upright, requiring more difficult and risky expansion. Risky because after surgical palatal closure, the resultant bridge of tissue across the palate is mostly scar tissue, which is quite inflexible. Stretching in expansion could cause problems with the palatal repair. If an oro-nasal fistula opens, it is very difficult to re-close surgically, certainly substituting a much more severe problem for the crossbite.

If it is absolutely necessary to attempt to correct a crossbite in the full primary dentition, the timing will be quite important, as would be true in any non-cleft patient. First of all, the treatment should not be started until the full primary dentition is developed, so that the mandibular dentition can serve as a guide for how much expansion will be necessary. If the crossbite is anterior, it must be remembered that the permanent teeth are developing above the primary incisors in the premaxillary segment. An anterior radiograph will reveal the relative positions of the primary incisors and the permanent tooth buds, and if the radiograph shows overlapping of the apex of the primary root with the permanent bud, it is too late to attempt the advancement of the primary incisors. This is because the primary incisors are lingually tipped, with their **apices** labial to the permanent tooth bud

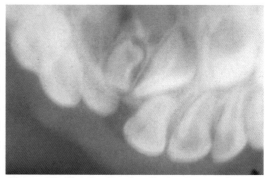

Figure 20-30: Occlusal radiograph to evaluate relative position of primary and permanent incisors in determining timing for early anterior crossbite correction. Also shows teeth erupting into alveolar graft site.

and when the primary incisor's crowns are tipped forward, the apices will move lingually, possibly colliding with the permanent buds and displacing them even further lingually. That could cause a more severe **anterior crossbite** when the permanent teeth erupt than if no early treatment had been attempted. Therefore, make sure the permanent tooth buds are above the apices of the primary teeth before treatment.

If it is a "dental" bilateral crossbite of the buccal segments, the buccal teeth will be quite upright or lingually inclined and the maxillary arch will appear quite constricted. This could have impact on speech and tongue posture because of the narrow palatal space and, certainly, compromise masticatory function as well. Expansion in this situation should be SLOW, and can be accomplished with the same type of mechanism previously described in infant orthopedics: the spring tension jack screw, or a standard jack screw activated just once every three days. This type of expansion will tip the upright or lingually inclined teeth buccally as opposed to moving the skeletal segments, will create less tension on the palatal repair in the process and should minimize the chance that the repair may fail, creating an oronasal fistula. Because of palatal scarring, this is not a self-retaining situation. There will be a strong tendency to relapse, and a cemented holding arch is the best means of retention.

The unilateral crossbite in the full primary dentition will usually not have the same speech impact and, even though masticatory function may be compromised, can usually go untreated until the mixed dentition.

3.6.4.2. The Transitional Dentition

3.6.4.2.1. Orthodontic Considerations

This is where the typical first phase of orthodontic treatment for the cleft lip and palate child will begin, the timing set by the exfoliation of the upper anterior primary teeth and eruption of the successors. The untreated problems of the primary dentition can often be corrected as part of this phase of treatment, and this phase should not extend longer than one year of active treatment. The retention of the accomplishments of this phase is usually prolonged, however, and may extend all the way to the start of the final, comprehensive phase of treatment.

One must remember that these patients have growth and development occurring determined by their basic genetic design, upon which has been superimposed the insult of a cleft of the lip and palate. We are dealing with the variability of a developing malocclusion worsened by the variability of the local and general effect of this orofacial anomaly. Generally, the more severe the defect, the greater the impact on the developing dentition. Obviously, a simple cleft of the **soft palate** only will not have the same effect on dental development as a bilateral cleft of the lip and palate. The final goal of orthodontic involvement for these patients must be the optimum result of the comprehensive phase of orthodontic treatment in the permanent dentition. This first phase of treatment should aid in the achievement of that goal and should provide interim improvement in the esthetics and function for the patient, as well.

Clefts of the soft or hard palate alone usually do not result in the need for a first phase of treatment. The cleft can extend as far forward as the incisive foramen and not penetrate the alveolus, largely removing the potential for affecting anterior tooth development and placement. Certainly, surgical closure of the palate can result in scarring, which may cause a tendency to narrowing of the palatal vault and resultant buccal segment crossbite, but this can usually be corrected in the full permanent dentition. Since the relapse tendency would be so great, treating this situation in the mixed dentition would only require prolonged retention and possible exhaustion of the patient cooperation that could be so much more important in the final phase of treatment.

By this time, the unilateral and bilateral cleft lip and palate patients present with **alveolar arch**es that have been separated and displaced, then molded back to arch form and sometimes beyond. There have been two or three surgical procedures in the area with the associated effects of the scarring on growth and tooth position, and the emotional and physical effects of almost continual medical, speech and dental treatment for the last six or seven years of their lives. As young children they are most concerned at this time with the esthetics of their developing permanent dentition and, though they may be tired of health professionals in general, are usually quite motivated to help in the correction of the situation. You should find anxious and cooperative patients and parents.

Buccal segment crossbite is the third most common orthodontic problem exhibited by the cleft lip and palate patient in the mixed dentition. Most of the time, the buccal segment crossbite in the bilateral cleft palate patient is symmetrically bilateral, involving all of the primary and permanent molars, where both right and left lateral segments have collapsed medially and require slow, reciprocal expansion. If the collapse has occurred more anteriorly, a hinged appliance may be used.

Again, prolonged retention will be necessary due to the high potential for relapse, possibly due to palatal scar tissue and/or reduced maxillary growth, and the cemented lingual holding arch is the retainer of choice.

Along with primary alveolar bone grafting to stabilize the maxillary bony segments, the mixed dentition presents an ideal time for the placement of an alveolar bone graft in conjunction with this first phase of orthodontic treatment. It can provide a bony nasal floor on the side of the cleft, help close an oro-nasal fistula if it exists and provide alveolar bone into which the lateral incisor, if present, and the canine can erupt. It should be timed so that the bone graft is placed within two months of the time of eruption or movement of the tooth into the area, or the grafted bone may resorb.

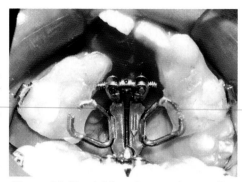

Figure 20-31: A hinged expansion appliance to accomplish more anterior expansion than posterior.

With the variability of the effect of this congenital insult and its early treatments on the developing child, there are many patients in whom the orthodontic problems are so minimal that the child requires no treatment during the mixed dentition. As early treatments become more sophisticated and less intrusive, this population of patients should, hopefully, increase as time goes by. Patients now do not even vaguely resemble patients of thirty years ago in the quality of their final treatment results. With our present understanding of our potential for interference with growth and the long term effect, procedures, especially surgical, have become generally more delicate, with less undermining of tissue during active growth, minimizing scarring where possible and achieving some spectacular esthetic and functional results. There may still be a basic lack of tissue and reduced growth potential with which to deal, but the body's determination for compensation during growth can often keep the effects minimized and the bony relations within acceptable limits.

In the mixed dentition patient with acceptable bony and tooth relationships, there are still orthodontic problems which may persist, but that may have been the case if they were not born with a cleft at all. Congenital absence of teeth is an example. If it has occurred in the buccal segment, we would deal with it as we would for any patient of this age. Do everything possible to maintain the primary tooth in the position as a natural space maintainer, and put off any action until the full permanent dentition. If the primary tooth is somehow lost, placement of your favorite type of space maintainer. If the congenital absence has occurred anteriorly, as it most often does at the lateral incisor position, and if the alignment of the other teeth is acceptable, placement of a removable upper appliance with a pontic is the treatment of choice. First, it improves the esthetics immediately and can aid in the child's self image development and second, it can help with speech by obturating an oro-nasal fistula, if present, and by providing a tooth in the space for improved **articulation**.

The development of crowding of the teeth in the mixed dentition is a common orthodontic problem in any young patient, whether born with a cleft lip and palate or not. Because of the insult to the maxilla with a strong tendency to maxillary constriction and secondary narrowing of the mandibular arch as well, crowding may present more of a problem in the cleft lip and palate patient. It can be seen, as usual, as a lack of **developmental spacing** in the primary dentition and, as the permanent anterior teeth being to exchange, some expansion or eruption guidance by removal of selected primary teeth may be necessary. Also, a **supernumerary tooth** that is blocking the eruption of one of the permanent teeth would be removed at this time. If the crowding is severe enough, eruption guidance may convert to **serial extraction** as the mixed dentition continues, with the removal of the first premolars. Then, as soon as there are enough permanent teeth present, on to the last, and comprehensive, phase of orthodontic treatment.

3.6.4.2.2. Surgical Considerations

Some, but not all, of the patients with cleft lip and palate develop a degree of maxillary deficiency. When it is minor, orthodontic movement of the teeth can sometimes mask the underlying skeletal disharmony. When it is moderate, a combination of orthodontic and standard orthognathic surgical procedures, such as a LeFort I maxillary osteotomy (advancement) at or near the time of skeletal maturity is the ideal treatment of choice. However, cleft palate patients with severe maxillary deficiency present a difficult challenge for the reconstructive team. These patients frequently exhibit vertical, horizontal and transverse maxillary **hypoplasia**. Severe soft tissue and palatal scarring from prior surgical repairs can affect blood supply and increase resistance to movement. Often, because of these restrictions, the traditional orthodontic/surgical approach would include performing mandibular setback surgery on a mandible that is normal in shape and position in an effort to improve occlusal relationships at the expense of esthetics. For these severe cases, maxillary **distraction osteogenesis** can offer significant advantages.

Distraction osteogenesis is a technique where bone can be gradually lengthened by slow controlled separation of surgically osteotomized bone segments. The exciting aspect of this approach is that the gradual nature of the movement allows the muscles and other soft tissues to expand and adapt to the new skeletal framework. Many feel that this allows for larger surgical movements and increases the stability of the surgical procedure.

The idea of bone distraction is not new. It was first developed for use in orthopedic leg length discrepancies in 1905 by Codivilla and modified by Abbot in 1927. However, the early attempts were fraught with complications and the technique was mostly abandoned until the 1950's when Ilizarov demonstrated a corticotomy with minimal disruption of the blood supply and a system of tension ring fixators that minimized complications significantly. Although its popularity in orthopedics grew rapidly, it wasn't until 1973 that Synder, et al., first applied the approach to mandibular lengthening in a dog. Another 20 years passed before McCarthy, et al., published, in 1992, the first report of mandibular lengthening for four children with mandibular deficiency (see Mandibular Distraction in the section relating to **Hemifacial Microsomia** following).

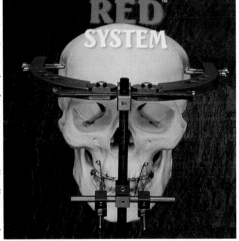

In 1997, Polley and Figueroa adapted the distraction technique for use in midface advancements. The Ilizarov Principle- "The Law of Tension-Stress : Tension forces stimulate histiogenesis" The technique of osteodistraction, whether it applies to the craniofacial bones or long bones, involves the following basic steps: 1.) an osteotomy in the area of bone deficiency; 2.) application of an external fixator; and 3.) initiation of expansion forces. Other factors that affect the development of new bone within the distraction site are: latency period, rate of distraction, rhythm of distraction, stability of the fixator, and the timing of fixator removal.

Figure 20-32 A: Shows the Rigid External Device developed by Polley and Figueroa in conjunction with KLS Martin, L.P. The total time of the distraction phase depends on the severity of the deformity and must be individualized to each patient.

The latency period refers to the period of time after the surgical procedure when fracture healing is allowed to occur before distracting forces are applied. This period typically lasts 5-7 days, but can be longer with older patients.

The rate of distraction refers to the number of activations per day and is typically 1.0 mm. However, some advocate up to 2 mm/day in younger children to avoid early consolidation and a slower rate of 0.5 mm/day in older patients to avoid fibrous unions.

The rhythm of distraction can be either once a day or divided into smaller increments throughout the day to maintain constant tension, which can favor histogenesis.

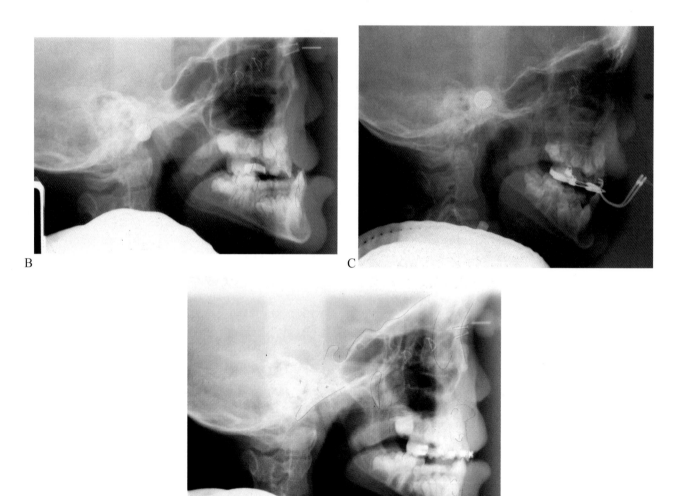

B

C

D

Figure 20-32 B-D: A series of cephalometric radiographs of a patient with severe maxillary deficiency illustrates the capabilities of the technique.

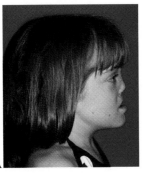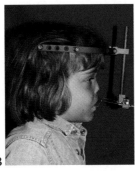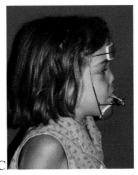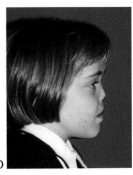

Figure 20-33A: A.) Shows the pretreatment profile of the same patient as in Figure 20-32. The deficiency is evident in vertical as well as horizontal planes. B.) Shows the appliance in place after 4 weeks of active distraction. Once the desired correction is achieved with the distracting phase, the appliance is left in place, ideally 6-8 weeks, to allow mineralization of the immature bone to occur. C.) After the appliance is removed, a removable face mask with elastic tension is used at night only for a period of time. The improvement is dramatic as shown in D.) Six weeks after face mask appliance removal.

The external device is bulky and looks uncomfortable, but the patients do surprisingly well with it. There are internal devices that are currently in development, but midfacial advancements with currently available internal devices are limited because of the difficulty in appropriately orienting the devices in the limited space. In addition, the fixation of the device may injure the developing dentition. Therefore, the external multidirectional devices are preferred as they allow more control over the distraction process.

3.6.4.3. The Permanent Dentition

3.6.4.3.1. Orthodontic Considerations

To a varying degree, depending upon the severity of the original cleft and the invasiveness of the needed previous treatments, all of the orthodontic problems previously described can be found with the emergence of the full permanent dentition. Namely, ectopic eruption, rotation of teeth, congenital absence, supernumerary teeth, crowding, maxillary and mandibular arch constriction, **posterior crossbite** and **anterior crossbite**.

The time just before the upper canine in the cleft area erupts also presents the third window of opportunity for the placement of an alveolar bone graft, if one hasn't been placed previously or has failed. This graft, placed at a time when the canine will be emerging or be moved into the area within two months, will often allow for a symmetry of orthodontic result not possible without continuity of the alveolus.

STARTING TIME

Typically, as with the non-cleft population, the comprehensive phase of orthodontic treatment for the cleft lip and palate patient can begin with the start of exfoliation of the second primary molars. At that time, the upper canines will usually be unerupted, which will allow the timing of possible placement of an alveolar graft to be performed during active treatment.

For diagnosis and treatment planning, in addition to complete medical and dental histories, clinical evaluation, facial and intraoral photographs and lateral and antero-posterior cephalometric radiographs, the orthodontist will also need:

3.6.3.5. FULL MOUTH PERIAPICAL RADIOGRAPHS

This series will accurately detail
>   --the presence of any active carious lesions and previous placement of restorations. This can be one good indication of the patient's susceptibility to caries and what may be expected after placement of fixed appliances.
>   --the integrity of the roots and possible predisposition to root resorption during orthodontic treatment.
>   --the integrity of the **supporting bone**, including periodontal ligament spaces, crestal bony heights and periodontal pocket formation. A copy of the family dentist's periodontal probing record would be helpful, as well.
>   --the presence and position of unerupted teeth. This would identify most congenitally absent, impacted or ectopically erupting teeth.
>   --the presence and location of supernumerary teeth.
>   --confirmation of **ankylosis** (submersion) of retained primary teeth.

3.6.3.6. PANORAMIC RADIOGRAPH

This view is very useful in confirming everything seen on the full mouth periapical radiographs, plus
>   --allowing evaluation of the form and symmetry of the condyles and fossae.
>   --identifying abnormalities in the surrounding areas, such as a deviation of the nasal septum.
>   --offering a better view for detecting and locating possible pathology (cysts, tumors, etc.), supernumeraries or ectopically eruption teeth.
>   --usually giving a better view for evaluation of the presence, location and eruption potential of the developing third molars.

Remember, treatment of a patient with an orofacial or craniofacial anomaly is not a unilateral affair. This is especially true with the cleft lip and palate patient. Now that formal records have been taken, the first thing that must be done is that communication should be made with the patient's plastic surgeon. The surgeon usually serves as the hub around which the team revolves and is usually also aware of planned treatment by other members of the team. The orthodontic treatment is important, but should be placed in the appropriate sequence of events. Without contact with the team at this time, a treatment plan may be adopted and carried out that is totally contradictory to future surgical plans, and the orthodontic treatment may have to be repeated or the needed surgery compromised. Either way, your patient suffers needlessly.

The goals for dental and orthodontic treatment should have a strong emphasis on the esthetic result. This does not mean that the functional result is unimportant, but a beautifully functioning result that is unesthetic will leave a very unhappy patient and family. A bright and symmetrical smile is very important to the patient's self image and to the evaluation of that patient by our society. The more secure that patient is about the projection of their smile, the better the acceptance and ultimate success of the patient. Simplistic, perhaps, but true.

We have stated before that the more severe the cleft, the more difficult it is to get a good esthetic and functional result. It is obvious that all cleft palate patients cannot be served by one treatment plan, but there are many things that they may have in common. For example, the relation of the upper incisors to the upper lip and to the face bear heavily on the symmetry and esthetics of the result, no matter what the cleft. One of the reasons that the placement of an alveolar bone graft at some point before or during the orthodontic treatment is so beneficial is that it removes the bony void of the cleft, providing alveolus into which teeth may erupt or be moved to allow the upper incisors to be centered in the face. If an alveolar bone graft had not been placed prior to this time, it should be included into the plan of treatment now. The ideal time is approximately two months before a tooth will erupt or be moved into the area.

Congenital absence or undersized crown formation of the lateral incisor in the cleft area is a common problem, no matter whether the cleft is unilateral or bilateral. Another of the goals of treatment, therefore, is to provide and maintain adequate space (matching the contralateral lateral) for the esthetic replacement or crowning of the tooth (or teeth), if root formation is adequate.

Another problem in common might be crowding of teeth in the maxillary and/or mandibular arches, requiring permanent tooth extraction as part of the orthodontic treatment plan. The goal, of course, is to be able to level, align and coordinate the arches, and excess tooth structure may have to be eliminated in the process. Which teeth to remove will depend on the needs of the individual case but, as a general rule, anteriors, canines and molars are preserved. Needed extractions may be in one or both arches and may be unilateral or bilateral.

If at all possible, the canine should be left in the canine position for the best functional and esthetic result. It is usually poorly shaped, too large and badly shaded to adequately substitute for a missing lateral incisor.

A goal of treatment should be not only to place the upper midline in the center of the face, but to align the lower midline to the upper, as well. This may necessitate some compromise in buccal segment relation on one or both sides. The aim in that case would be maximum occlusal contact for adequate function.

Of course, a goal of treatment for any orthodontic patient is to establish the best possible functional relation of the buccal segment teeth. We should strive for the ideal Class I bilateral **intercuspation** and get as close as possible, considering the patient's needs and limitations. The basic structural asymmetry of our cleft palate patient may dictate that one or both sides be a Class II relation, and we should then strive for maximum occlusal contact.

No matter what the severity of the cleft, the periodontal status of our patient should be monitored carefully during active orthodontic treatment. The presence of a **fixed orthodontic appliance** in any patient makes maintenance of good oral hygiene more difficult. We would suggest that the patient return to their family dentist for examination and prophylaxis more frequently than usual during active treatment to help monitor the health of the tissues, the oral hygiene and the diet. A progress panorex every six months or so would allow for assessment of any change in roots or supporting bone.

STOPPING TIME

A goal of treatment should definitely be to set a treatment time for any phase of treatment and abide by it. Get the job done as quickly and efficiently as possible. As with any patient, the motivation and attitude toward orthodontic treatment, no matter how noble the goals, diminishes rapidly as the projected end of treatment time is passed. Accept the fact that we can only treat any patient to the maximum of his or her potential, recognize the point where that maximum has been reached and end the active phase of treatment as quickly as possible.

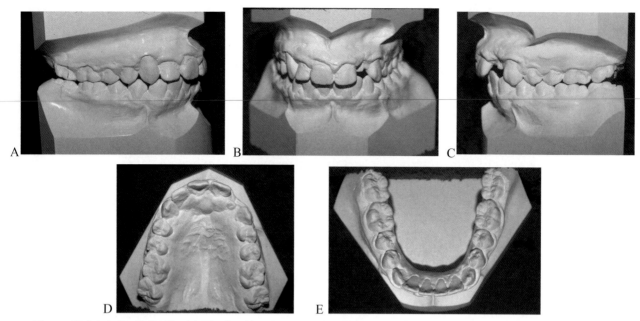

Figure 20-34 A, B, C, D, E: A.) Final study casts of patient in Figure 20-25. Right buccal segment. B.) Frontal view. Note improved premaxillary position and midline relation. C.) Left buccal segment. D.) Maxillary occlusal view. E.) Mandibular occlusal view.

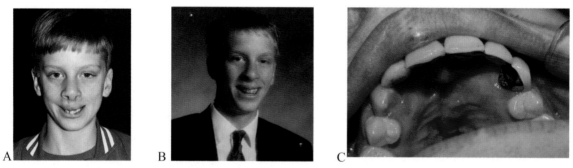

Figure 20-35 A, B, C: A.) Initial frontal facial view of patient in Figure 20-25. B.) Final frontal facial view showing orthodontic/orthopedic (non-surgical) repositioning of premaxilla so that upper central incisors are aligned with midline of face. C.) Later placement of Maryland Bridge to replace non-viable upper left lateral incisor.

As we have discussed previously, there is a strong tendency to rebound after tooth movement in the cleft lip and palate patient. Largely due to the lack of resiliency of palatal scarring, the corrected buccal segment crossbite can relapse with frightening speed. A patient with a removable maxillary retainer may find it impossible to replace it after leaving it out just a matter of hours and, by the time they return for adjustment, active treatment may be again necessary to regain the occlusal relation. Frequently ectopically placed and rotated teeth also offer a difficult area of retention, as they also have a strong tendency to move.

If there have been congenitally missing upper anterior teeth, a **removable appliance** with prosthetic teeth attached may be necessary until those teeth are permanently replaced but, as soon as feasible, the placement of fixed retention is best. Holding arches or bonded lingual wires can maintain width or rotations without need for dependence on patient cooperation, and without encroachment on articulation in speech. The term "semi-permanent retention" was meant for these patients, and can help assure that the worst kind of congenital orofacial defect can result, long term, in good function, esthetics and stability.

3.6.4.3.2. Surgical Considerations

Though it is not often seen in more recent times, extreme maxillary constriction may require combined orthodontic/orthognathic surgical expansion during active orthodontic treatment. Also, extreme maxillary hypoplasia may result in severe **retrusion** of the midface. This would require surgical maxillary advancement. Both of these possibilities and their timing must be pursued with the surgical members of the team.

4. THE PATIENT WITH HEMIFACIAL MICROSOMIA

When thinking about asymmetry, we must remember that it is a common presence in the development of any bilateral creature. It is impossible for a right side and a left side of any living structure to be identically configured, of necessity responding to different stimuli during growth and development. Again, we confront Wolf's Law of "form follows function." Classic studies have shown that development of the face is a perfect example. When frontal facial photographs have been sectioned in the midline with two right halves or left halves put together, the result looks little like the original photograph. Even the most pleasingly esthetic face will present with minor asymmetry. The problem is then, like most of our patient's other problems, the magnitude or degree of the situation.

Facial asymmetry can be divided into two basic categories: functional and structural. A "functional" asymmetry can usually be reversed, being caused by anything from transient swelling from an infection to the lateral mandibular shift associated with a unilateral buccal segment crossbite. Get rid of the cause and the symmetry will improve. A "structural" asymmetry, caused by an aberration in growth and development, is not reversible except by dramatic treatment effort. As we will see, this effort is usually made as early as possible because this is a progressive situation. The longer it goes on, the worse it gets. It gets worse not just from the lack of development of the affected parts, but from secondary change in associated parts as well. Hemifacial microsomia presents such a situation.

4.1 ETIOLOGY AND DESCRIPTION

Hemifacial Microsomia has also been called Temporo-Auromandibular Dysplasia, Craniofacial Microsomia, Lateral Facial Dysplasia, Facial Microsomia, First Arch **Syndrome**, First and Second Arch Syndrome, Oculoauriculovertebral Dysplasia, Otomandibular **Dysostosis**, Lateral Facial Dysplasia and Goldenhar Syndrome. The most popular belief is that the stapedial artery (from the second branchial arch) ruptures very early in fetal development and the magnitude of the resultant hematoma determines the severity of the result. The result usually has serious impact on the growth and development of the external ear, middle ear, facial muscles and other associated soft tissues, muscles of mastication, mandible and temporomandibular joint on the affected side. There may be a secondary effect on maxillary growth, as well. There may be partial or complete absence of the 7th nerve function and, in more severe cases (these perhaps more properly called "Craniofacial Microsomia") the orbit, zygomatic bone, squamous temporal bone and the frontal bone on that side may be affected.

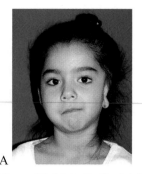
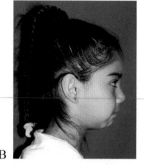
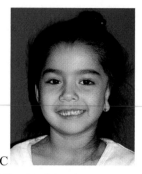

Figure 20-26 A, B, C: A.) Fontal facial view of patient with Hemifacial Microsomia. Note mandibular asymmetry to the left, cant of the lips up on the left and affected left ear. B.) Lateral profile view with some apparent mandibular retrognathia. C.) Frontal smile view showing the cant of the occlusal plane, up on the affected side.

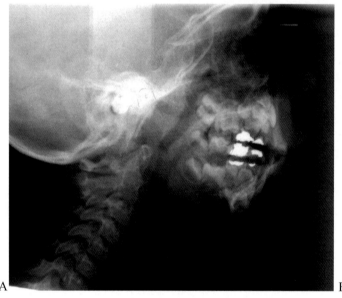
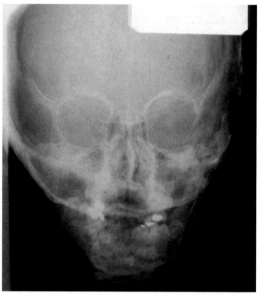

Figure 20-37 A, B: A.) Lateral cephalometric radiograph of same patient with Hemifacial Microsomia showing facial convexity with some apparent mandibular retrognathia. B.) Antero-posterior cephalometric radiograph showing asymmetry and reduction of mandibular height on the affected left side.

It is a progressive congenital deformity, worsening and causing more secondary effects as the patient grows. Unlike the facial asymmetry that is presented by the rarer overdevelopment of one side of the face, this facial asymmetry results from an under-development of the affected structures. On the affected side the ear lobe is deformed with possible skin tags, and the **external auditory meatus** may be absent, resulting in conductive hearing loss. Depending on the magnitude, the anatomy of the mandible may range from little aberration to unrecognizable. The same is true of the **glenoid fossa**, to the point where the temporomandibular joint on that side may be severely atypical or not exist at all, resulting in a limited range of mandibular movement, with limited range of excursion. Most of the mandibular effect is centered on the **condyle**, but the ramus may also be affected with **antegonial notching** and flattening of the angle. The mandibular form is narrowed, leaving reduced tongue space and apparent **macroglossia**. There is deviation of the chin toward the affected side. There is asymmetrical mandibular retrusion which, if severe enough, can even cause respiratory problems. The parotid gland may be missing and the muscles of mastication may be hypoplastic, resulting in flattening of the soft tissue on that side. If the pterygoid is affected, the result is a deviation toward the affected side on opening. The maxilla may be secondarily hypoplastic, resulting in a marked **cant** to the occlusal plane, higher on the affected side.

4.2 INCIDENCE

This is the second most common of the craniofacial **congenital anomalies**, with studies showing its occurrence from approximately 1 in 3500 to 1 in 5600 live births. It occurs with equal frequency in males and females, and 30% may be bilaterally affected.

4.3 CLASSIFICATION

The classification of Hemifacial Microsomia is directly related to the severity of the insult.

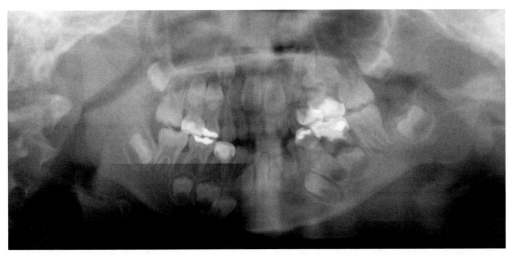

Figure 20-38: Panoramic radiograph to compare the anatomy of the same patient's (Figure 20-36 and 20-37) mandibular ramus and condyle on the unaffected right side compared to the affected left side.

TYPE I -- The mandibular ramus, condyle and glenoid fossa are well shaped, but small.

TYPE II -- The mandibular ramus is short and abnormally shaped, with atypical condyle, flattening of the angle and **antegonial notching**. The glenoid fossa is small, poorly formed and usually displaced.

TYPE III -- The mandibular condyle and ramus and the glenoid fossa are absent. There is no functioning temporomandibular joint. Munro prefers the name "Craniofacial Microsomia" for this congenital defect, and includes upper facial structures to add:

TYPE IV - The mandibular condyle, ramus and glenoid fossa are missing, with decrease in the vertical height of the zygoma, missing **zygomatic arch** and orbital involvement.

TYPE V - The most severe, with mandibular, glenoid fossa, zygomatic and orbital involvement and adding medial positioning of the squamous temporal bone and posterior rotation of the frontal bone on the affected side.

4.4 ASSOCIATED PROBLEMS

4.4.1. Psychosocial

The effect on the psychosocial development previously described for the cleft lip and palate patient applies to patients with other orofacial and craniofacial birth defects, as well. This is, again, why most craniofacial habilitation teams will try to institute surgical treatment as early as possible to improve facial esthetics before development of poor self image and negative social pressures begin to have their effect. In a study of 30 patients with hemifacial microsomia, Padwa, et al., found that there was diminished scholastic performance and, surprisingly, that children with symmetric facial deformity scored poorer than those with asymmetric deformity. It was suggested that the asymmetric face was possibly considered by the patient and others as normal with a superimposed deformity, whereas the face that was symmetrically affected was perceived as being completely deformed.

4.4.2. Growth and Development

Though approximately 50% of these patients show associated congenital heart problems and vertebral anomalies, the greatest impact on the development of all of them is from the effects of diminished growth of the affected parts. There is a basic lack of tissue, and this determines the shape and size of the developing mandible. Because of the lack of adequate mandibular growth, the asymmetry becomes progressively worse, gradually causing secondary distortion of development of associated areas of the midface. The longer treatment is delayed, the more difficult it is to gain the desired result. Hence, early surgery.

4.5 DENTAL PROBLEMS

Development and eruption of the teeth on the affected side has been found to be slower, with a higher incidence of congenital absence of the teeth as well, not only on the affected side, but in a population of the patients with hemifacial microsomia when compared to an unaffected control.

There is often a **telescoping crossbite** of the buccal segment on the affected side and, because of reduced mandibular arch size, severe crowding of the lower arch and mandibular **retrognathia**, marked Class II **malocclusion** with excessive overjet and **anterior open bite**. There is usually marked asymmetry of the **arch form** of both upper and lower arches. Because of the cant to the occlusal plane, the axial inclinations of the upper and lower anterior teeth are quite slanted when related to the **facial midline**, and there is usually considerable discrepancy between the upper and lower dental midlines.

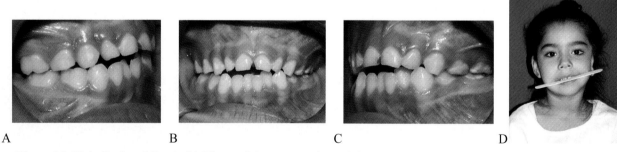

A   B   C   D

Figure 20-39 A, B, C and D: A-C.) Views of the same patient's (Figure 20-38) primary dentition. Basically Class I with slight anterior open bite. D.) Demonstration of the cant of the occlusal plane, up on the affected side.

The range of mandibular movement is seriously affected; not only limitation and deviation upon opening, but in lateral and protrusive excursions, as well. The lips may show restricted activity on the affected side, making access for oral hygiene and dental treatment difficult. There may be temporomandibular joint problems due to the **aberrant** form and function of the affected side, and this may cause a secondary effect on the unaffected side.

As with the cleft lip and palate patient, oral hygiene and patient motivation may be poor, with all the associated increases in occurrence of caries and periodontal problems. Response of the supporting tissues to orthodontic tooth movement must be monitored frequently, especially in areas where eruption of teeth is accomplished to correct the cant of the occlusal plane or close lateral open bites post-surgically. Often, this can result in elongation of clinical crowns and reduced bony root support with some associated instability and need for splinting or gingival grafting.

4.6 STRATEGIES FOR COORDINATING DENTAL AND SURGICAL TREATMENT

As was previously discussed in the segment on cleft lip and palate, orthodontic treatment must be planned and coordinated with other members of the team, especially the plastic surgeon.

A long-term treatment protocol is developed as early as the problem is identified, integrating the treatment plans of all team members involved with a tentative sequence of events that will ensure that a maximum result can be achieved with a minimum of confusion and counter-production. This is especially true in the patient with hemifacial microsomia because it is a progressive anomaly, and early intervention can prevent so many negative developments.

As the dentition develops, the orthodontist will work closest with the surgeon, if not in active treatment, then in surgical planning. This necessitates the most complete and early documentation of the patient's problem.

4.6.1. Documentation of the Patient's Problem

It involves, as was previously described in the segment on cleft lip and palate:
   a.) Pertinent Medical and Dental histories
   b.) Complete Clinical Examination
   c.) Oriented Profile and Frontal Facial Photographs. Specific to patients with hemifacial microsomia, the surgeon finds it most useful to have some method of measure in the photograph next to the patient, such as a ruler with easily visible markings held next to the face. Also, a frontal facial view with the orbits parallel to the floor and the patient biting on a tongue blade will effectively note the magnitude of the lateral cant of the occlusal plane.
   d.) Intraoral Photographs
   e.) Full Mouth Periapical Radiographs
   f.) Panoramic Radiograph
   g.) Oriented Lateral and Antero-Posterior Cephalometric Radiographs. Specific to patients with hemifacial microsomia is the difficulty to orient the head in the usual cephalostat. The displacement and abnormal form of the ear on the affected side make it difficult to use the ear rods. Goldsmith, et al., have shown a simple and effective means of setting the ear rod on the unaffected side and using the pupils of the eyes as a guide.
   h.) Study Casts. These should be able to be mounted on an articulator to allow for possible positioning of the mandible and construction of a surgical splint. If a surgical splint is needed, it should be made on duplicate casts to preserve the diagnostic models.

4.6.2. Setting of Goals, Team Coordination and Treatment Planning

There is no single "cook book" approach to treatment for these patients. There are five different classified types of patients with craniofacial microsomia, starting with very minor deformity, perhaps requiring no treatment or only orthodontic intervention, and ending with a congenital deformity involving the whole oro-facial complex that could require more than one phase of orthodontic treatment coupled with possible two jaw surgery. The overriding ideal goal of both surgical and orthodontic treatment is the earliest possible restoration of facial symmetry, with the midlines of the anterior dentition (especially the upper), the midline of the upper lip and that of the face all coincident and the cant of the occlusal plane aligned with the upper **lip line**.

4.6.2.1. The Primary and Transitional Dentitions

4.6.2.1.1. Orthodontic Considerations

To try to avoid the effects of the progression of the deformity, correction is begun between 2 to 5 years of age. In a child that young, most feel that surgical correction can be confined to the mandible, and the improvement that is established at that time has a good chance to persist. An attempt is made to create a new "functional matrix", which (again, Wolf's Law) can guide the developing form to a better relation and symmetry, if early enough, preventing secondary maxillary growth inhibition.

In the TYPE I patient, with minor deformity, this may be attempted with a functional orthodontic appliance, repositioning the mandible downward, forward and laterally to slightly overcorrect the dental midline relation.

In the TYPE II patient, with moderate deformity, a functional appliance may be tried, but the chance for success with the appliance alone is even less, with mandibular surgery of some type much more a certainty.

In the TYPE III patient, with the condyle, ramus and glenoid fossa absent, the functional appliance is circumvented and early surgery performed.

4.6.2.1.2. Surgical Considerations

In severe cases, there may be reconstruction of the ear at this age. The aim of jaw surgery would be to lengthen the short side of the mandible, either by placing a rib graft or by mandibular distraction osteogenesis, actually stimulating the growth of new mandibular bone. The rib graft is placed with the costal cartilage intact, simulating the condylar head and allowing a great potential for growth, although it is often unpredictable. This, with rebuilding of the glenoid fossa three dimensionally, will also create a functioning temporomandibular joint. The mandible is advanced on the affected side, creating a large lateral open bite, often in excess of 20 millimeters. The object is then to encourage the maxilla, which is high on the affected side, to grow vertically to level the lateral occlusal cant. Not eruption of the teeth on that side, but downward vertical maxillary growth. This may take one or two years and a lot of orthodontic guidance to accomplish.

Mandibular distraction osteogenesis is a technique where the mandible is gradually lengthened by the "normal healing process" following slow controlled separation of a surgical osteotomy site. The gradual nature of the bone lengthening allows the soft tissue envelope (nerves, muscle and blood supply) to expand as well, increasing the stability of the procedure. One of the main advantages of distraction is its ability to be used at a very young age. This is significant because, as stated previously, the midface adapts to the mandible in the early growth phases so that a disturbance in mandibular development results in decreased midface development as well. Use of early distraction can avoid secondary growth disturbances in the maxilla.

Mandibular distraction can have significant advantages for children with moderate Type I and Type II mandibles. However, a child with a severe Type III is unlikely to have sufficient bone to allow for a corticotomy and/or osteotomy and placement of pins for external or internal distraction devices. In such situations, conventional costochondral rib grafts remain the treatment of choice. Similarly, minimal mandibular deformities of Type I may be treated more appropriately with conventional **orthognathic surgery** at the time of skeletal maturity. McCarthy, et al., published, in 1992, the first report of mandibular lengthening in four children with mandibular deficiency.

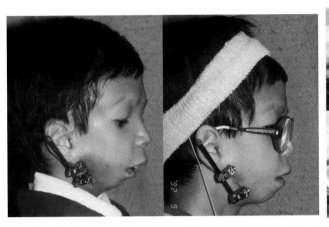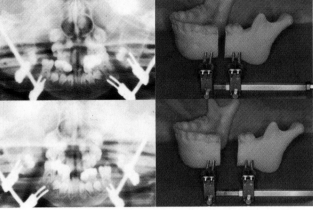

Figure 20-40 A, B: A.) Patient with severe micrognathia before (left) and after (right) bilateral mandibular distraction. B.) On the left: Radiographic view of a patient before (above) and after (below) bilateral mandibular distraction showing widening of the space in the mandibular body. On the right: Demonstration of the action of the distractor on the mandibular body.

Figure 20-40A and B shows a patient with severe **micrognathia** and the effect of bilateral unidirectional appliances, similar to the devices used by McCarthy.

For background on distraction osteogenesis, including history of development and a summary of treatment phases, see "surgical considerations" under the cleft lip and palate section.

On our team, the orthodontists are involved closely with this phase of treatment. First, we must remember that there will be times, as in the treatment of any of our patients, when patient cooperation, motivation and compliance will be absolutely critical to the success of the treatment. When we attempt early treatment phases that have little chance for success we deplete that patient's cooperation potential, and functional appliance therapy can take years. Loss of cooperation potential is usually not recoverable. The chance for success of early function treatment is not great because the patient in the pri-

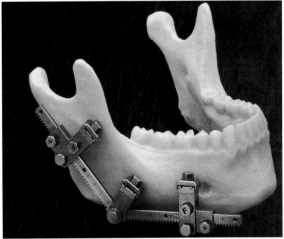

Figure 20-41: Shows a newer multi-directional appliance (KLS Marting, L.P.) with increased control of vertical and horizontal vectors. Although several internal devices are currently being used for mandibular lengthening, the multidirectional control needed for the more severe cases cannot yet be achieved with currently available internal devices.

mary dentition is very young and functional appliances tend to be bulky. Most young children would tend to play with the appliance or not wear it at all, instead of holding it steady in the proper position, which would obviously be necessary to affect any change in "functional matrix" and vertical maxillary growth. The constant need for admonition and monitoring by the parents places a strain on the entire family, in addition to interference by the appliance with the child's ability to communicate with parents and peers. With progression of the situation and canting of the occlusal plane in the mixed dentition, mandibular surgery would eventually be necessary anyway. As in cleft lip and palate treatment, we tend to avoid orthodontic (or functional orthopedic) treatment in the primary dentition, awaiting a time when we can set more specific goals with a shorter time frame and with higher chances of success.

If the severity and progression of the condition requires surgical placement of a rib graft in the late primary or early mixed dentition, the orthodontists on our team are involved in two ways: 1.) pre-surgical planning, and 2.) splint construction and placement of a post-surgical appliance that will maintain the new mandibular position and encourage the needed vertical maxillary growth. This will allow for closure of the lateral open bite created by surgery on the affected side, with associated improvement in the lateral cant of the occlusal plane.

First, there must be complete documentation of the pre-surgical situation. This includes duplicate study casts with wax bite, suitable for mounting on an articulator, lateral cephalometric radiograph with teeth in occlusion, antero-posterior cephalometric radiograph (oriented with pupils of the eyes parallel to the floor and the ear rod placed only in the unaffected ear), panoramic radiograph and facial and intraoral photographs. The facial photographs can have a ruler with clear markings held next to the head. The frontal view should have the pupils of the eyes parallel to the floor, and an additional view taken with the patient biting on a tongue blade to help evaluate the extent of the lateral cant of the occlusal plane.

Cephalometric evaluation is a very individual procedure. We each may use different vehicles to gain the same information for diagnosis and treatment planning. In this instance, the films may be digitized and computer predictions of one type or another may also prove useful to the surgeon. Since it is the surgeon who will be moving the parts, it is up to the orthodontist to provide whatever information the surgeon needs to develop the surgical plan. The surgeon will be your guide and will also probably be quite open to your suggestions. Once the plan is made, the study casts on the articulator can be manipulated to simulate the final tooth relation in the new mandibular position and a surgical splint made. The mandible is usually moved downward, forward and laterally to overcorrect the midline relation, usually creating a 15-16 mm anterior open bite and a 20-22 mm lateral open bite on the affected side. Depending on the surgeon's need, the mandibular positioning splint can be constructed in removable form with ball clasps to enable its easy attachment to the maxillary arch or in a form that can be wired into position.

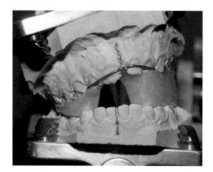 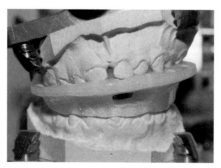 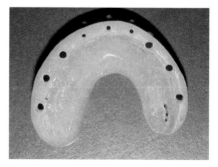

Figure 20-42 A, B and C: A.) Mandibular repositioning splint: removable type with ball clasps for retention. B. and C.) Mandibular repositioning splint: fixed type for intermaxillary wiring fixation.

The fabrication of a post-surgical orthopedic appliance, if desired, will involve mounting the duplicate set of the study casts on the articulator, using the surgical splint as a guide. A wax block is then shaped to relate the casts for shipment to the laboratory so that their positions can be duplicated on the lab articulator for fabrication of the first post-surgical appliance. This appliance, resembling an orthodontic finishing appliance (positioner) is made out of a moderately firm, flexible plastic designed to accomplish the following:

-- maintain and stabilize the post-surgical position.

--encourage vertical maxillary growth, undoubtedly with some tooth eruption, on the affected side to close the newly created open bite and improve the lateral cant of the occlusal plane.

--stimulate, exercise and strengthen the hypoplastic buccal musculature on the affected side, and

--allow for normal expansive maxillary and mandibular alveolar growth, without interference.

--The appliance is tooth borne on the unaffected side and tooth (mandibular) and tissue borne on the affected side.

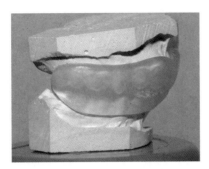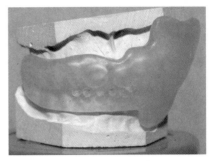

Figure 20-43 A and B: A and B.) Views of a post-surgical orthopedic appliance. Note the vestibular extensions for stimulation of the hypoplastic affected musculature.

The appliance is placed on the mandibular teeth and, as the mouth is closed, the extended vestibular shield on the affected side moves up to contact and stretch the vestibular tissue during exercise and to stabilize the appliance. The tooth contact through the appliance on the unaffected side should maintain their position (or, ideally, even gain some depression of the maxillary teeth), while the affected side of the maxilla is free to move vertically to re-establish contact of the teeth on the affected side. This vertical drop is made possible by the lab blocking out the maxillary teeth on the affected side prior to curing the appliance, leaving a void into which the unsupported maxillary teeth may move.

The accuracy of the height of the vestibular shield on the affected side must be assured by adding height to the upper and lower impression trays with beading wax to gain maximum stretch of the tissues and height of the vestibular fold during impression taking.

The appliance is to be worn as close to 24 hours per day as possible. The less it is worn, the more tooth eruption and mandibular rebound and the less actual vertical maxillary growth is involved in the closure of the open bite.

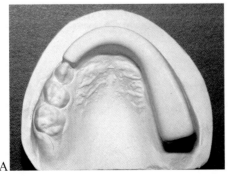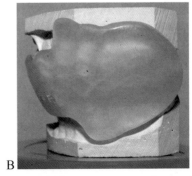

Figure 20-44 A,B: A.) View of laboratory model showing wax block to create space for maxillary teeth on affected side to erupt, closing the lateral open bite and improving the occlusal cant.
B.) Lateral view of the appliance showing space below the maxillary buccal teeth for eruption.

As viewed through the translucent wall of the appliance, when the maxillary teeth on the affected side have moved down to contact the appliance at the bottom of the void, the appliance is finished. The longer it takes, the better.

At that time, the lateral cant of the occlusal plane can be re-evaluated. If it is still excessive, an appliance may be used that is not as "invasive" into the patient's life as was the first. A lower removable appliance may be constructed with an acrylic block on the unaffected side.

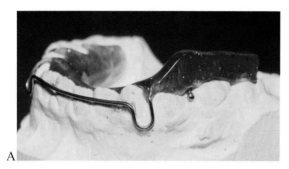 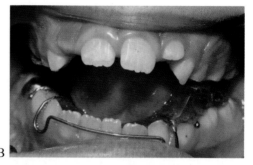

A   B

Figure 20-45 A,B: Views of a removable lower appliance with an acrylic pad on the unaffected side to create pressure on the maxillary dentition on the unaffected side and free the affected maxillary buccal segment to drop vertically with time and improve the occlusal cant.

This is much easier for the young patient to wear as often as needed because it does not interfere with their ability to communicate. Because the opening exceeds the **freeway space**, it should create continuous pressure on the maxillary buccal segment on the unaffected side and frees the other maxillary buccal segment to continue to drop vertically to improve the lateral cant of the occlusal plane.

4.6.2.2. The Permanent Dentition

4.6.2.2.1. Orthodontic Considerations

By the time the patient reaches the full permanent dentition, most of the progressive effects, both primary and secondary, will have been demonstrated. The female patients will be approaching maturity, with the natural diminution in growth that accompanies. By that time, the positive effects of early surgical and orthodontic interventions will also be seen. Some have had success continuing to try functional-type appliances if the occlusal cant is still prominent, advancing the short side with a fixed maxillary splint to stimulate additional vertical condylar growth on that side. The naturally diminished growth at that age and the invasiveness of the appliance into a patient's early teen years greatly reduce the chances for success. Once growth slows and stops, revisionary surgery still has a good chance of improving obvious facial asymmetry. From an orthodontic standpoint, fixed orthodontic appliances should have the best chance for improving tooth relations. Remember, at this point we can only treat the patient to the maximum of their potential. We must now do the most with the physical and emotional situation that is presented. It is important, with the team, to set a course that will get us out of this patient's still-developing life with the least interference and the best result that will be available to us.

The situation may certainly require compromise. The basal elements of bone and tissue, even with early interventions, may certainly still be lacking to a point where the "ideal" result cannot be achieved. This does not mean a failure in treatment. There will still be some degree of asymmetry. The mandible, the maxilla and all the associated hard and soft structures of the face may have been affected by hypoplastic growth to this point, leaving the teeth a base for support that is not only smaller than it should be, but displaced as well. Crowding of the teeth, possible telescoped crossbite of the buccal segment on the affected side, severe Class II skeletal relation on the affected side with the associated increase in overjet, overbite, midline shift and mandibular retrognathia may all be present. Tooth relations vary greatly because of differences in the degree of mandibular **arch length deficiency**. There may be deviation upon opening and closing due to difference in function of the joint on the affected side with some limited opening capability. One thing is fairly certain: because of reduced growth on the affected side, primarily the mandible and secondarily the maxilla, the tooth midline relation to the face will be off center. The upper teeth will be shifted toward the affected side.

Starting time for this comprehensive phase of orthodontic treatment, as with any of our adolescent patients, can be determined by the number of permanent teeth present. We usually point to the imminent loss of the last of the primary teeth so that treatment with fixed appliances will not be excessively lengthened by awaiting tooth eruption. This is a time for close coordination of orthodontic treatment plans with the surgeon. Do not ever plan to set out on a course of treatment without the knowledge and consent of the patient's surgeon. If there are surgical plans for the future, they must be coordinated with your orthodontic plans to avoid the need for later re-treatment or compromise in the potential of the result. Some delay in timing of the orthodontic treatment may even be necessary if there are surgical plans that would require growth to be finished, and an orthodontic/orthognathic surgical team treatment to be instituted later. At this time, the case would be documented with full orthodontic records as previously described. Before the orthodontic treatment plan is formulated, the records would be shared with the surgeon and a meeting, either in person or by phone, would follow, coordinating the last phases of treatment for this patient. Which treatment should be primary? Which secondary? What can the orthodontist do to help the surgeon and vice versa?

There is not just one orthodontic approach to treatment that can apply to all of these patients because of the huge variation found at this age. There is one constant, however, that should be kept in mind. Asymmetry is the problem, so symmetry should be the overall goal of treatment.   A symmetrical relation between the teeth, especially the upper anteriors, and the face and upper lip. The midline of the teeth as coincident with the midline of the face as possible. Because of the mandibular hypoplasia, the lower midline may not be able to follow, so that compromise in upper to lower midline relation is common. But, if the upper anteriors are aligned with the face and the upper lip, especially when the patient is smiling, the esthetics are improved greatly. Certainly, this can mean unilateral extraction in order to shift the midline, and compromise in buccal segment relation, especially on the affected side, is usually necessary, as well. Every attempt should be made to make this the last phase of orthodontic treatment for this patient.

4.6.2.2.2. Surgical Considerations

The timing for this treatment is usually past a chance for influencing growth. From an orthognathic surgical perspective, the goal of treatment is usually to advance the mandible, unilaterally or bilaterally. It is not uncommon, if the magnitude of needed advancement requires, that lower first premolars would be removed during the pre-surgical stage and the lower anteriors retracted to increase the overjet and allow for greater anterior placement of the chin. Of course, cosmetic surgical procedures could be considered at this time, also, for improvement of facial symmetry and further ear reconstruction.

5. THE PATIENT WITH **CROUZON'S** OR **APERT'S SYNDROMES**

Craniosynostosis is a term which means the premature fusion of a cranial suture. Premature sutural closure, with the resultant loss in its contribution to normal cranial growth, will cause the cranium and the **cranial base** to distort. As opposed to hemifacial microsomia, which becomes an asymmetrical distortion, craniosynostosis will usually result in a more symmetric pattern. Similar to hemifacial microsomia, it is a progressive distortion in growth, the degree of distortion here related directly to the degree of prematurity of the sutural fusion. It may happen later in fetal development than most craniofacial anomalies but, still, the earlier it happens the more far-reaching the effect which, again, accounts for the variability found in the population of afflicted patients.

Crouzon's and Apert's Syndromes both result from craniosynostoses, perhaps located somewhat differently in position but with similar enough cranial base and midface effect that, especially for the purposes of our dental discussion, we can consider them together.

5.1 ETIOLOGY AND DESCRIPTION

In Apert's Syndrome, the craniosynostosis is thought to involve the coronal suture, restricting the antero-posterior growth of the cranium. One result is retrusion of the midface with depression of the nasal bridge. In Crouzon's Syndrome, the premature fusion occurs lower, between the cranial and facial bones, with similar result, the retropositioning of the entire maxillary complex. In the Apert's patient, the anterior **fontanel** stays open, causing characteristic "bossing" or bulging of the frontal and temporal areas. Even more characteristic of Apert's Syndrome is the additional presence of deformities of the hands and feet, resulting in its other name, acrocephalosyndactyly.

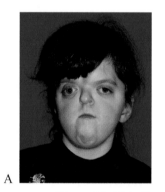 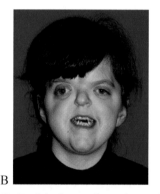 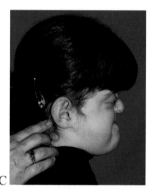

A   B   C

Figure 20-46 A, B and C: Facial views of a patient with Apert's Syndrome

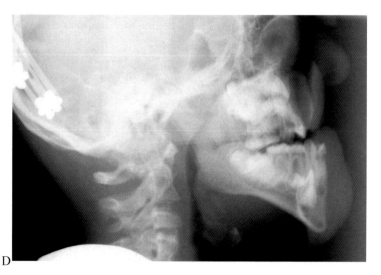 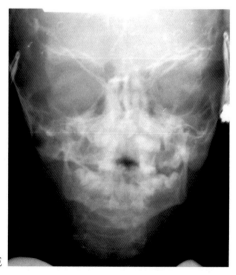

D   E

Figure 20-46 D and E: Lateral and antero-posterior cephalometric radiographs of the same patient.

The maxilla in these patients is hypoplastic in all three dimensions, causing the tip of the "beaked" nose to raise. The mandible, aside from a somewhat more vertical growth pattern, may be largely unaffected. The result is retrusion of the midface with a flat, sometimes concave face. This, because of hypoplasia of the maxilla, orbits and malar bones, is coupled with unusually wide separation of the globular eyes (**hypertelorism**). Stricker, et al., best described the oro-facial area, saying that "the mouth remains half open in the shape of an isosceles triangle. The upper lip is retracted, giving it a crossbow appearance. The cheeks are rounded while the dangling lower lip juts out. Maxillary retrusion is associated with a keel-shaped arch and dental crowding. Class III malocclusion with an open bite may be observed. The high palate is divided by a midline furrow with a **paramedian** fold on each side." In many cases, this central furrow extends posteriorly to end in a cleft of the soft palate. Though the mandible may be unaffected, the result is a relative **prognathism**, with pronounced bilateral buccal segment and anterior crossbites.

5.2 INCIDENCE

Apert first described his syndrome in 1906, Crouzon in 1912. It has been estimated that Crouzon's Syndrome, the third most common of the craniofacial birth defects, will occur once in 25,000 live births, whereas Apert's has been reported from 1:100,000 to 1:1,000,000 live births.

5.3 ASSOCIATED PROBLEMS

Many of the problems previously described for the cleft lip and palate and craniofacial microsomia patients can be applied to these patients, as well. These are all children with congenital orofacial and craniofacial deformity and, though the origin and physical effect may be different, the impact on growth and development, emotional and otherwise, can be quite similar.

5.3.1. Growth and Development

There are differences between patients with Crouzon's and Apert's Syndromes, but many more similarities. The cranial base similarities motivated Tessier to combine the syndromes, naming them "Croupert." The fact that the effects become progressively worse with age has long been known. The fact that the main facial impact is in its middle third, focused not necessarily on maxillary hypoplasia, but on maxillary retrognathia in relation to the cranial base, holds true for both syndromes. The mandible, though found to be secondarily directed somewhat more vertically in syndrome patients and somewhat shorter and narrower in the ramus, is relatively normal, creating a pseudo-prognathia because of the retrusion of the maxilla.

5.3.2. Breathing

The size of the nasopharynx is severely affected, with strong possibility of deviation of the nasal septum. This causes these patients to be mouth breathers, holding their mouths open and their heads in an extended position and posturing their tongues forward to allow increased air flow.

5.3.3. Psychosocial

These patients suffer the same problems in self image and psychosocial development as did those with the congenital orofacial and craniofacial deformities previously described (See Chapter 1). In a study of only Apert's patients, Campis found that with these patients as well, fast acceptance by the parents and the immediate family was critical in the quality of their development. Mental retardation has been associated with Apert's, but it was found that this has been reduced by the institution of early surgical procedures making room for more brain growth and intellectual development. Campis also found these children quite resilient, capable of good psychosocial adjustment even with early damaging experiences and that their self image improved greatly following surgery.

Other associated problems mentioned with Crouzon's and Apert's Syndromes are possible cleft of the lip and palate, increase in middle ear infections, cardiovascular problems, **ankylosis** of the joints, abnormalities in the vertebral column and early feeding difficulties because of shortness of the hard palate.

5.4 DENTAL PROBLEMS

Malocclusion is the most common dental problem shared by patients with Crouzon's or Apert's Syndromes. The small and retropositioned maxilla is tipped down posteriorly, bringing the molars into premature contact and resulting in an anterior open bite. The maxillary arch is v-shaped with extremely wide, bulging alveolar ridges, sometimes meeting in a deep medial groove. This groove can become a food trap, very hard for the patient to keep clean, especially if there are hand deformities as well. Early surgical procedures may have disrupted the developing tooth buds, resulting in abnormal roots or crowns. The tooth buds are in close approximation, some interfering with the eruption of others. Ectopic eruption of the upper first molars occurs in almost half of these patients. Radiographic identification of separate teeth is often impossible because of the congestion. Eruption guidance is often necessary, with removal of primary or even permanent teeth to allow for eruption of others. Sometimes the biggest problem is the decision of which teeth to remove and which to keep. Gingival tissue can be quite dense, with resultant delay in speed of tooth eruption. Supernumerary and pegged shaped teeth are not uncommon.

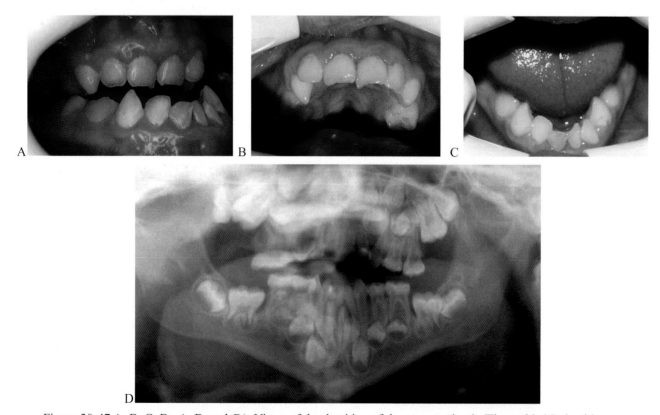

Figure 20-47 A, B, C, D: A, B, and C.) Views of the dentition of the same patient's (Figure 20-46) dentition. Note the Class III relation, asymmetry of the arches, crossbites and anterior open bite. D.) Panorex of this patient showing severe tendency to crowding and ectopic position of many of the unerupted permanent teeth.

There are buccal and anterior crossbites with a severe mandibular overjet and Class III malocclusion, often accentuated by the fact that the restricted nasopharynx size forces the patient to posture the mandible and tongue forward to gain additional air flow. The fact that these patients are mouth breathers, of course, will make any dental treatment more difficult. The use of cotton rolls to dry the field can make the patient quite uncomfortable, fearing that the airway will be blocked. High speed suction equipment is helpful.

Oral hygiene is most often poor. This, coupled with the wrong diet, as with any of our patients, can result in high incidence of caries and poor health of the supporting tissues. Dental recall every three months or so is necessary to monitor oral hygiene and periodontal status and to reinforce the need for continual and thorough home care, often with the help of a parent. Frequent prophylaxis and preventive sealants can be helpful, along with regular fluoride treatments. At home, electric toothbrush, floss holders and water flushing devices prove effective, especially for the patient with hand deformities.

5.5 STRATEGIES FOR ORTHODONTIC TREATMENT

5.5.1. Documentation and Diagnosis

Certainly, as with any other orofacial and craniofacial patient, coordination of treatment planning with other members of the patient's treating team is critical. When the patient is first seen by the team, complete documentation of the situation is necessary. This job usually falls to the orthodontists, who, as in the previous discussions, will provide study casts, intraoral and extraoral photographs, panoramic radiograph, lateral cephalometric radiographs (usually at rest and in occlusion) and antero-posterior cephalometric radiographs along with the appropriate tracings and evaluations. These patients will usually also receive CT scans or MRIs or both at that time to provide the involved members of the team with the greatest depth of information available. This is the time to set the sequence of treatment events for the patient, as far as the projection is possible. Priorities are set, and the members of the team establish the coordination and timing of treatments to ensure that unnecessary procedures are avoided, and that they compliment each other to gain the maximum success for the patient.

5.5.2. Setting of Goals, Team Coordination and Treatment

5.5.2.1. Planning

For patients with Crouzon's or Apert's Syndromes, aside from earlier dental involvement to supervise and protect the developing dentition, the first palliative treatment is usually surgical. The orthodontist can be of great help in the planning, not only providing the documentation, but with computer surgical prediction, as well.

Though some prefer to delay major surgery, if at all possible, until 9 years of age or older, in severe cases early high midface advancement (LeFort III) in the later primary or early mixed dentition can be safely performed and can increase the size of the nasopharynx, providing more space for the tongue and improving the air flow. This can also help protect the eyes and improve the facial esthetics and child's self image before school begins. Predictability of midface placement at this time is very difficult, and additional later surgery is usually necessary when growth is finished.

Active treatment of the malocclusion in the primary and early mixed dentition is usually avoided. This is usually a time, however, for selective extraction in eruption guidance to try to improve the chance for reasonable placement of the permanent teeth before later comprehensive orthodontic treatment. This may even require surgical uncovering of the crowns of some of the teeth to encourage their timely eruption.

If not done earlier, the loss of the last primary teeth with the patient between 9 and 12 years of age presents another opportunity for surgical midface advancement, this time possibly followed by a phase of orthodontic treatment. The mandible is still growing, which again makes it difficult to anticipate remaining growth potential and project a final maxillary position. The LeFort III is done with a downward rotation to reduce the **anterior open bite**, with care being taken not to elongate the upper incisors in relation to the upper lip. Rapid palatal expansion, sometimes surgically assisted, may be accomplished at this time.

As with any progressive growth disorder, if possible, comprehensive orthodontic treatment is best withheld until growth has ended so that a final and stable relation of the maxilla and mandible can be established without over-correction. This carries the final phase of treatment in these patients to their teens, when mandibular growth has finished. The orthodontist can monitor growth through lateral cephalometric radiographs taken and compared every six months or so, and when this shows no mandibular change the final phase of treatment can be started. Lack of growth allows the midface deficiency and the malocclusion to be treated at the same time. At this point, a low midface advancement (LeFort I) is usually performed, posteriorly impacted to reduce the anterior open bite, allowing autorotation of the mandible and increasing the prominence of the chin, establishing good incisor/lip relation and improving incisor overbite and overjet. The mandible may have developed a reverse curve of Spee, which may require two jaw surgery.

As with any orthodontic/orthognathic treatment, the orthodontist plays a key role in treatment planning, including surgical prediction, providing the full fixed orthodontic appliance and the presurgical tooth position to allow accuracy in surgical placement and the post-surgical finalizing and stabilizing that will assure the maximum result.

The authors sincerely hope that this material will prove useful to the reader in facing the "ultimate challenge" that is presented by diagnosis and treatment of a patient with a congenital orofacial or craniofacial anomaly. It is a challenge, not only in competence but in imagination. Your need to treat these patients, by the sheer lack of their numbers, will be infrequent, but it can represent the highest levels of intellectual stimulation and gratification you will experience professionally. As we have made clear, there is no one way to treat them because of the wide variability in the possible severity of the problems and the impact on the growth and development of the patients. There is usually a BEST way to treat them, however, and each patient may require a different treatment plan, coordinated differently with the other members of the treatment team. Unilaterally selecting a plan and sequence of treatment by any single member of the treatment team is a mistake. No one person can know all of the implications and possibilities. As the dentist, you will be very important, and not only your treatment but your diagnostic input will be critical to long term planning. All of your years of professional education, training and experience can be brought to bear, as well as your imagination and artistic sense. Both you and the patient benefit from your effort on their behalf.

The authors wish to express their deep thanks to Dr. Bruce Bauer and Dr. Pravin Patel, Department of Pediatric Plastic Surgery at Children's Memorial Hospital in Chicago for their expertise and input into the preparation of this chapter.

7. SUGGESTED READING

The Team Concept

American Cleft Palate/Craniofacial Association. Parameters for evaluation and treatment of patients with craniofacial anomalies. Prepared by the Grant Project Committee from resolutions approved at the Consensus Conference. May, 1991.

Kernahan, DA and Rosenstein, SW (eds.): Cleft Lip and Palate. A System of Management. Baltimore, Williams and Wilkins, 1990, pp 38.

Will, LA and Parsons, R: Characteristics of the new patients at Illinois cleft palate teams. Cleft Pal/Cranio J 1991; 28(4):378.

The Patient with a Cleft of the Lip and Palate

Kitamura, H: Evidence for cleft palate as a postfusion phenomenon. Cleft Pal/Cranio J April, 1991:28 (2).

Leonard, RN, Brust, JD, Abrahams, G and Sielaff, B: Self-concept of children and adolescents with cleft lip and/or palate. Cleft Pal/Cranio J 1991;28(4):347.

Noar, JH: Questionnaire survey of attitudes and concerns of patients with cleft lip and palate and their parents. Cleft Pal/Cranio J July, 1991;28(3):277.

Noar, JH: A questionnaire survey of attitudes and concerns of three professional groups involved in the cleft palate team. Cleft Pal/Cranio J January, 1992; 29(1):92-95.

Paynter, ET, Jordan, WJ and Finch, DL: Patient compliance with cleft palate team regimens. Jour Speech and Hearing Disorders, November 1990;55(4):740-750.

Paynter, ET, Edmonson, TW and Jordan, WJ: Accuracy of information reported by parents and children evaluated by a cleft palate team. Cleft Pal/Cranio J 1991;28(4):329.

Dorf, DS and Curtin, JW: Early cleft palate repair and speech outcome. Plast Recon Surg 1982;70:74.

Starr, CD: Dental and occlusal hazards to normal speech production. In Grabb, WC, Rosenstein, SW, Bzoch, KR (eds.): Cleft Lip and Palate. Surgical, Dental and Speech Aspects. Boston, Little, Brown, 1971.

Immamura N, et al. Comparison of the sizes of adenoidal tissues and upper airways of subjects with and without cleft lip and palate. Am J Orthod Dentofacial Orthop 2002;122:189-195.

Gray, S: Airway obstruction and apnea in cleft palate patients. In Bardach, J, Morris, HL (eds.): Multidisciplinary Management of Cleft Lip and Palate. Philadelphia, WB Saunders, 1990: pp 418.

Fields, HW and Sinclair, PM: Dentofacial growth and development. Jour Dent for Chil, Jan 1990;57(1):46-55.

Rosenstein, SW, Monroe, C, Kernahan, D, Jacobson, BN, Griffith, BJ and Bauer, B: The case for early bone grafting in cleft lip and cleft palate. Plast Recon Surg 1982;70(3):297.

Shaw, WC and Semb, G: Current approaches to the orthodontic management of cleft lip and palate. Jour of Royal Soc of Med, January 1990;83(1):30-33.

Subtelny, JD: Orthodontic principles in treatment of cleft lip and palate. In Bardach, J and Morris, HL (eds.): Multidisciplinary Management of Cleft Lip and Palate. Philadelphia, WB Saunders, 1990; pp 615.

Vargervik, K: Orthodontic treatment of cleft patients: Characteristics of growth and development/treatment principles. In Bardach, J and Morris, HL: Multidisciplinary Management of Cleft Lip and Palate. Philadelphia, WB Saunders, 1990:642.

Jacobson, BN and Rosenstein, SW: The cleft palate patient: Dental help needed. J Dent Child 1970;37:17.

Czerepak, C: The primary and mixed dentition: Dental considerations for the cleft lip and palate child. In Kernahan, DA, Rosenstein, SW (eds.): Cleft Lip and Palate. A System of Management. Baltimore, Williams and Wilkins 1990, p. 214.

Garn, SM, Osborne, RH, McCabe, KD: The effect of prenatal factors on crown dimensions. Am J Phys Anthropol 1979;51:665.

Ranta, R: A review of tooth formation in children with cleft lip/palate. Am J Ortho/Dentofacial Orthoped, July, 1986:90(1):11-17.

Werner, SP and Harris, EF: Odontometrics of the permanent teeth in cleft lip and palate: systemic size reduction and amplified asymmetry. Cleft Pal J, Jan 1989;26(1):56.

Dahllof, G, Ussisoo-Joandi, R, Ideberg, M and Modeer, T: Caries, gingivitis and dental abnormalities in preschool children with cleft lip and/or palate. Cleft Pal J, July, 1989;26(3).

Bragger, V, Schurch, E, Gusbert, FA and Lang, NP: Periodontal conditions in adolescents with cleft lip, alveolus and palate following treatment in a coordinated team approach. J Clin Perio 1985; 12:494.

Bragger, V, Schurch, E, Salvi, G, von Wyttenbach, T and Lang, N: Periodontal conditions in adult patients with cleft lip, alveolus and palate. Cleft Pal/Cranio J, March 1992;29(2):179.

Tan, AE and Henry, DJ: Periodontal implications of the adolescent cleft palate patient. Aust Dent J 1985;30:8.

Olin, WH: Orthodontic treatment in different stages of growth and development. In Bardach, J and Morris, H (eds.): Multidisciplinary Management of Cleft Lip and Palate. Philadelphia, WB Saunders, 1990.

Ranta, R: Orthodontic treatment alternatives for unilateral cleft lip and palate patients. In Bardach, J and Morris, JL: Multidisciplinary Management of Cleft Lip and Palate. Philadelphia, WB Saunders 1990, pp 637.

Verdi, FJ, Lanzi, GL, Cohen, SR and Powell, R: Use of the Branemark implant in the cleft palate patient. Cleft Pal/Cranio J, July 1991;28(3).

Curtin, G: The infant with cleft lip or palate: More than a surgical problem. Perinat Neonatal Nurs, January 1990;3(3):80-89.

Gnoinski, WM: Infant orthopedics and later orthodontic monitoring for unilateral cleft lip and palate patients in Zurich. In Bardach, J and Morris, HL: Multidisciplinary Management of Cleft Lip and Palate. Philadelphia, WB Saunders 1990; pp 578.

Huebener, DV and Marsh, J: Alveolar molding appliances in the treatment of cleft lip and palate infants. In Bardach, J and Morris, JL (eds): Multidisciplinary Management of Cleft Lip and Palate. Philadelphia, WB Saunders 1990: pp 601.

Jacobson, BN and Rosenstein, SW: Early maxillary orthopedics: a combination appliance. Cleft Pal J, October, 1965.

Jacobson, BN and Rosenstein, SW: Early maxillary orthopedics for the newborn cleft lip and palate patient: an impression and an appliance. Angle Ortho 1984; 54(3);247.

Jacobson, BN and Rosenstein, SW: Cleft lip and palate: the orthodontist's youngest patient. Amer J Ortho/Dentofacial Orthoped 1986; 90(1):63.

Richard, ME: Feeding the newborn with cleft lip and/or palate: the enlargement, stimulate, swallow, rest (ESSR) method. J of Ped Nursing 1991; 6(5):317.

Stricker, M, Van der Meulen, JC, Raphael, R and Mazzola, R: Craniofacial Malformations. New York, Churchill Livingstone, 1990.

Subtelny, JD: Orthodontic principles in treatment of cleft lip and palate. In Bardach, J and Morris, HL (eds.): Multidisciplinary Management of Cleft Lip and Palate. Philadelphia, WB Saunders, 1990: pp 615.

Keller, E and Jackson, IT: Treatment of skeletal deformities in the cleft palate. In Bardach, J and Morris, HL: Multidisciplinary Management of the Cleft Lip and Palate. Philadelphia, WB Saunders 1990: pp 515.

Ranta, R: Orthodontic treatment alternatives for unilateral cleft lip and palate patients. In Bardach, J and Morris, JL: Multidisciplinary Management of Cleft Lip and Palate. Philadelphia, WB Saunders 1990: pp 637.

Turvey, T: Commentary, in Verdi, FJ, Lanzi, GL, Cohen, SR and Powell, R: Use of the Branemark implant in the cleft palate patient. Cleft Pal/Cranio J July, 1991;28(3).

Eppley, BL and Sadove, AM: Management of alveolar cleft bone grafting -- State of the art. Cleft Pal/Cranio J May 2000; 37(3):229.

Monroe, CW, Griffith, BH, Rosenstein, SW and Jacobson, BN: The correction and preservation of arch form in complete clefts of the palate and alveolar ridge. Plast Recon Surg 1968; 41(2).

Rosenstein, SW, Monroe, C, Kernahan, D, Jacobson, BN, Griffith, BJ and Bauer, B: The case for early bone grafting in cleft lip and cleft palate. Plast Recon Surg 1982; 70(3):297.

El Deeb, M, Bevis, R and Gomez-Marin, O: Canines erupted through grafted alveolar cleft defects in patients with alveolar clefts: a pulp testing evaluation study. Cleft Pal J, April, 1989; 26(3).

Epker, BN and Fish, LC: Cleft lip and palate. In Dentofacial Deformities: Integrated Orthodontic and Surgical Correction. St. Louis, CV Mosby, 1986: pp 644.

Freihofer, P, van Damme, P and Kuijpers-Jagtman, A: Early secondary osteotomy-stabilization of the premaxilla in bilateral clefts. Jour Cranio-Maxillofacial Surg, January 1991;19(1):2-6.

Shaw, WC and Semb, G: Current approaches to the orthodontic management of cleft lip and palate. Jour of Royal Soc of Med, January 1990;83(1):30-33.

Vig, KWL and Turvey, T: Orthodontic-surgical interaction in the management of cleft lip and palate. Clin in Plast Surg 1985;12(4).

Vig, KW, Fonseca, RJ and Turvey, TA: Bone grafting of the cleft maxilla. In Bardach, J and Morris, HL: Multidisciplinary Management of Cleft Lip and Palate. Philadelphia, WB Saunders, 1990:543.

Aduss, H and Figueroa, A: Stages of orthodontic treatment in complete unilateral cleft lip and palate. In Bardach, J and Morris, HL (eds.): Multidisciplinary Management of Cleft Lip and Palate. Philadelphia, WB Saunders, 1990: pp 607

Ilizarov, GA: The Transosseous Osteosynthesis: Theoretical and Clinical Aspects of the Regeneration and Growth of Tissue. New York, Springer-Verlag; 1992

McCarthy, JG: Distraction of the Craniofacial Skeleton. New York, Springer-Verlag; 1999

Polley, JW, Figueroa, AA: Management of severe maxillary deficiency in childhood and adolescence through distraction osteogenesis with an external, adjustable, rigid distraction device. J Craniofac Surg, May 1997;8(3):181-186

The Patient with Hemifacial Microsomia

Calvert, M: Considerations in the management of craniofacial microsomia. Dental Update, March 1988;15(2):58-66.

Linder-Aronson, S: Early interceptive treatment of asymmetry. Proc Finn Dent Soc 1991;87(1):159-166.

Munro, IR: Treatment of craniofacial microsomia. Clin in Plast Surg, January 1987;14(1):177-186.

Poole, MD: Hemifacial microsomia. World Jour of Surg, July/Aug 1989;13(4):396-400.

Stricker, M, Van der Meulen, JC, Raphael, R and Mazzola, R: Craniofacial Malformations. New York, Churchill Livingstone, 1990.

Kaban, L, Moses, M and Mulliken, J: Surgical correction of hemifacial microsomia in the growing child. Plast and Recon Surg, July 1988; 82(1):9-19.

Mulliken, JB and Kaban, LB: Analysis and treatment of hemifacial microsomia in childhood. Clin in Plast Surg, January, 1987;14(1): 91-100.

Padwa, BL, Evans, CA and Pillemer, FC: Psychosocial adjustment in children with hemifacial microsomia and other craniofacial deformities. Cleft Pal/Cranio J, 1991;28(4)354.

Harvold, EP: The theoretical basis for the treatment of hemifacial microsomia. In: Harvold, EP, Vargervik, K and Chierici, G (eds.): Treatment of Hemifacial Microsomia. New York, Alan R. Liss, 1983:p. 1-37.

Marsh, JL, Baca, D and Vannier, MW: Facial musculoskeletal asymmetry in hemifacial microsomia. Cleft Pal J, 1989;26(4): 292.

Farias, M and Vargervik, K: Dental development in hemifacial microsomia. I. Eruption and agenesis. Ped Dent, June 1988;10(2): 140-143.

Sigal, MJ and Levine, N: Facial swelling and asymmetry in children: Systematic diagnosis and review. Canadian Dent Assoc J, October 1989;55(10):799-805.

Goldsmith, D, Sharzer, L and Merkman, M: Microvascular groin flaps in the treatment of hemifacial microsomia. Cleft Pal/Cranio J, January 1992; 29(1):44-71.

Poole, MD: Hemifacial microsomia. World Jour of Surg, July/August 1989; 13(4):396-400.

McCarthy, JG, Schreiber, J, Karp, N: Lengthening the human mandible by gradual distraction. Plast Recon Surg, January 1992; 89(1):1-10.

Molina, F, Ortiz Monasterio, F: Mandibular elongation and remodeling by distraction: a farewell to major osteotomies. Plast Recon Surg, September 1995;96(4):825-842.

Williamson, EH and Varela, J: Correction of mandibular asymmetry with the ligated anterior repositioning splint. Jour of Craniomand Prac, January 1990;8(1):30-34.

The Patient with Crouzon's or Apert's Syndromes

Bu, B, Kaban, LB and Vargervik, K: Effect of LeFort III osteotomy on mandibular growth in patients with Crouzon and Apert syndromes. Jour Oral and Max Surg, July 1989;47(7):666-671.

Jacobson R, Sarver DM. The predictability of maxillary repositioning in LeFort I orthognathic surgery. Am J Orthod Dentofacial Orthop 2002;122:142-154.

Kaplan, LC: Clinical assessment and multispecialty management of Apert Syndrome. Clinics in Plastic Surg, April 1991;18(2):217-225.

Kreiborg, S: Postnatal growth and development of the craniofacial complex in premature craniosynostosis. In Cohen, NM Jr (ed.): Craniosynostosis. Diagnosis, Evaluation and Management. New York, Raven Press, 1986: pp 157.

Stricker, M, Van der Meulen, JC, Raphael, R and Mazzola, R: Craniofacial Malformations. New York, Churchill Livingstone, 1990.

Cohen, MM Jr: Syndromes with craniosynostosis. In Cohen, MM Jr (ed.): Craniosynostosis. Diagnosis, Evaluation and Management. New York, Raven Press, 1986: pp 413.

Ferraro, NF: Dental, orthodontic and oral/maxillofacial evaluation and treatment in Apert Syndrome. Clin in Plast Surg, April 1991; 18(2): pp 291-307.

Kolar, JC, Munro, IR and Farkas, LG: Patterns of dysmorphology in Crouzon syndrome: an anthropometric study. Cleft pal J, 1988; 25(3):235.

Campis, LB: Children with Apert Syndrome: Developmental and psychologic considerations. Clin in Plast Surg, April 1991; 18(2): 409-416.

Sidhu, SS and Deshmukh, RN: Oro-dental anomalies in Apert's Syndrome. Indian Ped, May 1989; 26(5):501-504.

Tessier, P: Craniofacial surgery in syndromic craniosynostosis. In Cohen, MM Jr (ed.): Craniosynostosis. Diagnosis, Evaluation and Management. New York, Raven Press, 1986: pp 321.

McCarthy, JG, LaTrenta, GS, Breitbart, AS, Grayson, BH and Bookstein, FL: The LeFort III advancement osteotomy in the child under 7 years of age. Plast and Recon Surg, October 1990; 86(4): pp 633-646.

Mulliken, JB and Bruneteau, RJ: Surgical correction of the craniofacial anomalies in Apert Syndrome. Clin Plast Surg, April 1991; 18(2): pp 277-289.

Whitaker, LA and Bartlett, SP: The craniofacial dysostoses: Guidelines for management of the symmetric and asymmetric deformities. Clin Plast Surg, January 1987; 14(1): pp 73-81.

CHAPTER 21

Retention, Relapse and the Recurrence of Malocclusion

Manish Valiathan

Mark G. Hans

1. INTRODUCTION

Retention is the final phase of active orthodontic treatment where teeth are maintained in a healthy, functional, and esthetic position. The method of retention to be employed is best considered at the outset of treatment and incorporated in the treatment plan for each individual case. Successful resolution of malocclusion is based on a careful and accurate diagnosis and a treatment plan that addresses the etiology of the condition. Planning the regimen of retention to be employed should be based on the same principles. A lack of mention of retention may contribute in the loss of functional and esthetic improvements gained through years of effort by the clinician and patient. However,

minor changes generally occur as a result of physiologic maturational changes. In fact, such developmental changes occur regardless of orthodontic treatment and should be communicated to prospective patients. Major unacceptable changes following orthodontic treatment are "true" relapse.

The need for retention arises for several reasons, of which two biologic factors deserve special mention. First, during active tooth movement the **lamina dura** surrounding each tooth remodels to allow tooth movement to occur. During the first three months of the retention period the lamina dura is reformed. Second, retention is needed to counteract the inherent tendency of the aligned teeth to return to their original positions in the arch. The causes of this inherent tendency and methods to minimize the recurrence of the malocclusion have been issues of considerable clinical and investigative interest during the last century.

Expectedly, several viewpoints and philosophies have emerged. Kingsley and several subsequent investigators suggested that the final dental occlusion was the most important factor in determining the **stability** of the newly acquired dental position. Lundstrom focused on the importance of the **apical base** in maintenance of achieved occlusion, while Tweed suggested that uprighting the mandibular incisors over **basal bone** enhances stability. Rogers introduced the consideration of muscular balance as a factor in preventing **relapse** that found favor with many investigators. Branes stressed the importance of placing the dentition in excellent occlusion and retaining the teeth until the perioral musculature adapted to the new dental positions. If adequate time for adaptation were not allowed post-retention failure would result. Enlow defined relapse as " a histogenetic and morphogenetic response to some anatomical and functional violation of an existing state of anatomic and functional balance." Enlow does not accept the idea that **relapse** results from the mechanical recoil reaction of the periodontal membrane to forces it is subjected to, since the periodontal fibers have tremendous ability to remodel and accommodate virtually any tooth position if a regional state of anatomic and physiologic balance exists. Although all of these theories have merit, a comprehensive biologic understanding of relapse remains elusive. This is largely because the underlying causes of malocclusion are poorly understood. Therefore, this chapter relies on the "best available" clinical and scientific evidence to support the use of various retention strategies.

2. GENERAL FACTORS AFFECTING STABILITY

Among the many suggested factors mentioned that influence stability, three deserve further elaboration:
    1.) the involvement of the periodontal ligament fibers and gingival fibers
    2.) late mandibular growth, and
    3.) physiologic imbalance of local extrinsic forces acting on the corrected dentition.

The role of the periodontal ligament (PDL) as a "shock absorber" in occlusion is well established. Widening of the periodontal ligament space, disruption of the **collagen fiber** bundles that support each tooth, remodeling of **alveolar bone** and loss of the lamina dura are normal and required responses to orthodontic treatment. Following orthodontic treatment, restoration and reorganization of the arrangement of the PDL fibers and calcification of the lamina dura takes three to four months. Although some reorganization of the periodontal ligament would occur if teeth were attached to a passive archwire, reorganization is more effective and efficient after appliance removal. In addition to improved oral hygiene, retainers allow individual tooth response to occlusal forces and movement within their sockets relative to the rest of the dentition. The mild mobility present at the end of treatment disappears as reorganization of the supporting structures progresses. The reorganized PDL plays a part in the stability of individual dental units within the arches by contributing to the delicate balance of forces acting on the dentition to maintain equilibrium and hence a stable position. During the first three months of retention, unorganized gingival and PDL fibers lead to an increased susceptibility to tooth movement.

The gingival fibers are comprised of collagenous and elastic fibers. Chavrier, et al., and other investigators have demonstrated the dominant concentration of Type I collagen in gingiva (90%) and the lower levels of collagen type IV, V VI and VIII. These bundles of proteins provide strength and rigidity to the tissue. It appears that while having a high turnover rate, a physiological characteristic of tissues associated with high functional burdens, groups of collagen may be under common regulatory mechanisms. Based on the origins and insertions of these fibers, the dentogingival fibers and transseptal fibers are considered the most important. Yet the elasticity (a physical property related to relapse) of these fibers is very limited. The elastic fibers of the gingiva form about 6% of the total human gingival protein and provide the elastic properties of the tissue needed to adapt to pressure. The network of elastic fibers are composed of 1.) elastic fibers, the most important component in the elastic system, composed of the protein elastin and a glycoprotein at the periphery of the amorphous elastin protein 2.) elaunin, made of less mature elastin and 3.) oxytalan, a collection of microfibrils devoid of any elastic properties.

The structural integrity of the gingiva, which may play an important role in the tendency for relapse, is maintained by a family of extracellular proteoglycans such as chondroitinsulfate, dermatansulfate and heparansulphate that have a central core protein covalently bonded to a glycosaminoglycan (GAG). The currently identified glycoproteins of the gingiva, fibronectin, laminin and osteonectin, play important roles in cell **differentiation** and wound healing beside other functions. A better understanding of the ultrastructure of gingiva, coupled with the clinical observations of changes in gingival tissue during orthodontic treatment, has led to several histological studies. Epithelial hyperplasia is observed in extraction sites where teeth have been approximated and significant increases are observed in oxytylan and GAG levels.

Mechanical force systems studied on gingival **fibroblasts** *in vitro* have demonstrated an increase in the expression of the collagen type I gene and a decrease in the collagenase gene. Similarly, tension is known to alter the human skin and dermal fibroblast phenotype, the mRNA levels of procollagen, elastin levels and collagen concentration. Although similar metabolic changes that occur in gingival tissues as a result of mechanical forces are being vigorously investigated, whether the metabolic activity of the gingival tissues is normalized following force removal in unknown at the present time. What appears known is that collagenous fibers reorganize structurally in a four to six month period. However, the supracrestal elastic fibers of the gingiva take up to a year to structurally adapt to the new position of the teeth and recapture its ability to contribute to the stability of the dentition.

Studies on attempts to enhance retention by surgically sectioning the elastic supracrestal fibers surrounding severe rotations at the time of appliance removal has led to inconclusive results. Riedel found 19% of fibrotomized teeth rotating away from their original position. Edwards demonstrated the efficacy of this surgical procedure in the maxillary anterior segment rather than the more troublesome mandibular anterior region. He reported the procedure to be most effective in alleviating relapse during the first four to six years of post orthodontic retention. Edwards also demonstrated that dental rotational relapse was accompanied by the gingiva being relocated to its original pretreatment position. This finding led to the **hypothesis** that collagen fibers, the main structural component of the extra cellular matrix of gingiva, may be responsible for rotational relapse.

More recent studies by Redlich and colleagues have used Scanning Electron Microscopic (SEM) and Transmission Electron Microscopic (TEM) analyses on dogs to investigate the merits of supra crestal fibrotomies on the relapse of orthodontically treated teeth. These studies indicate that rotational relapse may not be due to stretched collagen bundles as might be indicated by their appearance under the light microscope. Instead, the ultra-structural data indicated that rotational relapse might be caused by the elastic fibers of the gingival tissue.

Growth is perhaps the orthodontist's best ally in several situations. However, while attempting to prevent relapse this is not always true. Retention of treated malocclusions that result from a pattern of skeletal growth are particularly challenging to the clinician. Skeletal growth patterns in all three planes of space tend to recur as growth continues. As transverse growth is "completed" first, long term transverse changes should be more stable than changes in the antero-posterior and vertical planes. However, relapse is likely in cases where significant arch expansion has occurred. Unfortunately, the amount of expansion that can be tolerated and retained by individual patients has not been determined. Continued growth patterns that contribute to a Class II, Class III, deep bite, or open bite are major causes for the recurrence of malocclusion. It is, therefore, important in children and adolescents to continue retention at least until growth levels have reduced to those observed in adult life. Rolf Behrents' studies at the Bolton Brush Growth Study Center have clearly demonstrated that remodeling of the craniofacial skeletal and soft tissue structures continues into adult life, leading to changes in dental alignment.

Forces acting on the dentition include those generated from occlusion, the tongue and cheek musculature, the gingival fibers and the fibers of the PDL. It is important to remember that the forces produced in orthodontic therapy necessarily require them to be greater than these naturally occurring forces. This means that orthodontists can move teeth into unstable positions within the oral cavity. Once the artificial orthodontic forces have been discontinued the naturally occurring forces, such as soft tissue pressures, remain and can lead to relapse, and may often be referred to as the "**rebound effect**."

Summary

Our poor understanding of the biologic factors that determine tooth position in the arch is the chief reason even the most diligent orthodontist cannot predictably achieve harmonious balance among the extrinsic forces acting on aligned dentition for a patient's lifetime. The prudent practitioner will therefore usually recommend that patients continue to wear retainers at night as long as the patient desires the teeth to be in ideal alignment. This has resulted in the full time **retention** period being followed by the limited use of removable appliances (one night per week) over a period of ten years or more by clinicians. In other words, the retention of teeth in their ideal positions within the arch should be considered a lifetime project.

3. RETENTION OF ANTERIOR-POSTERIOR CORRECTIONS

3.1 RETENTION OF CLASS II CORRECTIONS

Correction of Class II malocclusions results from differential jaw growth and may be accomplished using headgears, Class II elastics or functional appliances such as bionators, twin blocks and Herbst appliances, to name a few. **Headgear anchorage** is capable of influencing the normal downward and forward displacement of the maxilla. The dental effects of extraoral traction on the maxilla are the inhibition of mesial movement of the maxillary buccal segments, possible **extrusion** and distal tipping along with some bodily distal movement, while the mandible continues with its normal growth that may eventually result in a Class I occlusion. It is undesirable to leave the maxillary buccal segments distally tipped, as they tend to upright immediately following appliance removal.

Differential jaw growth of the maxilla and mandible causes the slower long-term relapse. The amount of growth remaining is a function of the age, gender and skeletal maturity of the patient. Altered jaw positions resulting from differential jaw growth contribute to the repositioning of the teeth. Instances where headgear and functional appliances have been utilized tend to demonstrate rebound growth accentuating the tendency toward deleterious differential growth. The tendency towards relapse may be curbed by continued headgear wear on a reduced basis (at night) in tandem with retainers that maintain dental corrections obtained. Although a retention strategy advocated to work, it does require substantial patient cooperation and motivation. Another method of retention is the use of a functional appliance such as an **activator**-bionator that essentially achieves the same results. As at the end of treatment, the patient has an ideal overjet. Construction bites for such appliances are taken without advancement of the mandible (Figures 21-1A-F illustrate correction of a Class II malocclusion treated with a twin block appliance, and Figures 21-2A-E illustrate the retention appliance for the same patient). The appliance is used only at night, and conventional retainers designed to maintain the dental corrections are used during the day. Although this may appear cumbersome to both clinician and patient, it is wise to remain guarded in patients who initially demonstrated severe skeletal problems.

Class II traction mechanics are necessary to correct Class II malocclusions. However, in the absence of a mandibular growth response, Class II elastics or functional appliances move the lower denture mesially to correct the malocclusion. Mesial movement causes **proclination** of the incisors. If this forward movement of the lower incisors alters the equilibrium between the lip musculature and tongue, post treatment relapse will occur. Following appliance removal lip pressure will upright the lower anteriors, causing lower anterior crowding and an increase in overjet.

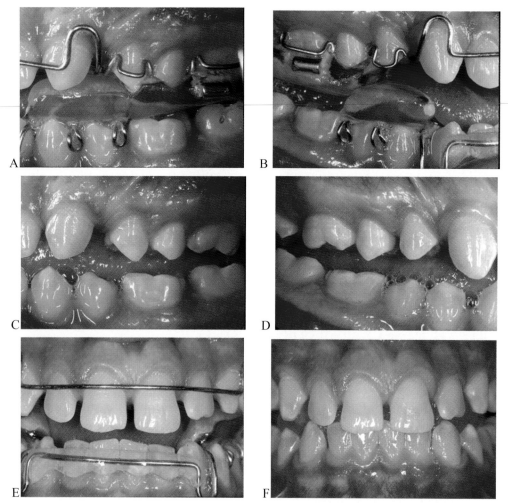

Figure 21-1 A-F: Retention of Early Class II Correction: A.) and B.) Twin block therapy in progress for a Class II malocclusion. C.) and D.) Post-Twin block treatment with the anticipated posterior open bite in a cooperative patient. E.) and F.) Frontal views of the patient with appliances in place and following phase I.

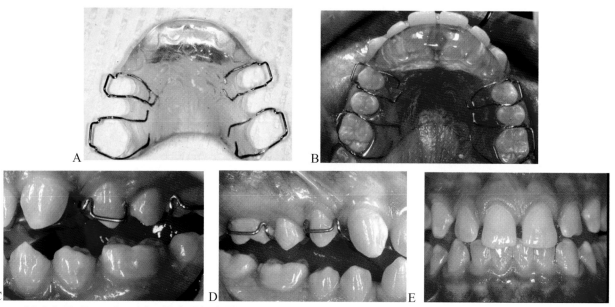

Figure 21-2 A-E: Retention After Twin Block Therapy. A.) and B.): Retention device following twin block therapy designed to hold the mandible in a forward posture. Note the indentations of the lower anteriors on the anterior palatal ramp of the retainer. C.) and D.) Retainer in place secured by Adams clasps on the first molars and first bicuspids. E.) Frontal view with the retainer in place. Note the non-coinciding midlines were not addressed in Phase I as it was caused by a dental asymmetry and not a skeletal asymmetry.

The big question for clinicians is "How much might the lower incisors be proclined and retained successfully?" As a general guideline, the cephalometric position of the labial surface of the lower incisor should not be increased during treatment. The exception to this guideline occurs in Class II division 2 malocclusions, where advancement of the retroclined lower incisors has been shown to be stable by Little, et al. However, this diagnostic and eventual biomechanical decision should be based on a careful assessment of the initial position of the lower incisors relative to the mandibular basal bone and the interincisor relationship.

3.2 RETENTION OF CLASS III CORRECTIONS

Adult cases presenting with a true Class III malocclusion caused by maxillary hypoplasia, mandibular prognathia or a combination of the two often require surgical correction of the skeletal **dysmorphogenesis** to obtain good facial esthetics and dental occlusion. In children, early correction of the skeletal imbalance is undertaken using functional appliances that aim to rearrange the skeletal components contributing to the malocclusion. Corrections should be obtained by alterations in the basal bones rather than the dentoalveolar segments. Cases corrected early by the use of palatal expanders and custom-made protraction headgears can be effective in the correction of mesio-occlusions with maxillary deficiency. Since Class III malocclusions often exhibit an increased incidence of maxillary transverse deficiency, McNamara and Turley recommend maxillary expansion prior to maxillary protraction.

Clinical evidence points to successful management in children treated between six and nine years of age, with patient cooperation being the most critical factor. Although a review of the literature indicates success with a maxillary protraction appliance, much uncertainty surrounds the long-term effectiveness and stability in the early intervention of Class III malocclusions. Following protraction of the maxilla, retention remains vital to maintain the effects of treatment. Petit discussed the use of a Frankel III appliance for retention following maxillary advancement with functional appliances. In a study designed to evaluate the effectiveness of maxillary protraction and the use of a Frankel III appliance for retention of post-protraction changes, Kulbersh, et al., concluded that Frankel III devices are an effective method to maintain the post-protraction, downward and forward position of maxilla. In fact, their findings indicate that there continues to be a positive change with the use of such a retention technique. The findings of Kulbersh, et al., corroborate the findings of McNamara, who reported an increase in lower anterior facial height along with forward repositioning of the maxilla in cases treated with a Frankel Class III. Turley recommends the overcorrection of the malocclusion until an overjet of 5mm is obtained, followed by three to six months of nighttime protraction facemask or Class III bionator use to minimize relapse. Turley also suggests that, depending on the amount of overcorrection and the relative amount of mandibular protrusion, additional retainer use may be warranted. However, no parameters or guidelines have been suggested to determine the regimen of retention to be used or their relative strengths and effectiveness.

Continued mandibular growth in cases of true Class III malocclusions is extremely difficult to control. The Class III malocclusion is often known to relapse due to continued mandibular growth. This has led many orthodontists to recommend treatment by surgical means after cessation of active growth. Application of a restraining force to the mandible (in the chin area) by means of a chin cup tends to rotate the mandible in a downward and backward direction, increasing the vertical height of the face. Class III functional appliances have been used with similar results. Mild Class III malocclusions corrected by orthodontic tooth movement may be retained by the use of a positioner.

4. RETENTION OF VERTICAL CORRECTIONS

4.1 RETENTION AFTER DEEP BITE CORRECTIONS

Deep bites are common traits in a variety of malocclusions and craniofacial patterns and are caused by the overeruption of the maxillary incisors, mandibular incisors or both. As emphasized earlier, careful diagnosis of the malocclusion is required to obtain ideal functional and esthetic results. Although the exact reason for overeruption of the incisors and the ensuing deep bites are not completely understood, maintenance of overbite appears related, in part, to establishing adequate torque or axial inclination of the incisors. When cases are finished with an upright interincisor relationship, as often observed in the extraction cases following space closure, they have a tendency to overerupt following active treatment. As the deep bite recurs, the lower incisal edges are in contact with the thicker palatal-cervical area of the maxillary incisors. This in turn results in lower incisor crowding or, more seldom, upper incisor spacing. It is not easy to achieve these levels of torque, which at best may be attained in an inordinate amount of time. As mentioned, inadequate torque would result in deepening of the bite and subsequent lower incisor crowding. The normal vertical facial growth pattern that occurs with age may contribute to the instability of vertical corrections. Studies on deep bites, commonly observed in Class II division 2 malocclusions, have demonstrated that the upright pretreatment maxillary and mandibular incisor positions tend to return to their original relationship. The works of Kim Tae-Woo and Canut confirm that the initial overbite is positively related to the post retention overbite. Although Riedel talked about overcorrection of the initial overbite to prevent vertical relapse, it does not appear that such a simple corrective measure can withstand the complex process of adult remodeling and growth that appears to be a major contributor in the relapse of overbites.

Retention of overbite correction can be accomplished by the use of a maxillary removable retainer with a built in anterior bite plane (Figure 21-3). This retainer design allows the lower incisor edges to contact acrylic if the bite begins to deepen. The appliance should be not be designed to actively disclude the posterior teeth.

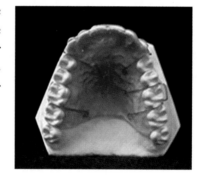

Figure 21-3: Modified maxillary Hawley retainer with an anterior bite plane for retention of a corrected overbite. Note the C clasp on the right and Adams clasp on the left.

4.2 RETENTION AFTER **ANTERIOR OPEN BITE** CORRECTIONS

In children and adolescents with acceptable facial balance, **anterior open bite**s are usually associated with active habits, such as digit sucking, that are frequently accompanied by a compensatory **tongue thrust**. In such cases, treatment and retention appliances should be designed to eliminate the habit and continually discourage the behavior from recurring (Figure 21-4). In severe cases of mouth breathing that contribute to an open mouth posture, further evaluation for partial nasal obstruction may be beneficial. An open mouth posture caused by mouth breathing or habits results in further elongation of the posterior teeth, particularly the upper molars, and leads to an increase in the lower anterior facial height. Open bites may also be caused by the depression of the anterior dentition caused by the presence of a physical barrier (a finger, etc.). Early correction of the condition is highly beneficial. The etiology of the open bite must be accurately diagnosed and treated if relapse of the potentially difficult malocclusion is to be controlled. Although the tongue habit was considered a principle etiologic factor in open bites, evidence to support this contention is inadequate. If the etiology of the open bite can be addressed and treated early, retention of the correction is possible. However, if the underlying case of the open bite is not corrected (as in a vertical growth pattern) the condition is likely to return. Correction of some open bites may be better addressed surgically in the late teens or early twenties.

One effective method of retaining an overbite correction is to use a high pull **headgear** to the upper molar area (to control the vertical) in conjunction with a removable retainer to maintain tooth position. Alternately, the use of a retainer with a posterior bite block maintains an intrusive force on the maxillary and mandibular posterior dentition, preventing further eruption and increase of the vertical dimension (Figure 21-5). The posterior bite blocks should be thick enough to impinge on the interocclusal **freeway space** and stretch the musculature. This will provide a masticatory force capable of opposing eruption. Variations in thickness of the bite blocks, varied designs with springs and magnets incorporated in them, and open bite bionators have all been used to prevent relapse of **anterior open bite** malocclusions. Retention of open bites present problems, as vertical growth continues into the late teens. As part of the long-term retention regimen, conventional retainers in the day with specially designed appliances (bite blocks or an open bite bionator) for nighttime wear are beneficial. The use of anterior labial or lingual elastics as a treatment and/or retention method must be adopted with caution, as the elongation of the dentition that occurs may be undesirable and unaesthetic.

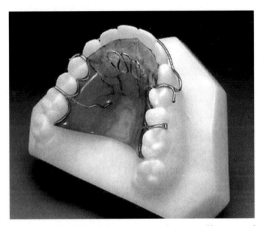

Figure 21-4: Modified upper Hawley appliance with ball clasps and an anterior tongue crib to prevent a tongue thrust habit from recurring.

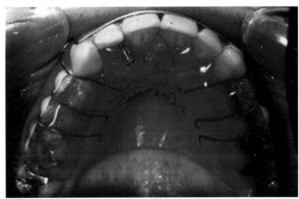

Figure 21-5: Modified upper Hawley retainer with a posterior bite block for retention of a corrected anterior open bite. Note the spring incorporated for correction of the lateral incisor rotation.

5. RETENTION OF **ARCH FORM** AND ARCH ALIGNMENT

The long-term outcome of orthodontic treatment is often measured by recording linear measurements from study casts. Study models may be compared from the commencement of treatment to the final result to the post-retention stage. Inter-arch measurements commonly recorded are the overjet, overbite, Angle's molar classification and anterior and posterior cross bites. Intra-arch measurements used are inter-molar width, inter-canine width, and, less frequently, inter-premolar width. Another method commonly adopted in recent years to evaluate the need for treatment, outcome of orthodontic treatment, and stability of orthodontic intervention has been the use of several different occlusal indices. While the **irregularity index** of Little assesses the labiolingual displacements of the six anterior teeth, the PAR (Peer Assessment Rating) index primarily deals with outcome assessments and takes into account maxillary anterior alignment, overjet, overbite, buccal occlusion and midline discrepancies. Indices are useful in assessment of the improvement in occlusion as a consequence of orthodontic treatment and may be used to evaluate stability over time. However, indices do suffer from inherent shortcomings.

The literature indicates that changes in arch form are critical in the long-term stability of treated cases. While the inter-canine and inter-molar widths may represent a position of muscular balance for the patient, the inter-premolar widths appear to be more amenable to change. Recent results from BeGole, et al., have reaffirmed and supported the **hypothesis** of Gardner and Chaconas from the 1970's, that expansion gained in the premolar regions of both arches are likely to be stable.

Long-term studies from the University of Washington and Saint Louis University (SLU) provide some of the best available data on stability of orthodontic treatment. Following extensive and continuous research over forty years focused on assessing stability and relapse in populations including premolar extractions, mandibular incisor extractions, non-extraction groups, expansion and non-expansion therapies and untreated samples, Little, et al., at the University of Washington have concluded that long-term alignment is highly variable and unpredictable. Both **arch length** and width tend to decrease with age leading to increases in dental crowding. Mandibular anterior alignment is the most likely region to demonstrate relapse. Less than 30% of the University of Washington cases showed good lower anterior stability, and nearly twenty percent demonstrated marked crowding several years after discontinuing retention.

The results from SLU and others are more encouraging. Cases included in these studies respected the initial **intercanine width** in the lower arch. In most studies, the intercuspid width has been found to decrease from post-treatment to post-retention. Post treatment relapse in this dimension is proportional to the amount of expansion during treatment. Gorman, in an interesting study, found that nearly 60% of the cases from the Seattle sample had undergone mandibular intercanine expansion of more than a millimeter. In a comparison of the Sandusky data to the Seattle material, Gorman found superior stability in the former sample. The Sandusky extraction sample was chosen from excellent finishes of Tweed and Merrifield's cases and included 85 finished cases. He concluded that 90% of the time acceptable results were maintained 10-15 years out of retention. It appears that the more desirable long term results may have been due, at least in part, to minimal **intercanine width** increase, complete correction of rotations and a longer retention period. Encouragingly, recent independent long-term follow up investigations have yielded more optimistic results than the Seattle material. It is noteworthy that in these studies, lower intercuspid width was maintained during treatment.

It also appears that changes in the original mandibular arch form tend to cause increased amounts of relapse. Several well-designed studies indicate that maintaining the original mandibular arch form is essential for long-term stability. In a long-term computer assisted study on the shape stability of the mandibular arch using thirty Class I, thirty Class II nonextraction cases and thirty untreated normal cases as controls, Felton and colleagues demonstrated that changes in the mandibular arch form are frequently unstable following nonextraction treatment. The investigators monitored the cases during treatment, during four years of retention and seven to nine years following retention. Nearly 70% of the cases evidenced significant relapse towards the original arch form. Given the tremendous variation in arch forms among individuals, and that prefabricated wires are useful only in 50% of the cases, it would follow that the use of prefabricated arch wires may not be beneficial to long-term stability and should be customized to the individual arch of the patient. Similarly, Franklin found satisfactory long-term results (12 years post retention) in the study of a 114 cases treated by the same clinician and concluded that maintenance of mandibular arch form and sound treatment principles contributed to the success in retention.

Some factors leading to relapse are under operator control. For example, incomplete corrections of all rotations in the original malocclusion predispose the case to relapse. This may be observed in cases from the sample of the University of Washington and in many treated cases of orthodontists. Only careful clinical examination and comparison of the models prior to debonding the case to the initial models detect these fine details. During the process of maturation of untreated occlusions, noticeable mandibular incisor crowding is observed during adolescence and young adulthood. Increased areas of crowding tend to be located primarily in areas of broken contact in both treated and untreated cases. Could slightly broken contact areas in both treated and untreated cases be the starting points for crowding to occur? It certainly would behoove clinicians to achieve complete correction of all rotations and reestablish contact areas by fabricating individualized **arch wires**. There is no evidence to support the claim that overcorrection of rotations during orthodontic treatment improves stability. Given the instability of a contact point and the potential for relapse, modest reshaping of the incisors while maintaining good anatomical contour is an accepted method to enhance stability.

Dugoni and colleagues recently demonstrated improved stability of the mandibular incisor region in nineteen of twenty-five cases treated in the early mixed dentition. The positive results may be indicative of the stage of development of the transseptal fibers. Kusters and colleagues have demonstrated that the transseptal fibers do not develop until the cementoenamel junctions of erupting teeth pass the bony border of the alveolar process. The derotation of teeth just after their emergence into the oral cavity implies correction before the transseptal fiber arrangement has been established. As the corrected teeth continue to erupt a more favorable arrangement of the transseptal fibers can develop. Could these findings be suggestive of the sequential removal of teeth, otherwise known as serial extractions, being beneficial from a standpoint of long-term stability?

Although minimal data exists on **serial extraction** cases that were not followed by comprehensive orthodontic treatment, Little, et al., demonstrated in a sample of fifty cases that did not have orthodontic treatment following serial extractions that at the ten year post-retention mark, the sample was more stable than premolar extraction cases treated with conventional appliances. Although different measurements were used, results reported by Persson, et al., found no significant differences between a group of patients where serial extractions were the sole treatment rendered and a group of untreated individuals with "normal occlusion". Both groups were evaluated thirty years following treatment and demonstrated a tendency to redevelop rotations and crowding. In a carefully designed and conducted study, Woodside, et al., chose twenty-two patients from the Burlington Growth Center who had undergone serial extractions of four premolars with no subsequent major orthodontic **mechanotherapy** for comparison with a matched, untreated, non-extraction sample. The pairs were matched for age, gender, facial height, skeletal balance between the maxilla and mandible and incisor irregularity. The authors concluded that post-retention crowding and mandibular incisor irregularity were independent of serial extraction treatment, and noted that it occurred to the same extent as the untreated, non-extraction sample.

6. EFFECTS OF EXTRACTION AND NON-EXTRACTION TREATMENT ON ARCH STABILITY

One of the both historic and contemporary debates in orthodontics has centered on the decision to extract permanent teeth in an effort to gain space, usually for the alignment of crowded teeth, retraction of anterior teeth and facial profile enhancement or to resolve a Bolton tooth size discrepancy. In the early period of the 1900's Calvin S. Case opposed Edward H. Angle, a champion of non-extraction therapy who believed that orthodontic appliances could enhance bone formation, that extraction procedures never overcame faulty muscular function and, therefore, orthodontic treatment should set out to remove the underlying cause of malocclusion while retaining a full complement of teeth. It was not until the development of gnathostatic evaluation of dental occlusion and the simultaneous introduction of **cephalometrics** by Broadbent that the shortcomings of a dominant non-extraction treatment could be evaluated. Tweed, one of Angle's staunch supporters and students, was so disillusioned at one point by post-treatment relapse that he strongly reflected on quitting his profession as an orthodontist. Out of

70% of all cases he had treated over a six and half year time period, during which time he followed the non-extraction philosophy, all but 20% of them had relapsed.

In a historic study that compared 100 extraction and 100 non-extraction cases examined twenty-five years post-retention, Tweed concluded that extraction cases were more stable. Innumerable studies have been published in an effort to understand the preferable course of treatment: extraction or non-extraction. As Brodie demonstrated, following a fanatical non-extraction philosophy in the belief that any substantial bone growth may be induced in tooth-bearing bones by tooth-borne appliances is undesirable. Brodie also provided vital evidence that once facial bone growth patterns are established, whether deemed desirable or otherwise, they cannot be altered, as they remain virtually constant and resistant to change. The answer is not to follow an extraction-based philosophy but to incorporate the principals of both, extraction and non-extraction treatment, to arrive at a carefully determined accurate treatment plan for individual patients. Conlin demonstrated in a study based on a large sample recalled for evaluation of long-term stability and facial esthetics that it is not necessary for extraction cases to lead to "dished-in profiles" or for non-extraction cases to create full faces. Notably, the great challenge to orthodontists is the need to make a sound diagnosis and an appropriate treatment plan that, when executed, results in superior stability. Just as no single treatment philosophy fits all patients and treatment plans need to be individualized, so do retention strategies that take into account the initial malocclusion.

In cases where extractions are required, a variety of extraction patterns have been adopted and documented, from lower incisor extractions and premolar extractions, to the removal of first or second molars. Proffit has advocated that premolar extractions limit the amount of lower anterior crowding and relapse following orthodontic treatment and assists in improved lip contours. While the latter claim has been disputed, it appears that irrespective of whether extractions are part of the treatment plan or not, relapse of an overbite as well as lower incisor crowding occurs following appliance removal. Little, et al., evaluating the mandibular anterior alignment in a sample of sixty-five patients treated with conventional edgewise appliances following the extraction of four first premolars, demonstrated that ten years post-retention only 30% of the premolar extraction therapy group retained good mandibular anterior alignment, while the rest of the sample demonstrated moderate to severe relapse. Although patients demonstrated a net improvement from the initial levels of crowding to the post-retention phase, Little concluded that the post-retention irregularity was unacceptable. Additionally, **arch width** changes established during treatment and post-retention arch length decrease correlated poorly with the amount of post-retention irregularity. The authors concluded that no single parameter such as gender, age, Angle classification, duration of retention or measurements made from study casts served as reliable indicators of future stability.

The sample examined, however, had a large age range (from 7 years to 18 years) and, although the sample was divided based on the Angle molar classification of malocclusion, the differences in skeletal morphology between patients was not accounted for. As Little pointed out, an additional flaw was the use of removable mandibular retainers that led to variable wear.

To further investigate and identify associations between long-term dental and skeletal changes in premolar extraction cases, Shields, et al., conducted a cephalometric study on fifty-four premolar extraction patients ten years out of retention. They reported that neither post-treatment and post-retention incisor positions nor specific cephalometric parameters were good indicators of incisor stability. Associations between cephalometric values and dental cast measurements were of limited value. The premolar extraction sample of Little was also compared to untreated normals by Sinclair and post-retention non-extraction cases by Glenn, et al. The post-retention irregularity observed in the extraction group was an astounding four times the untreated control group and twice the amount reported in the non-extraction group.

In an attempt to study the differences between post-treatment changes in the extraction and non-extraction groups and to determine the relationship between these groups and lower incisor irregularity, Rossouw, et al., studied a random sample of 88 individuals consisting of 56% of non-extraction patients and 44% of extraction cases. Cephalometrics and study casts were used to assess treatment and post-treatment effects at three stages: initial, post-treatment and post-retention, in all three planes of space. Expectedly, significant differences were observed in the pre-treatment comparison of lower incisor irregularity, mandibular canine width, several of the occlusal variables such as overjet, molar as well as canine relations, and overbite. Additionally, there existed soft tissue differences at the commencement of treatment. At the final post-retentive observation, minimal and statistically insignificant differences were observed between the two groups with regard to lower incisor irregularity and most other measurements made. The authors concluded by stressing the importance of an accurate diagnosis and meticulous orthodontic care in order to achieve the best possible functional, esthetic and stable results.

Shapiro, in a study of 80 orthodontic patients (58 extraction and 22 non-extraction) observed an arch length decrease following the retention phase. This phenomenon was observed regardless of the extraction or non-extraction treatment choice made. Swanson, et al., attempted to find factors that may have been associated with rotational relapse observed. Variables analyzed included the gender, age, **Angle classification**, arch length changes and growth of the jaws. Although none of the factors mentioned were found associated with the rotational relapse observed, the amount of rotational correction undertaken during treatment was directly proportional to the rotational relapse noted. No associations were found between the rotational relapse observed and premolar extractions.

From the data available, it appears that mandibular incisor irregularities continue to increase well after cessation of active growth and varies tremendously. Such changes are not exclusive to orthodontically treated individuals, but presents in untreated controls as well. In modern day orthodontics there is a distinct tendency to pursue non-extraction therapy. In order to gain arch length, expansions of both arches, distalization of the posterior segments and mild to moderate flaring of the anterior teeth are commonly employed procedures. The argument simply stated is, do such mechanics provide patients with stable results or are extractions to gain space superior from the standpoint of long-term stability?

7. PALATAL EXPANSION AND STABILITY

Rapid palatal expansion (RPE) or rapid maxillary expansion (RME) is the current accepted treatment of choice in cases with skeletal transverse deficiencies. The treatment aims to widen the midpalatal suture by forcing a lateral shift of the two horizontal processes of the maxilla. In the first available report on palatal expansion undertaken, Angell addressed the need to retain the altered arch form by using a retainer. Studies since on the effects and long-term results of rapid palatal expansion have documented the tendency for relapse despite retention schedules employed. The amount of relapse occurring post-expansion has been a major area of investigation, with studies reporting a wide range from 30% to 90% relapse being suffered. The relapse of transverse deficiencies following treatment comprises skeletal as well as dental components. Dental units tipped laterally during expansion tend to rebound medially following appliance removal.

But how much of the expansion obtained is in fact dental and therefore prone to relapse (lateral tipping of the dentition) and how much is actual skeletal separation of the suture? How do we recognize (remember, the appropriate diagnosis of a clinical condition is a prerequisite for long-term stability) a skeletal transverse deficiency and measure the treatment outcome? Commonly used dental casts are not the best method for evaluation of skeletal discrepancies or treatment outcome for skeletal deficiencies. The presence or absence of posterior crossbites and measurements made from the dental landmarks on study casts (typically located on the occlusal surfaces of the posterior teeth) are at best indicators, but certainly are not concrete representations of skeletal discrepancies.

Ricketts advised the use of the postero-anterior cephalogram to distinguish between the width of the dental arches, the alveolar segments and the basal bones. A large number of clinicians use the postero-anterior radiographs primarily to detect skeletal asymmetries. Despite advanced imaging being available, the postero-anterior cephalogram remains the most readily available radiograph for identification of skeletal transverse discrepancies. In conjunction with Rocky Mountain, Ricketts developed an index for evaluation of transverse skeletal problems. The index is the observed maxillomandibular difference subtracted from the expected maxillomandibular difference. The observed maxillomandibular difference is calculated by subtracting the maxillary width (measured from the left and right intersections of the maxillary tuberosity and the zygomatic buttress) from the mandibular width (measured from the right and left **antegonial notches**). The value is then compared to the expected maxillomandibular difference that is established for different Caucasian age groups.   However, use of this method to diagnose, evaluate the need for maxillary expansion, and study the effects of expansion has not gained popularity because of the difficulty associated with reliably identifying landmarks on antero-posterior cephalograms, although this inherent shortcoming of cephalometrics is overlooked in our zeal to scrutinize lateral cephalograms.

Clinicians are known to significantly over-expand the maxilla in anticipation of the relapse known to occur (up to 50% of overcorrection). Krebs, in a study using metallic implants, demonstrated in young children that the forces required to induce skeletal expansion are less. He also reported and about 50% of the expansion obtained is skeletal with the remaining 50% was the result of dental tipping and alveolar bending. In adolescents, on the other hand, the investigator demonstrated 35% skeletal expansion and 65% dental tipping. Expansion is typically followed by a phase of retention, during which time filling in of immature bone in the widened suture takes place as a healing response while the tipped dental units revert back to their original positions.

Krebs suggested that the RPE results, being more stable in younger children, indicate that suture recovery, which is also age related, plays a major role in stability. Haas concluded that ossification of the sutural margins requires sixty to ninety days. Vardimon, et al., recently demonstrated in their investigations on the different retention requirements at diverse suture sites in cats that the anterior suture region requires a greater duration of retention than the intermolar region. The authors concluded that the clinical use of occlusal radiographs to determine the amount of retention required to complete mineralization is advisable, and that better retention may be achieved if the anterior region is retained twice the amount of time the posterior region is retained.

It appears that minimizing maxillary arch form alteration is important for stability. However, there are instances where the upper arch form has to be modified to coordinate it with the lower arch. An example of such a situation would be in a Class II division 1 malocclusion. The long-term consequences of such changes have revealed that rounding of the maxillary arch during treatment is prone to returning to the original tapered form following retention. The greater the treatment effect, the greater the post - retention changes observed. However, considerable individual variation has been noted. Maintaining modifications in the arch form are not easy to accomplish in the long run. Therefore, indiscriminate lateral expansion and tipping of the dentition in an effort to produce a full smile is fraught with the danger of relapse. Similarly, retention of incorrectly or inadequately diagnosed over-expanded maxillary arches has been shown to result in gingival recession and periodontal problems. This suggests that after expansion a period of physiologic rebound should be allowed to insure that arch width is not artificially maintained at unhealthy levels.

8. THIRD MOLARS AND RELAPSE

Post-pubertal late mandibular crowding in treated and untreated subjects is multifactorial in origin. It is imperative that the stability of orthodontic treatment be scrutinized against the backdrop of natural-ly occurring changes in untreated samples. Since John Hunter's demonstration that mesial migration of the dentition is a normal physiologic process, it is generally accepted that human dentition and occlusion are dynamic in nature and continually change during the course of life. Most obvious is the change in alignment of the lower arch, which may be crowded in the early mixed dentition, less so in the late mixed dentition, and then resorts to increased crowding after eruption of the second molars around the age of twelve. Since minimal skeletal growth occurs in the anterior portion of the mandible, the changes may be in part due to dentoalveolar alteration.

Richardson demonstrated that the lower incisors tend to procline approximately thirteen degrees rela-tive the **mandibular plane** between five and eleven years of age. Also, the increase in inter-canine width caused by dentoalveolar development prior to and during incisor eruption assists in space cre-ation and a transient alleviation of crowding in the mandibular anterior region. But what causes the crowding of the lower anterior region to become more pronounced with time? The role of the third molars has been extensively debated in this regard. Although some authors have attributed the presence of the third molars to decreased long-term mandibular stability, a larger volume of literature indicates little role of third molars in the long-term stability of lower incisor alignment.

Well-designed studies have failed to demonstrate that third molars exert pressure on the dentition mesial to them. However, in these studies, lateral expansion of the intercuspid area had occurred during treat-ment, predisposing the sample to lower anterior crowding irrespective of the presence or absence of the terminal molars. Also, few nonextraction cases were included in the sample in which the third molars had erupted. It is well documented that the eruption of the mandibular first molars occurs in a mesial and occlusal direction and continues as the third molars emerge in the oral cavity. A recent study, based on the archives of the implant studies of Bjork, has also demonstrated the individual eruption patterns of maxillary incisors and molars till the age of twenty-five years and does not terminate at that time.

Richardson demonstrated the significantly reduced mesial movement of the first molars in second molar extraction cases. The removal of second molars effectively isolates the third molar forces from the rest of the arch. It was also evidenced that following eruption of the second molar there was sig-nificant increase in the space for the third molars by forward movement of the second molars when compared to the control group, where no increase in mandibular anterior crowding was observed.

It is unclear whether the state of eruption or impaction of the mandibular third molars, which may con-ceivably have an effect on the mesial forces associated with it, plays a role in the severity of late mandibular crowding. Schwarze, using photodocumentation techniques and computer analysis of three-dimensional tooth movement, demonstrated less mesial movement of the first molars when the third molars were extracted between twelve and twenty-two years of age.

The etiology of late crowding of the mandibular arch is multifactorial and is associated with the amount and direction of late mandibular growth, soft tissue maturation, **apical base** differences, incisor posi-tion relative to the basal bone, occlusal status, tooth morphology and size, muscle forces involved in physiologic function, degenerative tissue changes and the periodontal changes with age. These factors act in different combinations with varying effects and intensity. As Richardson pointed out, one of the challenges in post-retention studies remains the wide range of treatment ages pooled in the samples studied.

The controversy surrounding the relative merits of extraction of third molars to alleviate late lower inci-sor crowding are far from resolved. Present studies of third molars are not optimally designed to establish any direct relationship between third molar eruption and increased mandibular crowding. In the absence of further scientific evidence, the extraction of third molars for the purpose of preventing lower incisor relapse is not justified.

9. APPLIANCE DESIGNS AND RETENTION

Every completed orthodontic case requires a period of retention.   Based on the factors discussed in this chapter the following general plan for retention is suggested.

Duration: Full time retention (twenty or more hours per day) is best advised for the first three months after appliance removal. During this time the lamina dura is reforming and rapid rebound of teeth is possible. This initial intense period of retainer wear should be followed by a period of nine months when the retainers are worn the majority of the time (twelve or more hours a day). During this time, the collagenous and elastic fibers of the PDL and gingiva reorganize. This first year of retention should be followed by night-time (six or more hours of wear) for at least an additional year.

General Rules for Appliance Design

During retention the teeth should be free to flex individually as **alveolar bone** responds to the heavy loads during mastication. This requirement may be met by the use of removable retainers that are removed during meals or by a fixed retainer that is not too rigid.

Removable retainers

Important aspects in the fabrication of removable retainers are obtaining accurate impressions, immediate pour up in stone, debubbling of the casts, an appropriate appliance design and proper fabrication. The initial diagnostic criterion that dictates the treatment rendered must be kept in mind while planning the design of the retainer. Undoubtedly, the use of the maxillary (Figures 21-6 and 21-7) and mandibular Hawley (Figures 21-8 and 21-9) designs introduced in 1919 remains the most popular. The labial bow (usually extending from canine to canine) provides the clinician with the ability to control to some extent the maxillary and mandibular anteriors.

In extraction cases, several designs of clasps and labial bows avoid passing through extraction sites, as they tend to wedge open the space. The use of a short labial bow (from lateral incisor to lateral incisor), or the use of circumferential maxillary retainers (Figures 21-10 21-11) provides the benefit of minimizing occlusal interference. Alternately, the labial bow may be soldered to the bridge of the Adams clasp. The use of the U loops in the labial bow is extremely useful, as it allows the clinician to adjust and manipulate the appliance as desired. While providing palatal (upper retainer) or lingual (lower retainer) acrylic coverage that aids in the retentive ability of the appliance, the presence of clasps on the molars and occasionally on the premolars adds to the ability to secure the appliance. Traditional Adams clasps (Figure 21-12) provide excellent retention of the appliance. However, the clinician may select clasps based on the occlusal interference it could cause and the **clinical crown** height of teeth. Circumferential clasps, eye clasps, arrowhead clasps and ball clasps (Figures 21-13 thru 21-19) provide adequate retention in cases where Adams clasps may not be suited. The use of more than one clasp adds to the retentive ability of the appliance.

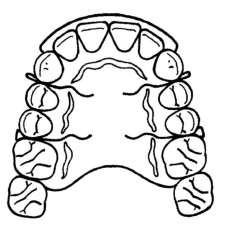

Figure 21-6: Traditional maxillary Hawley retainer design with triangular clasps.

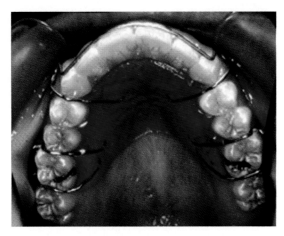

Figure 21-7: Traditional maxillary Hawley retainer with Adams clasps.

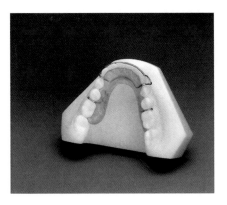

Figure 21-8: Lower Hawley appliance with ball clasps.

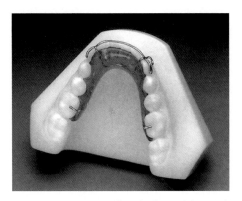

Figure 21-9: Lower Hawley design with attachments to prevent canine rotations and occlusal rests to prevent molar eruption.

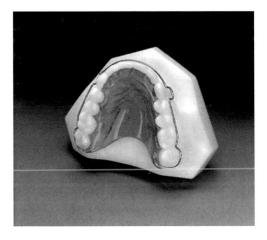

Figure 21-10: Wrap-around retainer appliance

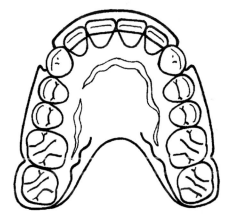

Figure 21-11: Wrap around retainer design avoids occlusal interference.

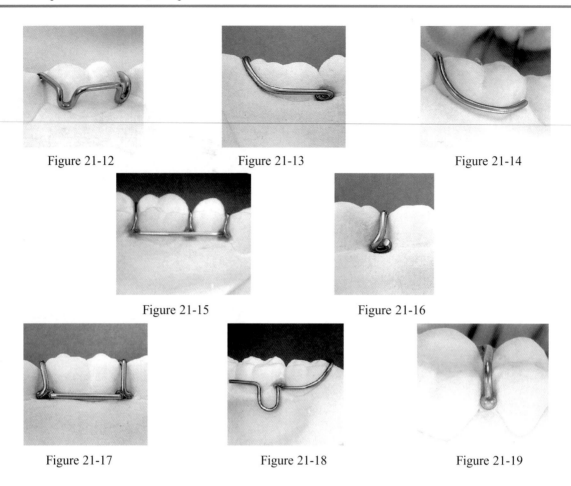

Figure 21-12   Figure 21-13   Figure 21-14

Figure 21-15   Figure 21-16

Figure 21-17   Figure 21-18   Figure 21-19

Clasp Designs. Figure 21-12: Traditional Adams clasp. Figure 21-13: "L" clasp, used in cases of tight occlusal contact with the eye providing good stability. Figure 21-14: "C" clasp design. Figure 2-15: Long modified Adams clasp design engages two teeth for additional retention. Figure 21-16: Eye clasp. Figure 21-17: Modified Adams clasp. Figure 21-18: Modified lingual clasp avoids inter-occlusal contact. Figure 21-19: Ball clasps provide excellent retention.

In instances where a tooth or multiple teeth are missing, the Hawley appliance may have pontics incorporated in the design (Figure 21-20). Care should be taken to avoid palatal impingement and maintain the esthetics of the region until more permanent restorative measures are taken. As discussed earlier, incorporating bite plates in retainers assists in controlling a rectified vertical discrepancy. The upper Hawley retainer is stronger than the lower design by virtue of the bulk of the appliance.

A commonly used retainer that provides excellent retention and may be used for mild corrections that have occurred as a result of relapse is the spring aligner (Figure 21-21). Similar in appearance and design to the Hawley retainer, the spring aligner provides additional protection against relapse with labial coverage of the teeth by clear acrylic. Often, the acrylic extends from canine to canine, as it is more difficult to get proper engagement of the appliance to the posterior segments (which results from undercuts). Although the appliance may be used routinely as a retainer, it can be used to actively correct mild relapses that commonly occur in the lower anterior region.   In such cases, an accurate wax set-up where individual teeth are sectioned and set on the arch to mimic the desired result should follow the dental impressions. An exact measure of the amount of interproximal reduction required may be obtained in this manner. Cases that demonstrate moderate amounts of relapse should be not be treated with the spring aligner unless a significant compromise is acceptable to patient and clinician.

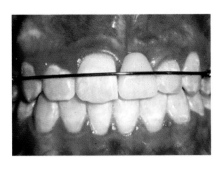

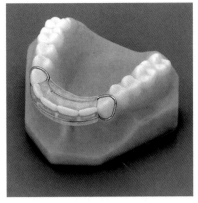

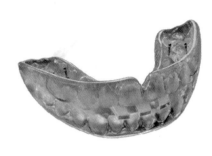

Figure 21-20: Use of a pontic to maintain space for a missing central incisor. Note the midline disparity accepted as a result of a Bolton tooth size discrepancy.

Figure 21-21: Upper spring aligner with acrylic coverage on the labial aspect to assist in correction of mild rotations.

Figure 21-22: Positioner appliance for upper and lower dentition

Tooth positioners (Figure 21-22) can also be used during the retention phase of treatment. The advantages of this appliance are its resistance to fracture and its "massaging" effect on gingival tissue. However, it is a bulky appliance that obstructs speech and chewing, and is typically worn a considerably shorter period of time, which may not be beneficial to the overall retention strategy. It can be used as a finishing appliance, but clearly does not assist in the correction of rotations or torque management. Positioners may be more useful in the retention of Class II or III conditions because they actively couple the upper and lower teeth. For optimum effect and retention, a positioner should be made on mounted casts using a facebow transfer.

While removable appliances do not interfere with maintaining oral hygiene, the need for patient compliance may be considered a shortcoming. Additionally, the retaining component of the anterior teeth, a point contact of wire on the labial surface and acrylic approximating the lingual cervix, requires frequent adjustments as the appliances tend to get loose and the mechanical constraints to tooth movement are reduced.

Thermoplastic Retainers

With the advent of clear, thin thermoplastic materials a new class of retention appliances has gained favor with some clinicians in the last decade (Figure 21-23). These retainers have several advantages for patients and practitioners. First, they are fabricated on a dental study cast in less than thirty minutes from start to finish. Second, they are almost invisible in the mouth and therefore teeth appear brilliant by reflecting light that falls on them. Third, they are thin and rarely interfere with speech. Fourth, no adjustments are required with the appliance, hence saving the clinician chairside time. Finally, they are easily cleaned and provide good stability of retained areas of the arch.

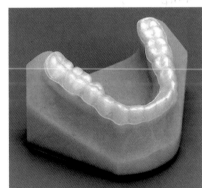

Figure 21-23: Commonly used lower Tru-tain retainer that is easy to fabricate and esthetic.

Three disadvantages have also been reported. First, they do not allow **settling of the occlusion** (when designed to cover the entire arch). Second, since they cover the occlusal surfaces there is some masticatory wear, which reduces the longevity of the appliance in the mouth. And third, by virtue of being a **removable appliance**, patient cooperation becomes important. However, with an understanding of these limitations thermoplastic retainers are an integral part of modern retention strategies.

Sheridan, et al., popularized the "Essix" retainers with the design incorporating only the anterior teeth. The fabrication of the thermoplastic retainers is simple. Following accurate impressions and pour up in die stone, the model is debubbled and extreme undercuts are removed using a light cured composite gel. Care must be taken to retain adequate undercuts to ensure good retention of the appliance. A coat of separating medium is advisable prior to thermoforming, which is then undertaken in a pressure sensitive thermoforming unit such as the Biostar from Great Lakes Orthodontics, Ltd. A 0.75 mm or 0.030 inch thermoplastic copolyester is used in the fabrication of the retainer.

During the thermoforming process, the thickness of the plastic film is reduced from 0.030 inches to 0.015 inches. The plastic sheet is then cut away from the cast, extending about two millimeters of the plastic cervical to the free gingival margin on the labial aspect. The appliances are typically seated the day of **fixed appliance** removal. The appliances should require firm pressure over the incisal edges for proper seating, and the initial pressure experienced by the patient will dissipate over time. The retainer ought to be cleaned with a soapy cotton swab tip, as toothpaste tends to dull their brilliance.

Fixed Retainers

Direct bonded retainers are usually wires bonded to the lingual aspect for its superior esthetics and ability to retain teeth in their positions in challenging clinical situations. The retainer derives its retention from the mechanical interphase of the twists in the wire and the composite resin. The flexible wire allows the physiologic movement of teeth during mastication, essential to reorganization of the gingival fibers and PDL, and reduces the stress concentration on the composite.

Following accurate impressions (prior to debonding), and pour up in stone, the flexible retainer wire is carefully adapted to the lingual aspect of the model to provide passive and good contact with the critical areas of the dentition. Before placement, the wire must be checked in the patient's mouth to ascertain the contact the wire makes with the teeth. Following acid etching of the surfaces involved, the retainer wire is placed in the region desired and may be secured while bonding by use of dental floss that runs interdentally from the lingual to the to the labial aspect. Following preliminary securing of the wire with light cure composite resin, passiveness of the wire is rechecked. The bulk of adhesive may now be added and finishing can be accomplished by the use of tungsten carbide burs (Nos. 7006 and 7408). Flossing can be done using a floss threader. Fabrication and placement of the fixed retainer by this indirect-direct method provides the best results. Alternately, the fabricated fixed retainer may be bonded indirectly.

The most common scenarios where fixed retention is adopted are in the retention of the lower canine-to-canine region (given its propensity to relapse) (Figures 21-24 and 21-25), cases where space needs to be maintained (Figures 21-27 and 21-28), corrected midline diastemas (Figure 21-27), and occasionally in the upper anterior region when significant vertical alignment of the incisal edges was undertaken (Figure 21-26). In most instances, the wire does not need to be bonded to each independent tooth in the segment retained. For example, when the wire is in good contact with the lower incisors and canines, bonding to the terminal teeth in that segment (canines) is sufficient. Patients are quick to observe a fractured bond and may be scheduled immediately for a short repair appointment. The results of follow up studies in the use of fixed retainers are encouraging. However, clinicians need to watch for gingival inflammation and poor oral hygiene that may be associated with the regions of the fixed retainers.

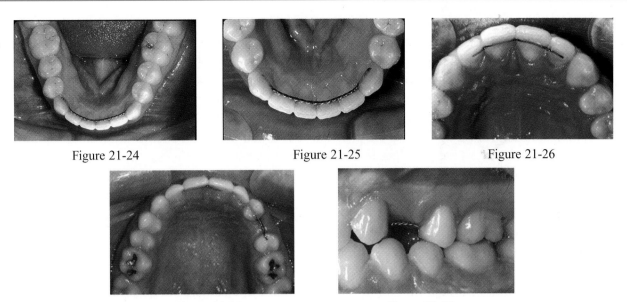

Figure 21-24   Figure 21-25   Figure 21-26

Figure 21-27   Figure 21-28

Figure 21-24: lower bonded retainer from cuspid to cuspid. Figure 21-25: lower bonded retainer from canine to canine demonstrating the intimate contact of the spiral wire with the lingual surface of the teeth. Figure 21-26: fixed bonded retainer from upper 2-2, undertaken in cases where potential for space reopening or crowding is high and in cases where significant vertical alignment of the incisal edges was undertaken. Figure 21-27: occlusal view of an upper fixed retainer between the central incisors and upper left canine (first bicuspid substitution) and second bicuspid. Figure 21-28: close up of the bonded spiral wire retainer used to maintain space in the buccal segment.

In conclusion, given our knowledge about the etiology of relapse, its consequences, and the methods available to prevent the recurrence of malocclusion, there is a real need to customize retention regimes for each patient based at least on their original malocclusion.

10. LOOKING AHEAD

The extensive data published on stability, retention and relapse does not provide us with all the answers clinicians require. It is fair to say that most issues discussed in this chapter are far from resolved, as the data analyzed to date has led to opinions that vary on treatment modalities with regard to long-term stability (extraction versus non-extraction, expansion versus no expansion), and the various retention strategies. Most samples analyzed have been retrospective samples, automatically introducing a selection **bias**. Similarly, the degrees of crowding typically associated with extraction treatment groups tend to bias studies attempting to directly compare them to non-extraction groups. Therefore, the conclusions of such studies may not be representative of the outcome. The idealistic solution would be to design studies that use long-term randomized prospective samples. The difficulties such efforts pose are well recognized.

Perhaps the next best solution would be to meta-analyze data available which would provide a method of examining large collections of results from independent studies for the purpose of integrating findings as done by Burke, et al., who analyzed twenty-six previous studies on mandibular intercanine widths and reported that, regardless of diagnostic and treatment modalities, intercanine width typically is expanded during active treatment and lost following retention. Such efforts to increase the sample size may provide stronger statistical support for conclusions. Additionally, the method of analysis may demonstrate underlying patterns and identify significant relations between specific exposures and outcomes.

It is perhaps just as important that orthodontists understand the range of variations that exist in nature "normally". The literature for the most part emphasizes the need to obtain certain esthetic standards of occlusion. Attempts to link occlusal relations to physiologic dysfunctions remain inconclusive. It is likely that there exists in nature a large range in inter-arch relations measured by overjet, overbite and a host of similar measurements. If we are caught up in seeking occlusal relations that may be just a subset of perfectly acceptable physiologic alternatives, are we setting ourselves up for future frustration? Relapse to any one of the normal relations may be a biologically acceptable and likely outcome. Yet, satisfying our patients by providing the best esthetic result possible and treating their chief complaint remains the most critical service we provide. Retaining such corrections, then, must be part of our treatment objectives. This dilemma is not presented to excuse clinicians whose prime goal is to attain a self-gratifying standard of occlusal beauty with scant regard for the foundations of biology and the principles of occlusion and who merely indulge in satisfying patient's expectations. Instead, this is for the young clinician and investigator to seek out the biologic factors that determine tooth position, the physiologic boundaries of acceptability and, ultimately, the determinants of occlusion. The phenomenon and control mechanisms of tooth eruption, tooth position in the arch following eruption, remodeling and the biochemical physiology of gingival and periodontal fibers, tissue fluid dynamics, the range of asymptomatic functional occlusion, and the narrow or wide range of esthetic acceptability will provide us with the breakthrough and understanding needed to individualize treatment for each patient and set standards best suited for her/him. We will remain obligated to educate patients and understand and satisfy their expectations in such an endeavor.

The issues that confronted us at the end of the twentieth century will be quite different than those we can expect to face in the first part of the twenty-first. Health care technology has changed our perspectives about life, death, and our understanding of illness. Procedures such as *in vitro* fertilization, organ transplantation, and genetic testing all have had an impact. It is inevitable that the effects of these advances will impact dentistry and orthodontics. This is partly because oral health is an important component for the **quality of life**, and even after the human genome has been decoded the death rate remains one per person!

Dentistry in the next century will continue to develop new approaches to treat and cure conditions, but a new emphasis will emerge toward enhancement. This will include treatment of problems before their symptoms appear while patients are seemingly healthy, and treatments that don't target conditions but will allow us to control them. With these technologies used to enhance our lives will come new issues about who will have access to them and how they will be paid for, questions about when their risks are outweighed by their benefits.

Instead of waiting for orthodontic relapse to eventually take its toll, treatments may be used to provide potential cures while people are still relatively malocclusion free. Gene therapy used to prevent genetically linked heart disease and cancer may find its way into the orthodontic arena to determine patients at greater risk for relapse than others or provide clinicians with alternative therapies. But these treatments will have risks, so the possibility of permanent cures will have to be weighed against the risks of the therapies themselves. Also, to realize these benefits will require early (pre-symptomatic) testing — again raising questions of cost and access. This will create a serious problem for "optional" enhancement technologies, such as intelligence-enhancing or memory-extending gene therapy or drugs.

Gene therapy is on the cusp of becoming effective. This bodes huge impact, since these are therapies that provide permanent cures at the molecular level. Questions will arise around how serious an illness or condition must be to warrant the use of gene therapy, and whether to use the technology not to cure, but to enhance performance. Since such therapies will work at the genetic level, we'll need to decide whether they should be used on children, or wait until adulthood. This will be easier for decisions about treating conditions that have effects in childhood but much more difficult for decisions about other uses, such as enhancing height or athletic ability, orthodontics, or treating late onset diseases.

All this means that this century promises remarkable possibilities. We need to be sure we look ahead, find answers, try to understand their costs and ask whether we can afford to pay them lest we muddle through this new century older but no wiser than we were in the last one.

Acknowledgements: The authors would like to thank TP Orthodontics®, Indiana, Dr. Gary Wolf, Norwalk, Ohio and Dr. Douglas Amberman of CWRU for their pictorial contributions.

11. SUGGESTED READINGS

Introduction

Markus MB: A review and consideration of the problem of retention. Am J Orthod Oral Surg 1938; 24:203.

Tweed CH: Indications for extraction of teeth in orthodontic procedure. Am J Orthod Oral Surg 1944; 30:405-408.

Tweed CH: Why I extract teeth in the treatment of certain types of malocclusion, Alpha Omega, 1952.

Rogers AP: Making facial muscles our allies in treatment of retention. Dental Cosmos; 1922, 7.

Barnes RE: The early expansion of decidous arches and its effect on the developing permanent dentition. Am J Orthod 1956; 42:83-97.

Enlow DH: Morphologic factors involved in the biology of relapse. J Charles H. Tweed Foundation 1980; 8:16-23.

General Factors Affecting Stability of the Treated Dentition.

Behrents RG: A treatise on the continuation of growth in the aging craniofacial skeleton. Ann Arbor, University of Michigan, Center of Human Growth and Development, 1984.

Reitan K: Principles of retention and avoidance of post-treatment relapse. Am J Orthod 1969; 55:776-790.

Boese LR: Fiberotomy and reproximation without lower retention, nine years in retrospect: Part I Angle Orthod 1980; 50(3):88-97.

Chavrier C, Couble ML, Magloirre H, Grimaud JA: Connective tissue organization of healthy human gingiva. Ultrastructural localization of collagen types I-III-IV. J Periodont Res 1984; 19:221-9.

Everts V, Niehof A, Beertsen W: Type VI collagen is associated with microfibrils and oxytalan fibers in the extracellular matrix of periodontium, mesenterium and periosteum. J Periodont Res 1998; 33:118-125.

Hynes RO: Fibronectins. New York, Springer-Verlag, 1990.

Edwards JG: The prevention of relapse in extraction cases. Am J Orthod 1971; 60:128-141.

Redlich M, Palmon A, Zaks B, Edel J, Rayzman S, Shoshan S: The effect of mechanical force on transcription levels of collagen type I and collagenase in cultured gingival fibroblasts. Arch Oral Biol 1998; 43: 313-316.

Edwards JG: A long-term prospective evaluation of circumferential supracrestal fibrotomy in alleviating orthodontic relapse. Am J Orthod 1988; 93(5):380-387.

Redlich M, Rahamim E, Graft A, Shoshan S: The response of supragingival collagen to orthodontic rotation movement in dogs. Am J Orthod 1996; 110:247-255.

Retention of Anterior-Posterior Corrections

Turley P: Orthopedic correction of Class III malocclusion with palatal expansion and a custom protraction headgear. J Clin Orthod 1988; 22:314-325.

McNamara JA: An orthopedic approach to the treatment of Class III malocclusion in young patients. J Clin Orthod 1987; 21:598-608.

Kulbersh VP, Berger J, Kersten G: Effects of protraction mechanics on the midface. Am J Orthod Dentofac Orthop 1998; 114:484-491.
McNamara JA, Huge SA: The functional regulator (FR3) of Frankel. Am J Orthod 1985; 88:409-24.

Turley PK: Orthopedic correction of Class III malocclusion: retention and phase II therapy. J Clin Orthod 1996; 30 (6):313-324.

Retention of Vertical Corrections

Lewis P: Correction of deep overbite: A report of three cases. Am J Orthod 1987; 91:342-345.

Kim TW, Little RM: Postretention assessment of deep overbite correction in Class II division 2 malocclusion. Angle Orthod 1999; 69 (2):175-186.

Canut JA, Arias S: A long-term evaluation of treated Class II division 2 malocclusion: a retrospective study model analysis. Eur J Orthod 1999; l21 377-386.

Retention of Arch Form and Arch Alignment

Little RM: The irregularity index: A quantitative score of mandibular anterior alignment. Am J Orthod 1975; 68:554-563.

Richmond S, Shaw WC, O'Brien KD, Buchanan IB, et al: The development of the PAR index (Peer Assessment Rating: Reliability and validity). Eur J Orthod 1992; 14:125-139.

Sandowsky C, Sakols EI: Long-term assessment of orthodontic relapse. Am J Orthod 1982; 82:456-463.

BeGole EA, Fox DL, Sandowsky C: Analysis of change of arch form with premolar expansion. Am J Orthod Dentofac Orthop 1998; 113:307-315.

Little RM, Riedel RA, Artun J: An evaluation of changes in mandibular anterior alignment from 10 to 20 years postretention. Am J Orthod 1988; 93:423-428.

Little RM: Stability and relapse of dental arch alignment. Retention and Stability in Orthodontics, ed. C. J. Burstone and R. Nanda, Philadelphia, W. B. Saunders Co., pp 97-106, 1993.

Sadowsky, C: Long term stability following orthodontic therapy, Retention and Stability in Orthodontics, ed. C. J. Burstone and R. Nanda, Philadelphia, W. B. Saunders Co., pp 107-113, 1993.

Zachrisson BU: JCO Interviews on excellence in finishing. J Clin Orthod 1986; 20:460-482, 536-556.

Sinclair PM, Little RM: Maturation of untreated normal occlusions. Am J Orthod 1983; 83:114-123.

Tuverson DL: Anterior interocclusal relations. Am J Orthod 1980; 78:361-393.

Dugoni SA, Lee JS, Varela, Dugoni AA: early mixed dentition treatment: Postretention evaluation of stability and relapse. Angle Orthod 1995; 65:311-320.

Kusters ST, Kuijpers-Jagtman AM, Maltha JC: An experimental study in dogs of transseptal fiber arrangement between teeth, which have emerged in rotated and non-rotated positions. J Dent Res 1991; 70:192-197.

Little RM, Riedel RA, Engst ED: Serial extraction of first premolars-Postretention evaluation of stability and relapse. Angle Orthod 1990; 60:255-262.

Persson M, Persson E, Skagies S: Long-term spontaneous changes following removal of all first premolars in Class I cases with crowding. Eur J Orthod 1989; 11:271-282.

Woodside GD, Rossouw PE, Shearer D: Postretention mandibular incisor stability after premolar serial extractions. Semin Orthod 1999; 5:181-190.

Sadowsky C, Schneider BJ, BeGole EA, Tahir E: Long-term stability after orthodontic treatment: Nonextraction with prolonged retention. Am J Orthod 1994; 106:243-249.

Gorman JC: The effects of premolar extractions on the long-term stability of the mandibular incisors. Retention and Stability in Orthodontics, ed, CJ Burstone and R. Nanda, Philadelphia, W. B. Saunders Co., pp. 81-95, 1993.

Franklin GS, Rossouw PE, Woodside DG: A longitudinal study of dental and skeletal parameters associated with stability of orthodontic treatment (abstr.), Am J Orthod 1996; 109:109.

Paquette DE, Beattie JR, Johnston LE: A long-term comparison of nonextraction and premolar extraction edgewise therapy in "borderline" Class II patients. Am J Orthod 1992; 102: 1-14.

Felton JM, Sinclair PM, Jones DL, Alexander RG: A computerized analysis of the shape and stability of mandibular arch form. Am J Orthod 1987; 92: 478-483.

Effects of Extraction and Non-extraction Treatment on Arch Stability

Little RM, Riedel RA, Artun J: An evaluation of changes in mandibular anterior alignment from 10 to 20 years postretention. Am J Orthod 1988; 93:423-428.

Kokich VG, Shapiro PA: Lower incisor extraction in orthodontic treatment. Four clinical reports. Angle Orthod 1984; 54:139-153.

Williams R: Single arch extraction-upper first molars or what to do when non-extraction treatment fails. Am J Orthod 1979; 76:376-393.

Richardson ME, Mills K: Late lower arch crowding: The effect of lower second molar extraction. Am J Orthod 1990; 98: 242-246.
Shapiro P: Mandibular dental arch form and dimension. Am J Orthod 1974; 66: 58-70.

Sinclair PM, Little RM: Maturation of untreated normal occlusions. Am J Orthod 1983; 83:114-123.

Glenn G, Sinclair PM, Alexander RG: Nonextraction orthodontic therapy: Posttreatment dental and skeletal stability. Am J Orthod Dentofac Orthop 1983; 92:321-328.

Palatal Expansion

Ricketts RM: The wisdom of the bioprogressive philosophy. Sem Orthod 1998; 4:201-207.

Vardimon AD, Brosh T, Spiegler A, Lieberman M, Pitaru S: Rapid palatal expansion: Part 1. Mineralization pattern of the midpalatal suture in cats. Am J Orthod Dentofacial Orthop 1998; 113:371-8.

Vardimon AD, Brosh T, Spiegler A, Lieberman M, Pitaru S: Rapid palatal expansion: Part 2. Dentoskeletal changes in cats with patent versus synostosed midpalatal suture. Am J Orthod Dentofacial Orthop 1998; 113:488-97.

Aelbers CMF, Dermaut LR: Orthopedics in orthodontics: Fiction or reality-a review of the literature, Part I. Am J Orthod 1996; 110:513-519.

Dermaut LR, Aelbers CMF: Orthopedics in orthodontics: Fiction or reality-a review of the literature, Part II. Am J Orthod 1996; 110:667-671.

Sarnas KV, Bjork A, Rune B: Long-term effect of rapid maxillary expansion studied in one patient with the aid of metallic implants and roentgen stereometry. Eur J Orthod 1992; 14:427-432.

De La Cruz AR, Sampson P, Little RM, Artun J, Shapiro PA: Long-term changes in arch form following orthodontic treatment and retention. Am J Orthod 1995; 107:518-530.

Third Molars and Relapse

Little RM: Stability and relapse of dental arch alignment. Br J Orthod 1990; 17:235-241.

Hagberg C: The alignment of permanent mandibular incisors in children. A longitudinal prospective study. Eur J Orthod 1994; 16:121-129.

Richardson ME, Gormley JS: Lower arch crowding in the third decade. Eur J Orthod 1998; 20:597-607.

Richardson ME: A review of changes in lower arch alignment from seven to fifty years. Semin Orthod 1999; 5:151-159.

Ades A, Joondeph D: A long-term study of the relationship of third molars to mandibular dental arch changes. Am J Orthod Dentofac Orthop 1990; 97:323-335.

Iseri H and Solow B: Continued eruption of maxillary incisors and first molars in girls from 9 to 25 years, studied by the implant method. Eur J Orthod 1996; 18:245-256.

Zachrisson BU: Important aspects of long-term stability. J Clin Orthod 1997; 9:563-583.

Appliances for Retention

Espen HD, Zachrisson BU: Long-term experience with direct bonded lingual retainers. J Clin Orthod 1991; 10:619-630.
Looking ahead

Burke SP, Silveira AM, Goldsmith LJ, Yancey JM, Stewart AV, and Scarfe WC: A meta-analysis of mandibular intercanine width in treatment and postretention. Angle Orthod 1997; 68 (1):53-60.

CHAPTER 22

The Adverse Effects of Orthodontic Treatment

William F. Hohlt

Judith B. Rose

1. INTRODUCTION

Achieving a pleasing cosmetic orthodontic result with acceptable function is not accomplished without risks. It is the responsibility of the orthodontist to inform the patients and/or their parents of the potential for undesirable sequelae that may occur during and after orthodontics. An Informed Consent currently represents the standard of care in modern day orthodontics. Being made aware of the risks and hazards of orthodontic treatment allows the patients and/or their parents to make an educated decision on the pursuit of orthodontic treatment.   Information is presented to educate rather than to alarm and it allows consent to be given or withheld for any orthodontic procedure.

The major risks involved in orthodontic treatment are:

- Tooth decay and enamel decalcification
- Periodontal disease
- External apical **root resorption**
- Patient injuries from orthodontic appliances
- Length of treatment
- Temporo-mandibular joint disorders
- Aspiration or ingestion of orthodontic appliances
- Injury from dental instruments
- Abnormal wear of tooth structure and debonding fractures
- Nickel allergy
- **Bacteremia** after orthodontic banding
- Pain and discomfort
- Impacted third molar teeth may still

occur
- Tooth mass discrepancies may not be resolved
- Extraction of teeth and supplemental **orthognathic surgery** may be necessary
- Abnormal growth patterns of the jaws
- Teeth with questionable vitality may be adversely affected
- Post-treatment changes in alignment

2. TOOTH DECAY AND ENAMEL DECALCIFICATION

There is nothing more disheartening than to debond and/or deband a well-treated orthodontic case only to find "tell-tale" signs of enamel decalcification or tooth decay. In a 1992 longitudinal clinical study by Robert Boyd, it was found that 20% to 30% of adolescents who had ineffective plaque removal during orthodontic treatment would develop significant enamel decalcification. The adolescents in this study were raised in an environment where fluoride was present in the water and they had a very low incidence of smooth surface caries before orthodontic treatment.

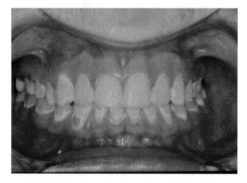

Figure 22-1: Decalcification and tooth decay associated with poor oral hygiene during orthodontic treatment.

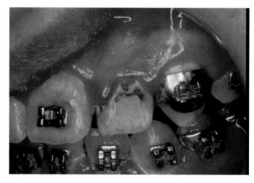

Figure 22-2: Decalcification and tooth decay associated with poor oral hygiene during orthodontic treatment.

The University of the Pacific investigated methods of enhancing the effectiveness of plaque removal in adolescent patients and devised the following guidelines:

1.) Decalcification can be reduced by adding small amounts of fluoride to saliva in the form of over-the-counter 0.05% neutral sodium fluoride rinses or twice daily rinses of 0.4% stannous fluoride gels.

2.) Powered toothbrushes such as Braun-Oral B, Rotadent, Interplak and Sonicare all remove plaque more effectively than conventional toothbrushes and thereby reduce decalcification.

3.) An additional reduction in smooth surface decay can occur if subjects use fluoride toothpaste such as Colgate Total but do not rinse with water after brushing, which would dilute the fluoride.

4.) Gingivitis and bacterial counts associated with plaque can also be reduced with the use of 0.12% chlorohexidine rinses.

Band cementation using glass ionomer cements seems to prevent band wash-out decalcification. Although it is not ADA approved, European orthodontists have been painting recognized decalcification with fluoride resins such as a 5% sodium fluoride varnish.

Of course, regular visits to the family dentist f̶
ical fluoride should occur at least every six m̶
Finally, if all attempts to motivate the non-com̶
treatment should be terminated and all orthodo̶

3. PERIODONTAL DISEASE

In 1989, a longitudinal study was published in the ̶
Orthopedics (AJO/DO) by a research team at the U̶
prehensive orthodontic treatment in adults who had re̶
ly healthy adults and adolescents. The results of that st̶
the periodontal tissues occurred in adult periodontal pati̶
vided adequate preventative measures that included p̶
orthodontic treatment period.

̶plication of top-
̶ntic treatment.
̶que fail, then

̶tofacial
̶ com-
̶ntal-
̶ to
̶o-

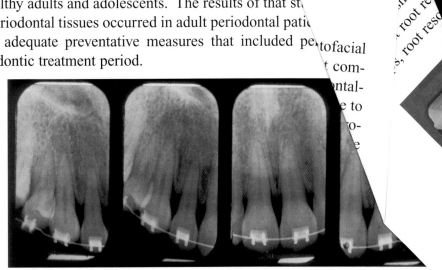

Figure 22-3: Crestal bone loss occurring with orthodontic treatment associated wit̶

The same study indicated that, generally, adults had significantly less plaque accumu̶
ier gingival tissues than adolescents during treatment. The results also showed that health̶
be treated orthodontically without significant periodontal breakdown. However, the study fu̶
that approximately 20% to 30% of the adolescents had inadequate plaque removal during treatn̶
they also lost significant periodontal bone support during this period.

Effective plaque control before, during and after orthodontic treatment is imperative. It is the responsibility of the orthodontist to educate the patient about proper oral hygiene technique. It is the responsibility of the parents and the family dentist as a team to motivate the adolescent patient about the
importance of good oral hygiene and monitor his/her progress.

Gingival recession relating to the effects of **proclination** of the mandibular incisors on periodontal status is controversial. A study was done by Ruf, Pancherz, et al., in 1998 that utilized 98 patients with
Class II malocclusions who were treated with a fixed Herbst appliance for an average of seven months.
All of the subjects exhibited good oral hygiene. Analysis included 392 lower incisors. The average age
of the participants was 12.8 years. The results of this study showed that the average proclination was
8.9 degrees. There was no significant difference found in the amount of gingival recession before treatment, nor was there significant difference after treatment.

Being aware of the amount of the **attached gingiva** around the lower incisors may be a better indicator
for predicting gingival recession. Patients who have attached gingiva that is less than 2mm in width are
generally candidates for gingival grafting before orthodontic treatment as a preventative measure for
gingival recession during and after treatment.

SORPTION (EARR)

urs in all disciplines of dentistry, but it is most commonly seen in
rable sequela of treatment. Root resorption can result in permanent
ot apex. The cause is multifactorial and is still poorly understood, i.e.,
plicating factors in root resorption include the types of tooth movement
o move teeth, trauma, tooth devitalization, **ectopic eruption** of adjacent
d **bruxism**. Root resorption during orthodontic treatment is more likely
gns of previous root resorption prior to orthodontic treatment. It is inter-
orption seems to occur only during active orthodontic treatment. Once the
rption ceases.

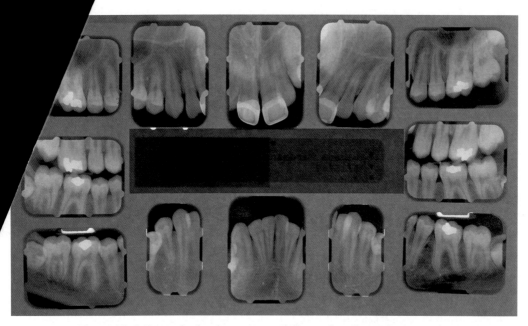

Figure 22-4: Pre-orthodontic treatment full-mouth radiographs.

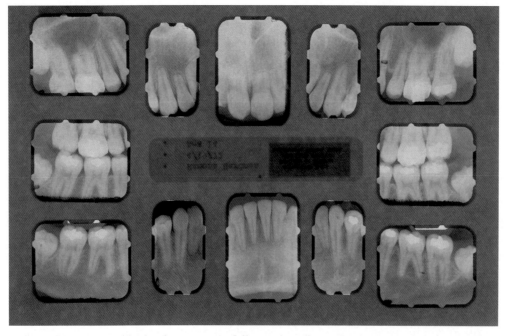

Figure 22-5: Post-orthodontic treatment full-mouth radiographs demonstrating EARR of
incisors.

In a study conducted by Parker and Harris that was reported in the AJO/DO, 110 orthodontic cases were studied longitudinally and retrospectively. These 110 cases were selected from a Tweed standard edgewise practice, a Begg light wire practice and a Roth prescriptive straight-wire practice. The subjects in the study were all adolescents at the start of treatment. Their root formation was complete and there was no history of trauma. They all had Class I molar relationships and all had four premolars extracted prior to treatment. Before and after lateral cephalograms were analyzed to determine the presence of root resorption. The conclusions of the study were that incisor tooth movements are strong statistical predictors of the amount of root resorption experienced during treatment. The specific direction of the movement differentially enhances the extent of the external apical root resorption. The combination of intrusive movement and lingual root torque was the strongest predictor of external apical root resorption. In contrast to the previously mentioned indicator, bodily retraction in a posterior direction, **extrusion** or lingual crown tipping had no discernable influence on root resorption.

Heredity, not just the amount or type of force used, plays a major role in determining the actual clinical severity of external apical root resorption in orthodontic treatment, according to various studies. Newman, in a 1975 study published in the AJO/DO, suggests family clustering of external apical root resorption. However, the pattern of inheritance was not clear. In 1997, Harris, et al., explored the **hypothesis** of genetic influence on external apical root resorption for the first time using the sib-pair model and reported that moderately high heritability (**h**^{2}) was present. While this study clearly indicated susceptibility being familial, it could not determine the extent of the familial component being genetic versus environmental factors that the sibs may have in common.

Research at the Indiana University School of Dentistry confirmed the greatest extent of orthodontics-associated external apical root resorption occurred in the maxillary incisors. They also confirmed the familial nature of the tendency. Heritability studies at Indiana indicate that orthodontics-related root resorption is influenced, for the main part, by previously unknown genetic factors and, to a lesser extent, by occlusal variables such as overjet and overbite. In addition they have, for the first time, shown a genetic marker to be associated with an increased risk of orthodontics-associated root resorption. Al-Qawasmi and Hartsfield from Indiana University have also discovered a different chromosome area where another genetic marker for orthodontics-associated root resorption appears to be located. Their research is ongoing to further identify genetic determinants for increased susceptibility to external apical root resorption.

An impacted canine is sometimes associated with the root resorption of adjacent teeth. The most commonly affected tooth is the maxillary lateral incisor. Maxillary canine impaction occurs in approximately 1% to 2% of the population, and females are affected almost twice as often as males. Of these impacted canines, approximately 80% to 90% are palatal and 10% to 20% are labial. Early detection of an ectopically erupting canine is the key to prevention. Ericson and Kurol found that if canine impaction is suspected, extraction of the deciduous canine before the age of 11 will allow for normal eruption of the permanent canine 91% of the time. This finding is dependent on the crown of the impacted canine being distal to the lateral incisor. If the crown of the impacted canine is mesial to the lateral incisor, natural eruption will occur 64% of the time.

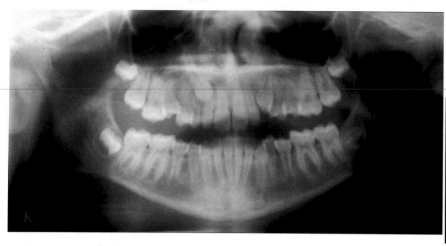

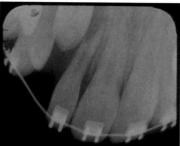

Figure 22-6: Impacted maxillary canine in close proximity to lateral incisor apex.

Figure 22-7: Apical root resorption associated with impacted canine.

During comprehensive orthodontic treatment, progress panographic radiographs should be taken annually and supplemental periapical radiographs should be taken of the maxillary and mandibular anterior teeth every six months. If apical root resorption is diagnosed, the patient should be informed. The patient should be advised that continued tooth movement could result in additional resorption that could compromise the longevity of the tooth or teeth involved. In cases of severe root resorption, it is advisable to discontinue orthodontic treatment and to splint the affected teeth to reduce mobility.

5. PATIENT INJURIES FROM ORTHODONTIC APPLIANCES

Headgear has been widely used in orthodontics since its introduction by Kloehn in the early 1900s. Early headgear attachments utilized elastic straps that were connected directly to the outer bow, or elastic connections from the head attachment to the outer bow. In 1975, the American Association of Orthodontists issued a special bulletin to its membership regarding headgear safety. The California State Society of Orthodontics in 1984 recommended that all headgear be a safety type and that all force mechanisms be a breakaway type.

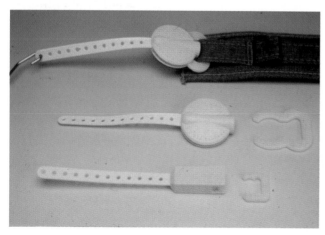

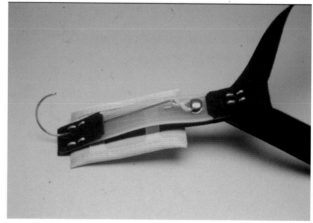

Figure 22-8: Safety release mechanisms on head gear attachment

Figure 22-9: J-hook headgear.

Its use for **anchorage** control and growth modification demands patient compliance in wearing the headgear from eight to twelve hours per day. Utilizing various types of headgear such as cervical, occipital, Interlande, and J-hook appliances can regulate the force delivery. Anytime the headgear delivers an upward and posterior force, there is danger of face-bow rebound toward the face and eyes if the appliance is pulled out of the headgear tubes and released. Reports of eye injuries resulting from headgears have been published. Although this type of injury is rare, there is a high morbidity to the eyes if they are affected.

In order to increase safety to the patient during headgear use, manufacturers have made two modifications. One modification is a release mechanism and the other is a safety inner bow. The release mechanism releases the neck strap or head strap from the face bow if any excessive anterior force is placed on the face bow. Studies have demonstrated that it takes 5.33 pounds to 32.83 pounds at a mean extension of 0.84 inches to 2.93 inches to dislodge the inner bow. The safety inner bow is designed to prevent the headgear from coming out of the tubes accidentally, which reduces the possibility of causing injury.

Whenever a headgear appliance is delivered to the patient, the patient and/or the patient's parent should be precisely instructed on the hours the headgear is to be worn. There should be clear instruction on the potential danger of the patient being stuck in the face or eye during the wearing of the appliance or during the process of putting on or taking off the headgear. It should be noted to them that wearing headgear during sleep decreases the danger that might exist in contrast to wearing the appliance during the daytime at school or at play.

6. LENGTH OF TREATMENT MAY VARY FROM ESTIMATE

During the initial consultation and treatment plan review with the patient and/or the patient's parent, an estimate of the time that is necessary to treat the malocclusion is presented. It is very important to emphasize that the suggested treatment time is an estimate and that many factors can impact this presentation. These factors should be explained as loose bands and brackets, poor oral hygiene, failed appointments, failure to wear headgear or intraoral elastics, and inadequate growth of the jaws. The first phase of treatment should generally be limited to one year or less. Comprehensive treatment of adolescent or adult malocclusions should take approximately twenty-four to twenty-eight months. Three months prior to the end of orthodontic treatment a panographic radiograph should be taken so that second order corrections can be recognized and accomplished, instead of at the end of the estimated time frame.

7. TEMPOROMANDIBULAR JOINT DYSFUNCTION (TMD)

According to William R. Proffit in his textbook, "Contemporary Orthodontics", the number of people with moderate degrees of malocclusion in the United States is between 50% to 75%. This number far exceeds the number of people in the same population that have TMD symptoms, which is between 5% and 30%. He also states that stress induced diseases such as ulcerative colitis very rarely occur in conjunction with TMD symptoms. This would indicate that in the great majority of orthodontic patients, there is little correlation between TMD and malocclusion.

In a 1998 Angle Orthodontist publication, Deguchi, et al., studied the TMD-related effects of chin-cup therapy on patients with Class III malocclusion. They found that no TMD symptoms were present in 67% of the 160 patients studied that were treated with chin cup therapy. Evidence of TMD was found in 16% of the patients during chin cup use, in 9% during active treatment and in 6% after active treatment. Spontaneous pain was found most often during active treatment. Clicking of the jaw occurred more often during the retention phase.

During active orthodontic treatment, it is advisable to monitor the temporomandibular joint monthly to check for range of motion, pain and noise. If symptoms are present, it is advisable to discontinue the use of such appliances as headgear and intra-oral elastics. It is then indicated to place the patient on anti-inflammatory, non-steroidal drugs, moist heat, and a soft diet. In some cases, construction of flat plane splints or anterior repositioning splints is indicated if internal derangement of the joint is suspected.

8. ASPIRATION OR INGESTION OF ORTHODONTIC APPLIANCES

Although it is a rare occurrence, orthodontic appliances have been ingested or aspirated during the banding/bonding or debanding/debonding procedures. Fixed canine-to-canine retainers occasionally come loose and can easily be swallowed. Such accidents should not be ignored. For medical and legal reasons, the practitioner should take aggressive steps to locate the aspirated or ingested object. In the case of the minor patient, the parents should be notified of the potential danger and advised to report any adverse symptoms such as fever, cramping, or difficulty in breathing to the orthodontist. If there is the slightest possibility of aspiration or ingestion of an **orthodontic appliance**, the patient should be referred to a hospital emergency facility for the appropriate chest and/or gastrointestinal radiographs. Ingested appliances normally are passed through the gastrointestinal tract within an eight-hour period. Aspirated objects must be retrieved.

9. INJURY FROM DENTAL INSTRUMENTS

It is possible for a patient to be inadvertently poked, scratched or lacerated when dental instruments are used in the mouth. Use of thumb rests while using band pushers and use of disc shields while using diamond discs can prevent injury. The practitioner needs to use common language when instructing the young patient about the procedure about to be performed. They need to be advised of the danger and consequences of not remaining still and they need to be instructed to not jerk or push the orthodontist's hands away.

Sometimes the long wire spans extending from the first molars to the incisors will slowly irritate the buccal vestibule, giving the appearance of a cut. Placing buccal tubing on the unsupported arch-wire section can prevent this irritation. Transpalatal arches and lingual arches can occasionally embed into the adjacent soft tissue to such an extent that they require surgical removal under local anesthesia. However, in most cases just removal of the wire for a few days will allow healing, then careful readjustment will suffice.

10. ABNORMAL TOOTH WEAR AND DEBONDING FRACTURES

When porcelain type brackets occlude with tooth enamel, abnormal tooth wear can occur due to the difference in hardness between porcelain and enamel. There have been reports of attrition, enamel flaking, and tooth fractures when clear or tooth colored brackets are debonded. The practitioner must pay strict attention to the manufacturer's debonding instructions to diminished such damage.

The removal of excess adhesive flash around the clear bracket base seems to be most important when debonding. When a banded tooth has a large dental restoration, extreme care must be used when using a band remover during the debonding procedure. If there is a potential for a cusp fracture, the band should be split with a high-speed dental instrument along the mesiobuccal line angle. Abnormal wear of the tooth structure can occur if the patient grinds excessively. This wear can be diminished if the patient wears a night guard while sleeping.

11. NICKEL ALLERGY

Several metallic alloys such as cobalt-chromium, nickel-titanium, beta-titanium, and stainless steel are used in contemporary orthodontic treatment. The majority of these alloys have nickel as one of their components, varying from 8% in stainless steel to 50% in nickel-titanium. It is estimated that 4.55% to 28.5% of the population have hypersensitivity to nickel. Females seem to have a higher prevalence of allergy to nickel because of contact with detergents, jewelry, especially earrings, and other metallic objects.

In 1998, a study of 170 patients was conducted at the Bauru Dental School in Sao Paulo, Brazil, to determine prevalence of allergy to nickel. The patients were divided into three groups and given nickel patch tests and a questionnaire before orthodontic treatment, during orthodontic treatment, and post orthodontic treatment. The results of this study were similar to the findings for the general population. The results showed an allergic reaction in 28.3% of the study subjects, of which 23% were female and 5.3% were male. There was no significant difference in the prevalence of contact dermatitis among the three groups. This study suggests that orthodontic therapy with conventional stainless steel appliances does not initiate or aggravate a nickel hypersensitivity reaction. Titanium is realized as one of the most inert metals to human tissue. Orthodontic brackets and wires are currently on the market for patients who have a known allergy even though the results of the Bauru study would indicate that it is not warranted.

12. BACTEREMIA AFTER ORTHODONTIC BANDING

Bacteremia associated with dental procedures such as tooth extraction, periodontal operations, endodontic procedures and tooth brushing lasts from ten minutes to thirty minutes and is clinically unimportant to healthy individuals. However, **bacteremia** is a **risk factor** in patients with prosthetic cardiac valves, previous bacterial endocarditis, surgically constructed systemic-pulmonary shunts, history of rheumatic fever and other valvular dysfunction, hypertrophic cardiomyopathy, mitral valve prolapse with valvular regurgitation, synthetic vascular grafts, and prosthetic joints.

Since orthodontic banding procedures can induce bleeding, it is advisable to prescribe prophylactic antibiotics thirty minutes before commencing with a procedure whenever the pre-treatment medical history demonstrates one of the at-risk disorders. The current American Heart Association guidelines recommend the administration of two grams of amoxycillin one hour before the dental procedure for adults and 50mg/kg PO for children. If the patient is allergic to penicillin, clindamycin should be substituted using the dosage for adults of 600mg and for children 20mg/kg PO one hour before the procedure. However, the March 2000 issue of the Journal of the American Dental Association concluded that there is little or no scientific basis for the use of antibiotic prophylaxis in dentistry. It was felt that the risk of inappropriate use of antibiotics and the widespread antibiotic resistance to bacteria was a far more important deterrent than any possible perceived benefit. The practitioner must exercise common sense and good clinical judgment regarding this issue. Maintaining a "rather be safe than sorry" attitude toward antibiotic coverage can easily be argued when it comes to placing the patient's systemic health at unnecessary risk.

13. PAIN AND DISCOMFORT

It is normal to experience mild pain and discomfort for the period of twenty-four hours to forty-eight hours after routine orthodontic adjustments. Most patients will not require any medication for the discomfort. However, there are cases where the discomfort is enough to require the use of over-the-counter non-steroidal anti-inflammatory agents such as ibuprofen (Advil®), naproxen sodium (Aleve®), or acetaminophen (Tylenol®). On rare occasions, additional pain relief can be accomplished by administering controlled substances such as Tylenol® with ¼ grain to ½ grain codeine, or Darvocet-N-100®.

There are other situations when taking 200 mg of Advil® thirty minutes before a procedure is performed will make the experience more comfortable. A good example of the use of this type of pre-medication would be at the initial stage of the placement of headgear.

Patients or their parents should be instructed to inform the orthodontist if the severe pain lasts more than twenty-four hours. In these unusual cases, the forces placed on the teeth may be reduced or discontinued. An example of a case when force reduction is necessary would be when there is failure of palatal sutures to open when sutural expansion is attempted on patients over fifteen years of age.

14. IMPACTED THIRD MOLAR TEETH MAY STILL OCCUR

One of the most common misconceptions in dentistry is the idea that third molar eruption is the cause of mandibular incisor relapse. Nowhere in dental literature can this cause and effect relationship be proven. It is normal for the third molar to erupt between the age of seventeen years and nineteen years. During this same period of maturation, the mandible is completing its downward and forward rotation into the obicularis oris muscular complex. This last minute growth displacement may prove a better explanation for mandibular anterior teeth collapse rather than the eruption of the third molars.

Annual radiographs should help the practitioner decide if there is enough space present for the normal eruption of the third molars. The indications for extraction are true impaction, lack of opposing occlusion, and associated soft or hard tissue pathology. In current practice, implants are placed in the retro-molar area of the mandible to enable the second and third molars to be moved anteriorly for long distances without sacrificing anterior anchorage. In the case where the second premolars are congenitally missing or when the first molars have large restorations or questionable endodontic therapy, it is advisable to not extract the third molars.

15. TOOTH MASS DISCREPANCIES MAY NOT BE RESOLVED

When the occlusion is perfect, the teeth are proportional in size. If large maxillary teeth are combined with small mandibular teeth, overjet will exist. Reciprocally, if large mandibular incisors are combined with small maxillary incisors, maxillary spacing will occur. In some occlusions small maxillary incisors will necessitate the leaving of diastemas mesial and distal to the lateral incisors. According to Profitt, 5% of the American population has some degree of disproportion that is defined as a **tooth size discrepancy** or tooth mass discrepancy. The most common tooth affected by this discrepancy in the Caucasian race is the maxillary lateral incisor. Premolars are the most discrepant in African Americans.

Small lateral incisors can be built up by the use of restorative bonding procedures or the use of porcelain laminates to correct the problem. Reduction of tooth mass can be accomplished by slenderizing the teeth using lightening strips. Diamond discs can also be used to help dental arches become proportional. Pre-treatment wax setups help diagnose the discrepancy as well as individual tooth measurement and performing a **Bolton analysis**. It is appropriate for the practitioner to explain the tooth mass discrepancy before orthodontic treatment rather than post-treatment.

16. EXTRACTION OF TEETH AND SUPPLEMENTAL ORTHOGNATHIC SURGERY MAY BE NECESSARY

Sometimes the amount of dental crowding is so great that teeth have to be extracted in order to create needed space for alignment. Changes in orthodontic treatment in the 21st Century such as doing fewer extractions than was done in the 20th Century may be at the expense of long term **dental arch** stability. Dental arch expansion, bonded brackets, and high tech orthodontic wires have been instrumental in making borderline extraction cases into non-extraction cases.

Since the 1980's, new and sophisticated oral surgery procedures have been vastly improved, allowing major changes in the movement of facial bones into a balanced esthetic position. Skeletal malocclusions can be corrected by treating the skeletal component that is disproportionate as well as treating the dental malocclusion. **Orthognathic surgery** performed by the **maxillofacial** surgeon/orthodontist team makes these major changes in skeletal malocclusions possible. However, these extensive procedures can bring added risks such as anesthetic death, trismus, condylar sag, infection, non-bony union, hemorrhage, temporomandibular joint dysfunction, swelling paresthesia, and skeletal component relapse. It should be noted that the most common sequela of surgical mandibular protraction or retraction is paresthesia of the lower lip. Also, skeletal component relapse happens more often in large surgical corrections. The greater the correction made, the greater the chance for relapse.

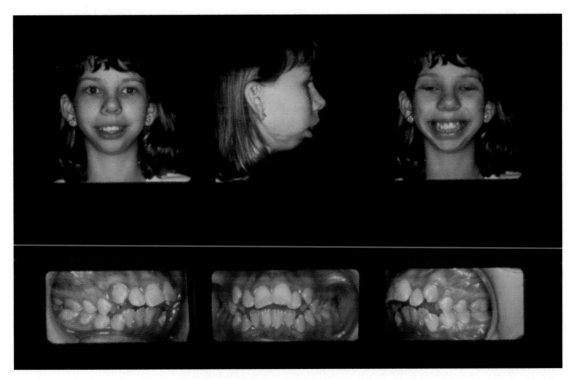

Figure 22-10: Pre-surgical correction of severe Class II malocclusion.

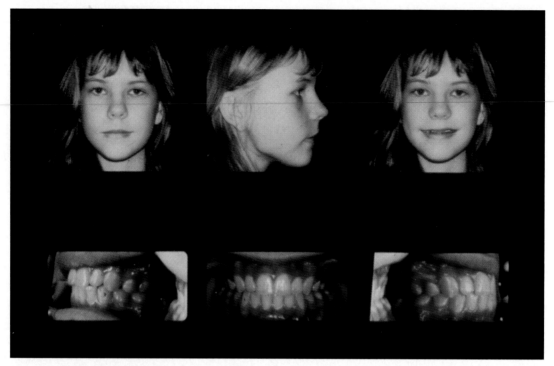

Figure 22-11: Post-surgical correction of same severe Class II malocclusion.

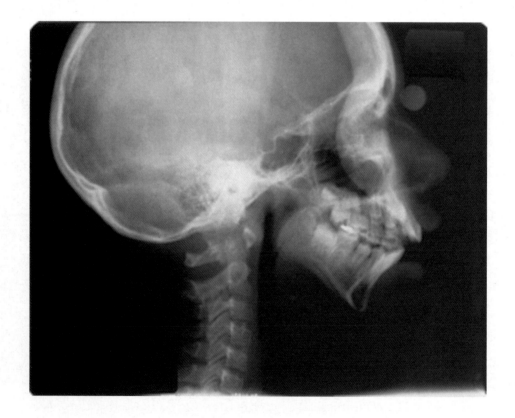

Figure 22-12: Pre-surgical correction headplate of severe Class II
malocclusion.

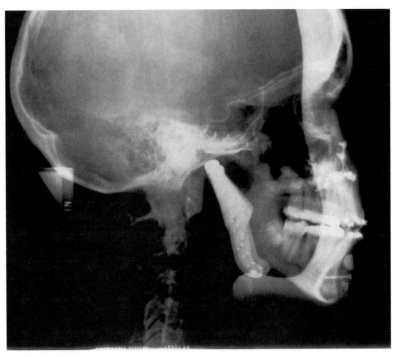

Figure 24-13: Post-surgical correction headplate of severe Class II malocclusion.

17. ABNORMAL GROWTH PATTERNS OF THE JAWS

Excessive or insufficient growth of the jaws may limit the orthodontist's ability to achieve the desired final result of orthodontic treatment. It is possible for Class III malocclusions to return after treatment when there is late mandibular growth. For optimal correction of Class II malocclusions, it is necessary to have horizontal growth vectors rather than vertical displacement of the mandible. Generally, there is more mandibular rotation in the growth pattern for males than there is for females.

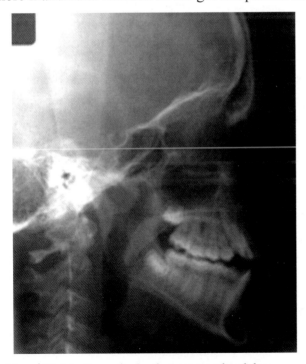

Figure 22-14: Pre-orthodontic treatment headplate demonstrating anterior open bite.

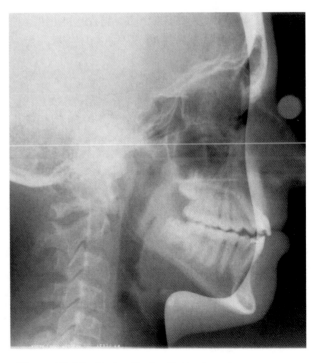

Figure 22-15: Post orthodontic treatment demonstrating relapse of open bite treatment.

Undesirable growth patterns and changes are a biological process that cannot be adequately predicted and are beyond the orthodontist's control. Prediction of the growth of the maxillary and the mandibular jaws is available utilizing sophisticated computer softwear programs. However, it must be noted that they are not 100% reliable. Excessive or insufficient growth may require supplemental orthognathic surgical procedures to achieve the desired esthetic treatment objective.

18. TEETH WITH QUESTIONABLE VITALITY MAY BE ADVERSELY AFFECTED

In theory, light continuous orthodontic forces placed on a healthy tooth should have little effect on the dental pulp. Tooth movement is a reaction brought about through compression and tension in the periodontal ligament. This

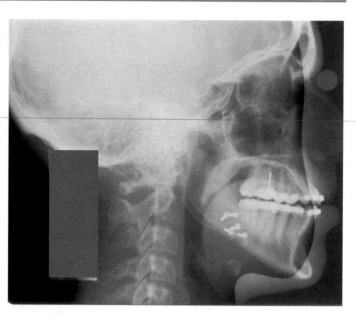

Figure 22-16: Final surgical correction due to abnormal mandibular growth.

movement has little effect on the dental pulp other than possibly a transient inflammatory reaction or mild pulpitis. Light continuous forces will move the teeth very slowly to allow the nerves and vessels to reorganize in their new positions. Abrupt dental movements related to heavy continuous dental forces will cause indirect or back side resorption. This may allow the dental apex to move so abruptly that the blood supply to the tooth is compromised.

When orthodontic tooth movement aggravates a latent pulpal injury causing the necessity of endodontic therapy, there is usually a previous history of dental trauma or a large dental restoration. A tooth that has been successfully treated endodontically will move in the same manner as a healthy tooth. Attempts to move a non-vital endodontically untreated tooth will cause an acute exacerbation. The practitioner should give careful attention to clinical symptoms such as discoloration, pain, and radiographic changes during treatment. Electric vitality testing during active orthodontic treatment can give a false negative result.

At Indiana University, the utilization of implants for anchorage in the retromolar area demonstrated that second and third molars can be successfully moved eight millimeters anteriorly causing no interruption in vitality. The employment of light continuous forces during orthodontic treatment cannot be overemphasized.

19. POST-TREATMENT CHANGES IN ALIGNMENT

It is not unusual for teeth to change their position after orthodontic treatment. The most common type of possible change is the first order rotation that occurs in the first twenty-four hours after debonding. Supracrestal fiberotomies and over-correction of the first order rotations are usual methods of combating this type of relapse. Patient compliance in the wearing of the retainers will also minimize change.

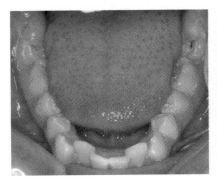

Figure 22-17: Pre-orthodontic treatment.

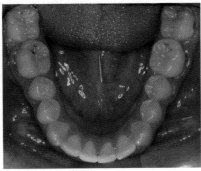

Figure 22-18: Completion of orthodontic treatment.

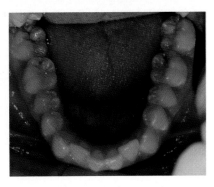

Figure 22-19: Post-orthodontic treatment relapse.

Throughout anyone's lifetime, their occlusion can change due to various factors. The most common factors inducing change are growth, para-oral habits, mouth breathing, and eruption of the third molars. Para-oral habits will allow maxillary incisors to flare and can possibly cause transverse changes in the maxillary width. Mouth breathing will allow for molar eruption and the possible development of an anterior open-bite. Third molars are frequently and erroneously blamed for relapse when the real culprit is late growth of the mandible combined with forward rotation into the orbicularis oris complex.

In some cases, retention after orthodontic treatment can be indefinite. In most cases, it is necessary to wear retainers 24 hours per day for six months. This regimen can be eased into wear only during sleeping hours after that period of time. The orthodontist should monitor the treatment retention every three months to be aware of subtle changes. If there is change in the early phases, it is more easily reversed. In some cases, fixed retention is indicated, especially if there is a possibility of patient non-compliance in the use of the removable retainer. Maxillary midline diastemas can be permanently closed with a fixed wire splint on the lingual.

All patients will react differently during the orthodontic retention period. Some will be almost religious in the practice of wearing the retainers while others will be completely remiss. Other patients may be so excited by the esthetics of the finished treatment they become obsessive in their compliance. Then, there is the same type of excitement generated by pleasing esthetics when the patient wants nothing marring the appearance of the "perfect" teeth. It is therefore the standard for the practitioner to carefully monitor the finished treatment during the retention period to make minor corrections and to encourage patient compliance.

In conclusion, it is the responsibility of the orthodontist to assure there is a clear explanation of the above-mentioned risk factors associated with orthodontic treatment. This information should be presented at the pretreatment consultation with the patient and/or the patient's parents. The discussion should be in language that can easily be processed by a layperson. There should be time allowed for necessary questions and answers. The patient and/or parent should be given an open invitation to ask questions at any time during the orthodontic treatment. There should be discussion of the consent to treat form and appropriate signatures should be obtained. After adequate discussion, the practitioner should make an entry in the patient's records that this consent was signed and a copy should be in the chart.

20. SUGGESTED READINGS

Tooth Decay, Enamel Decalcification and Periodontal Disease

Boyd, R L., Enhancing the value of orthodontic treatment: Incorporating effective preventative dentistry into treatment. Am J Ortho Dentofacial Orthop 2000: 117,(5)5:601-603.

Loesche, Walter J., Dental Caries: A Treatable Infection, ADD Publications, Grand Haven, Michigan, 1993.

Nelson P A., Artun J., Alveolar bone loss of maxillary anterior teeth in adult orthodontic patients. Am J Orthop 1997:111(3):328-334.

Riolo, C. S., Kulbersh,R., Riolo, M. L., and Haerian, H.A. Periodontal Pathogen Levels in an Adolescent Population Before and During Fixed Orthodontic Appliance Therapy, Craniofacial Monograph Series, #31, In Orthodontic Treatment: The Management of Unfavorable Sequelae. The University of Michigan, Ann Arbor, Michigan, 1996

Ruf S., Hansen, K., Pancherz, H., Does orthodontic proclination of lower incisors in children and adolescents cause gingival recession. Am J Orthop 1998: 114(1):100-106.

Todd M A., Staley, R N., Kanellis, M J., Donly, K J., Wefel, J S., Effect of a fluoride varnish on demineralization adjacent to orthodontic brackets. Am J Ortho Dentofacial Orthop 1999: 116 (2):159-167.

Vorhies, A B., Donly, K J., Staley, R H., Wefel, J S. Enamel demineralization adjacent to orthodontic brackets bonded with hybrid glass ionomer cements. An in vitro study. Am J Ortho Dentofacial Orthop 1998: 114(6):668-674.

Wenderoth C J., Weinstein, M., Barislow, A J., Effectiveness of a fluoride-releasing sealant in reducing decalcification during orthodontic treatment. Am J Orthop 1999: 116(6):629-634.

External Apical Root Resorption

Al-Qawasmi RA, Hartsfield Jr JK. Everett ET, Flury LL, Liu L, Foroud TM, Marci JV, Roberts WE. Genetic predisposition to external apical root resorption in orthodontic patients; Linkage and association of interleukin 1B gene. Jm J Orthod Dentofac Orthop 2002 in press.

Baumrind S., Korn E., Boyd R L., Apical root resorption in orthodontically treated adults. Am J Orthod Dentofac Orthop 1996: 110:311-320.

Beck B W., Harris E F., Apical root resorption in orthodontically treated subjects: Analysis of edgewise and light wire mechanics. Am J. Orthod Dentofac Orthop 1994: 105:350-361.

McNab S., Battistutta D., Taverne A., Symons A L., External apical root resorption following orthodontic treatment. Angle Orthod, 2000, Vol. 70, No. 3, 227-232.

Parker R J, Harris E F., Directions of orthodontic tooth movements associated with external apical root resorption of the maxillary incisor. Am J Orthop 1998: 114(6):677-683.

Shellhart W C., Jasper S., Abrams H., Wilson T., Case Report: Management of significant incisor root resorption associated with maxillary canine impaction. Angle Orthod 1998: 68(2)L, 187-192.

Harris E F., Kineret S E., Tolley E A. A heritable component for external apical root resorption in patients treated orthodontically. AmJ Orthod Dentofac Orthop 1997:111:301-309.

Personal communication. Indianapolis, IN. November 26, 2001.

Patient Injuries from Orthodontic Appliances

American Association of Orthodontists, Your Orthodontic Treatment, Informed Consent for the Orthodontic Patient brochure 1990.

Stafford G D., Caputo A A., Turley P K. Characteristics of head-gear release mechanisms: Safety implications 1998 Angle Orthod:68(4):319-326.

Temporomandibular Joint Disorders

Deguchi T., Uematsu S., Kawahara Y., Mimura H. Clinical evaluation of temporomandibular joint disorders (TMD) in patients treated with chin cup. 1998 Angle Orthod: 68(1)91-94.

Abnormal Tooth Wear and Debonding Fractures

American Association of Orthodontists, Your Orthodontic Treatment, Informed Consent for the Orthodontic Patient. Brochure: 1990.

Nickel Allergy

Janson G R P., Dainesi E A., Consolaro, A., Woodside D G., de Freitas M R. Nickel hypersensitivity reaction before, during and after orthodontic therapy. Am J Ortho Dentofacial Orthop 1998:113,(6):655-660.

Bacteremia After Orthodontic Banding

American Dental Association and the American Academy of Orthopedic Surgeons, JADA 1997:128, 1004-1007.

Erverdi N., Kadir T., Oskan H., Acar A. Investigation of bacteremia after orthodontic banding. Am J Orthod Dentofac Orthop 1999: 116, No 6:687-690.

Fournier A., Payant L., Bouclin R. Adherence of Streptococcus mutans to orthodontic brackets. Am J Orthod Dentofac Orthop 1998:114,(6):687-690.

Tong D C., Rothwell B R. Antibiotic prophylaxis in dentistry: A review and practice recommendations. JADA 2000;131:366-374.

Tooth Mass Discrepancies

Adelsperger J.M., Comparison of the incidence of Bolton tooth mass discrepancy in African-American and Caucasion populations. Indiana University School of Dentistry, Masters Thesis: 1998.

Bolton W., The clinical application of a tooth-size analysis. Am J Ortho 1992:48, 504-529.

Abnormal Growth Changes of the Jaw

Bjork A., Skieller V. Normal and abnormal growth of the mandible. A synthesis of longitudinal cephalometric implant studies over a period of 25 years. European J of Ortho 5 1983:1-46.

Rickets R M., A four-step method to distinguish orthodontic changes from natural growth. JCO 1995:IX, No IX:4:208-228.

Sinclair P M., Little R M. Maturation of untreated normal occlusions. Am J Ortho 1983:83(2):114-123.

GLOSSARY

Edited by: Michelle J. Thornberg
Elizabeth A. Van Tubergen

A

Aberrant. Deviating from the usual type or natural of tissue or straying from the normal way (behavior).

Accessional teeth. The 12 permanent teeth that develop posterior to the primary and succeedanous teeth. They accede the primary teeth with six in each arch, i.e., permanent first molars, permanent second molars, and third molars.

Accessional teeth. The permanent teeth which erupt posterior to the primary teeth.

Achievement tests. Tests that measure what a child has already learned in a particular academic subject or subjects.

Actin. Structural intracellular filament involved in muscle contraction.

Activator. A myofunctional appliance (Andresen, Bimler, Monobloc, Frankel, Twin Block etc.) A removable type of orthodontic appliance which acts as a passive transmitter of force, produced by the function of the activated muscles, to the teeth and alveolar process which are in contact with it.

Addiction. A person's dependence on a drug or a behavior in order to feel physically or psychologically at ease.

Adolescence. The period of biologic, cognitive, and psychosocial transition from childhood to adulthood, defined to begin at 13 years of age.

Adult orthodontic treatment. Treatment rendered to the dentition that is present after cessation of growth that would affect orthodontic treatment.

Agenesis. Lack or failure of development, such as of a body part.

Aggressive. Behavior that takes the form of verbal insults or social rejection is called relational aggression. The peer group shuns aggressive-rejected children, because they are overly confrontational.

Allogenic cell sourcing. Procurement of cells from an individual within the same species as the eventual recipient.

Allogenic transplantation. Transplantation of an organ or tissue that is donated by another individual within the same species as the recipient.

Alveolar arch. The archial measurement of the alveolar process. This joins the tooth to the basal bone (arch) and thus can be a compromise in size and shape between the basal arch and the dental arch.

Alveolar bone. The ridge of bone on the surface of the body of the maxilla and mandible. This term is applied to the tooth-bearing part of the mandible and maxilla as it contains the tooth sockets.

Alveolar bone proper. A thin lamina of bone that surrounds and supports the roots of the teeth and serves as attachment of the principal fibers of the periodontal ligament.

Alveolar crestal bony height. The height of the alveolar bone between the teeth.

Alveolar crest fibers. Those principal fibers of the periodontal ligament extending between the alveolar crest of the alveolar bone and the neck of the tooth.

Alveolar fundus. The base or bottom of the alveolar bone proper lining the tooth socket.

Alveolar ridge [alveolar process]. The bony ridge or raised thickened border on each side of the upper and lower jaw that contains the sockets of the teeth. Called also "alveolar process."

Anatomic crown. The true crown; that portion of the tooth covered by enamel.

Anchorage. The nature and degree of resistance to displacement offered by an anatomical unit when used for the purpose of affecting tooth movement.

Cervical anchorage. Anchorage in which the back of the neck is used for resistance through means of a neck strap.

Extraoral anchorage. Anchorage in which the resistance unit is outside the oral cavity, such as cranial, occipital, or cervical anchorage.

Intermaxillary anchorage. Anchorage in which the units in one jaw are used to effect tooth movement in the other jaw.

Intramaxillary anchorage. Anchorage in which the resistance units are all situated within the same jaw.

Intraoral anchorage. Anchorage in which the resistance units are all located within the oral cavity.

Multiple anchorage (reinforced anchorage). Anchorage in which more than one type of resistance units are utilized.

Occipital anchorage. Anchorage in which the top and back of the head are used for resistance through means of headgear.

Reciprocal anchorage. Anchorage in which the movement of one or more teeth is/are balanced against the movement of one or more opposing teeth.

Simple anchorage. Dental anchorage in which the resistance to the movement of one or more teeth comes from the resistance to tipping movement of the anchorage unit.

Angiogenesis. The formation of new capillary blood vessels from pre-existing capillaries or venules.

Angiogenic. The ability to induce or catalyze angiogenesis.

Angle classification system. A classification system devised by Dr. E.H. Angle in 1900 to describe the anteroposterior relationships of the permanent first molars, which was then used to define dental malocclusions as well as normal occlusion. Even though this system is not without criticisms, it remains the most popular classification system used today.

Angle's Classification of malocclusion. Classification of different types of malocclusions introduced by Edward H. Angle "based on the mesiodistal relationship of the teeth, arches, and jaws as shown by the relationship of the permanent molars on their eruption and locking".

Class I. Normal relationship of jaws. The mesiobuccal cusp of the maxillary first molar occludes in the buccal groove of the mandibular first permanent molar.

Class II. Distal relationship of the mandible. The distobuccal cusp of the maxillary first permanent molar occludes in the buccal groove of the mandibular first molar.

Division 1 Labioversion of the maxillary incisor teeth.

Subdivision. Unilateral condition.

Division 2. Lingioversion of maxillary central incisors.

Subdivision. Unilateral condition, right or left, i.e., Class II division I, subdivision left (or right).

Class III. Mesial relationship of mandible. The mesiobuccal cusp of the maxillary first molar occludes in the embrasure between the mandibular first and second permanent molars.

Subdivision. Unilateral.

Angle of convexity. It is measured at point A as the inferior angle between the linear Nasion-A point (N-A) and A point-Pogonion (A-Pog). It naturally decreases with growth and development. The normal adult value is 0 degrees with a range of (-) 9 degrees to (+) 9 degrees. If Pogonion is posterior or behind N-A line, the angle is positive with measurements over (+) 5 degrees indicating a convex skeletal profile and 0 degrees measurements between to (+) 5 degrees indicating a straight skeletal profile. If the angle is negative with Pogonion anterior or in front of N-A line, the angle is negative and indicates a concave skeletal profile. The skeletal value is smaller than the soft tissue angle of convexity by 8 degrees to 11 degrees.

Angle FMA. Frankfort mandibular plane angle (FMA) is the inferior–anterior angle between Frankfort horizontal plane and mandibular plane (Down's mandibular plane drawn from the inferior border at menton tangent to the posterior border of the mandible). It naturally decreases with growth and development. The adult norm is 25 degrees $\pm$ 3 degrees. A high FMA after childhood is 30 degrees or more and indicates a skeletal openbite tendency while a low FMA at 20 degrees or below indicates a skeletal deepbite tendency. It is not a measurement of growth pattern as much as it assists in the decision to treat orthodontic cases extraction or non-extraction, i.e., higher angle cases lean toward extractions while low angle cases favor non-extraction.

Angle IMPA (Incisor Mandibular Plane Angle), or /1 to mandibular plane. It is the superior-posterior angle between Down's mandibular plane and the long axis of the root of the most facial mandibular incisor. The adult norm is 90 degrees $\pm$ 7 degrees. It measures the degree of inclination of the mandibular incisors from the basis mandibuli. Thus angles IMPA along with FMA create two of the three angles of the Tweed Triangle. The third angle is the Frankfort Mandibular Incisor Angle (FMIA).

Angles SNA, SNB, and ANB. SNA is the inferior-posterior angle between S-N line to N-A line. It usually does not change with growth and development. The adult norm is 82 degrees $\pm$ 4 degrees. It shows the anterior-posterior position of the maxilla in relation to cranial base. SNB is the inferior-posterior angle measured from S-N line to N-B point line. It normally increases with growth and development. The adult norm is 80 degrees $\pm$ 4 degrees. It shows the anterior-posterior position of the mandible in relation to cranial base. ANB is the calculated difference of SNA minus SNB. It naturally decreases with growth and development. The adult norm is (+) 2 degrees $\pm$ 2 degrees. The ANB angle expresses the antero-posterior relationship of the mandible to the maxilla. A large positive value is associated with skeletal Class II malocclusions while negative values are associated with skeletal Class III malocclusions, i.e., mandibular prognathia and/or maxillary retrognathia.

Angle 1/ to SN (U1 to SN). It is the inferior-posterior angle between SN plane and the long axis of the root of the most facial maxillary permanent central incisor. It naturally increases as the incisors erupts. The adult norm is 104 degrees $\pm$ 4 degrees. It indicates the inclination of the maxillary incisor to cranial base with proclination as higher value and retroclination or upright as lower value.

Ankyloglossia. Restricted movement of the tongue, which may result in speech difficulty.

Ankylosed. Stiffened; bound by adhesions; fused; denoting a joint in a state of ankylosis; rigid fixation of a tooth to the surrounding bony alveolus as a result of periodontal ossification.

Ankylosis. Fusion of the two bones where they articulate, but also occurs in the dentition when there is a fusion with the cementum of the teeth and the alveolar bone. The failure of a tooth to erupt due to this fusion or an abnormal relationship between the tooth and the alveolar bone; can be related to related to repair after trauma.

Ankylosis (joint). Abnormal fixation and immobility of a joint. The ankylosis may be fibrous or bony.

Ankylosis (tooth). Abnormal fixation and immobility of a tooth, (a) clinically by a tooth which is below the occlusal plane which may elicit a different sound in response to percussion, (b) may show radiographic evidence of union between alveolar bone and dentin and invading alveolar bone, (c) histologically by union between radicular dentin and invading alveolar bone.

Anlage. A theoretically earlier stage before even the recognizable or primordial features of an organ or part have appeared.

Anodontia. Congenital absence of one or more teeth because of failure of the teeth to form; it may be partial or total. It is usually associated with an absence or deficiency of the epidermal glands.

Anomalies of teeth. They are patterned after tooth growth and development with anomalies of numbers (supernumerary or congenital absence), size and shape (microdontia/macrodontia, dilaceration, attrition, anomalous permanent maxillary lateral incisors, and gemination (two crowns/one root) / fusion (two crowns/two roots) concrescence (two teeth joined at cementum), and eruption/position/exfoliation (ectopic eruption, transposition, impaction, ankylosis, retained primary teeth without successors, crossbite and rotations).

Anorexia nervosa. A serious eating disorder in which a person restricts eating to the point of emaciation and possible starvation.

Antegonial notch. The concave curve at the distal part of the lower border of the mandible immediately anterior to the gonial angle of the mandible.

Antegonical (notch). The highest point of the notch or concavity of the lower border of the ramus where it joins the body of the mandible.

Antegonial notching. The increase in curvature of the lower border of the mandibular body just anterior to the angle of the mandible.

Anterior border of the ramus. This is defined as the intersection of the functional occlusal plane (FOP) with the anterior border of the ramus.

Anterior cranial base. Anatomically, the anterior cranial fossa.

Anterior component of force. The resultant mesially-directed horizontal force vector created by the forces of mastication on the slightly mesially angulated permanent teeth.

Anterior crossbite. A malocclusion in which one or more of the upper anterior teeth occlude lingually to the mandibular incisors; the lingual malpositions of one or more maxillary anterior teeth in relation to the mandibular anterior teeth when the teeth are in centric relation occlusion.

Anterior Downs point. The midpoint of the line connecting landmarks 6 and 7 (LIE and UID). This represents the anterior point through which Downs Occlusal Plane passes.

Anterior nasal spine. The tip of the median, sharp bony process of the maxilla at the lower margin of the anterior nasal opening.

ANS (anterior nasal spine). A cephalometric landmark the tip of the anterior nasal spine as seen on the x-ray film in normal lateralis.

Anterior open bite. No vertical overlap of the maxillary and mandibular anterior teeth, and/or there is no contact of the anterior teeth.

Antibody. An immunoglobulin molecule that reacts with or binds to the substance (antigen) that induced its synthesis. These proteins are produced by plasma cells.

Antigen. A substance that is recognized as foreign by the body.

Antimere. The symmetrically opposite tooth.

Antisocial behavior. An action, such as hitting or insulting, that is intended to hurt another person.

A Point. The most posterior point on the curve of the maxilla between the anterior nasal spine and supradentale.

Apical base. The base bone portion of maxilla and mandible upon which the teeth and alveolar bone rest. The anatomic and morphological area of the alveolar bone on a level with the apices of the teeth. Orthodontists have suggested that this is an important factor to maintain when correcting a malocclusion for optimal stability.

Apices. Plural for apex, the end of a tooth root.

Apical cementum. Cementum positioned on the apical region of the tooth root.

Appliance, orthodontic. A mechanism for the application of pressure to the teeth and their supporting tissues to produce changes in the relationship of the teeth and/or the related osseous structures.

> **Extraoral appliance.** An appliance that utilizes the top and back of the head and/or neck for anchorage or a resistance unit.

> **Fixed appliance.** An appliance that is cemented to the teeth or attached by means of an adhesive material.

> **Removable appliance.** An orthodontic appliance that the patient can insert and remove from the mouth.

Appositional growth. Growth by layered incremental deposition on boney surfaces.

Aptitude tests. Tests designed to measure potential rather than actual accomplishment.

AR (articulare). A cephalometric landmark; the point of intersection of the posterior border (ramus) of the mandible and the inferior surface of the occipital bone as seen in a lateral head film.

Arch circumference (arch perimeter). The distance measured from the distal surface of the primary second molar (or mesial surface of the permanent first molar) around the arch over the contact points and incisal edges in a smoothed curve to the contralateral point.

Arch (dental). The curved composite structure of the natural dentition.

Arch depth. The linear distance from the midpoint of a line from the mesial surfaces of the permanent first molars or the distal surfaces of the second primary molars or second premolars, to the midline at a point of the central incisors. In the mixed dentition, it naturally decreases in the lower arch without orthodontic intervention.

Arch form. The shape and contour of a dental arch and/or an orthodontic wire formed to conform to the shape of that arch or a wire formed to reshape the dental arch form..

Arch length. Arch length should be thought of as the same as arch perimeter or arch circumference, though it has been erroneously equated with arch depth.

Arch length discrepancy. The difference between the available space and required space, and could exhibit a deficiency or crowding versus excess or spacing. Also is influenced by the individual tooth sizes.

Arch width. The measurement taken across the arch as measured between contralateral teeth.

Arch perimeter. (Arch Circumference).

Arch Perimeter or Arch circumference. The mesiodistal dimension around the arch from mesial of the permanent first molar to its contralateral tooth. Methods to determine accurate measurement in the transitional or permanent dentition are difficult to attain. Individual adjacent tooth differences should be considered without changes in arch form. Some measure the arches in four segments; left incisors, left canine-premolars, right incisors, and right canine-premolars.

Articulare, anterior. The point of intersection of the inferior surface of the cranial base (clivus) and the averaged right and left posterior (neck) surfaces of the mandibular condyles.

Articulare (Articulare, posterior). The point of intersection of the inferior cranial base surface and the averaged posterior surfaces of the mandibular condyles.

Articular disc. Of the temporomandibular joint; the fibrous disc that separates the joint into upper and lower cavities.

Articular eminence. A bony bump on the inferior surface of the temporal bone which is continuous anteriorly with the articular fossa, upon which the mandibular condyles ride as the mandible opens.

Asperger's syndrome. A disorder in which a person has many symptoms of autism, despite having near normal communication skills.

Association. An association is present, if the probability of occurrence of an event or characteristic depends upon the occurrence of one or more other events or characteristics.

Association, apparent. Non-causal associations due to chance, bias, and failure to control for extraneous variables.

Attached gingiva. The connection of the gingival tissue to the alveolar bone at the base of the gingival crevice.

Attachment. The enduring emotional tie that a person forms with another. Following, approaching, and other proximity-seeking behaviors are intended to place an individual close to another person to whom he or she is attached. Clinging, resisting being put down, and other contact-maintaining behaviors are intended to keep a person near another person to whom he or she is attached.

Attention Deficit Hyperactivity Disorder (ADHD). A behavior problem in which the individual has great difficulty concentrating, is often excessively excitable and impulsive, and is sometimes aggressive.

Arch length available. Space present for the permanent teeth around the dental arch from first permanent molar to first permanent molar.

Arch length required. Sum of mesiodistal widths of the permanent teeth from first permanent molar to first permanent molar.

Arch length deficiency. Difference between available and required arch lengths.

Arch wire. A wire utilized in the application of orthodontic force to teeth.

Asymmetrical. Dissimilarity in corresponding parts on opposite sides of the face and cranium. A dental arch or face may not be symmetrical.

Authoritarian parenting. The style of child rearing in which the parents show little affection or nurturance for their children; maturity demands are high and parent-child communication is low.

Authoritative parenting. The style of parenting in which the parents set limits and enforce rules but do so more democratically than do authoritarian parents.

Autism. A severe disturbance of early childhood characterized by inability or unwillingness to communicate, poor social skills, and diminished imagination.

Autogenous. Originating or derived from sources within the same individual.

Autologous cell sourcing. Procurement of cells from a different anatomical location within the body of the eventual recipient.

Autologous transplantation. Transplantation of an organ or tissue that is taken from a different anatomical location within the body of the eventual recipient.

Axon. The nerve fiber extension that sends impulses from one neuron to the dendrites of other neurons.

B

Babinski's reflex. Oral-motor reflex that is present at birth and persists until 3 – 4 months of age. Stroking of the palm of the infant's hand elicits mouth opening, eye closing, head moving forward and centering on the sagital midline. May also be seen in older individuals with frontal lobe damage and as such represents one of several "frontal release" signs.

Bacteremia. The presence of bacteria in the blood.

Band, orthodontic. A thin strip of metal closely adapted to the crown of a tooth.

Basal arch. The arch formed by the configuration of the corpus mandibular or maxillaries itself. It is the archical measurement of the apical base, and whose dimension would probably be unaltered by the loss of all the permanent teeth and the resorption of the alveolar processes.

Basal bone. (See apical base)

Basion. The most inferior, posterior point on the anterior margin of the foramen magnum.

Bias. Deviation of results from the truth.

Bias, information. A flaw in measuring exposure or outcome data that results in a different quality of information between comparison groups.

Bias, selection. Error due to systematic differences in characteristics between those who take part in a study and those who do not.

Bioactive factors. Molecules such as cell adhesion peptides or proteins, polypeptide growth factors, and plasmid DNA that elicit a biological response, and are typically used to induce a specified cell activity.

Bioactivity. A measure of the ability of a delivered molecule to elicit its intended biological response. This is typically influenced by the methods for encapsulation and delivery of the molecule.

Biologic width. Comprised of the supracrestal attachment apparatus from the crestal bone to the depth of the sulcus with an average length of 2.04 mm.

Bimaxillary dentoalveolar protrusion. The condition occurs when the anterior teeth of both jaws are positioned forward of the normal limits of the basal bone.

Bimaxillary dentoalveolar protrusion. The positioning of the entire dentition forward with respect to the facial profile.

Bimaxillary dentoalveolar retrusion. The anterior teeth of both jaws are posterior to the normal limits of the basal bone.

Bimaxillary prognathism (protrusion). Both jaws protrude forward of the normal limits of the face.

Bimaxillary protrusion. The excessive forward projection of both the maxilla and the mandible in relation to the cranial base.

Bimaxillary retrognathism (retrusion). Both jaws are posterior to the normal limits of the face.

Biologic age. The maturational age, or skeletal age, not the chronologic age.

Biteplate. A removable appliance that incorporates a plane of acrylic designed to occlude with the opposing anterior teeth.

Bite splint. Usually a removable acrylic appliance which is worn on the occlusal aspect of one arch to manage temporomandibular joint disorders, minimize trauma to the occlusion or reduce para-functional irritation to the orofacial musculature.

Bo (Bolton point). A cephalometric landmark; the most superior point in the upper curvature of the retrocondylar fossa. It is just posterior to the occipital condyle.

Bodily movement of a tooth. When force is applied through the center of resistance the tooth moves in a bodily fashion. All parts move the same amount in the same direction.

Body image. Refers to adolescents' mental conception of, and attitude toward, their physical appearance.

Body Mass Index (BMI). A measure of obesity in which a person's weight in kilograms is divided by one's height squared in meters.

Bolton Analysis (Discrepancy). A tooth size analysis named after its creator Wayne. Bolton, to measure the proportion of tooth size discrepancies in the mesial distal dimension between the maxillary and the mandibular teeth. Two analyses exist to measure either the anterior ratios (canine to canine) or the overall ration (permanent first molar to permanent first molar).

Bone. Mineralized animal tissue consisting of an organic matrix of cells and fibers of collagen impregnated with mineral matter, chiefly calcium phosphate and calcium carbonate.

Bone age, or skeletal age, or physiologic age. It is a radiographic evaluation of the hand, cervical spine foot to determine the extent of bone growth potential remaining for an individual. It compares favorably with height but not weight. Under 10 years of age, they do not correlate well to chronologic age, mental age, or dental age.

Bone Morphogenetic Proteins (BMPs). A class of proteins belonging to the transforming growth factor beta family having cartilage or bone-inducing potential.

B Point. The point most posterior to a line from Infradentale to Pogonion on the anterior surface of the symphyseal outline of the mandible. B Point should lie within the apical third of the incisor roots. When there is no curvature in this region and determination of B Point is not possible by the above method, it is chosen with the aid of preceding or succeeding films because erupting teeth obscure mandibular concavity on occasion.

Breathing reflex. An involuntary physical response that ensures that the infant has an adequate supply of oxygen and discharges carbon dioxide.

Branchial. Bar-like, developmentally resembling the gills of a fish.

Brachycephalic. (Euryprosopic) A description of an individual that has a larger than average cranial width and usually presents with a broad square head shape and a low mandibular plane angle. (Having a cephalic index of 81.0-85.4). It is the opposite of dolichocephalic.

Brachyfacial. Individual that has a a broad square face with a strong chin, flat lip posture, low mandibular plane and a straight profile.

Bracket. A small metal attachment that is soldered or welded to an orthodontic band or bonded directly to the teeth, serving to fasten that arch wire to the band or tooth.

Bruxism. A habit of grinding, clenching, or clamping the teeth, usually during the sleeping hours. The force so generated may damage both teeth and/or supporting structures.

Buccal. Pertaining to or adjacent to the cheek. (Buccally, in the direction of the cheek).

Buccal crossbite, buccoversion, telescopic occlusion, or scissors bite. This occurs when the lingual cusps of the maxillary posterior teeth occlude completely buccally to the buccal cusps of the mandibular posterior teeth, frequently resulting in a functional shift of the mandible completely away from the affected area.

Buccoversion. The displacement of a tooth from the normal line of occlusion toward the cheek.

Bulimia nervosa. An eating disorder in which the person engages repeatedly in episodes of binge eating followed by purging through induced vomiting or the abuse of laxatives.

Bullying. The repeated, unprovoked, systematic effort to inflict harm on another person through physical, verbal, or social attack.

Bundle bone. Specialized bone lining the tooth socket into which the fibers of the periodontal ligament penetrate; synonymous with the radiographic term "lamina dura."

C

Callus. The hard, bonelike substance that develops between the ends of a fractured bone.

Cant. An inclination or tipping; a slope or set to one side.

Cast. (study or diagnostic) A positive replica of the form of the teeth and tissues made from an impression.

Cell-based approach. Tissue engineering approach in which cells are either transplanted directly (with or without a material carrier), or allowed to grow and form tissue for a period of time *in vitro* prior to implantation.

Cellular cementum. That part of the cementum that covers the apical half to two-thirds of the root of a tooth. It is usually opposed to a layer of acellular cementum. It contains cementocytes embedded in the calcified matrix.

Cementicles. Calcified spherical bodies composed of cementum, either lying free in the periodontal ligament, attached to the cementum or embedded in it.

Cementoblast. The connective tissue cell type responsible for the formation of cementum.

Cementocyte. A cell found in the lacunae of cellular cementum, from 8 mm to 15 mm in diameter with a wide variety of shapes from round to oval to flattened. Numerous cytoplasmic processes extend from its free surfaces.

Cementoenamel junction. Represents the boundary between enamel and cementum that lies at the cervix of the tooth. These two tissues may overlap or be slightly separated.

Center of the spheno-occipital synchondrosis. The midpoint of the cartilaginous union of the anterior end of the basilar portion of the occipital bone and the posterior surface of the body of the sphenoid bone. In cases where the synchondrosis is not readily apparent, it is located by comparison with either previous or subsequent cephalograms.

Central ray. The line or beam of x rays arising from the anode or source of radiation in an x ray machine, which is parallel to the horizon or is level.

Centric occlusion. A static reproducible position of the mandible in which there is maximal contact of the inclined planes of the opposing teeth with balanced, unstrained relationship in the temporomandibular articulation.

Centric Occlusion (CO). Mandibular position dictated by maximum and habitual intercuspation of the upper and lower teeth; variously referred to as intercuspal position (IC), habitual centric, usual occlusal position. The condylar position may or may not be in harmony with centric relation (CR). Because of this, the term habitual occlusion is preferable. Historically, a gnathologic and articulator oriented term.

Centric Relation (CR). A gnathologic term, signifying optimal condyle-articular eminence-glenoid fossa relationships, determined by muscle balance and not by tooth intercuspation. Changing concepts no longer accept the most retruded, rear-most or hinge-axis definition, originally derived from prosthetic articulators. To the orthodontist, the condylar position can vary somewhat, but is generally recognized as high on the posterior surface of the articular eminence. Lack of harmony of centric occlusion and centric relation status is particularly important in diagnosis of TMD problems.

Cephalic index. An anthropometric ratio of head width to head length. Cephalic index = Maximum head width*100/ (maximum head length).

Cephalometric analysis. The process by which one evaluates the relationship between the soft tissue, teeth, and skeleton; an attempt to measure geometrically the form and growth of the face in a manner that more readily provides comparisons to known standards or idealized norms. These analyses afford the clinician the ability to diagnose abnormalities in craniofacial form and growth, plan orthodontic treatment goals, predict craniofacial growth, and assess the results of orthodontic treatment.

Cephalometric analysis. A study or analysis of the skeletal and dental relationships used in orthodontic case analysis, as calculated from cephalograms.

Cephalometer (cephalostat). An instrument for positioning the head to produce oriented, reproducible, lateral and posteroanterior, submentovertex, oblique or anteroposterior headfilms.

Cephalometrics, cephalometry. Measurements of the craniofacial structures, either directly on the skull, or through the use of oriented, reproducible lateral and posteroanterior (PA, etc.) roentgenograms. The measurement of the bones of the cranium utilizing a fixed, reproducible position for the exposure of lateral anteroposterior skull roentgenograms. Study of the measurements of the head using specific reference points.

Cephalometric radiograph. (roentgenogram, cephalogram, head film or image) An x-ray image of the anatomic structures of the head with precise reproducible positioning of the film and x-ray source.

Cephalometric tracing. A tracing of the teeth, facial bones, and anthropometric landmarks made directly from a cephalometric radiograph and used as a basis for a cephalometric analysis.

Cephalometry. The science of measuring the head in living individuals.

Cervical appliance. An extraoral appliance that uses the back of the neck for anchorage or as a base for traction.

Cervical headgear. An extraoral device or headgear used to control anchorage where a heavy wire attaches to bracket tubes on the permanent first molars and a neck strap is attached adjacent to the cervical spine. This device tends to erupt first molar and move them distally.

Child abuse. Deliberate actions that are harmful to a child's well-being.

Child maltreatment. Intentional harm to, or avoidable endangerment of, anyone under age 18 years.

Child neglect. Failure to appropriately meet a child's basic needs.

Chin cap. An extraoral appliance applying pressure to the chin, designed to exert an upward and backward force on the mandible.

Circumferential sulcus fiberatomy. Surgical excision of the free gingival fibers and the transceptal fibers to reduce rotational relapse.

Chlorohexidine. A prescription mouth rinse used to lower bacteria counts in dental plaque manufactured by Procter and Gamble called Peridex.

Chondrocranium. Cartilaginous skull; the embryonic skull before ossification.

Chronologic age. Record of time elapsed since birth.

Cleft lip. A congenital facial malformation characterized by non-fusion of the embryologic processes that form the lip, usually of the upper lip in the area of the lateral incisor(s).

Cleft palate. A congenital fissure of the soft and/or hard palate, either partial or complete, that may extend between the premaxilla and lateral maxillary processes.

Clinical crown. That portion of the crown exposed above the gingiva and visible in the oral cavity.

Clinical eruption. Emergence into the oral cavity of the crown of a tooth, and is the portion of the crown which can be observed clinically.

Clinoid processes. The lesser wings of the sphenoid at the superior surface of the Sella Turcica.

Clivus. The portion of the cranial base from Sella to Basion.

Closed bite. Excessive vertical overlap of the anterior teeth.

Collagen. White fibers of the periodontal ligament, tendon, skin or other connective tissue. A fiber is composed of fibrils bound together with interfibrillar cement. The fibrils, in turn, are formed from ultramicroscopic filaments. An albuminoid found in connective tissue, bone and cartilage and notable for high content of the amino acids glycine, proline, and hydroxyproline.

Collagen fiber. A high molecular weight protein composed of a number of structural types that vary in diameter from less than 1μ m to about 12 mm and are usually arranged in bundles.

Columella of the nose. The anterior, lower part of the nasal septum.

Compact bone. Hard external, more highly calcified than the cancellous portion of bone.

Complete clefts. Cleft of the primary and secondary palates characterized by complete separation of the tissue parts.

Complete crossbite. Found when all the teeth in one arch are positioned either inside or outside to all the teeth in the opposing arch.

Complete mandibular buccal crossbite. Present when all the mandibular teeth are buccally positioned to all the maxillary teeth if the mandibular arch is wider than the maxillary arch.

Complete mandibular lingual crossbite. Present when all the mandibular teeth are lingually positioned to the maxillary teeth due to a narrower mandibular arch than the maxillary arch.

Complete maxillary buccal crossbite. Occurs when all the maxillary teeth are buccally positioned to the mandibular teeth.

Complete maxillary palatal crossbite. Present when all the maxillary teeth are palatal to the mandibular arch.

Comprehensive orthodontic therapy. Treatment usually utilizes fixed orthodontic appliances. Adjunctive procedures such as extractions, maxillofacial surgery, nasopharyngeal surgery, myofunctional or speech therapy and restorative or periodontal care, may be coordinated disciplines. Treatment may incorporate several phases with specific objectives at various stages of dentofacial development.

Conductive approach. A tissue engineering approach in which a material construct is implanted into a physiological location and designed to encourage conduction of tissue-forming cells onto itself.

Condylar plane. Condylion- Orbitale. CO-OR.

Condyle. Rounded surface at the articular end of the mandible.

Condylion. The most posterior superior point on the curvature of the average of the right and left outlines of the condylar head. Determined as the point of tangency to a perpendicular construction line to the anterior and posterior borders of the condylar head. The CO point is, therefore, located as the most superior axial point of the condylar head rather than as the most superior point on the condyle.

Congenital anomalies. Developmental defects existing at or dating from birth.

Confounding. Distortion of the estimated effect of an exposure on an outcome, caused by the presence of an extraneous factor associated both with the exposure and the outcome.

Controls, friend. Persons used as comparison who are friends of cases.

Controls, hospital. Persons used for comparison who are drawn from the population of patients in a hospital.

Controls, neighborhood. Persons used for comparison who live in the same locality as cases and, therefore, may resemble cases on environmental and socioeconomic criteria.

Coronoid process. The most superior point of on the average of the right and left outlines of the coronoid process. Determined as the point of tangency to a perpendicular drawn to the plane of the anterior border of the ramus.

Correction of crossbite. Orthodontic or orthopedic treatment designed to address abnormal buccolingual or labiolingual interdigitation of teeth.

Cranial. Pertaining to the bones covering the brain on the superior end of the body.

Cranial base. The endochondral bone that forms the anteroinferior aspect of the brain case; lower portion of the skull consisting the floor of the cranial cavity. The bony support for the brain, separating the cranial from the facial region.

Cranial index. The relationship established by the measurement of the length of the cranium from the forehead to the back of the skull as compared with the width of the head between the ears.

Craniofacial. Relating to or involving both the cranium and the face.

Craniometry. The direct measurement of the head and dry skull and is used to arrive at the cranial index to classify the different head shapes found in a human population.

Craniosynostosis. Premature fusion of the sutures of the skull, usually occurring before birth and leads to deformity of the skull.

Crepitus. A grating or crackling sound or sensation.

Cribriform. Bone containing perforations or numerous foramina.

Crossbite. A malrelation between the maxillary and mandibular teeth when they occlude with the antagonistic tooth/teeth in an opposite relationship to normal due to labial, buccal, or lingual deviation of tooth position or to abnormal jaw position. They can involve one or more teeth and may be present in the anterior and/or the posterior teeth.

Crowding. The condition in which teeth have inadequate space for their normal alignment; they assume altered positions such as bunching of the teeth, overlapping, displacement in various directions, torsiversion, etc.

Curve of Spee. Vertical positions of the teeth in relation to the occlusal plane which take on the appearance of an arc or curve when laterally viewed.

D

Debanding (debonding). The removal of fixed orthodontic appliances.

Deciduous (Primary). Pertains specifically to the first dentition.

Deciduous dentition. Primary teeth or first-formed set of teeth that undergo exfoliation to provide space for the permanent teeth. Primary dentition is the preferred term.

Deglutition. The act of swallowing.

Degradable/Degradability. A biological material is said to be degradable if the material can be chemically degraded over a biologically relevant time scale. In tissue engineering it is desirable to tune the degradation time so that material degradation and new tissue formation occur in concert.

Demineralization. To remove minerals such as calcium or hydroxyapitate from dental enamel associated with poor oral hygiene; a disease state, not hypocalicification.

Dendrites. Nerve fiber extensions that receive the impulses transmitted from other neurons via their axons.

Dental arch. The relationship between the combined sizes of the crowns of the teeth as measured through the contact points of the teeth. This represents a balance between the muscle forces of the tongue and lips, the buccal wall functions, and the positions of the teeth.

Dental crossbite. A malocclusion with maxillary teeth occluding lingual to mandibular due to tipping of teeth as opposed to malposition of an entire skeletal maxillary segment(s).

Dental lamina. Thickened epithelial cells of odontogenic origin along the maxillary and mandibular arches. They begin as isolated areas and ultimately form a contiguous plate of epithelium evident in embryos at 37 days.

Dentigerous. Containing or bearing teeth (cyst, for example).

Determinant. Any factor, whether event, characteristic, or other definable entity, that brings about change in a health condition or other definite characteristic.

Development. Progress toward maturity; increase in complexity.

Developmental Language Disorders (DLD). Clinically heterogeneous group of disorders characterized by selective impairment of speech and/or language development, with relative sparing of other developmental domains.

Developmental spacing. Space found between the primary teeth, helpful in accommodating the difference in size of the erupting permanent teeth.

Diagnosis. The process of determining health status and the factors responsible for producing it.

Diagnostic or prognostic set-up. A three dimensional technique to visualize space concerns in the permanent dentition, which traditionally has involved cutting the teeth off a working cast and resetting them into a more desirable position.

Diastema (Diastemata). The space between two teeth in the dental arch. However, this term generally refers to the space found between the maxillary central incisors even though the more accurate term would be a maxillary midline diastema.

Differentiation. Growth associated with or having a distinguishing character or function from the surrounding structures or from the original type; specialization.

Digital image. An image composed of numbers derived from the 'on/off' or '0/1' procedures used for digital data.

Direct bonding. Adhesion of a bracket directly to the surface of a tooth.

Disease. A condition that alters or interferes with the normal state of an organism and is usually characterized by the abnormal functioning of one or more of the host's systems, parts or organs.

Disorder. Disturbance or departure from normal health function.

Distal. Away from the midline following the curvature of the dental arch.

Distoclusion or disto-occlusion. (Angle Class II) The occlusal relationship described by Dr. E.H.Angle where the mesio-buccal cusp of the maxillary permanent first molar occludes anteriorly to the buccal groove of the mandibular permanent first molar. Two types of this type of occlusion are defined (Division I and Division II) depending upon the angulation of the maxillary incisor teeth. Dr. Angle considered the term "disto-occlusion" to be an appropriate synonym for Class II since it suggested a distal positioning of the mandible (see Angle's classification).

Displacement. Change in position of a bone due to growth at its border or movement of an adjacent bone. Change in attachment when one element, radical, or molecule is removed and is replaced by another.

Distoversion. A tooth that is in the arch form but located farther from the midline of the face then it would normally be found.

Distraction osteogenesis. The formation of new bone caused by slow separation of surgically separated segments after nitial callus formation. The *de novo* formation of bone tissue between two vascular corticotomy surfaces undergoing gradual distraction.

Divergency. The divergency of the face can be determined by mentally drawing a line from Glabella to Pogonion and observing is relationship with Frankfort plane. When the angle is greater than 90 degrees, the face is considered to have an anterior divergency. When the angle is less than 90 degrees, the face is considered to have a posterior divergency.

Division. Angle Classification used to describe different anterior tooth alignments of Class II malocclusion.

Dolicocephalic. (Leptoprosopic) an individual that has a narrower cranial width and usually presents with a long narrow head shape and high mandibular plane angle opposite of brachycephalic. (Having a cephalic index of 75.9 or less).

Dolicofacial. An individual that is characterized by a long, narrow face with a high mandibular plane angle, convex profile, poor chin development, and an anterior-posterior face height imbalance.

Downs occlusal plane. Anterior Downs Point-Posterior Downs Point. ADP-PDP

Drift. Dental; the change in position of a tooth due to remodeling (apposition on one side and resorption on the other); movement of a tooth to a position of greater stability. Mesial drift refers to medial movement of a tooth or teeth anteriorly toward the midline.

Drug use. The ingestion of a drug, regardless of the amount or affect of ingestion.

Drug abuse. The ingestion of a drug to the extent that it impairs the user's well being.

DSM-IV. The fourth edition of the Diagnostic and Statistical Manual of Mental Disorders, developed by the American Psychiatric Association, the leading means of distinguishing various emotional and behavioral disorders.

Dysarthria. Articulation disorder refers to a physical dysfunction of the muscles of speech production.

Dyslexia. A learning disability in reading.

Dysmorphogenesis. Development of a structural defect.

Dysostosis. Defective formation of bone.

Dysplasia. Abnormality in development; disharmony between component parts. Frequently it is a result of an abnormality of growth and development.

E

Early mesial shift. The shift that can occur in the buccal segment at age six to seven years of age if the mandibular primate space is present, or other interdental spaces, so that during the eruption of the permanent first molars they can shift from an end to end relationship to a Class I relationship. It is not a common event.

Eccentric growth. Dental; process whereby one part of the developing tooth germ remains stationary, while the remainder continues to grow. This leads to a shift in its center.

Ectopic. A tooth that develops in or erupts into an abnormal position.

Ectopic eruption. Teeth erupting away from their normal positions are considered to be ectopic. This most likely involves the maxillary first molars and the incisors, although any tooth can be involved. Ectopic eruption can lead to premature resorption of adjacent primary teeth and loss of available arch length.

Edentulous. Without teeth, having lost the natural teeth.

Edgewise appliance. A fixed, multibanded/ bonded appliance using an attachment bracket developed by Dr. E.H. Angle. The bracket slot receives a rectangular arch wire horizontally which gives precise control in all three planes of space.

Environment. External factors interacting with the genotype.

Effect. The result of a cause.

Effect modification. A factor modifies the effect of a putative causal factor under study. Effect modification is detected by varying the selected effect measure for the factor under study across levels of another factor.

Efficiency. The effects or end results achieved in relation to the effort expended in terms of other factors such as time, money and resources.

Egocentrism. The tendency to perceive events and interpret experiences exclusively from one's own, self-centered perspective.

Elastic ligature. Threadlike material which stretches. May be tied from a tooth to an arch-wire or from tooth to tooth to gain movement of these units.

Electromyography. The recording of the electrical activity of muscles.

Emotional regulation. The ability to manage and modify one's feelings, particularly feelings of fear, frustration, and anger.

Enamel core. A structure connecting the enamel knot to the enamel navel.

Enamel knot (primary knot and secondary knots). A collection of epithelia cells associated with the inner enamel epithelium of the enamel organ of a developing tooth near the developing cusp tips. It is a transient structure responsible for the production of signaling molecules that control the development of both the enamel epithelium and papilla.

Endochondral. Relating to the type of formation of bone formed within cartilage and replacing it.

Endosseous implants. Implants that are embedded in bone and fixed throughout the entire length of the implant. The various implant types are screw, blade, and cylinder.

Enlargement. In cephalometry; the image of the head is enlarged, because the source of the x rays is a point from which the rays diverge. The farther the source is from the head, the less will be the enlargement, and the farther from the head the film is the more will be the enlargement.

Equilibrate. Modification of teeth by selective occlusal grinding to optimize occlusion.

Epigenetic. Embryonic development by gradual change. Interactions during embryonic development that alter the activity of genes without changing their stucture; events that are the inevitable consequences of genetic specification such as proteins, cell and tissue interactions.

Epidemiology. The study of distribution and determinants of health-related states or events in specified populations, and the application of this study to control of health problems.

Eruption. A developmental phenomenon that moves a tooth from its crypt position, through the alveolar process in a path that is not always straight, into the oral cavity and into occlusion with its antagonist. Appearance of teeth in the oral cavity; a stage coordinated with root growth and maturation of tissues surrounding the tooth.

E SPACE. The difference in mesiodistal width between the larger primary second molar and its successor (the second premolar). Usually it is limited to the lower e space with an average (+) 3 mm value. If it does occur, it is usually associated with late mesial shift. The maxillary e space is not commonly used and is less, at an average of (+) 1.5 mm.

Esthetic lines, or E-lines, for both the upper and lower lips. The esthetic line or plane is drawn from the tip of the nose to soft tissue pogonion. Perpendicular distances are measured in millimeter ($\pm$ 0.5 mm) from the most prominent points on the upper and lower lips to the E-line. If the lips are ahead of this line, the value is positive. If the lips are behind this line, the value is negative. The normal adult upper E-line value ranges from (-) 2 mm to (-) 4 mm while the normal adult lower E-line ranges measurements from 0 mm to (-) 2 mm. In general, males have more negative values than females. The significance relates the position of the lips to the nose and chin. A larger chin usually creates a more esthetic balance than from a larger nose.

Etiology. Causative or circumstance agent of medical or dental conditions.

Ethmoid registration point. Intersection of the phenoidal plane with the right and left averaged upper outline of the greater sphenoid wing.

Eustachian tube. A bony and cartilaginous tube connecting the middle ear with the nasopharynx and whose function is to equalize air pressure on both sides of the tympanic membrane.

Exfoliate. To shed or eliminate something, such as scales from the surface of the body, or loss of teeth from the jaws.

Exposure. Factor to which a group or individual was exposed.

Exposure odds ratio. The ratio of the odds in favor of exposure among the cases to the odds in favor of exposure among the controls.

External auditory meatus. The passage leading from the opening of the external ear to the eardrum.

Extrafusal fibers. The contractile cells of muscles.

Extrusion (vertical). The overeruption or migration of the tooth beyond its normal occlusal position.

F

Facial angle. It is the inferior-posterior angle between facial plane (N-Pog) and Frankfort horizontal. It naturally increases with growth and development. The norm adult value is 90 degrees $\pm$ 4 degrees. This measurement represents the anteroposterior divergence of the chin in relation to the face. A small facial angle represents a retrognathic and/or small mandibular corpus while a large facial angle represents a prognathic and/or large corpus or chin. The skeletal facial angle is smaller than the soft tissue facial angle by an average of 3 degrees.

Facial asymmetry. A reduction of similarity or proportion between the right and left sides of the face or the craniofacial skeleton.

Facial midline. The line that is considered to be a line drawn perpendicular to the interpupillary line from Glabella to the tip of the nose, passing through the midpoint of the philtrum of the upper lip, and the midline of the chin.

Factor. An event, characteristic, or other definable entity that brings about a change in a health condition or other defined outcome.

Fibroblasts. A cell type that is elongated, ovoid, spindle shaped or flattened and found in connective tissue or periodontium and forms or destroys connective tissue fibers.

First order positions (horizontal). The faciolingual or buccolingual relationship of the crown of a tooth to the line of occlusion as described by Dr. E.H. Angle. This is also casually referred to an "in-out" position.

Fine motor skills. Physical abilities that require precise, small movements, such as tying shoes.

Finishing. A stage of treatment toward the end of comprehensive orthodontic care in which the teeth are placed in their final detailed positions.

Fontanel. Any of the spaces located at the junction of the coronal, frontal and sagittal sutures which are closed by membranous and cartilaginous structures between the uncompleted angles of these bones and the neighboring bones of a fetal or young skull.

Force. Implied exertion of power causing a tooth or other object to move against resistance.

Forced eruption. Orthodontic movement of a tooth in coronal (vertical) direction through the application of continuous forces to cause changes in the architecture of the soft tissue and bone.

Frankfort plane. – Porion – Orbitale. PO- OR.

Free gingiva. That portion of the gingiva that surrounds the tooth and is not directly attached to the tooth surface; the outer wall of the gingival sulcus.

Frenectomy. The surgical removal or repositioning of a frenum. Performed to enhance the stability of a corrected diastema or to alleviate a tongue-tie.

Freeway space. Interocclusal clearance when the mandible is at physiologic resting position. (See postural resting position)

Frenum. Midline fold of mucous membrane that limits movement of an organ or part.

> **Labial.** The band of tissue which passes from the inside of the lip to a point midway between the central incisors.

> **Lingual.** The band of tissue which passes from under the tongue to the lingual aspect of the midpoint of the lower jaw.

Frontal cephalometric radiograph. A posterior anterior cephalometric radiograph taken with the subject oriented in the cephalometer.

Frontal plane. (Coronal plane) an imaginary plane that passes longitudinally through the body perpendicular to the median plane dividing the head into the back and front.

Frontomaxillary nasal suture. The junction of the frontal, maxillary, and nasal bones.

Functional crossbite. Occurs when there is an occlusal interference that requires the mandible to shift either anteriorly and/or laterally in order to achieve maximum occlusion.

Functional corrector. A removable orthodontic appliance, utilizing oral and facial muscle forces to move teeth and possibly change relationship of dental arches, as developed by Frankel.

Functional jaw orthopedics. Utilization of muscle forces to effect changes in jaw position and tooth alignment by removable appliances (See activator).

Functional occlusal plane. Premolar Mesial Contact Point- Upper Molar Distal Cusp Tip.

Furcation. An anatomic area of multirooted tooth where the individual roots leave the common root stock.

Fusion. A union by or as if by melting together.

G

Gag reflex. Present at birth. Level of sensitivity is variable between individuals but tends to decrease with age. Stimulus to the posterior 1/4 to 3/4 of the tongue or the posterior pharyngeal wall elicits constriction and elevation of the pharynx.

Gateway drugs. Drugs - usually tobacco, alcohol, and marijuana - whose use increases the risk that a person will later use "harder drugs".

Gene mapping. Identification of the chromosomal location of an individual gene.

Generalizability. A study is generalizable if it can produce unbiased inferences beyond the subjects in the study.

Genetic. Relating to genetics or ontogenesis.

Genioplasty. A surgical procedure performed either intra- or extra-orally to correct deformities in the area of the mandibular symphysis.

Genome mapping. A research program designed to identify the chromosomal location of all genes in the genome of a particular species.

Genotype. The genetic make-up or constitution of an individual organism.

Gingiva. The soft tissue surrounding the necks of teeth. It is composed of two parts; the masticatory mucosa, which faces the oral cavity, and the sulcular (crevicular) epithelium, which faces the cheeks and the attachment epithelium facing the tooth. The gingiva is composed of fibrous tissue covered by mucous membrane, and it covers the alveolar processes of the maxilla and mandible.

Gingival sulcus. The shallow V-shaped trench around each tooth bounded by the tooth surface on one surface and the epithelial-lined free margin on the other.

Gingivectomy. The surgical excision of excessive unattached gingival tissue.

Gingivo-labial sulcus. The tissue trough between the lips and the alveolus.

Glabella. The height of curvature of the bone overlying the frontal sinus. In cases where this point is not readily apparent, the overlying soft tissue is used to locate it.

Glenoid fossa. The depression in each lateral wall of the skull with which the mandible articulates.

Glossectomy. Excision or amputation of a segment or all of the tongue.

Gnathion. The most anterior-inferior point on the contour of the bony chin symphysis. Determined by bisecting the angle formed by the mandibular plane and a line through Pogonion and Nasion.

Gnathology. The study of functional and occlusal relations of the teeth.

Go (gonion). A cephalometric landmark; the most outward point of the mandibular angle at the junction of the ramus and body.

Golgi tendon organs. Sensory endings in the tendons of muscles.

Gonial angle. Angle between the lower border and posterior ramus of the mandible.

Gonial intersection. The intersection of the mandibular plane with a plane through articulare, posterior and along the portion of the mandibular ramus inferior to it.

Gonion. The midpoint of the angle of the mandible. Found by bisecting the angle formed by the mandibular plane and a plane through articulare posterior and along the portion of the mandibular ramus inferior to it.

Goodness of fit. The match between the child's temperamental pattern and the demands of the environment.

Gross motor skills. Physical abilities that demand large body movements, such as climbing, jumping, or running.

Growth. Increase in size.

Growth factors. Chemical substances that induce cells to initial DNA synthesis.

Guided Tissue Regeneration (GTR). Approach to new tissue formation in which cells involved in formation of the tissue of interest are encouraged to conduct onto a degradable or non-degradable material construct, while cells that interfere with the process of tissue formation are intentionally excluded from the region.

Guidance of eruption. The process of removing or discing primary teeth in the transitional dentition to relieve minor clinical crowding. These cases are associated with non-extraction therapy of succedaneous teeth. Crossbites and openbites need to be resolved along with this process. Conservation of mandibular arch perimeter is very important with space maintenance and prevention of late mesial shift or loss of mandibular e space. Permanent teeth should not be disced on their proximal surfaces in the transitional dentition.

H

Hard palate. Anterior part of the palate, forming the roof of the mouth, consisting of the bony palate covered above by the respiratory mucosa of the floor of the nose and below by the keratinized stratified squamous oral mucosa of the roof of the mouth. The hard palate contains palatine vessels and nerves, adipose tissue, and mucous glands.

Haversian bone. Compact bone containing tubular channels with blood vessels, nerves, and bone cells with concentrically located lacunae that are termed the Haversion system or osteon.

Hawley retainer. A removable wire and acrylic appliance used as a stabilizing appliance or, with modifications, to move teeth.

Headfilm. An oriented, reproducible cephalometric film.

Headgear. A removable extraoral appliance used as a source of traction to apply force to the teeth and jaws.

Healthy worker effect. A phenomenon observed initially in studies of occupational diseases. Workers usually exhibit lower overall death rates than the general population, because the severely ill and chronically disabled are ordinarily excluded from employment.

Hemifacial. Involving or affecting one lateral half of the face.

Homeobox-containing genes. Regulatory genes that contain a highly conserved motif (the homeobox) encoding a DNA-binding domain (homeodomain). One type of homeobox-containing genes are the Hox genes.

Homeobox genes. A class of highly conserved DNA sequences involved in the control of development, spatial orientation and patterning. A gene that manifests itself at an early stage of development.

Hyalinization. The result of compression of the periodontal ligament in which all the vascularity and most cells are lost from the zone, creating a glass-like appearance. As a result, tooth movement will cease.

Hypernasal. Incomplete seal between the velum and the posterior pharyngeal wall during a plosive sound resulting in air escaping through the nose. "Cleft palate speech."

Hyperteliorism. Excessive width between two bodily parts or organs (as with the eyes.)

Hyperdivergent skeletal pattern. A pattern in which there is an excessive divergence of the skeletal planes.

Hypodivergent skeletal pattern. A skeletal pattern in which the skeletal planes are more parallel to each other.

Hypodontia (oligodontia). (See oligodontia).

Hypophyseal fossa. (See Sella Turcica).

Hypoplasia. A condition of arrested development in which an organ or part remains below the normal size or in an immature state.

Hypothesis. A supposition arrived at from observation or reflection, that leads to refutable predictions.

I

Iatrogenic. An adverse condition resulting from the activities of a health professional's therapeutic effort.

Idiopathic root resorption. Root resorption of unknown cause.

Immunoglobulins. Serum proteins that function as antibodies and are responsible for humoral immunity.

Impaction. Position of a tooth in the alveolus so that it is incapable of eruption into the oral cavity. Impaction may be due to crowding of teeth that results in a lack of available space for eruption. Teeth being driven into the alveolar process or surrounding tissues as a result of trauma.

Impaction of the bony segments. The resultant alignment of maxillary arches in the cleft lip and palate when the lateral segment(s) are close and trapped behind the premaxillary segment.

Incidence rate. The rate at which new events occur in a population. The numerator is the number of new events that occur in a defined period; the denominator is the population at risk of experiencing the event during this period, sometimes expressed as person-time.

Incisal papilla. The elevation of attached, palatal, mucosal tissue covering the foramen of the incisive or nasopalatine canal located along the midsagittal plane of the palate.

Incisive foramen. The oral opening of the incisive canal behind the maxillary central incisors through which exit the nasopalatine nerve and a branch of the greater palatine artery.

Incisor liability. The mesiodistal width differences between the smaller primary incisors and the larger permanent incisors as a group of four.

This liability is more in the maxilla and more in boys. Maxillary incisor liability in girls averages (-) 6.5 mm and in boys (-) 7.5 mm. Mandibular incisor liability in girls averages (-) 5.0 mm and in boys (-) 5.5 mm.

Incomplete clefts. Cleft of the primary and secondary palates characterized by the presence of a tissue bridge located anywhere along the cleft.

Induction period. The period required for a specific disease to produce the disease in a host.

Inductive approach. Tissue engineering approach in which bioactive factors, either soluble or surface immobilized, are introduced into a physiological location in order to induce a desired biological response, i.e., tissue formation.

Inductive factors. Bioactive factors that are intended to induce the formation of a particular tissue.

Inferior zygoma. The lowest point on the average of the right and left outlines of the zygoma.

Infradentale. The anterior superior point on the mandible at its labial contact with the mandibular central incisor.

Infraorbital ridge. The bony border beneath the orbit.

Infraversion. A tooth that has not erupted to the occlusal plane.

Insecure attachment. Characterized by the infant's fear, anger, or seeming indifference toward the caregiver.

Intercanine width. The linear measurement taken across the arch between the canines.

Intercuspation. The buccal interlocking of the teeth; the cusp-to-fossa relation of the maxillary and mandibular posterior teeth to each other.

Interdisciplinary treatment. Treatment that involves more than one specialty in dentistry.

Interincisal angle (angle U1 to LI or 1/1). It is the posterior angle between of the long axes of the root of the maxillary and mandibular central incisors. The adult norm is 135 degrees $\pm$ 10 degrees. The preschool intercisal angle of primary incisors (a/a) averages 150 degrees. As the incisors become more proclined, the intercisal angle decreases while if the incisors become more upright as with Class II division 2 malocclusions the interincisal angle becomes larger.

Intermolar width. The linear measurement taken across the arch between the first molars.

Intermaxillary. Between the arches, from one arch to the other.

Intermaxillary elastics. The use of elastic traction between the upper and lower teeth.

Interocclusal clearance. (See freeway space, and postural resting position)

Intrafusal fibers. (See "Muscle spindles").

Intramaxillary elastic traction. The use of elastic traction within the same arch to achieve space closure.

Intramembranous bone. Bone formation within or between connective-tissue membranes. It does not replace cartilage as does endochondral bone.

Instrumental aggression. An action whose purpose is to obtain or retain an object desired by another.

IQ tests. Aptitude tests, which were originally designed to yield a measure of intelligence, calculated as mental age divided by chronological age, multiplied by 100.

Irregularity index. Determined by measuring the linear displacement of the anatomic contact points of each mandibular incisor from the respective points of the adjacent teeth and the sum of these displacements represents the relative degree of anterior irregularity.

J

JackscreW. A threaded device used in appliances for the movement of teeth or arch segments.

K

Key ridge (Zygomaxillare). A cephalometric landmark; the most inferior point on the zygomatic ridge.

Kohlberg's Level of Moral Reasoning. Kohlberg's first level of moral reasoning, preconventional moral reasoning, emphasizes obedience to authority in order to avoid punishment (stage 1) and being nice to other people so they will be nice to you (stage 2). (Kohlberg's second level of moral reasoning, conventional moral reasoning, emphasizes winning the approval of others (stage 3) and obeying the laws set down by those in power (stage 4). Kohlberg's third level, postconventional moral reasoning, emphasizes the social and contractual nature of moral principles (stage 5) and the existence of universal ethical principles (stage 6). Compared with boys and men, girls and women are more likely to develop a morality of care that is based on comparison, nurturance, and concern for the well-being of others. Compared with girls and women, boys and men are more likely to develop a morality of justice based on depersonalized standards of right and wrong.

L

Labial. Of or pertaining to the lip. (Labially, facing or in the direction of the lips.)

Lability. Rapidly changing emotions, emotional instability, emotions that are inordinately changeable.

Labioversion. Used to describe an incisor or canine that is outside the arch form and is located toward the lips.

Lamina dura. Radiogaphic term describing the hard compact bone layer lining the dental alveoli.

Late mesial shift. The shift that can occur in the buccal segment at age 11 to 14 years, independent of the incisor liability resolution, with the mandibular e space used as the permanent first molar shifting from an end to end relationship to Class I. It does not always occur. Mesial shift of the permanent first molar into the normally excessive posterior leeway space following eruption of the permanent cuspid and the premolars.

/1 to APog (LI to A-Pog line). a distance in millimeter (+ 0.5 mm). It is measured from the incisal edge or tip of the most facial mandibular incisor to the line from point A to pogonion. If the edge of the incisor is ahead of the line, it is a positive value. If the edge is behind the line, it is a negative value. The normal adult is 0 mm to (+) 1 mm with a range from (-) 2 mm to (+) 3 mm. It indicates the protrusion of the lower incisor relative to the lower third of the face. It is an indicator of the stability of the lower incisor after treatment. Class III malocclusions naturally give an unusually high value.

/1 to NB (LI to NB). in degrees and millimeters. It is the inferior-posterior angle between N-B line and the long axis of the root of the most facial mandibular permanent central incisor ($\pm$ 1 degrees with $\pm$ 0.5 degrees error of measurement). The adult norm is 25 degrees $\pm$ 3 degrees. It indicates the inclination of the mandibular incisor relative to the mandible. The distance of /1 to NB is a millimeter measure ($\pm$ 0.5 mm) of procumbency from the most facial surface of the mandibular incisor to N-B line. The adult norm is (+) 4 mm $\pm$ 2 mm. It indicates the relative forward (procumbent) or backward (retrocumbent) positioning of the mandibular incisor to N-B line. If the incisor is ahead of N-B line, the value is preceded by a plus or positive sign while if it is posterior, it is negative. A negative value rarely occurs.

Lateral cephalometric headfilm. An oriented reproducible lateral headfilm of the head.

Learning disability. A difficulty in a particular cognitive skill that is not attributable to an overall intellectual slowness, a physical handicap, a severely stressful living condition, or a lack of basic education.

Leeway space (posterior). The difference in size between the primary canines and molars and their permanent successors. The average leeway space in the maxilla is 1.3 mm per side and in the mandible is 3.1 mm per side.

Leveling and alignment. The initial phase of comprehensive orthodontic treatment using fixed appliances designed to change the line of intercuspation from a curve to a straight line; to align the teeth in the same plane.

Levels of Knowledge:

In-depth. A thorough knowledge of concepts and theories for the purpose of critical analysis and the synthesis of more complete understanding.

Understanding. Adequate knowledge with the ability to apply.

Familiarity. A simplified knowledge for the purposes of orientation and recognition of general principles.

Levels of Skill:

Proficient. The level of skill beyond competency. It is that level of skill acquired through advanced training or the level of skill attained when a particular activity is accomplished with repeated quality and a more efficient utilization of time.

Competent. The level of skill displaying special ability or knowledge derived from training and experience.

Exposed. The level of skill attained by observation of or participation in a particular activity.

Ligature. A wire or other material used to secure an orthodontic attachment or tooth to an arch wire.

Limited tooth movement. Tooth movement not involving the entire dentition. It may be directed at the only existing problem, or at only one aspect of a larger problem in which a decision is made to defer or forgo more comprehensive therapy.

Lingual. Relating to or associated with the tongue; on the tongue side of a tooth or bone.

Lingual crossbite. The lingual displacement of the mandibular affected tooth or teeth as it relates to the antagonistic tooth or teeth.

Lingual symphyseal point. A constructed point used to determine symphyseal width at Pogonion. The SYMP Point is located at the intersection of a construction line through Pogonion and parallel with the mandibular plane with the posterior border of the mandibular symphysis.

Linguoclusion or linguoversion. An occlusion in which a tooth or group of teeth have lingual position with respect to normal; used to describe a tooth that is inside the arch form and located toward the tongue.

Lip incompetence. The inability of the patient to have the lips contacting in the rest position without showing any muscular strain.

Lip line. The amount of tooth and/or gingival tissue that is exposed at rest.

Lower incisor apex. The root tip of the mandibular central incisor. When the root is not yet completed the midpoint of the growing root tip is marked.

Lower incisor incisal edge. The incisal tip of the mandibular central incisor.

Lower incisor lingual bony contact point. The lingual contact of alveolar bone with the mandibular central incisor. Generally corresponds with the lingual CEJ.

Lower molar distal CEJ. The posterior cemento-enamel junction of the mandibular first molar.

Lower molar distal contact point. The posterior contact point of the mandibular first molar.

Lower molar distal cusp tip. The posterior cusp tip of the mandibular first molar.

Lower molar mesial CEJ. The anterior cementoenamal junction of the mandibular first molar.

Lower molar mesial contact. The mesial contact or height of contour of the mandibular first molar relative to the functional occlusal plane.

Lower molar mesial cusp tip. The anterior cusp tip of the mandibular first molar.

M

Macroglossia. Enlargement of the tongue, usually due to local lymphangiectasia or to muscular hypertrophy; megaloglossia; pathological and commonly congenital enlargement of the tongue.

Macrognathia. Excessive size of the jaw.

Malalignment. The displacement of a tooth or teeth from a normal position in the dental arch.

Malocclusion. A deviation from the accepted relation of teeth. Abnormality in the coming together of the teeth; a deviation in the relationship of the teeth within or between the dental arches that impacts or has the potential to impact the dental, physical or psychological well being of an individual.

Mandible. Horseshoe-shaped bone forming the lower jaw and articulating, by its upturned extremities, the condyles, with the temporal bone on either side. The mandible is composed of the body and the ramus that is located posteriorly. The body includes the alveolar process that contains the teeth.

Mandibular dental midline. Determined by drawing a line from the proximal contacts of the central incisors perpendicular to the mandibular occlusal plane and noting its relationship with the facial midline, the maxillary dental midline, and the midline of the chin.

Mandibular dentoalveolar retrusion. (Retrognathism) the anterior teeth of the lower jaw are posterior to the normal limits of the basal bone.

Mandibular dentoalveolar protrusion. (Prognathism) the lower anterior teeth are positioned forward of the normal limits of the basal bone.

Mandibular plane. Menton – Gonial Intersection. ME-GOI.

Mandibular prognathism. (Protrusion) the lower jaw protrudes forward of the normal limits of the face.

Mandibular primate space. The space in the arch between the mandibular primary canine and the mandibular primary first molar. If present, it assists in early mesial shift from end to end permanent first molar toward a Class I molar relationship.

Mandibular retrognathism. (Retrusion) the lower jaw is posterior to the normal limits of the face.

Mastery play. Any form of play in which a skill is practiced until one is proficient at it.

Mastication. Process of chewing food in preparation for swallowing and digestion.

Maxillary dental midline. Determined by drawing a line perpendicular to the maxillary occlusal plane through the proximal contacts of the central incisors and noting its relationship to the philtrum of the upper lip.

Maxillary dentoalveolar Retrusion. retrognathism) the anterior teeth of the upper jaw are posterior to the normal limits of the basal bone.

Maxillary primate space. The space in the arch between the maxillary primary canine and the maxillary primary lateral incisor. If present, it assists in resolution of maxillary incisor liability.

Maxillary prognathism. (Protrusion) the upper jaw protrudes forward of the normal limits of the face.

Maxillary retrognathism. (Retrusion) the upper jaw is posterior to the normal limits of the face.

Maxillary sinus. Paired sinus cavities occupying the space beneath the floor of the orbit and above the roots of the posterior maxillary teeth.

Maxillofacial. Of, relating to, treating or affecting the maxilla and the face.

Me (menton). A cephalometric landmark; the most inferior point on the symphysis of the mandible, as seen on the lateral cephalometric roentgenogram.

Mechanotherapy. Orthodontic treatment by mechanical forces, acting on the dentofacial complex.

Meckel's cartilage. The initial skeletal component of the first pharyngeal arch. It is the supporting cartilage of the mandibular arch in the embryo.

Median plane. (midsagittal plane) An imaginary plane that passes longitudinally through the middle of the head and divides it into right and left halves.

Mental retardation. A pervasive and permanent delay in cognitive development.

Menton. The most inferior point on the symphyseal outline.

Mesenchyme. Loose, undifferentiated embryonic type of connective tissue that is usually of mesodermal origin but is a mixture of mesodermal and neural-crest derivatives in the head and neck region.

Mesial drift. An inherent disposition of teeth to drift mesially even before they are in occlusion; gradual movement of a tooth or teeth anteriorly toward the midline.

Mesiocclusion or mesio-occlusion. (Angle Class III) The occlusal relationship described by Dr. E. H.Angle where the mesio-buccal cusp of the maxillary permanent first molar occludes distally to the buccal groove of the mandibular permanent first molar. Dr. Angle considered the term "mesio-occlusion" to be an appropriate synonym for Class III since it suggested a mesial positioning of the mandible.

Mesiodens. A supernumerary tooth appearing in an erupted or unerupted state between the two maxillary central incisors.

Mesioversion. A tooth that is in the arch form but located nearer the midline of the face then it would normally be found.

Mesocephalic. (Mesoprosopic) an individual that falls between the brachycephalic and dolicocephalic pattern and has an average cranial width whose facial features appear well balanced in all of the orientation planes (having a cephalic index between 76.0 and 80.9).

Micrognathia. An abnormally small jaw.

Microsomia. Abnormal smallness of the body.

Microglossia. Smallness of tongue.

Migration. Movement of a tooth or teeth out of normal position.

Mixed dentition (transitional dentition). The state of possessing primary and secondary teeth simultaneously.

Mixed dentition space analysis or mixed dentition analysis. A method to evaluate the amount of space available in the arch for succeeding permanent teeth and for any necessary occlusal adjustments.

Monobloc. (See activator).

Morphogenesis. The development process that creates the shape and form of an organ. The branching process that occurs during salivary-gland development is an example of morphogenesis.

Motor unit. A contractile unit of muscle consisting of a single axon and the muscle fibers it innervates.

Mouth guard. An elastoplastic removable appliance, used to protect teeth and investing tissues in contact sports.

Mu. Greek unit designating the scientific notation of one an one-millionths, 10^{-6} of the metric unit of a meter.

Multidisciplinary. An approach to treatment involving many and varied health professionals.

Muscle fiber. A mature, contractile muscle cell in which the nuclei are situated immediately under the cell membrane.

Muscle spindles (intrafusal fibers). Muscle fibers modified for sensing the stretch in muscles.

Myelination. The process in which axons are coated with myelin, a fatty substance that speeds neural communication.

Myelin The insulating substance of nerve fibers formed by layers of cell membrane wrapped around nerve fibers and formed by Schwann cells.

Myoblasts. Mononucleated cells which will fuse together to the contractile cells of muscle.

Myofascial Of or relating to the fascia of muscles as origin of pain.

Myofunctional. The role of muscle function in the etiology or correction of orthodontic problems.

Myosin. The contractile filament in muscle cells that contains myosin ATPase.

Myosin ATPase. The enzyme involved in converting ATP into AMP, which provides the energy required for muscle contraction.

Myotubes. Immature contractile muscle cells in which the nuclei are lined up in the center of the cell.

Null mutation. Both alleles for a specific gene locus are non-functioning or inactive ("double knockout").

N

O

Na (Nasion). A cephalometric landmark; the junction of the nasal and frontal bones as seen on the profile of the cephalometric roentgenogram.

Nasion. The junction of the frontonasal suture at the most posterior point on the curve at the bridge of the nose.

Naris. One of the orifices of the nasal cavity; nostril. May be the anterior internal or posterior naris.

Nasopharynx. The space formed by the junction of the posterior nasal cavity and the throat.

Neonatal biobehavioral states. State 1 Deep sleep; State 2 Light sleep; State 3 Drowsy awake; State 4 Quiet alert; State 5 Active alert; and State 6 Crying.

Neuron. Nerve cell; the main component of the central nervous system.

Neural crest. Ganglionic crest; a band of ectodermal cells that appear along either side of the line of closure of the embryonic neural groove. With the closure of the neural groove to form the neural tube, these bands then lie between the developing spinal cord and the superficial ectoderm. They later separate into cell groups that constitute the primordia of the ganglia of cranial and spinal nerves. Other derivatives migrate ventrally to induce formation of various other tissues.

Neutral occlusion. (Angle Class I) The occlusal relationship described by Dr. E. H. Angle where the mesio-buccal cusp of the maxillary permanent first molar occludes in the buccal groove of the mandibular permanent first molar.

Neutroclusion. (Class I, Angle) (See Angle classification).

Object constancy. The concept that objects retain their identity, despite changes in their appearance or movement caused by shifts in the observer, the object, or the context.

Object permanence. The concept that objects continue to exist even when they can not be seen, touched, or heard.

Obturator. A prosthetic device that closes or blocks up an opening (as a fissure in the palate).

Occlusal adjustment. Procedure designed to selectively reshape the occlusal surface of teeth to eliminate dental interferences.

Occlusal map. A patient specific arch form fabricated by the clinician for the purpose of maintaining the individual's arch form and for identifying and measuring space requirements within that individual's arch form.

Occlusion. Relation of the functional contact of the maxillary and mandibular teeth during activity of the mandible.

Odontoid process. The finger like process of the second cervical vertebra that passes through the first cervical vertebra.

Offset. When the x-ray images of the proximal surfaces of the teeth do not superimpose upon one another anteroposteriorly, their images are said to be offset horizontally. When the images of the occlusal surfaces do not superimpose vertically, they are said to be offset vertically.

Oligodontia (hypodontia). Having fewer than the normal number of teeth. This term usually refers to a congenital absence of teeth. Congenitally missing teeth with permanent teeth more common than primary teeth and a decreased frequency starting from third molars to second premolars, and to maxillary lateral incisors. Marked oligodontia means many missing teeth. Partial anodontia (part of nothing is still nothing) is a poor substitute for oligodontia.

Open bite. (Negative overbite) no vertical overlap of the maxillary and mandibular teeth; failure of certain teeth to come into occlusal contact in any excursion of the mandible.

Op (Opisthion). A cephalometric landmark the most posterior point on the posterior margin of the foramen magnum. The posterior midsagittal point on the posterior margin of foramen magnum.

Or (orbitale). A cephalometric landmark; the most inferior point on the lower border of the left orbit. The lowest point on the average of the right and left borders of the bony orbit.

Orofacial. Of or relating to the mouth and face.

Oronasal fistula. An incomplete opening connecting the mouth and nasal cavity.

Orthognathic. Having normally related jaws and a straight profile.

Orthognathic face. (Straight) a line that is drawn and is approximately 90 degrees to the Frankfort plane with no divergency.

Orthopedic forces. Rather strong forces used in orthodontic treatment. Forces are usually over two pounds.

Orthognathic surgery. Surgery to alter relationships of teeth and/or supporting bones, usually accomplished in conjunction with orthodontic therapy.

Osteointegration. A direct structural and functional connection at the light microscope level between living bone and at the surface of a load-carrying implant.

Ostectomy. The excision of a bone or portion of a bone.

Osteoblasts. Bone-forming cells derived from mesenchyme. They form the osseous matrix in which they may become enclosed to become osteocytes.

Osteoclasts. Larger multinucleated cells derived from monocytes with abundant acidophilic cytoplasm, formed in bone marrow and functioning in the absorption and removal of osseous tissue.

Outcomes. All the possible results that may stem from exposure to a causal factor, or preventive or therapeutic interventions; all identified changes in health status arising as a consequence of the handling of a health problem.

Overbite (positive overbite) (vertical). The measurement of the vertical overlap between the maxillary and mandibular incisors. This measurement is expressed in more commonly in percent overlap than in millimeters.

Overjet (horizontal). Describes the distance between the labial surface of the mandibular incisors and the incisal edges of the maxillary incisors.

Overregularization. Occurs when children apply rules of grammar when they should not. It is seen in English, for example, when children add "s" to form the plural even in irregular cases that form the plural in a different way.

P

Palatal crossbite. The palatal displacement of the maxillary affected tooth or teeth as it relates to the antagonistic tooth or teeth.

Palatal plane. Anterior Nasal Spine – Posterior Nasal Spine. ANS-PNS

Palatine rugae. Transverse ridges located in the mucous membrane of the anterior part of the hard palate. They extend laterally from the incisive papilla. They have a core of dense connective tissue.

Palate. The hard and soft tissues dividing the oral from the nasal cavity.

Palate, primary. That part of the palate formed from the median nasal process. The first palate to form, which is anterior to the secondary palate.

Palate, secondary. The palate proper, formed by fusion of the lateral palatine processes of the maxilla.

Panoramic x-ray film. Radiogram taken to give a panoramic view of the entire upper and lower arch as well as the temporomandibular joint.

Palmomental reflex. Present at birth. May persist into adulthood in some individuals. Stroking of the hand elicits wrinkling of the mentalis muscle.

Papilla(e). (See incisive papillae)

Palpilla(e) palatine. A convexly rounded and elliptically shaped pad of soft tissue lying posteriorly to the upper central incisors.

Paramedian. Situated adjacent to the midline.

Parenchyma. The functional elements of an organ rather than the supporting framework (stroma) of the organ.

Peer pressure. Refers to the social pressure to conform to one's friends in behavior, dress, and attitude. It may be positive or negative in its effects.

Peg shaped lateral incisor. A morphological diminuation in the size and shape of the maxillary lateral incisor tooth, which can adversely affect individuals' occlusion and esthetics.

Perforating fibers. Penetrating connective tissue fibers by which the tooth is attached to the adjacent alveolar bone. These bundles of collagen fibers penetrate both the cementum and alveolar bone.

Peridontium. The supporting structures of the teeth.

Periodontal ligament. The connective tissue attaching the teeth to the alveolus. It includes collagenous fibers arranged in bundles, between which are loose connective tissue, blood vessels ,and nerves. Tissue surrounding the root of a tooth which holds or connects the tooth to the bone.

Periodontal screening & recording. Endorsed by American Dental Association of Periodontology, PSR, is a rapid, effective method to screen patients for periodontal disease and summarize necessary information with minimum documentation. PSR is a complete periodontal probing of each tooth and is performed by assessing all six sites of the tooth (mesiofacial, midfacial, distofacial, and the corresponding linual/palatal surfaces). However, instead of the timeconsuming charting associated with comprehensive full-mouth periodontal examination, the mouth is divided into sextants and only the deepest probing depth of each sextant is recorded in the patient's record.

Perioral muscles. The musculature of the lips.

Permissive parenting. The style of parenting in which the parents make few demands on their children, yet are nurturant and accepting, and communicate well with their children.

Person-time. Incidence rates (see incidence rate) are calculated of over a specified period of time. Time period is selected by the investigators for a specific study. The demoninator of incidence rate formula is the sum of the times each person had the possibility of developing the outcome, which is also referred to as person-time. The reason that the time contributed by each person is calculated is that subjects may be observed for different lengths of times in a study, for instance due to loss to follow up.

Personality. Refers to the emotions, behaviors, and attitudes that make an individual unique.

Phasic bite reflex. Present at birth and persists until approximately 6 months of age. Stroking the gum elicits rhythmic vertical biting motions of the jaw.

Pharyngeal-arch cartilages. One of the cartilages formed in a pharyngeal arch of the embryo.

Pharyngeal arches. One of a series of mesodermal thickenings between the phyarngeal clefts, appearing in higher forms only vestigially. During embryonic stages they contribute to the formation of the face, jaws, and neck.

Pharyngeal flap. Surgical attachment of the soft palate to the posterior pharyngeal wall, leaving lateral openings to limit escape of air during speech.

Phenotypic variation. The variation in physical expression.

Philtrum of the lip. The vertical groove on the median line of the upper lip.

Phobia. An exaggerated and irrational fear of an object or experience.

Physiologic (biologic) width of the PDL. Width which it attains when the tooth is in function.

Piaget. Jean Pierre Piaget (1896-1980); Swiss child psychologist; through his studies of children developed extensive theory for cognitive development; considered one of the most influential thinkers in child development and child psychology.

Pincer grasp. When the thumb and forefinger are used together to hold an object.

Plosive. Designating a speech sound produced by a total blockage of the breath stream followed by an explosive release.

PM Vertical (PMV). Pterygo-Maxillary Fissure, Inferior – Ethmoid Registration Point. PTME-SE.

Po (Pogonion). A cephalometric landmark; the most anterior point of the bony chin.

Point A. (subspinale) A cephalometric landmark; the most posterior midline point on the premaxilla between the anterior nasal spine and prosthion.

Point B. (supramentale) A cephalometric landmark; the most posterior point in the anterior mandibular profile curvature between infradentale and Pogonion.

Pogonion. The most anterior point on the contour of the bony chin. Determined by a tangent through Nasion.

Pog to NB. As a distance in millimeter ($\pm$ 0.5 mm). It is the perpendicular distance from Pogonion to N-B line. The adult norm is (+) 2 mm $\pm$ 2 mm. It is rarely positive in children under eight to 10 years of age and is usually larger in males than females. Its significance is the prominence of the bony chin. It does not necessarily correlate well with the prominence of the soft tissue chin. If Pogonion is behind N-B line, it is a negative value.

Population, target. The group from which a study population is selected.

P (porion). (anatomical) A cephalometric landmark; noting the superior edge of the external auditory meatus.

P (porion). (mechanical) A point 4-1/2 mm. Above the center of the ear rods as seen on the lateral head film.

Posterior border of the ramus. This is defined as the intersection of the functional occlusal plane with the posterior border of the mandibular ramus.

Posterior crossbite. One or more posterior teeth locked in an abnormal relation with the opposing teeth of the opposite arch; can be either buccal or a lingual cross-bite and may be accompanied by a shift of the mandible.

Posterior Downs Point. The midpoint of the line connecting landmarks 18 and 19 (LMT and UMT). This represents the posterior point through which Downs Occlusal Plane passes.

Posterior leeway space. The mesiodistal width differences between the primary canine/both primary molars and the permanent canine/both premolars. This space is usually positive in the exchange and more so in the mandible. Maxillary posterior leeway space ranges from (+) 1 mm to (+) 1.5 mm while mandibular posterior leeway space ranges form (+) 4 mm to (+) 5 mm.

Posterior nasal spine (PNS). (posterior nasal spine) The bony posterior projection of the horizontal portion of the palatine bone at the midline; the most posterior point at the sagittal plane on the bony hard palate.

Posterior open bite. No contact between the maxillary and mandibular posterior teeth in occlusion.

Power. The ability of a study to demonstrate an association if it exists. The power of a study is determined by several factors, including the frequency of the condition under study, the magnitude of the effect, study design, and sample size.

Preoperational thought. Piaget's term for the cognition of children between the ages of approximately 2 and 6 years. Refers to fact that children between these ages have not yet learned to use logical principles in their thinking.

Precision. The quality of being sharply defined through exact detail.

Premaxillary segment. The median anterior part of the maxillary bones.

Primary palate. The maxillary structure anterior to the incisive foramen.

Primate space. The interdental space occurring mesial to the primary canines in the maxilla and distal to the canines in the mandible.

Proclination. The labial tipping of the anterior teeth.

Procumbency. Leaning forward, usually related to the upper and lower anterior teeth.

Prognathic. A forward relationship of either or both of the jaws relative to the craniofacial skeleton.

Prognathic face. (Anterior divergent) is considered to be an anterior divergent face.

Prognathism. The projection of one or both jaws beyond the upper part of the face; skeletal protrusion that can occur in the maxilla or mandible.

Project Headstart. A preschool program that was initiated in 1965 in response to a perceived need to improve the educational future of low-income children.

Prosocial behavior. Any act, such as sharing or cooperating, performed to help other people without the expectations of reward or repayment.

Pr (prosthion). A cephalometric landmark; the most anterior point of the maxillary alveolar process at the midline.

Prosthion. The midpoint of the line connecting the most superior point of the radiopacity generated by each of the two ear rods of the cephalostat.

Protrusion. Indicating teeth or other maxillary and mandibular structures that are anterior to generally accepted standards.

Protrusion. (Retrusion) The terms used more frequently to represent skeletal relationships as well as the position of the teeth as they relate to the maxillary and mandibular basal bone.

Proxy measures. Information gathered from other family members about a person.

Pseudo Class II or Class III malocclusion. The malocclusion is a Class I malocclusion masking as a Class II in the molar relationship (pseudo Class II), i.e., early loss of maxillary primary second molar, or pseudo Class III, i.e., early loss of mandibular primary second molar or a shift of a Class I anterior crossbite malocclusion in retruded contact to a Class III molar in maximum intercuspation.

Pterygo-maxillary fissure, inferior. The most inferior point on the average of the right and left outlines of the pterygo-maxillary fissure.

Pterygo-maxillary fissure, superior. The most superior point of the average of the right and left outlines of the pterygo-maxillary fissure.

Q

Quality of life. The degree to which persons perceive themselves able to function physically, emotionally, and socially.

R

Radicular. Concerning a root.

Ramus. The vertically oriented portion of the mandible that joins the tooth-bearing part of the mandible to the condyle, which articulates with the temporal fossa of the skull.

Ramus. General term to designate a smaller structure given off a larger one or into which a larger structure divides.

Ramus of mandible. Quadrilateral process projecting superiorly and posteriorly from the body of the mandible.

Random error. Variation of measurements from the true values by chance. The degree to which the results obtained by a measurement, procedure can be replicated.

Reactive aggression. Aggressive behavior that is an angry retaliation for some intentional or incidental act by another person.

Rebound effect. The elastic recoil of the gingiva, the periodontal ligament, and the musculature that results in relapse of tooth and jaw position following orthodontic treatment.

Reflex. An automatic action or movement in response to an external stimulus and mediated involuntarily through the nervous system.

Reflexes. Involuntary physical responses to specific stimuli. A reflected action or movement; the sum total of any specifice involuntary activity.

Cheyne-Stokes. A type of breathing characterized by rhythmic variations in intensity that occur in cycles: rhythmic acceleration, deepening, and stopping of breathing movements.

Hering-Breuer. The nervous mechanism that tends to limit respiratory excursions. Stimuli from the sensory endings in the lungs (and perhaps in other parts) pass up the vagi and tend to limit both inspiriation and expiration during ordinary breathing.

Jaw. An extension-flexion reflex that is initiated by tapping the mandible downward. The masseter and other elevators of the mandible are the first stretched; then reflex flexion-contraction elevates the mandible by flexion of elevator muscles while there is a simultaneous stretching (extension) or the depressor muscles of the mandible.

Pathologic. Those reflexes observed in the abnormal or inappropriate motor responses of controlled stimuli initiated in the sensory organ that is appropriate to the reflex arc. They may be initiated in the superficial reflexes of the skin and mucous membrane; in the deep myotatic reflexes of the joints, tendons, and muscles; and in the visceral reflexes of the viscera and other organs of the body. The pathologic reflexes are thus syndromes of abnormal responses to otherwise normal stimuli.

Stretch. One of the most important features of tonic contraction of muscle. It is the relex contraction of a healthy muscle that results from a pull. It has been found that stretching a muscle by as little as 0.8% of its original lenth is sufficient to evoke a reflex response.

In speech. In normal speech, the action of the respiratory apparatus during exhalation, which provides a continuous stream of air with sufficient volume and pressure (under adequate voluntary control) to initiate phonation. The stream of air is modified in its course from the lungs by the facial and oral structures, giving rise to the sound symbols that are recognized as speech.

Regainer. (space) Appliance used in an attempt to regain space in the dental arches.

Relapse. The change in tooth position, towards their former location, following active orthodontic therapy.

Relative risk. The ratio of the risk of disease or death among the exposed to the risk among the unexposed.

Releveling. Orthodontic procedure often necessary after orthodontic space closure of extraction site, to correct the plane of occlusion, or after banding or bonding the second molars.

Remodeling. Altering of the structure by reconstruction. The continuous process of turnover of bone carried out by osteoblasts and osteoclasts.

Removable appliance. (See appliance).

Required space. Sum of mesio-distal widths of individual permanent teeth from first permanent molar to first permanent molar.

Replantation. The replacement of a tooth that has been displaced from the alveolus, usually a result of traumatic injury.

Reproducibility. A test or measurement is reproducible, if the results are identical or closely similar each time it is conducted.

Reproximation. (See stripping).

Resection. Surgical excision of a considerable portion of an organ (i.e., maxilla or mandible), to produce spatial changes of these and related structures.

Resection. (root) The surgical removal of the apical portion of the root of a tooth.

Resorb. To absorb again; to lose substance, as in the resorption of a tooth.

Resorption. The loss of bone or cementum by phsyiologic or pathologic means, due to the activity of multinucleated giant cells, the osteoclasts. It may occur anywhere along the surface of the root or tooth socket in response to caries, trauma, loss of a primary tooth or orthodontic treatment.

Response rate. The number of people participating in a study divided by the total number of people who would have participated if all had consented to participate in the study.

Rest position. (See postural resting position, free way space).

Retainer. An appliance used for maintaining the corrected positions of the teeth. May be fixed or removable.

Retention. The final phase in active orthodontic treatment where teeth are maintained in a healthy, functional, and esthetic position by using a variety of mechanical appliances. That passive treatment period following active orthodontic correction during which retaining appliances may be used to maintain or stabilize the teeth in the new position into which they have been moved.

Retraction. Posterior movement of teeth, usually with an orthodontic appliance.

Retroinclination. Lingual tipping of the anterior teeth.

Retrognathia. Facial disharmony in which one or both jaws are posterior to normal in their craniofacial relationships, usually referring to the mandible; recession of one or both jaws.

Retrognathic face. Considered to be a posterior divergent face.

Retrognathism. A skeletal retrusion.

Retrusion. A condition in which a tooth or the jaw is posterior to its proper occlusal position. Indicating teeth or other maxillary and mandibular structures that are posterior to normal, or to the accepted standard.

Reversal lines. Lines separating layers of bone deposited in a resorption site from the scalloped outline of Howship's lacunae of osteoclasts. The latter is obliterated by the action of osteoblasts or cementoblasts. Deposition of new hard tissue leaves a visible line where the reversal of resorption took place.

Rigid fixation. Stabilization of two bony segments, using metal plates or screws to eliminate movement between the parts.

Risk factor. An aspect of personal behavior or life-style, an environmental exposure or inherited characteristic that is known to be associated with health related conditions.

Rooting reflex. A reflex which helps babies find a nipple, causes them to turn their heads and start to suck when something brushes against their cheek near their mouth. Present at birth and persists until at least 3 to 4 months.

Root resorption. Dissolution of the root of a tooth by addition of osteoclasts. May occur anywhere along the surface of the tooth root in response to caries, trauma, or the loss of a primary tooth. (External) Loss or blunting of apical portion of the root of a tooth. (Internal) Loss of dentin from the inside (pulpal) part of the root area.

S

Sarcolemma. The surface membrane of muscle cells.

Sarcoplasmic reticulum. An intracellular system of membranes involved in transmitting contractile stimulus from the neuromuscular junction to contractile filaments within a muscle cell.

Sagittal plane. Median plane in the anteroposterior direction, which divides the left and right sides of the head equally.

Sample size determination. The process of deciding, before a study begins, how many subjects should be studied. The factors that need to be taken into account; the prevalence or incidence of the condition being studied, the estimated or putative relationship among the variables in the study, the power that is desired, and the allowable magnitude of Type I error.

Sampling. The process of selecting a number of subjects from all the subjects in a particular group.

Scaffold. A highly porous material construct intended to support the growth of the desired tissue or organ.

Scissor-bite. The presence of one or more of the adjacent posterior teeth are either positioned completely buccally or lingually to the antagonistic teeth and exhibit a vertical overlap.

Secondary palate. The maxillary structure posterior to the incisive foramen.

Second order positions (vertical). The mesial or distal inclination of the crown or root of a tooth to the line of occlusion as described by Dr. E.H. Angle. This is also casually referred to as a "tip" or "angulation" position of the tooth.

Secure attachment. Is one in which the infant derives comfort and confidence from the secure base provided by a caregiver.

Selective attention. The ability to screen out distractions and concentrate on relevant information.

Self-awareness. A person's sense of self as being distinct from other people that makes possible many new self-conscious emotions, including shame, guilt, embarrassment, and pride.

S (sella). A cephalometric landmark; the center of the pituitary fossa (sella turcica).

SE (spheno-ethmoidal suture). A cephalometric landmark designating the junction of the sphenoid and ethmoid bones in the anterior cranial base.

Sella-nasion plane. Sella – Nasion. S-N.

Sella Turcica. The hypophyseal fossa in the center of the cranium in the sphenoid bone that contains the pineal gland; center of the pituitary fossa of the sphenoid bone, determined by inspection.

Separation. The process of gaining slight spaces between the teeth preparatory to adapting and cementing bands.

Separation anxiety. The individual, usually a child, fear of being left by the loved one, usually the mother or other caregiver. In normal development separation anxiety emerges in infants at about 8 or 9 months, peaks at about 14 months, and then gradually subsides.

Sensitivity. Proportion of the truly diseased persons in the screened population who have been identified as diseased by the screening test.

Serial extraction. The process of removing permanent teeth in the middle transitional dentition along with selected primary teeth. It is limited usually to Class I malocclusions with balanced faces and severe mandibular arch perimeter discrepancies (over the mesiodistal width of a premolar at 7 mm). There should be no crossbites or openbites. It is not indicated in Class II or Class III patterns without active orthodontic tooth movement. The classic pattern is seen with first premolar removal upon their eruption. The second pattern is seen with non-restorable permanent first molars in the transitional dentition. One should plan that all serial extraction cases need corrective orthodontic therapy in the adolescent dentition. Extraction of a single permanent tooth in the transitional dentition is not indicated; symmetrical extractions predominate with rarer unilateral extractions of both molars.

Setting up anchorage. Orthodontic procedure designed to establish receptors of responsive forces delivered by the activation of orthodontic appliances.

Settling of the occlusion. The natural tooth movement that occurs as teeth adapt to their new intra-arch positions and inter-arch relations (occlusion), following appliance removal. Such settling movements may be desirable or undesirable.

Setup, diagnostic. Traditionally a procedure in case analysis involving cutting off and repositioning of teeth in the desired positions on a plaster cast. Orthocad and emodel offer alternatives.

Six keys to normal occlusion. Dental alignment and intercuspation exhibited by well occluded dental arches.

Skeletal crossbite. A malocclusion with maxillary posterior teeth occluding lingual to the mandibular due to malposition of the entire skeletal segment(s).

Smile line. The amount of tooth and/or gingival tissue that is exposed upon smiling.

SO (spheno-occipital synchondrosis). A cephalometric landmark designating the cartilagenous joint located between the sphenoid and occipital bones.

Social smile. A smile of pleasure in response to a human face or voice, first appears at approximately 6 weeks of age.

Soft palate. The membranous and muscular fold suspended from the posterior margin of the hard palate and partially separating the mouth cavity from the pharynx.

Somatic growth. The growth pattern of the body in general.

Space closure. Procedure designed to reestablish the contact points along the perimeter of the dental arches.

Space deficiency. A situation where the sum total of the widths of the individual teeth is greater than the arch perimeter.

Space excess. A situation where the sum total of the widths of the individual teeth is less than the arch perimeter.

Specificity. Proportion of truly nondiseased persons who have been identified as nondiseased by the screening test.

Spee, curve of. The anatomic curvature of the mandibular occlusal plane beginning at the tip of the lower cuspid and following the buccal cusps of the posterior teeth, continuing to the terminal molar.

Splint. A rigid appliance used to connect and mutually support teeth or bones. A removable form is often used to temporarily relieve occlusal interferences in functional disorders of the temporomandibular joint and related musculature.

Stability. The ability to maintain a position, i.e., withstand force or stress without alteration of position.

Steiner chevrons. Steiner chevrons are used as compensation in the positions of the permanent maxillary and mandibular incisors due to apical base discrepancies with predictions to estimate future changes in ANB and Pogonion. As the apical bases separate (toward Class II), the maxillary incisor uprights in angulation and is positioned posterior while the mandibular incisor proclines in angulation and becomes procumbent in distance. As the apical bases cross (toward Class III), the reverse occurs with the maxillary incisor procumbent and proclined while the mandibular incisor becomes more retroclined and retrocumbent. This compensation is more in the maxilla than the mandible. The greater the bony chin the more the lower incisor can be positioned forward. This change in incisor angulation is called dentoalveolar compensation for an apical base discrepancy.

Stops. Bends in or wires soldered to an arch wire to limit passage through a bracket or tube.

Stripping of teeth. Removal of tooth structure or restorative material from the mesial or distal surfaces of teeth, usually to alleviate crowding, utilizing abrasive strips

Succedaneous. The permanent or second teeth that replace the 20 deciduous or primary (first) teeth.

Succedaneous teeth. The 20 permanent teeth that develop beneath the 20 primary teeth. They succeed the primary teeth with 10 in each arch, i.e., permanent central and lateral incisors, permanent canines, and first and second premolars.

Successional lamina. Portion of the dental lamina lingual to the developing primary teeth. It gives rise to the enamel organs that differentiate into permanent teeth.

Successional teeth. The permanent teeth that replace primary teeth.

Sucking reflex. The involuntary tendency of newborns to suck anything that touches their lips. This reflex fosters feeding.

Suicidal ideation. Refers to thinking about committing suicide, usually with some serious emotional and intellectual overtones.

Supernumerary teeth. Extra teeth usually malformed and erupting ectopically; teeth in excess of the normal number and usually unerupted.

Supporting bone. Bone tissue functionally related to the roots of the teeth. It surrounds, protects and supports the tooth roots through the alveolar bone proper.

Supradentale. The most anterior inferior point on the maxilla at its labial contact with the maxillary central incisor.

Supraocclusion. (over-eruption) Teeth that have erupted beyond the occlusal level of the contiguous teeth or beyond their normal alveolar level.

Supraversion. The term used to describe a tooth that is over erupted.

Suture. (bony) The junction of two bones, as in the skull and face.

Swallowing. The act of passing food from the mouth into the esophagus tube leading to the stomach. A complicated neuromuscular action.

Symbolic thought. Thinking that involves the use of words, gestures, pictures, or actions to represent other objects, behaviors, or experiences.

Symmetrograph. A transparent grid placed atop the occlusal surface of a dental cast to detect any symmetries of shape or form. In particular, individual tooth malpositions, rotations or tipping as well as crown form anomalies can easily be visualized this way.

Symphysis. The anterior junction of the right and left sides of the mandible. Although most species with bony mandibles have a connective tissue symphyseal suture, humans fuse by one year after birth.

Symphysis. The anterior midpoint area of the mandible. Designating the union of the two lateral halves of the mandible.

Synapse. The junction or narrow gap at which the axon of a sending neuron meets the dendrites of a receiving neuron. The narrow gap between the terminal bouton of the neuron and the dendrite or cell body of another.

Synchondrosis. A type of cartilaginous joint that usually is temporary. The intervening hyaline cartilage ordinarily converts to bone before the person reaches adult life.

Synchrony. The coordinated interaction between caregiver and infant that helps infants learn to express and read emotions.

Syndrome. A group of signs and symptoms that occur together and characterize a particular abnormality.

Systematic error. Systematic (one-sided) variation of measurements from the true values.

T

Tangent. The mathematical junction of a line and a curve.

Temperament. The set of innate tendencies, or dispositions, that underlie and affect each person's interactions with people, situations, and events.

Temporomandibular joint. Joint formed between the condyle of the mandible and the mandibular fossa concavity of the temporal bone.

Temporormandbular ligaments. Four ligaments on the medial surface, the sphenomandibular; on the posterior surface, the stylomandibular; on the lateral surface, the temporomandibular and the capsular.

The "big five". The five major clusters of personality found in adults, including extroversion, agreeableness, conscientiousness, neuroticism, and openness.

Theory of mind. An understanding of mental processes, that is, of one's own or another's emotions, perceptions, intentions, and thoughts.

Third order position (twist or torque). The inclination of the crown or root of a tooth to the line of occlusion as described by Dr. E.H. Angle. The labial lingual/buccal lingual is casually referred to as the "torque" of a tooth.

Thumb-sucking. (finger-sucking) An infantile oral habit that is fairly normal and common early in a child's development but may persist and cause deformation of supporting bony tissue and abnormal function.

Tipping. A tooth movement in which the angulation of the long axis tooth is altered.

Tissue engineering. The emerging field of tissue engineering is concerned with the development of natural biological surrogates that restore, maintain, or improve upon tissue structure and function.

Tissue regeneration. The natural renewal of a tissue or organ that has lost structure and/or function.

TMD. Temporomandibular joint dysfunction.

Tongue crib. An appliance used to control visceral (infantile swallowing and tongue thrusting and to encourage the mature or somatic tongue postures and function.

Tongue thrust. The infantile pattern of the suckle-swallow in which the tongue is placed between the incisor teeth or alveolar ridges during the initial stage of swallowing, resulting sometimes in an anterior open bite.

Tooth crypt. Space filled by the dental follicle and developing tooth in the alveolar process.

Tooth size discrepancy. A disproportionate relationship between the sums of the mesiodistal measurements of the maxillary teeth and the mandibular teeth. Lack of harmony of size of individual teeth or groups of teeth when related to others within the same arch or the opposing arch.

Torque. A torsion force applied to a tooth to maintain or produce a crown or root movement.

Torsiversion. A tooth that is rotated on its axis.

Total leeway space. The mesiodistal width differences between the 10 primary teeth in one arch as compared to the 10 succedeous teeth in that arch. This total differential, which excludes diastemata, is worse in the maxilla and with boys. Maxillary total leeway space in girls averages (+) 6 mm and in boys (+) 7.5 mm. Mandibular total leeway space in girls averages 0 mm and in boys (+) 1.5 mm.

Total porosity. The total porosity, or void volume of a porous construct is defined as the percent of the total volume of the material that is enclosed within pores.

Tracing. (cephalometric) An overlay drawing on a cephalometric head film, designating specific structures and landmarks from which planes and angles can be made.

Tragus of the ear. The small projection in front of the external opening of the ear.

Transitional Dentition. The stage of the development of the dentition in transition between the primary and permanent dentitions. The usual period is six to 12 years of age.

Translation. The movement of a tooth through alveolar bone without change in axial inclination.

Transposition. Teeth positioned out of their normal sequence in an arch.

Transport vesicles. Vesicles for the transport of materials from one intercellular compartment to another compartment, e.g., from the rough endoplasmic reticulum to the Golgi apparatus.

Transverse plane. An imaginary plane that passes through the head at right angles to the median and frontal plane dividing the head into upper and lower halves.

Transversion. (Transposition) the teeth are in the wrong sequential order. An example of this is present when the maxillary first premolar assumes the position of the canine and the canine assumes the position of the premolar.

Turnover. Quantity of material metabolized or processed in the body or tissue within a given length of time.

Tweed triangle. A triangle described by Charles H. Tweed and defined by facial and dental landmarks on a lateral cephalometric film, using the Frankfort Horizontal Plane as a base and intended for use as a guide in the evaluation and planning of orthodontic treatment.

Types I and III collagen. Two of the fibrillar collagens that form collagen fibrils after secretion into the extracellular milieu. Type I collagen is the most common form, accounting for about 90% of the collagen of the body. It is found in bone, tendon, and skin. Type III collagen is found in loose connective tissue, blood vessels, and the haematopoetic and lymphoid tissues, and it is associated with the connective tissue side of the basement membrane.

Type IV collagen. The type of collagen associated with the basement membrane.

U

Underbite. A non-technical term applied to mandibular underdevelopment, or to excessive maxillary development, e.g., Angle Class III occlusion.

Undermining resorption. (See resorption) A type of bone resorption which occurs when forces are heavy enough to produce a cell-free zone in the compressed periodontal membrane.

Upper incisor apex. The root tip of the maxillary central incisor. In cases where the root is not yet completed, the midpoint of the growing root tip is marked.

Upper incisor incisal edge. The incisal tip of the maxillary central incisor.

Upper incisor lingual bony contact point. The lingual contact of alveolar bone with the maxillary central incisor. This point generally corresponds with the lingual cementoenamel junction (CEJ).

Upper molar distal CEJ. The posterior cemento-enamel junction of the maxillary first molar.

Upper molar distal contact point. The posterior contact, or height of contour, of the maxillary first molar.

Upper molar distal cusp tip. The posterior cusp tip of the maxillary first molar.

Upper molar mesial CEJ. The anterior cementoenamal junction of the maxillary first molar.

Upper molar mesial contact. The mesial contact, or height of contour of the maxillary first molar relative to the functional occlusal plane.

Upper molar mesial cusp tip. The anterior cusp tip of the maxillary first molar.

Utility. The value of a particular event, action or state.

Uvula. The posterior portion of the soft palate (Velum).

V

Validity. An expression of the degree to which a measurement measures what it purports to measure. The degree to which the inference drawn form a study, warranted when account is taken of the study methods, the representativeness of the study sample, and the nature of the population from which it is drawn.

Validity, internal. The subject and control groups are selected and compared in such a manner that the observed differences between them on the dependent variables under study may be attributed only to the hypothesized effect under investigation, apart from sampling error.

Validity, external. A study is externally valid or generalizable if it can produce unbiased inferences regarding a target population.

Variable expressivity. The various degrees of expression of a gene in individuals in which the gene is expressed. Penetrance and variable expressivity qualify gene expression. Sometimes an individual may carry a gene that normally results in its expression (an autosomal dominant inheritance pattern) but it is not expressed. Such genes are said to be non-penetrant. The expression of a gene can be mimicked by the environment (phenocopy) or by a different gene (genocopy, or genetic heterogeneity).

Velo-pharyngeal. Of or relating to the soft palate and the pharynx.

Velopharyngeal insufficiency. Anatomic deficiency in the soft palate or superior constrictor muscle, resulting in the inability to achieve valving or closure.

Velopharyngeal seal. Closure between oral and nasopharyngeal cavities.

Vermilion zone of the lip. Transitional zone between the skin of the lip and the mucous membrane of the lip, known as the red zone. Color due to thin epithelium, the presence of eleiden in the cells, and superficial blood vessels apparent in humans.

Vertical Maxillary Excess (VME). Excessive vertical growth of the maxilla, either anteriorly or posteriorly. This condition frequently is seen in conjunction with a downward and backward rotation of the mandible and hyper-eruption of the teeth. Occasionally referred to as a "gummy smile" in lay terms.

Vestibular space. The part of the mouth cavity outside the teeth and supporting tissues.

Visceral swallowing. (infantile, see tongue thrust) immature swallowing habit of an infant.

Viscerocranial. Those parts of the facial cranial skeleton that are of pharyngeal arch origin.

Visual Treatment Objective or "VTO". A predictive analysis used by the orthodontist to predict both antero-posterior and vertical changes that will occur as a result of changes in the denture bases and positions of the teeth subsequent to treatment, usually including orthognathic surgery.

Vomer. The base of the nasal septum; the flat, unpaired bone located in the midline of the face, shaped like a trapezoid, and forming the inferior and posterior portion of the nasal septum. It articulates with the spheroid, ethmoid, two maxillary, and two palatine bones.

W

Withdrawn-rejected children. Children shunned by the peer group because of their withdrawn and anxious demeanor.

Wolf's Law. Form follows function.

Working memory. The part of memory that handles current, conscious mental activity.

Y

Y-Axis (SGN/FH). It is the inferior-anterior angle between Frankfort horizontal an Sella-Gnathion line (the line from the center of the pituitary fossa or sella turcica junction of middle and posterior cranial bases to the outer-inferior point of the mandible). It normally does not change with growth and development. The adult norm is 59 degrees $\pm$ 4 degrees. It expresses the combined vertical and sagittal growth effects of the anterior mandible. A high value indicates a vertical growth pattern while a low value indicates a more horizontal growth pattern.

Z

Z-angle. It is the inferior-posterior angle between Frankfort horizontal and the line from soft tissue pogonion up to the most protrusive lip as determined from the chin. It can be measured from either lip, whichever is the more protrusive. This angle naturally increases with growth and development. Normal child values are 78 degrees $\pm$ 5 degrees while normal adult values are 80 degrees $\pm$ 5 degrees.

Zygomatic arch. The cheek bone. The bone which braces the maxilla laterally and is connected with it by the zygomatico-maxillary suture and to the frontal bone by the zygomatico-frontal suture and to the temporal bone by the zygomatico-temporal suture.

B

C

E

Ectopic eruption: 142, 146, 184, 267, 276, 284, 296, 300, 343, 419-420, 462-463, 533, 544, 549, 565, 571, 588, 620, 636, 647

Edentulous: 433, 518, 527-528, 542, 558, 647

Edgewise appliance: 647

Effect modification: 647

Effectiveness: 12, 51, 252-253, 261, 426, 490, 541, 599, 618

Efficacy: 45, 54, 56, 261, 355, 596

Efficiency: 240, 253-255, 257, 450, 490, 541, 647

Egocentric: 11, 267

Electromyography: 109, 647

Embryological organization of the face: 61-62

Development of the primary palate: 61, 69

Development of the secondary palate: 61, 71

Earliest stages of embryonic development: 61-62

Formation, merging and fusion of facial growth centers: 66

Pharyngeal arch formation: 61, 64

emodel™: 352-353, 355-356

Emotional age: 268

Emotional development: 2-3, 13, 17, 20, 45, 541

Development of emotional security: 2, 14

Emotional regulation: 2, 15

Emotions: 2, 12-13, 15, 19-20, 25, 39, 44

Emotional regulation: 647

Enamel knot: 137, 140, 647

Enamel organ: 136-138, 374, 378

Endosseous implants: 647

Environment: 4, 16, 19-20, 32, 41, 82, 138, 179, 187, 190-191, 195, 224, 241, 247-248, 342, 371, 384, 405, 418, 475, 477, 481, 534-535, 618, 647, 650, 670

Epidemiological methods: 247

Epigenetic: 135, 138, 140, 180, 371, 647

Epithelial buds: 136

Epithelial swelling: 136

Epithelial thickenings: 136

Equilibrate: 647

Error

Random: 247, 253, 255, 257, 605

Systematic: 246-247, 257, 299, 335, 511, 592

Eruption

Ectopic: 138, 142, 146, 169, 184, 267-268, 276, 284, 296, 300, 343-344, 359, 418-420, 462-463, 466, 504, 533, 544, 546, 549, 565, 571, 588, 620

Sequence: 13, 52, 81, 137-138, 142-143, 146, 148-150, 160, 168, 179, 265, 267, 271, 275, 277, 284, 294, 296, 298, 300, 308, 320, 367, 444, 449, 456-457, 459, 461, 464, 510, 514, 529, 534, 541, 564, 572, 579, 589-590

Stages: 3, 17, 50, 61-62, 73, 78, 91, 136-137, 139-141, 147, 160, 195, 206, 213, 225, 265, 421, 428, 434, 438, 510, 527, 591-592, 605

Theories: 120, 138, 142, 307, 311, 511, 536, 595

Eruption of teeth: 108, 156, 181, 184, 420, 462, 476, 578

Esthetic lines: 273, 648

Ethmoid registration point: 648, 661

Etiologic classification: 249

Etiologic sites that can contribute to malocclusions: 179-180

Number of teeth: 179, 181

Periodontal tissues: 107, 179, 181, 187

Size of teeth: 179, 181, 183, 446

Eustacian tube: 648

Exfoliate: 455, 458

Exposure: 38, 175, 254-256, 258, 260, 303, 381, 386, 393, 395, 504, 521, 550

Exposure odds ratio: 255, 648

External auditory meatus: 576, 648, 661

Extrafusal fibers: 96, 648

Extrusion: 131, 182, 186, 198-199, 201, 203, 226, 282, 443, 469, 492, 495, 499, 501, 515, 521, 527-528, 532, 549, 597, 621, 648

F

Facial angle: 273-274, 285, 292, 402, 648

Facial asymmetry: 166, 320, 367, 504, 513, 531, 575-576, 584, 648

Facial growth: 66, 90, 107-108, 111, 113-122, 124, 132, 134, 161, 247-248, 267, 269, 283, 334, 339, 388, 401, 429, 439, 509, 600

Facial midline: 166, 169, 276, 278, 322, 578, 648, 655

Facial skeleton: 88, 100, 179, 187-188, 191, 247, 265, 338, 446, 460, 473

G

H

I

Q-R

T

U-V

W-Z